THE **KIDNEY BOOK**

THE KIDNEY BOOK

EDITORS

TERENCE KEE YI SHERN

JASON CHOO CHON JUN

WOO KENG THYE

TAN CHIEH SUAI

SINGAPORE GENERAL HOSPITAL, SINGAPORE

World Scientific

NEW JERSEY · LONDON · SINGAPORE · BEIJING · SHANGHAI · HONG KONG · TAIPEI · CHENNAI · TOKYO

Published by

World Scientific Publishing Co. Pte. Ltd.
5 Toh Tuck Link, Singapore 596224
USA office: 27 Warren Street, Suite 401-402, Hackensack, NJ 07601
UK office: 57 Shelton Street, Covent Garden, London WC2H 9HE

British Library Cataloguing-in-Publication Data
A catalogue record for this book is available from the British Library.

THE KIDNEY BOOK
A Practical Guide on Renal Medicine

ISBN 978-981-12-8397-0 (hardcover)
ISBN 978-981-12-8422-9 (paperback)
ISBN 978-981-12-8398-7 (ebook for institutions)
ISBN 978-981-12-8399-4 (ebook for individuals)

For any available supplementary material, please visit
https://www.worldscientific.com/worldscibooks/10.1142/13613#t=suppl

Epigraph

Uraemia — a poison chalice

So let it be told
How in the early days
The pioneers struggled, strived

To save a few lives
Of patients suffering from renal failure
They did not have the knowhow
But knew that in countries
Like the UK and USA, even then
There was dialysis and transplant
To keep these patients alive

Our health care was basic
Only to save that life, once
If acutely, but long term
We did not have the wherewithal
But if others can do it, so can we

Such was the pioneering spirit of our founders
The early fathers who had the courage
They dared to face the odds and come to a solution
And while they pondered and dreamed

Before their very eyes they saw
Young man and young women
Perish one by one.

Who would sing for the lonesome one
Who would care for the lonesome one
Let me be the one, aye aye sir
So, I would strive for the lonesome one
He's the one who has lost both wit and brain

Alas if you had only
Seen him two weeks ago
Vomiting now, no appetite
Eyes dazed like in a stupor

Go near to him
And catch the fish monger's smell
Alas for him, he has lost both self and soul
His skin covered in sores and scabs
Scratching, bleeding, tearing tissue
To relieve the pruritic scourge

In renal failure your whole body
The skin itches like hell
You scratch and scratch to quell that itch
Life has indeed forsaken him

His doctor told him its uraemia
Meaning he has urine in his blood
Swollen all over — face, limbs, bloated abdomen
He could hardly breathe, lungs swollen with fluid
A deep sighing respiration, acidotic

He is starting to fit now, slowly into coma fade
His sunset eyes rolling upwards
A few more turns, spastic rigidity
And he lies still, for dead

The nurse pulls the sheet
A mortuary cover over him
Another death, another digit we cannot prevent
Despite all our heroic deeds

How did they do it, in all the developing countries
Throughout the developed world
Why can't we do the same
Meanwhile, the newly dead join the rest

So many and still counting
100 cases of end-stage renal disease a year, 1975
How do we pick up the pieces
End this ravage, or at least slow it if we cannot prevent.

The monkey trembles on the tree trunk
Its fear shakes the trembling leaves
As they fall to the ground
Each leaf a life

Do we still call ourselves doctors
Why can't we save these lives
When others can
Dialysis and transplantation, that is the cure

We must do it, it's humanly possible
If others can do it, so can we

Pursue that dream, a quest for life
Transform into reality
A new remedy to save these lives
Through dialysis and transplantation
And thus was born, "**A *Tale from the Attic***"

Professor Woo Keng Thye
14th Jan 2023

Dedication

We would like to dedicate this book to

Our pioneers, who against all odds, laid the foundations of Nephrology in Singapore.

Our teachers, whom without them, we would not be what we are today.

Our trainees, who remind us that we must build a better future than today.

Our nurses, allied health professionals, and administrative staff for making care complete.

Our families, who supported us in our career and aspirations.

And finally, our patients, who are the purpose of what we do yesterday, today, and tomorrow.

Terence Kee, Jason Choo, Woo Keng Thye, Tan Chieh Suai

Contributors in Order of Presentation

Woo Keng Thye, MBBS, MMed, FAMS, FRACP
Emeritus Consultant
Glomerulonephritis Program, Department of Renal Medicine
Singapore General Hospital

Terence Kee, MBBS, MRCP, FAMS, FRCP, FACP, FASN, GDipHML
Senior Consultant
Kidney Transplantation Program, Department of Renal Medicine
Singapore General Hospital

Jason Choo, MBBS, MCRP, FAMS, FRCP, FASN
Senior Consultant
Glomerulonephritis Program, Department of Renal Medicine
Singapore General Hospital

Tan Chieh Suai, MBBS, MRCP, FAMS, FRCP
Head of Department and Senior Consultant
Interventional Nephrology Program, Department of Renal Medicine
Singapore General Hospital

Tan Hui Zhuan, MBBS, MMed, MRCP, FAMS
Consultant
Glomerulonephritis Program, Department of Renal Medicine
Singapore General Hospital

Kanagasabapathy Kamaraj, MBBS, MCRP, FRCP
Consultant
Pancreas Transplant Program, Department of Renal Medicine
Singapore General Hospital

Tan Chee Wooi, MBBS, MRCP
Associate Consultant
Interventional Nephrology Program, Department of Renal Medicine
Singapore General Hospital

Lath Narayan, MBBS, FRCR
Senior Consultant
Department of Diagnostic Radiology
Singapore General Hospital

Cai Jiashen, MBBS, MRCP
Senior Resident
Senior Residency Program in Renal Medicine
Singapore Health Services

Kwek Jia Liang, MBBS, MRCP, FAMS
Senior Consultant
Chronic Kidney Disease Program, Department of Renal Medicine
Singapore General Hospital

Nigel Fong, MBBS, MRCP
Senior Resident
Senior Residency Program in Renal Medicine,
Singapore Health Services

Kog Zheng Xi, MBBS, MRCP
Senior Resident
Senior Residency Program in Renal Medicine,
Singapore Health Services

Wong Jiunn, MBBS, MRCP, MMed
Senior Consultant
Mineral Bone Disease Program, Department of Renal Medicine
Singapore General Hospital

Ivan Lee, MBBS, MRCP
Senior Resident
Senior Residency Program in Renal Medicine,
Singapore Health Services

Carolyn Tien, MBBS, MRCP, FAMS
Associate Consultant
Kidney Transplantation Program, Department of Renal Medicine
Singapore General Hospital

Chan Choong Meng, MBBS, MRCP, FAMS, FRCP, FACP (Hon)
Senior Consultant
Chronic Kidney Disease Program, Department of Renal Medicine
Singapore General Hospital

Liew Zhong Hong, MD, MRCP
Associate Consultant
Critical Care Nephrology Program, Department of Renal
Medicine
Singapore General Hospital

Wong Kok Seng, MBBS, MMed, MCRP, FAMS, FRCP, FRACP
(Hon)
Senior Consultant
General Nephrology Program, Hypertension,
Department of Renal Medicine
Singapore General Hospital

Alvin Tng, MBBS, MMed, MRCP, FAMS
Consultant
Interventional Nephrology Program,
Department of Renal Medicine
Singapore General Hospital

Riece Koniman, MBBS, MRCP
Consultant
Critical Care Nephrology Program,
Department of Renal Medicine
Singapore General Hospital

Jasmine Chung Shimin, MBBS, MRCP
Senior Consultant
Department of Infectious Diseases
Singapore General Hospital

Liew Ian Tatt, MBBS, MMed, MRCP
Consultant
Kidney Transplant Program, Department of Renal Medicine
Singapore General Hospital

Irene Mok, MBBS, MMed, MRCP, FAMS
Senior Consultant
Glomerulonephritis Program, Department of Renal Medicine
Singapore General Hospital

Cynthia Lim, MBBS, MRCP, FRCP
Senior Consultant
Glomerulonephritis Program, Department of Renal Medicine
Singapore General Hospital

Phang Chee Chin, MBBS, MRCP, FAMS
Consultant
Haemodialysis Program, Department of Renal Medicine
Singapore General Hospital

Sheryl Gan, MBBS, MRCP, FAMS
Senior Consultant
Haemodialysis Program, Department of Renal Medicine
Singapore General Hospital

Liu Pei Yun, MBBS, MMed, MRCP, FAMS
Consultant
Haemodialysis Program, Department of Renal Medicine
Singapore General Hospital

Lina Choong, MBBS, MMed, FAMS
Senior Consultant
Haemodialysis Program, Department of Renal Medicine
Singapore General Hospital

Tan Ru Yu, MBBS, MRCP, FAMS, MMedStats
Senior Consultant
Interventional Nephrology, Department of Renal Medicine
Singapore General Hospital

Gan Chye Chung, MBBS, MRCP, FRCP
Consultant
Faculty of Medicine
University of Malaya, Kuala Lumpur, Malaysia

Pang Suh Chien, MBBS, MRCP
Consultant
Interventional Nephrology, Department of Renal Medicine
Singapore General Hospital

Elizabeth Oei, MBChB, MRCP
Consultant
Peritoneal Dialysis Program, Department of Renal Medicine
Singapore General Hospital

April Toh Jiapei, MBBS, MRCP
Senior Resident
Senior Residency Program in Renal Medicine,
Singapore Health Services

Htay Htay, MBBS, MMed, MRCP, FRCP
Senior Consultant
Peritoneal Dialysis Program, Department of Renal Medicine
Singapore General Hospital

Marjorie Foo, MBChB, MRCP, FAMS, FRCP, FASN
Senior Consultant
Peritoneal Dialysis Program, Department of Renal Medicine
Singapore General Hospital

Mathini Jayaballa, MBChB, FRACP
Consultant
Peritoneal Dialysis Program, Department of Renal Medicine
Singapore General Hospital

Teo Su Hooi, MD, MRCP
Senior Consultant
Critical Care Nephrology, Department of Renal Medicine
Singapore General Hospital

Manish Kaushik, MBBS, MRCP, FAMS
Senior Consultant
Critical Care Nephrology Program,
Department of Renal Medicine
Singapore General Hospital

Tan Han Khim, MBBS, MD, FAMS, FRCP
Senior Consultant
Critical Care Nephrology Program,
Department of Renal Medicine
Singapore General Hospital

Ho Quan Yao, MBBS, MMed, MRCP, FAMS
Consultant
Kidney Transplant Program, Department of Renal Medicine
Singapore General Hospital

Sobhana D/O Thangaraju, MBBS, MRCP, FAMS
Senior Consultant
Kidney Transplantation Program, Department of Renal Medicine
Singapore General Hospital

Lim Rou Wei, PharmD, BCPS
Principal Clinical Pharmacist
Department of Pharmacy
Singapore General Hospital

Lee Guozhang, MBBS, MMed, MRCP, FAMS
Consultant
Department of Internal Medicine
Singapore General Hospital

Natalie Woong Liling, MBBS, MMed, MRCP
Consultant
Department of Internal Medicine
Singapore General Hospital

Sim Mui Hian, PharmD, BCPS
Principal Clinical Pharmacist
Department of Pharmacy
Singapore General Hospital

Lee Puay Hoon, PharmD, BCPS
Senior Principal Clinical Pharmacist
Department of Pharmacy
Singapore General Hospital

Tan Sheau Kang, MSc Nutrition and Dietetics,
BSc Biomedical Sciences
Principal Dietitian
Department of Dietetics
Singapore General Hospital

Pindar Yu Poo Yee, MSc Health Sciences, MSc Nutrition
and Dietetics
Certified Nutrition Support Clinician
Senior Principal Dietitian
Department of Dietetics
Singapore General Hospital

Denise Ann Tsang, MBBS, MRCP
Senior Resident
Department of Dermatology
Singapore General Hospital

Oh Choon Chiat, MBBS, MSc, MRCP, FRCP
Senior Consultant
Department of Dermatology
Singapore General Hospital

Faith Wong, BA, BSc, MSW
Principal Medical Social Worker
Department of Medical Social Services
Singapore General Hospital

Goh Soo Cheng, BA, MSW
Master Medical Social Worker
Department of Medical Social Services
Singapore General Hospital

Crystal Lim, BA, MSW, MA Bioethics, PhD Social Work
Master Medical Social Worker
Department of Medical Social Services
Singapore General Hospital

Foreword

Welcome to *The Kidney Book* — a comprehensive guide designed to assist you in the diagnosis, treatment, and management of common renal conditions.

The kidneys play a pivotal role in maintaining homeostasis within the body, filtering waste products, regulating electrolyte balance, contributing to blood pressure control and performing multiple endocrine functions. The discovery of dialysis and transplantation has converted end stage renal disease, which was once a terminal disease, into a chronic illness. Navigating the intricate landscape of renal medicine can be a challenging endeavour.

As part of the 50th Anniversary celebration of the establishment of renal medicine in Singapore, this handbook has been meticulously crafted in 2023 to serve as your reliable companion in the understanding and management of the myriad renal disorders that can profoundly affect our patients' lives.

We have designed this handbook to be a concise, accessible, and invaluable resource. Whether you are preparing for exams, seeing patients on the wards, or seeking a quick reference at the point of care, this handbook is tailored to meet your needs.

May your journey through the realm of renal medicine be both fulfilling and enlightening.

Associate Professor Tan Chieh Suai
Head and Senior Consultant
Department of Renal Medicine
Singapore General Hospital

Preface

The Department of Renal Medicine at the Singapore General Hospital is the oldest and largest renal unit in Singapore. It had its humble beginnings in 1961 when pioneering doctors such as Professor Khoo Oon Teik and Dr Lim Cheng Hong delivered the first haemodialysis treatment to a British soldier who had suffered acute kidney injury from a motor-cycle accident. This was soon followed by the establishment of a chronic haemodialysis unit in 1968 and the first kidney transplant was performed in 1970. As services for patients with kidney diseases grew, the Department of Renal Medicine was officially established in 1973 with Dr Lim Cheng Hong as its founding head of department. Peritoneal dialysis was subsequently introduced in 1980 and since then the renal unit has grown by leaps and bounds to become a world-class, academic renal unit. This book is produced in the year 2023 to celebrate the 50th Anniversary of the Department and to consolidate the years of experience and knowledge that the department has accrued from many generations of nephrologists and other healthcare professionals.

This book is called *The Kidney Book* to recognise that kidney care is provided by an entire village of healthcare professionals and not only by physicians. It provides a multidisciplinary practical guide to the clinical management of common kidney conditions, procedures and situations encountered by physicians, residents, nurses, and other healthcare professionals involved in the day-to-day care of patients with kidney diseases. Being a book aimed at assisting in the daily clinical care of patients, it is written by nephrologists and allied health professionals in a deliberate point-by-point format with tables, algorithms, and figures to summarise important clinical practices and procedures that would be easy to refer to.

Consistent with our strong collaborative and patient-centric values at the Singapore General Hospital, we are extremely grateful to our co-authors from various sub-specialties and other disciplines who have agreed to contribute chapters to this book. We are deeply appreciative of their efforts as well as their consensus on keeping this book as practical as possible. We would also like to thank our many other physicians, nurses and allied health professionals in our department who have not written a chapter but continue to work tirelessly to provide the best care and journey for our patients who struggle with kidney diseases.

We hope that readers of this book will find it practically useful as well as a tool for learning and revision. *The Kidney Book* will also stand out among other similar books in that it is one of the few books written in English on nephrology from Asia. It will therefore appeal to the kidney community in this part of the world.

Associate Professor Terence Kee
Senior Consultant, Department of Renal Medicine
Director, Kidney Transplant Program
Singapore General Hospital

Contents

Glomerulonephritis 255

Haemodialysis 309

General Nephrology

Woo Keng Thye

Chapter 1

Pebbles From the Grand Round

Introduction

The renal grand rounds were a grand affair on every Monday morning, where the entire department from consultants and nurses to allied health professionals would gather at the high dependency renal unit to wait for Professor Woo Keng Thye to start his grand round. During the grand rounds, the medical officers would present the patients they were looking after in an eloquent manner, having prepared their script the evening before and being ready to answer questions posed by Professor Woo. If the medical officers did not know the answers to the questions, Professor Woo would then turn to the registrars where the expectations were higher for them. So in order to 'protect' their registrars, the medical officers would have studied the evening before and in most instances, answered Professor Woo's questions with poise and accuracy. This is a fondly remembered selection of questions and answers in Professor Woo's own words.

Terence Kee

Question 1

When treating patients with urinary tract infection, how soon would bacteria be killed after antibiotics administration? When would symptoms disappear and how long would pyuria last?

Answer 1

Bacteria would be killed within hours. Symptoms go off after 24 to 48 hours. Pyuria goes off by the end of 1 week. That is why we review patients in a week's time at the outpatients. If pyuria persists after 1 week, it means either the antibiotic was not appropriate or the infection was in the upper urinary tract (e.g., pyelonephritis) and the patient would require an intravenous pyelogram or a CT pyelogram.

Question 2

How do scars in the kidney form in patients with UTI?

Answer 2

Scars may occur in patients with chronic pyelonephritis, by which we mean chronic atrophic pyelonephritis because of vesico-ureteric reflux. Acute pyelonephritis does not cause scarring, unless there is acute papillary necrosis associated with the urinary tract infection. For scars to form, two conditions are necessary. First there must be the presence of infected urine. Then there must be intrarenal reflux or grade IV reflux occurring, so that the infected urine can get into the kidney during micturition when there is retrograde flow of the infected urine to allow scarring to occur. If urine is rendered sterile using prophylactic antibiotics, scars will not form.

Scars occur first in the upper pole, next the lower pole, and then the mid pole, hence the irregular scarring we see in chronic pyelonephritis. Scars once formed will progress inexorably until the kidney becomes shrunken and contracted. Compensatory hypertrophy occurs in the other kidney due to glomerular hyper-filtration, hence the presence of unequally sized scarred kidneys in patients with chronic pyelonephritis, compared to the bilateral and symmetrical contraction kidneys of equal size we see in patients with chronic glomerulonephritis.

Question 3

How do you tell whether a patient has Type I renal tubular acidosis (distal RTA) or Type II renal tubular acidosis (proximal or classic RTA) by the bedside?

Answer 3

Check the urine pH of the patient. If the patient has RTA and the serum bicarbonate is less than 15 mEq/l (i.e., severe metabolic acidosis) and if the urine pH is still more than 5.3, this patient has distal RTA because a patient with Type I distal RTA, no matter how severe the acidosis is, will never be able to acidify their urine to a pH of 5.3 or less.

This contrasts with a patient with proximal or Type II RTA where he is severely acidotic but would be able to acidify his urine and bring the urine pH to 5.3 and below. This is because a patient with Type II RTA or proximal/classic RTA cannot absorb his usual load of 65% bicarbonate filtered through the proximal tubule, as in the case of someone without RTA. The patient with Type II classic or proximal/classic RTA can only absorb up to 40% of his filtered load of bicarbonate as there is a defect in his bicarbonate absorption mechanism. So the extra 20% filtered bicarbonate is now presented at the distal tubule. The distal tubule has its normal bicarbonate load of 20% to be absorbed, but the additional 20% spill over from the proximal tubule overwhelms the distal tubular mechanism for absorption of bicarbonate, competing with the H^+ ions for excretion of $NH4^+$ and titratable acidity. The limit of the distal tubule is 20% bicarbonate absorption, so the extra 20% from the spill over by the proximal tubule now renders the pH of the urine at the distal tubule above 5.3, reflecting the inability to acidify the urine.

So, check the urine pH of patients with RTA when they are very acidotic. If urine pH is 5.3 and below, it means the patient has Type II or proximal/classic RTA, in contrast to patients with Type I or distal RTA who would not be able to acidify their urine no matter how acidotic they are.

Question 4

What is acute nephritic-nephrotic syndrome and its clinical significance?

Answer 4

When a patient has nephrotic syndrome, which is a triad of oedema, proteinuria more than 3 g/day, and low serum albumin less than 30 g, and if he also passes blood in the urine (i.e., gross haematuria), then he has acute nephritic-nephrotic syndrome. In Singapore, one of the conditions to be excluded is lupus nephritis, because patients with acute nephritic-nephrotic syndrome often have mesangiocapillary glomerulonephritis (MCGN), which is very common in patients with systemic lupus erythematosus (SLE). Idiopathic MCGN is very uncommon in Singapore compared to lupus nephritis.

Histologically, patients with MCGN would have subepithelial and subendothelial deposits on light microscopy. So, if any patient is found to have subepithelial and subendothelial deposits on light microscopy, one should suspect lupus nephritis and investigate for SLE. In lupus nephritis, the immunofluorescence on renal biopsy would also show a full house immunofluorescence pattern with the presence of IgG, IgA, IgM, C1q etc, which would further support a diagnosis of lupus nephritis in addition to the electron microscopy findings of subepithelial and subendothelial deposits.

Question 5

What is a telescoped urine specimen and what is the clinical significance?

Answer 5

A telescoped urine, not telescopic, is when the urine shows all the formed elements of urine such as red blood cells, white blood cell casts, and the urine test for albumin is positive. This is a full house urinary finding as if one is looking through a telescope and visualises a complete view of whatever is happening in the urine. When confronted with such a full house picture of the urine, one must exclude lupus nephritis as the usual patient with glomerulonephritis should not have a full house view. He is likely to have red blood cells signifying haematuria but not white blood cells signifying pyuria.

In lupus nephritis, the tubular cells are also affected, hence the presence of tubulointerstitial nephritis with pyuria as lupus nephritis also involves the glomeruli as well as the tubules. This explains why patients with lupus nephritis have Type I RTA and less often Type II RTA, because the autoantibodies present in SLE cause tubular injury resulting in RTA. So, with lupus nephritis, a full house immunofluorescence goes hand in hand with full house urine microscopy, which signifies active lupus nephritis and indicates the need for therapy. Once treated, the active sediment as seen in full house urine microscopy subsides and we find a bland urinary sediment with occasional red blood cells and traces of protein, but no pyuria. The immunosuppressant can be reduced as the proteinuria would be decreased, the anti-DNA titre would be lower, and serum complements back to normal levels.

Question 6

What is synpharyngitic haematuria?

Answer 6

Synpharyngitic haematuria means the patient is passing blood in the urine (i.e., gross haematuria) while having sore throat (pharyngitis) or some form of upper respiratory tract infection. The word synpharyngitic means the patient is having pharyngitis at the same time or simultaneously as he is passing blood in the urine. This is characteristic and diagnostic of IgA nephritis which is the commonest glomerulonephritis in Singapore as well as the world.

This contrasts with patients with post-streptococcal glomerulonephritis (PSGN) or post-infectious glomerulonephritis. In PSGN, the patient has a sore throat and a few weeks later finds that he passes blood in the urine and notices that he has puffy face or facial oedema associated with ankle oedema. However, the sore throat was a few weeks ago. When the patient with PSGN had sore throat a few weeks ago, the infection gave rise to immune complexes which get deposited in the kidney. It is an immuno-logical reaction and takes a few weeks to develop. Some weeks later the effects of the kidney immunological injury manifest, and these immune complexes cause PSGN which manifests with renal symptoms like gross haematuria, oedema, hypertension, protein-uria, and renal impairment.

This manifestation of PSGN contrasts with IgA nephritis, where another episode of sore throat or some other upper respi-ratory tract infection triggers a shower of immune complexes which get deposited in the kidney, bringing about another episode of haematuria with gross haematuria and proteinuria, hence the synpharyngitic haematuria.

Question 7

How do you manage recurrent haemorrhagic cystitis in a young woman?

Answer 7

Recurrent haemorrhagic cystitis in a young woman usually means this condition is related to sexual intercourse, often referred to as honeymoon cystitis. As the term suggests, it involves a young bride who encounters sexual intercourse with her partner for the first time. However, women can also get this each time or often following sexual intercourse presumably as they have not been made aware of the precautions to avoid the situation. This occurs in married couples too where either one partner or both are nervous and, in their anxiety, lack the natural sexual secretions which lubricate the sexual orifices. The result is that when the penis is introduced into the vagina, penetration does not occur smoothly and sometimes the penis lingers outside the vagina near the anal orifice and in so doing introduces bacteria into the urethra. The bacteria then enter the urinary bladder, causing cystitis which usually results in acute inflammation within the bladder and is often associated with dysuria and bleeding, hence the haemorrhagic cystitis.

To prevent haemorrhagic cystitis, the patient must practise 3 things as part of the routine of sexual hygiene. First, within 15 minutes of sexual intercourse, the patient should empty her bladder as this flushes out any offending bacteria that have entered the bladder. Second, before sexual intercourse, prolong the period of foreplay through kissing or stroking, touching the genitalia to excite the partner so that secretions from the sexual organs will flow freely to provide lubrication which aids penetration. If either partner is dry, KY jelly can be used. Third, post coitally, take 1 tablet of nitrofurantoin, half a tablet of cotrimoxazole, or 125 mg of cefuroxime as part of the routine of sexual hygiene to prevent infection. This must be done soon after sexual intercourse. If infection still occurs despite this, then take 1 tablet every night whether having intercourse or not. At the end of 6 months or 1 year, review the situation and if improved, then reduce to post coital prophylaxis.

Question 8

A patient with diabetes has urine microscopy showing dysmorphic red blood cells. How do you approach the problem?

Answer 8

A patient with diabetes should not have dysmorphic red blood cells in the urine. The presence of dysmorphic red blood cells means the patient has a non-diabetic nephropathy like focal segmental glomerulosclerosis or minimal change disease with or without associated diabetic nephropathy. If there is proteinuria, this could be the result of non-diabetic kidney disease, diabetic nephropathy, or both. The only way to resolve this is to do a kidney biopsy to confirm the presence of another glomerular disease apart from diabetic nephropathy, especially if there is heavy proteinuria which could be due to primary focal segmental glomerulosclerosis, a progressive nephropathy that can respond to treatment unlike diabetic nephropathy. The renal biopsy may show the presence of Kimmelstein-Wilson (KW) nodules indicating diabetic nephropathy as well as a non-diabetic nephropathy, likely focal segmental glomerulosclerosis, which is also the commonest type of glomerulonephritis associated with diabetic nephropathy. Patients with diabetic nephropathy usually have other features, such as diabetic retinopathy which occurs in 90% of patients with diabetic nephropathy. The third feature is the presence of peripheral neuropathy. This triad usually occurs in patients diagnosed with diabetic nephropathy. The fourth feature is diabetic vasculopathy, hence the importance of palpating the peripheral blood vessels in the physical examination of the patient.

The histological diagnosis would be diabetic nephropathy if the biopsy shows the KW lesion with its typical nodular glomerulosclerosis. KW lesion carries a bad prognosis and is associated with heavy proteinuria and eventual progression to renal failure, with poor response to therapy. Nowadays, with sodium-glucose transport protein 2 (SGLT2) inhibitors, patients with diabetic nephropathy with proteinuria may be able to retard the progression to end-stage kidney disease by reducing the effects of glomerular hyperfiltration causing proteinuria. SGLT2 has been shown to be useful in both diabetic and non-diabetic choronic kidney disease (CKD). In one of our recent publications, we have shown that diabetic retinopathy is associated with the presence of KW lesions in the kidneys and there is a greater likelihood of the patient developing end-stage kidney disease with these two lesions present. Among all the non-diabetic kidney diseases, we have also shown that focal segmental glomerulosclerosis is most commonly associated non-diabetic kidney disease, which occurs in Type 2 diabetes mellitus.

Question 9

What is the impact of primary focal and segmental glomerulosclerosis (FSGS) over the past decade?

Answer 9

We have published a study on the demographics and clinical outcome influencing the response of patients with primary FSGS between 2008 to 2018. The patients ($n = 150$) were analysed for their clinical, laboratory and histological characteristics including features that could influence disease progression and clinical outcome. There were two categories of patients, those with nephrotic syndrome (NS; $n = 62$) and those without NS ($n = 88$).

For patients with FSGS without NS, the indices for progression involved them having significantly more tubular interstitial and blood vessel lesions in addition to their glomerular pathology compared to patients with NS. Patients with NS responded to immunosuppressive therapy more favourably compared to the non-NS group, though both groups responded with decreasing proteinuria. The NS group had better 10 years survival of 92% versus 72% for the non-NS group (log rank 0.002). The 10 years survival for the whole group ($N = 150$) was 64%. Our data suggest that in FSGS, one of the significant components of the disease is vascular and tubular damage apart from the underlying glomerular pathology resulting in varying responses to immunosuppressive therapy, distinct from those with NS who responded to immunosuppressive therapy with stabilisation of renal function, and these patients also had less blood vessel and tubular lesions.

Question 10

How do you approach the problem of acute on chronic kidney injury?

Answer 10

The patient may reveal a history of previous symptoms of renal impairment, hypertension, or urinary tract infection. Urine microscopy may show red blood cells, casts, or protein. The urinary protein usually ranges from 1 to 2 g/day in these cases. A renal biopsy should confirm the diagnosis of pre-existing glomerulonephritis. In patients with "acute on chronic" renal failure, the acute elements causing acute kidney injury may be dehydration, sepsis, uncontrolled hypertension, obstruction, and nephrotoxic antibiotics as well as contrast agents and non-steroidal anti-inflammatory drugs. When considering obstruction, one should exclude obstruction to the urological tract as well as thrombosis of renal veins and arteries.

Based on a diagnosis of acute renal failure (ARF) in a series of 92 cases from 1976 to 1982, infections accounted for 30%, pregnancy-related ARF for 13%, and glomerulonephritis for 10%. In another series of 48 ARF cases from 1985 to 1989, septicaemia accounted for 23 cases, drugs and poisoning for 4, and glomerulonephritis for 3. Using a definition of acute kidney injury (AKI), there were 173 cases from June 2009 to May 2010, and 34% were due to dehydration, 27% due to sepsis, and 10% due to drugs. In the older system using ARF instead of AKI, mild degrees of ARF which are more readily reversible like those due to dehydration and drugs may not have been captured under the definition of ARF, hence the present term AKI is all encompassing and has a wider spectrum which accounts for the large number of cases with AKI compared to those with ARF.

Reference

Woo KT (2011). *Clinical Nephrology 3rd ed.* World Scientific Publishing, Singapore.

2 Assessment of Kidney Function

Tan Hui Zhuan

Introduction

- Glomerular filtration rate (GFR) is accepted as the best overall measure of kidney function and the kidney's ability to carry out its excretory, endocrine, and metabolic functions.
- The estimation of the GFR is used clinically to assess the degree of kidney impairment, follow disease progression, and inform clinical decisions.

Assessment of GFR

Glomerular filtration rate

- GFR is defined as the sum of the filtration rates in all functioning nephrons.
- True GFR is a physiological property that cannot be measured directly in humans.
- The normal value is approximately 140 to 173 litres/day/1.73 m^2 (90 to 120 mL/min/1.73 m^2), with considerable variation due to age, gender, body size, physical activity, diet, pharmacotherapy, and physiological state (e.g., pregnancy).

- GFR is assessed using:

  - Measured GFR, using urinary or plasma clearance of an exogenous filtration marker — remains a reference standard

  - Estimated GFR, using blood levels of endogenous filtration markers — commonly used in routine clinical settings

Estimation of GFR

- Estimated GFR (eGFR) using blood levels of endogenous filtration markers is recommended for the initial evaluation of GFR.

- Creatinine is the most used and widely available endogenous filtration marker.

- The 2021 Chronic Kidney Disease Epidemiology Collaboration (CKD-EPI) equation is recommended over other creatinine-based estimating equations, such as the 2009 CKD-EPI equation, the Modification of Diet in Renal Disease (MDRD) study equation, or the Cockcroft-Gault equation.

- Of note, the 2021 CKD-EPI equation does not include a term for race.

- Clinical laboratories should use creatinine assays that are calibrated to the international standard.

- Despite standardisation of serum creatinine assays, GFR estimates remain imprecise because of variation in non-GFR physiological determinants of serum creatinine which affects its generation, tubular secretion, reabsorption, and extrarenal elimination.

- Cystatin C is another endogenous filtration marker but is less commonly available for routine use.

Limitations of creatinine-based eGFR

- Clinical settings in which eGFR is less accurate include:
  - Extremes of body size or mass
  - Diet and nutritional status (e.g., high protein diet, use of creatine supplements)
  - Usage of certain medications — drugs can affect the serum creatinine level by competing with creatinine secretion at the level of kidney tubule (e.g., histamine H2 antagonists, poly-ADP ribose polymerase (PARP) inhibitors), and certain tyrosine kinase inhibitors interfering with the assay
  - Non-steady states such as acute kidney injury where changes in serum creatinine often lag behind changes in true GFR
- Measured GFR (mGFR) can be performed as a confirmatory test in specific circumstances when a more accurate assessment of GFR is required for clinical decision making (e.g., evaluation of a living donor candidate).
- Type of confirmatory test to perform depends on the availability and clinical setting.
- Equations have been developed to estimate GFR in the non-steady state, but none of these have been validated in comparison with mGFR.

References

Poggio ED, Rule AD, Tanchanco R, *et al.* (2009). Demographic and clinical characteristics associated with glomerular filtration rates in living kidney donors. *Kidney Int* **75**(10): 1079–1087.

Stevens LA, Coresh J, Greene T and Levey AS (2006). Assessing kidney function — measured and estimated glomerular filtration rate. *N Engl J Med* **354**(23): 2473–2483.

Zarogiannis SG, Liakopoulos V and Schmitt CP (2017). Single-nephron glomerular filtration rate in healthy adults. *N Engl J Med* **377**(12): 1203.

3 Haematuria and Proteinuria

Kanagasabapathy Kamaraj

Introduction

- Microscopic haematuria and/or albuminuria/proteinuria are commonly detected during routine health assessment, enlistment for military service, medical insurance, or pre-employment screening.

- The presence of haematuria and proteinuria together significantly increases the likelihood of significant kidney disease.

Proteinuria

- Under normal circumstances, less than 150 mg of protein appear in the urine because

  - the negatively charged glomerular capillary basement membrane acts as a barrier to large molecular weight (MW >20,000 Daltons) and negatively charged proteins

  - tubular epithelium reabsorbs lower MW proteins filtered out into the tubular lumen

- In healthy individuals, 60% of urinary protein are plasma proteins (mainly albumin) while 40% are from the tubular epithelium (mainly Tamm-Horsfall protein which is secreted by the thick ascending limb of the loop of Henle).

- Proteinuria can be differentiated according to
  - Temporal features — transient or persistent
  - Body position — orthostatic or non-orthostatic
  - Pathogenesis (Table 3.1)
  - Type of protein (albuminuria or low molecular weight proteinuria)
  - Amount excreted in the urine (nephrotic >3–3.5 g/day, non-nephrotic <3 g/day, or low grade <1–2 g/day)
  - Clinical significance

Table 3.1:   Different Types of Proteinuria

Type of Proteinuria	Physiology
Glomerular	Increased filtration of proteins (large molecular proteins like albumin and immunoglobulin) through the glomerular capillary basement membrane, which typically occurs in glomerular diseases.
Tubular	Increased excretion of proteins (low molecular weight proteins like beta-2-microglobulin) that are normally reabsorbed by the proximal tubules. This typically occurs in tubulointerstitial diseases.
Overflow	Overproduction of specific proteins, leading to increased glomerular filtration and excretion which overwhelms the ability for proximal tubules to reabsorb these proteins.
Orthostatic	Mechanism unclear — proteinuria increases when the patient is in an upright position and ambulating but decreases when lying down. It is common among adolescents, < 1 g/day and is benign.
Post-renal	Mechanisms unclear but occurs in inflammation of the urinary tract infection (e.g., infection, stone, or tumours of the urinary tract)

Measurement of proteinuria

- Measurement of proteinuria is not only important in the diagnosis of kidney disease but also assists in determining the response to treatments and kidney prognosis.

Urine dipstick test

- Dipstick analysis of urine is a useful semi-quantitative screening tool for proteinuria — trace (10–20 mg/dL), 1+ (30 mg/dL), 2+ (100 mg/dL), 3+ (300 mg/dL), and 4+ (1000 mg/dL).
- Urine dipstick detects mainly albumin but is vulnerable to false positive and false negative results (Table 3.2).

Timed urine collections

- The amount of urinary protein detected by urine dipstick needs to be quantified with actual measurement of urinary protein.

Table 3.2:   False Positive and False Negative Results for Urine Dipstick Detection of Proteinuria

False Positive for Proteinuria	False Negative for Proteinuria
• Highly alkaline urine	• Diluted urine
• Highly concentrated urine	• When the predominant protein excreted is not albumin (e.g., Bence Jones protein in multiple myeloma)
• Macroscopic haematuria	
• Prolonged dipstick exposure to urine	
• Cleaning compounds (quaternary ammonium)	
• Detergents	
• Iodinated contrast	
• Antiseptics (e.g., chlorhexidine, benzalkonium chloride)	
• Dye (e.g., phenazopyridine)	

- Urine collections over 24 hours are the gold standard to quantify protein and albumin concentration in the urine. It is often the initial evaluation test for proteinuria. A normal 24-hour urine total protein level is <150 mg/day.

- However, these collections are cumbersome and may not be accurate if the patient under- or over-collects urine. The adequacy of the collection can be assessed by comparing the 24-hour urine creatinine concentration to the expected urine creatinine concentration.

Daily urinary excretion of creatinine

Male   –   20–25 mg/kg or 177–221 μmmol/kg
Female   –   15–20 mg/kg or 133–177 μmol/kg

- 24-hour urine collection of albumin is also available — normally, 24-hour urine albumin is <30 mg/day. Micro- and macro-albuminuria is defined by urine albumin 30–300 mg/day and >300 mg/day respectively.

Spot urine measurements

- Urine albumin or total protein as a ratio to urine creatinine concentration has been shown to be comparable to timed urine collection and is more convenient for patients.

- However, there are limitations when interpreting urine albumin to creatinine ratio (UACR) or urine protein to creatinine ratio (UPCR) as follows:

  - UACR and UPCR may under- or overestimate albuminuria and proteinuria if the urinary creatinine excretion is significantly higher or lower than the average urinary creatinine excretion (1000 mg/day). UACR and UPCR in muscular individuals may be underestimated due to the high creatinine excretion from muscle (> 1000 mg/day) whereas elderly or cachectic individuals with low muscle mass may have overestimated UACR and UPCR.

■ UACR and UPCR undergo diurnal variation and can vary from day to day. A first morning sample most closely estimates 24-hour protein excretion. It is also best to collect spot urine samples at the same time each day if it is being used to monitor patients' progress.

Clinical Significance of Different Types of Proteinuria

• Proteinuria can be associated with several conditions and more than one clinical condition causing proteinuria may occur at the same time (Table 3.3).

Table 3.3:   Clinical Associations of Proteinuria

Type of Proteinuria	Clinical Association

Isolated, asymptomatic proteinuria < 3 g/day	• This may be benign and transient in the absence of haematuria, occurring in situations such as:
	  ■ Exercise
	  ■ Fever
	  ■ Urinary tract infection
	  ■ Cardiac failure
	• Patients presenting with isolated and asymptomatic proteinuria <3 g/day should have urinary protein measurement repeated to confirm its persistence.
	• If persistent, orthostatic proteinuria should be excluded (e.g., a normal urine PCR on the first morning void but an elevated urine PCR on the second void confirms the diagnosis).

(Continued)

Table 3.3:   (*Continued*)

Type of Proteinuria	Clinical Association
	• If orthostatic proteinuria is excluded, then further evaluation for glomerular or tubulointerstitial disease is required.
Microalbuminuria Normal albumin excretion: < 30 mg/day 24-hour urine albumin: 30–300 mg/day Urine albumin: creatinine ratio: 30–300 mg/g or 3.4 to 34 mg/mmol	• May be the earliest sign of diabetic/chronic kidney disease • Risk factor for cardiovascular disease and mortality • Associated with endothelial dysfunction • Angiotensin-converting enzyme inhibitors or angiotensin receptor blockers are used to treat diabetics or hypertensive individuals with microalbuminuria
Glomerular proteinuria > 3 g/day	• Urinary protein excretion of > 3 g/day is usually due to glomerular disease • When associated with hypoalbuminaemia, hyperlipidaemia, and oedema, it is called nephrotic syndrome
Tubular proteinuria < 2 g/day	• Associated with tubulointerstitial disease • Glomerular diseases can also be associated with tubular proteinuria because increased urinary protein also causes tubulointerstitial inflammation and injury
Overflow proteinuria	• Associated with specific urinary proteins ■ Ig light chains/Bence Jones protein (multiple myeloma) ■ Myoglobin (rhabdomyolysis) ■ Haemoglobin (haemolysis) ■ Lysozyme (acute myelomonocytic leukaemia)

Management of proteinuria

• Patients may be referred because of either a positive urine dip-stick or urinary measurement of urinary protein or albumin.

- A detailed history and physical examination are required, especially looking for:

  - Past laboratory reports to determine if proteinuria is new or old

  - Confounding factors — exogenous protein supplementation, fever, cardiac failure, exercise, orthostatic proteinuria

  - Presence of systemic disease

  - Family history of kidney disease

  - Medication chart, especially those associated with glomerulonephritis (e.g., non-steroidal anti-inflammatory drugs) or tubulointerstitial nephritis (e.g., antibiotics)

- Repeat measurement for proteinuria/albuminuria, ideally a 24-hour urine collection for protein or albumin together with renal panel and urine microscopy for haematuria/pyuria.

- If repeat test shows proteinuria without abnormal kidney function or haematuria/pyuria, exclude orthostatic proteinuria.

- If orthostatic proteinuria is excluded, evaluate for urinary tract infection (especially if there is pyuria), paraproteinaemia (urinary light chains), and primary kidney diseases (especially if there is abnormal kidney function and haematuria).

- An ultrasound of the kidney, ureter, and bladder is also useful to exclude structural causes and assess suitability for kidney biopsy, if indicated.

Haematuria

- Haematuria is generally defined by the presence of 3 or more red blood cells per high power field in a spun urine sediment. Urine dipstick can also detect haematuria but a

Table 3.4:   Causes of Haematuria

Glomerular causes	**Tumours**
IgA nephropathy	Renal, ureteral, and bladder tumours
Thin glomerular basement membrane disease	Bladder and ureteral polyps
Alport's syndrome	Prostate tumour
Other types of glomerulonephritis	Vascular malformation
Renal parenchymal	**Urinary tract**
Polycystic kidney disease	Calculi
Medullary sponge kidney	Infection
Sickle cell disease/trait	Vascular malformation
Papillary necrosis	Urethral and meatal stricture
Renal infarction	Schistosoma haematobium
Renal arteriovenous malformation	
Drugs	**Infections/Inflammation**
Over anticoagulation with warfarin, heparin	Pyelonephritis
Aspirin	Prostatitis
Cyclophosphamide	Cystitis e.g. Adenovirus, BKV
	Urethritis
	Tuberculosis
Other causes	
Systemic bleeding disorders	
Trauma	
Exercise haematuria	
Hypercalciuria/hyperuricosuria	

positive dipstick test for haematuria may also be due to other factors such as myoglobinuria, haemoglobinuria, or contaminants (e.g., semen, cleansing agents).

- Haematuria may be defined by its visibility (microscopic or macroscopic) or its source (glomerular or lower urinary tract) (Table 3.4).

Macroscopic haematuria

Haematuria that is visible to the naked eye as red or brown urine and may be associated with the passage of blood clots. It may be confused with menses (in women) and urinary excretion of heme due to haemolysis or rhabdomyolysis.

Microscopic haematuria

Haematuria that is invisible to the naked eye and can only be seen by microscopy. Microscopic haematuria is more commonly encountered than macroscopic haematuria.

Management of haematuria

- Patients are often referred because of either a positive urine dipstick or urine microscopy result showing haematuria.
- Repeat test for haematuria using urine dipstick and microscopy — if the dipstick is positive but microscopy is negative for red blood cells, consider other diagnoses such as myoglobinuria or haemoglobinuria.
- Take a detailed history, looking for possible causes of haematuria, especially:
  - Past laboratory reports to determine if haematuria is new or old
  - Exclude confounding factors — menses, recent exercise, infection, trauma/instrumentation, sexual intercourse
  - Risk factors for malignancy — smoking, cyclophosphamide, occupational history for risk factors of urologic cancers

- Review medication chart for drugs that can increase bleeding risks
- Family history of urinary abnormalities or kidney diseases

- If urine microscopy is still positive for haematuria, further evaluation is required such as:
  - Renal panel
  - Full blood count
  - Coagulation profile
  - Urine culture if there is suspicion of urinary tract infection such as symptoms/signs, positive nitrite on urine dipstick, pyuria on urine microscopy
  - Urine phase contrast to detect dysmorphic red blood cells and/or red blood cell casts, suggestive of glomerular haematuria
  - Urine protein measurement (e.g., 24-hour urinary total protein)
  - Cystoscopy, especially for macroscopic haematuria and risk factors for malignancy — some guidelines also suggest an age cut-off for cystoscopy evaluation of haematuria, such as 35 years and older (American Urological Association 2012 guidelines) or 40 years and older (Canadian Urologic Association 2009).
  - Computed tomography of kidneys, ureters, and bladder — ultrasound is an alternative for pregnant women
  - Kidney biopsy is indicated in those with dysmorphic red blood cells, proteinuria, and abnormal kidney function

- When no cause is found for haematuria, patients should be followed up at least annually while the haematuria remains persistent. Repeat work-up may be required when there is a change in condition (e.g., macroscopic haematuria, development of proteinuria).

References

Davis R, Jones JS, Barocas DA, *et al.* (2012). Diagnosis, evaluation and follow-up of asymptomatic macrohematuria (AMH) in adults: AUA guideline. *J Urol* **188**(6 Suppl): 2473–2481.

Niemi MA and Cohen RA (2015). Evaluation of microscopic hematuria: A critical review and proposed algorithm. *Adv Chronic Kidney Dis* **22**(4): 289–296.

Wingo CS and Clapp WL (2000). Proteinuria: potential causes and approach to evaluation. *Am J Med Sci* **320**(3): 188–194.

Wollin T, Laroche B and Psooy K (2009). Canadian guidelines for the management of asymptomatic microscopic hematuria in adults. *Can Urol Assoc J* **3**(1): 77–80.

4 Imaging of the Kidney and Urinary Tract

Tan Chee Wooi, Lath Narayan

Introduction

- Imaging is one of the useful tools in daily clinical care for a patient with kidney disease. Over the past 100 years, imaging has evolved rapidly from weak X-ray machines to a multitude of modalities (e.g., ultrasonography, computed tomography, magnetic resonance imaging, catheter angiography, scintigraphy with nuclear medicine agents, positron emission tomography).

- Understanding the diagnostic utilities and limitations of each imaging modality facilitates optimal evaluation of patients with specific clinical presentation.

Diagnostic Imaging

Plain radiograph

- Kidney-ureter-bladder (KUB) X-ray is the most common X-ray imaging used to identify urinary calculi (Figure 4.1) and calcification in kidney parenchyma (nephrocalcinosis) (Figure 4.2). It can also delineate gas when present in large quantity, e.g., in emphysematous infections.

- Radiation exposure is about 35x of a CXR.

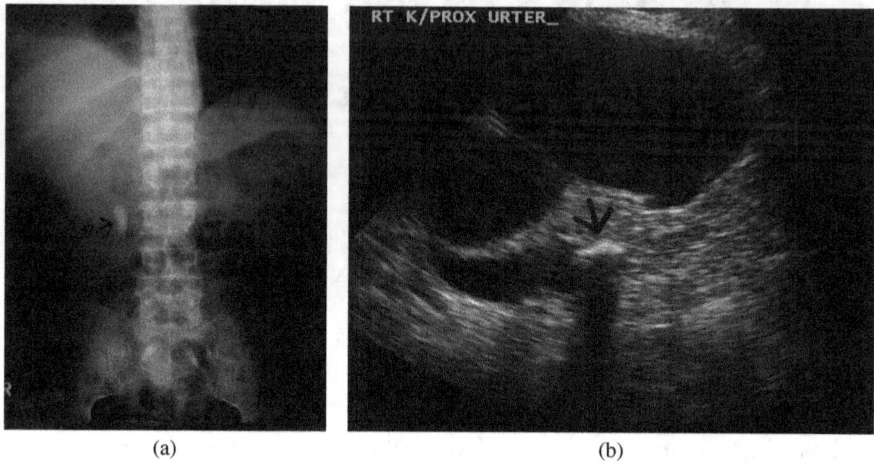

(a)   (b)

Figure 4.1: Patients with right loin to groin pain. (a) X-ray KUB shows calcified right ureteric calculus, which on (b) the US is seen as an echogenic focus with shadowing (black arrow). There is also severe right hydronephrosis.

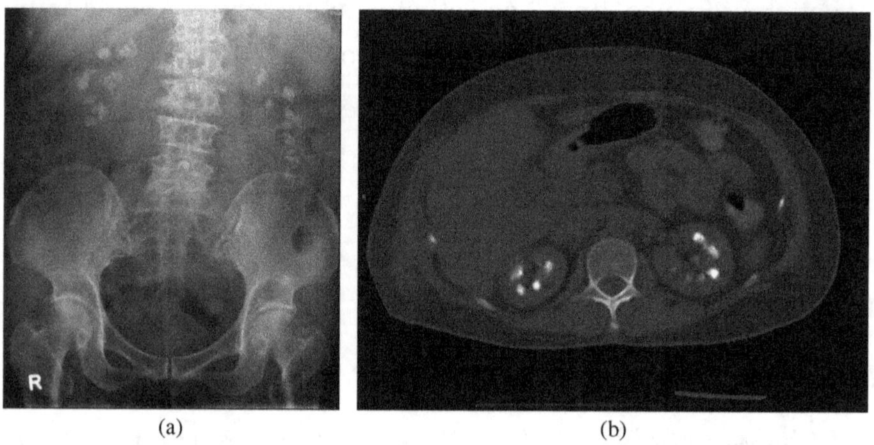

(a)   (b)

Figure 4.2: (a) X-ray KUB and (b) Non-contrast CT KUB showing medullary nephrocalcinosis.

- Kidneys appear bigger on X-ray than on ultrasound (due to distance magnification).

- Most of urinary calculi (90%) are radio-opaque except uric acid and xanthine.

Table 4.1:   Causes of Nephrocalcinosis

Area of Distribution	Causes

Medullary	• Disturbances in calcium regulation
	  ▪ Hyperparathyroidism
	  ▪ Vitamin D toxicity
	  ▪ Idiopathic hypercalciuria
	  ▪ Sarcoidosis
	  ▪ Multiple myeloma
	• Tubular disease
	  ▪ Renal tubular acidosis (Type 1)
	  ▪ Tubulopathies, e.g., Bartter's syndrome
	• Others — medullary sponge kidney or papillary necrosis

Cortical	• Usually due to trauma or cortical necrosis

- Nephrocalcinosis, previously known as Anderson-Carr kidney or Albright calcinosis, refers to the deposition of calcium in the parenchyma of the kidney and is caused by conditions that cause hypercalcaemia, hyperphosphataemia and hypercalciuria (Table 4.1).

Ultrasound

- Most frequently used imaging modality in the evaluation of kidneys and urinary tracts. It can assess:

  - Kidney size — The normal size of kidneys is 10–14 cm for (males) and 9–13 cm for females (Table 4.2).

  - Presence or absence of urinary tract obstruction or hydronephrosis

  - Able to evaluate renal structure and characterise renal masses (cystic vs. solid)

Table 4.2: Causes of Small and Large Kidneys on Ultrasound

	One Kidney	Both Kidneys
Small kidney(s)	• Congenital • Renal artery stenosis	• Smooth texture — chronic kidney disease • Irregular texture — infection (e.g., tuberculosis), reflux nephropathy, congenital dysplastic syndrome
Large kidney(s)	• Renal masses, e.g., tumours, cysts	• Polycystic kidney disease • Diabetes nephropathy (early phase) • Cystic kidney disease

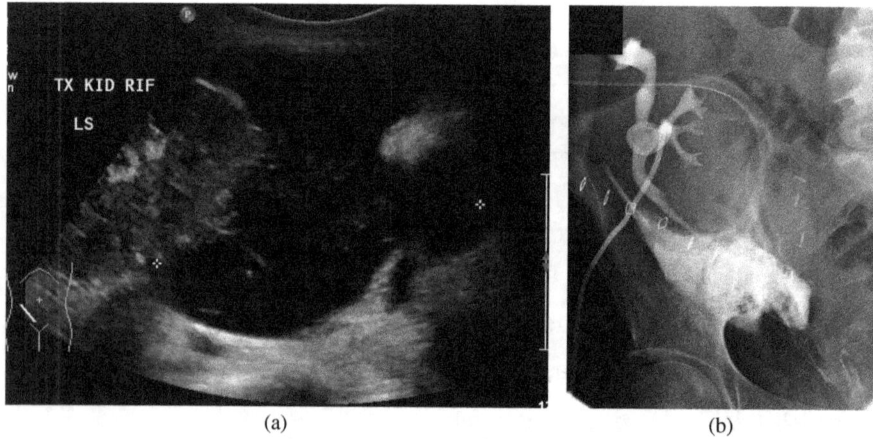

(a)   (b)

Figure 4.3: (a) Peri-graft colllection near lower pole, anechoic with some debris on ultrasound, (b) Anterograde pyelogram shows a leak of urinary contrast into the collection, confirming a urinoma. Surgical ureteric re-anastomosis was performed with subsequent resolution.

- Identify perinephric fluid collections (Figure 4.3)
- Bladder structure
- Prostate size
- Provide real-time images (e.g., renal biopsy guidance)

Contrast-enhanced ultrasound

- Ultrasound (US) using intravenous administration of a contrast agent, microbubbles containing sulphur hexafluoride gas for enhancement. The contrast agent is not nephrotoxic and is excreted by the pulmonary system. Therefore, it is useful in patients with impaired kidney function.

- Contrast-enhanced ultrasound (CEUS) is able to characterise kidney lesions and stratifies the risk of malignancy according to the Bosniak classification (Table 4.3 and Figures 4.4 and 4.5).

Table 4.3:   Bosniak Classification of Cystic Kidney Masses*

Class	Description	Workup	Risk of Malignancy (%)
1	Benign simple cyst • thin wall • no septation/calcification/ solid components	Nil	0
2	Minimal complex cyst • thin septa or calcification • well marginated	Nil	0
2F	Minimal complex cyst • multiple thin septa • calcification can be thick or nodular • high attenuation lesion	Surveillance	5
3	Indeterminate cystic mass • thickened irregular walls or septa with enhancement	Partial nephrectomy	50
4	Clearly malignant cystic mass	Partial/Total nephrectomy	100

*Bosniak 2019 version proposed to include features from an MRI but has not undergone widespread validation.

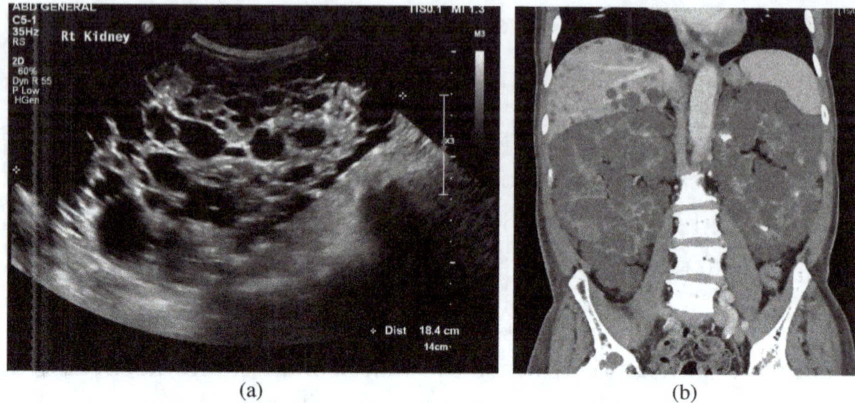

Figure 4.4: Patient with adult polycystic kidney disease. Both kidneys are enlarged with numerous cysts, as seen on (a) the US as anechoic lesions and (b) cystic density lesions on contrast-enhanced CT. Also note the cysts in the liver on CT.

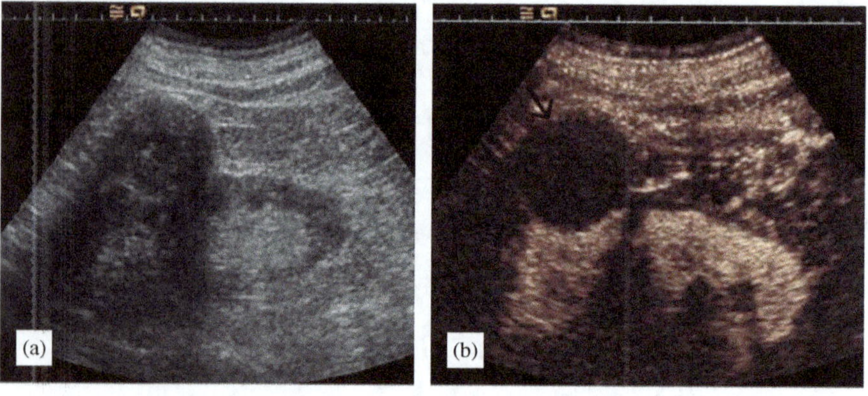

Figure 4.5: (a) Exophytic complex renal mass on ultrasound with differentials of a tumour versus complicated cyst. Due to impaired kidney function, contrast-enhanced CT or MRI were not indicated, (b) instead CEUS was performed which showed the lesion to be avascular, indicating a complicated cyst. Note the enhancement of normal renal parenchyma on CEUS.

Doppler ultrasound

- Doppler US is based on the frequency shift of the sound wave caused by moving objects; hence, it can be used to assess arterial and venous blood flow of native and transplanted kidneys.

- Renal arteries arise from proximal abdominal aorta, just below the origin of superior mesenteric artery. Accessory renal artery is in 20–30% of the population.

- Renal veins are located anterior to the ipsilateral renal artery, and both vessels course anterior to the renal pelvis before entering the renal hilum.

- Indications for a Doppler US are

  - Renal artery stenosis (Figure 4.6)

  - Renal vein thrombosis

  - Kidney masses with tumour invasion of the renal veins

  - Renal arterial aneurysms

  - Post-intervention complication (post-kidney biopsy)

  - Arteriovenous fistulas (AVFs), arteriovenous malformations (AVMs) (Figure 4.7)

- Doppler US renal artery interpretation

  - Peak Systolic Velocity (PSV)

    - normal values are 60–100 cm/s. If PSV >200 cm/s, suggestive of RAS

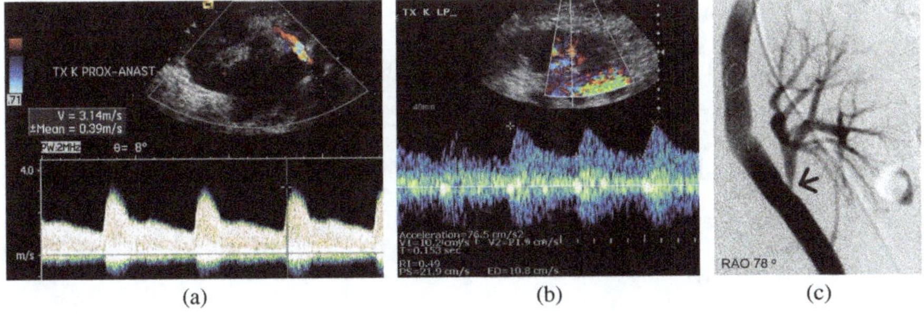

Figure 4.6:   Patient with kidney graft dysfunction due to renal artery stenosis. Doppler at anastomosis shows (a) focal "aliasing" with increased peak systolic velocity (314 cm/sec), and (b) intraparenchymal waveforms showing "parvus tardus" with increased acceleration time (77 msec), (c) catheter angiography confirms significant stenosis at anastomosis due to kink.

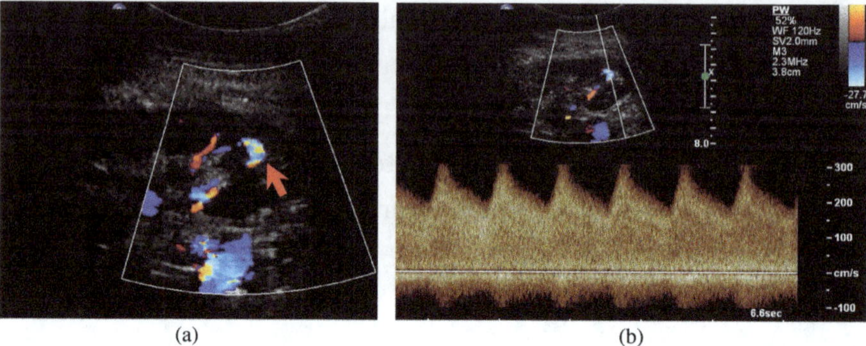

Figure 4.7: Post-renal biopsy AV fistula at the lower pole. (a) Colour doppler shows the area of aliasing which (b) on spectral doppler shows high velocities (up to 300 cm/sec) and spectral broadening.

- measured at the renal artery origin, mid portion, and hilum
- doppler-to-vessel angle of 60 degrees or less is mandatory to ensure that velocity information is accurate

- Renal aortic ratio (RAR)
  - normal value is <3.5
  - determined by the ratio of PSV in the renal artery and PSV in the aorta

- Resistive index (RI)
  - normal range is 0.5 to 0.7
  - determined by dividing the difference between the PSV and end-diastolic velocity by the PSV
  - high RI is a sign of increased peripheral vascular resistance and is a nonspecific finding

- Waveform
  - Acceleration time (AT) (time of the start of systole to peak systole) <70 msec
  - Acceleration index (AI) (slope of the systolic upstroke) >3 m/s

- Tardus parvus is seen downstream to the site of stenosis (tardus: slow upstroke or prolonged AT, while parvus: small systolic amplitude/peak (AI))

Computed Tomography

- Computer reconstruction of X-ray images from multiple angles, producing "cross-sectional" images of the body. There are several types of computed tomography (CT) (Table 4.4).

Table 4.4:   Types of Computer Tomography

Non-contrast CT	Indications
CT KUB (Figure 4.8)	• Mainly for an assessment of stone disease
Contrast-enhanced CT	**Indications**

CT urography or intravenous urography (Figures 4.9 and 4.10)	• Multiphasic, usually unenhanced, and post-contrast (nephrographic and excretory phase scans)
	• Demonstrates collecting system, ureter, and bladder on an excretory phase
	• Superior to traditional intravenous pyelography
	• Useful for
	   – urothelial mass
	   – obstructive uropathy
	   – urothelial surveillance
	   – ureteric stricture

CT angiogram (CTA) (Figure 4.11)	• Demonstrates renal vasculature
	• Superior to US Doppler
	• Useful for
	   – Diagnosis of renal artery stenosis in determining the level and extent of stenosis
	   – Providing information to guide subsequent treatment planning

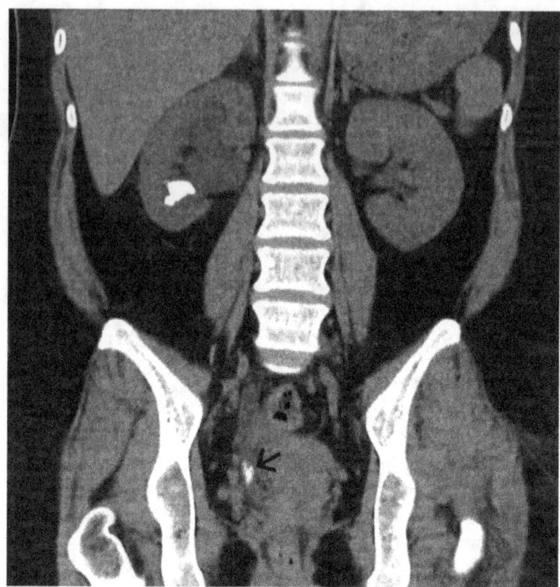

Figure 4.8:   Non-contrast CT KUB shows right renal calculus and distal right ureteric calculus (black arrow), resulting in right hydronephrosis.

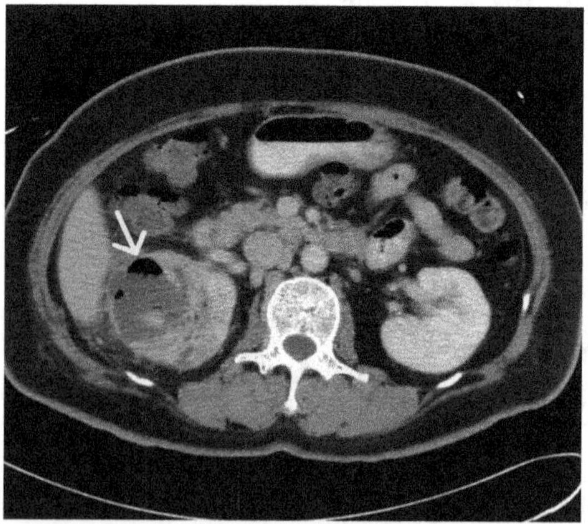

Figure 4.9:   Contrast-enhanced CT in a patient with fever showing right kidney abscess, containing pockets of gas, parenchymal swelling, and adjacent fat stranding.

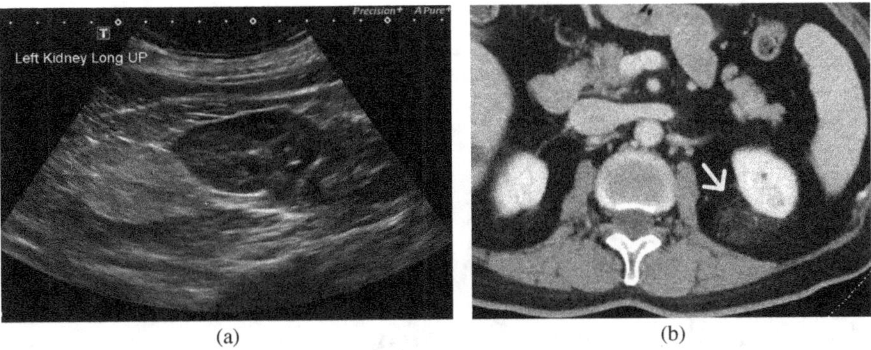

(a)   (b)

Figure 4.10:   Renal angiomyolipoma. (a) Ultrasound shows an exophytic echogenic mass at the upper pole of the left kidney, (b) Contrast-enhanced CT confirms a mass with predominant fatty density.

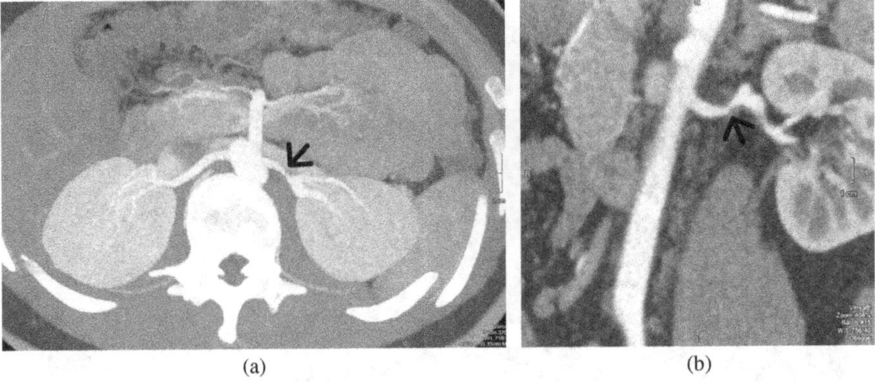

(a)   (b)

Figure 4.11:   Young hypertensive. CT angiography (CTA): (a) Axial maximum intensity projection (MIP) image and (b) Coronal reconstruction image shows severe stenosis of the mid segment left renal artery (black arrows), likely fibromuscular dysplasia.

- Has a better resolution with faster and better characterisation of renal masses.

- Indications:

  - Further characterisation of renal masses — can differentiate a simple cyst from a tumour (e.g., Bosniak class 2F)

  - Staging of tumours — helps in prognostication and a treatment plan

- Urinary calculi
- Renal collection/perirenal collection/abscess
- Retroperitoneal pathology
- Obstructive uropathy — degree and cause of obstruction
- Renovascular disease

Magnetic Resonance Imaging

- Uses electromagnetic radiation (radiofrequency waves) to create images from hydrogen protons in water present in body tissues (Figure 4.12). There is no patient exposure to ionising radiation as compared to CT.

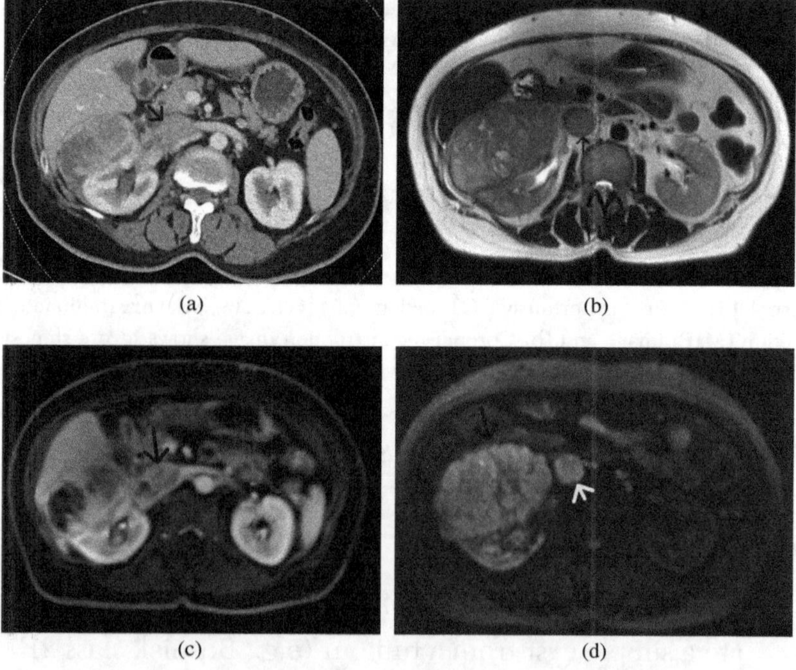

Figure 4.12:   Patient with haematuria. (a) Axial contrast-enhanced CT, (b) MRI axial T2, and (c) Post-gadolinium images shows a heterogenously enhancing right renal mass, invading right renal vein and inferior vena cava (black arrows), which are consistent with renal cell carcinoma, (d) diffuse weighted (DWI) MR image shows a mass and tumour thrombus in the inferior vena cava with bright signal.

- Magnetic resonance imaging (MRI) is an alternative to CT for specific patient populations:
  - Allergies to iodinated contrast
  - Special population where exposure to radiation should be minimised — pregnant women and children
  - Patients with impaired kidney function
- Gadolinium-based agents are the most common contrast agent used in MRI imaging, but there is a risk for nephrogenic systemic fibrosis (NSF).

Nephrogenic systemic fibrosis

- Nephrogenic systemic fibrosis (NSF) is a rare but painful and devastating skin complication of gadolinium and can progress to involve internal organs (muscle, heart, lung).
- The dermopathy present with symmetric, dark red patches and burning, itching, and severe pain over affected areas. It initially involves the lower legs and forearms and progresses to peri-articular tissue, which can lead to contractures and impaired mobility.
- Internal organs can be involved where scarring leads to a restriction of individual organ function.
- A diagnosis of NSF is made when there is a history of gadolinium exposure and a diagnostic full thickness skin biopsy showing thickened collagen bundles, mucin deposition, proliferation of fibroblast, and elastic fibres but no sign of inflammation.
- Prevention is the key, as there is no effective treatment for NSF.
- ACR (American College of Radiology) classifies gadolinium-based agents into 3 groups relative to the risk of NSF:

  Group 1: Agents associated with the greatest number of NSF cases — Omniscan®, Magnevist®, OptiMARK®

Table 4.5:   Guidelines for the Use of Gadolinium Contrast in Patients with Kidney Diseases

Kidney Disease	Guideline
End-stage kidney disease on dialysis	• Review indication for an MRI scan with gadolinium. • Explore alternative imaging modalities, e.g., contrast-enhanced CT. • Group I gadolinium contrast agents are contraindicated. • If an MRI with gadolinium is needed, schedule an MRI before the scheduled dialysis and use group II gadolinium contrast agents.
Patients with chronic kidney disease (estimated glomerular filtration rate <30 mL/min/1.73 m²)	• Group I gadolinium contrast agents are contraindicated — use group II agents instead. • No role to perform dialysis for the removal of gadolinium contrast agent.

Group II: Agents associated with few, if any, unconfounded cases of NSF — MultiHance®, Gadavist®, Dotarem®, Clariscan®, ProHance®

Group III: Agents for which data remains limited regarding NSF risk but for which few, if any, unconfounded cases of NSF have been reported — Eovist® / Primovist®

• Patients with kidney disease are at high risk for NSF (Table 4.5).

Nuclear renal scans or renal scintigraphy

• Scintigraphy provides functional and structural information (Table 4.6).

Table 4.6:   Types of Renal Scintigraphy

Type of Nuclear Scintigraphy	Clearance	Utility	Indication
Technetium-99m diethylenetriamine pentaacetic acid (DTPA)	Analogous to inulin — cleared by glomerular filtration and is not reabsorbed or secreted by tubules	• Estimation of the glomerular filtration rate	• Imaging of kidney perfusion • Imaging of kidney function, especially in kidney donor • Captopril renography (DPTA/MAG3) — in renal artery stenosis, a positive scan will show asymmetry of size or function, delayed time to peak activity, and cortical isotope retention
Technetium-99m-labelled agent mercaptoacetyltriglycine (MAG3)	95% cleared by proximal tubular secretion and thence useful for patients with low glomerular filtration rates (5% cleared by glomerular filtration)	• Estimation of effective renal plasma flow • Higher extraction fraction than DPTA, better for imaging obstructed kidneys or kidneys with poor function	• Imaging of kidney function • Generate renogram curves, which show the transit of tracer through the kidneys • Evaluate for urinoma
Technetium-99m-dimercaptosuccinic acid (DMSA)	Filtered by glomerulus and reabsorbed — binds and is retained in proximal tubules of the cortex	• Imaging of the kidney cortex and parenchyma • Not useful for the evaluation of the excretory function	• Evaluate the kidney cortex, such as regions of cortical scarring or pseudotumours • Congenital abnormalities, e.g., horseshoe kidney or ectopic kidney • Chronic pyelonephritis or vesicoureteral reflux

References

ACR Manual on Contrast Media. (2020). ACR Committee on Drugs and Contrast Media. https://www.acr.org/-/media/ACR/files/clinical-resources/contrast_media.pdf

Al-Katib S, Shetty M, Jafri SM, *et al.* (2017). Radiologic assessment of native renal vasculature: A multimodality review. *Radiographics* **37**(1): 136–156.

Taffel MT, Nikolaidis P, Beland MD, *et al.* (2017). ACR Appropriateness Criteria® renal transplant dysfunction. *J Am Coll Radiol* **14**(5S): S272–S281.

Warren KS and McFarlane J. (2005). The Bosniak classification of renal cystic masses. *BJU Int* **95**(7): 939–942.

5 Sodium Disorders

Cai Jiashen, Kwek Jia Liang

Introduction

- Sodium disorders, such as hyponatraemia and hypernatraemia, reflect disruptions in the delicate balance of water and sodium in the body. The kidneys, along with other osmoregulatory mechanisms, play a central role in maintaining water and sodium balance.

Sodium Balance

- The renin-angiotensin-aldosterone system (RAAS) and the atrial natriuretic peptide (ANP) system are crucial in regulating sodium (Na^+) levels and are influenced by extracellular fluid (ECF) volume and effective arterial blood volume (EABV).

  - RAAS: When EABV decreases, renin is released, leading to the production of angiotensin II. Angiotensin II then stimulates the release of aldosterone from the adrenal glands, promoting Na^+ reabsorption in the kidneys.

  - ANP: When EABV increases, ANP is released by the heart and increases kidney excretion of Na^+ and inhibits the effects of aldosterone.

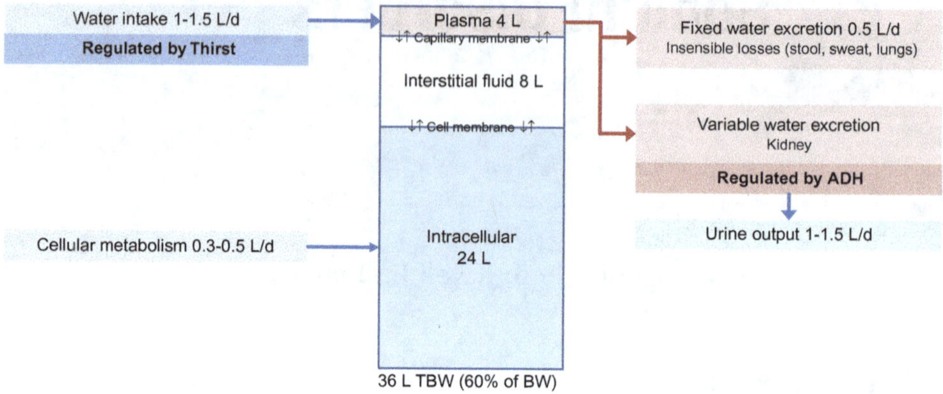

Figure 5.1:   Normal water balance (assuming body weight of 60 kg)

Water Balance

- Water balance in the body involves the intricate interplay between anti-diuretic hormone (ADH) and the sensation of thirst (Figure 5.1).

  - ADH: ADH is produced by the hypothalamus and released by the posterior pituitary gland in response to increased serum osmolality or decreased EABV. ADH acts on the renal-collecting ducts to increase water reabsorption. Suppression of ADH release serves as a primary protective mechanism against water retention and the development of hyponatraemia.

  - Thirst: The sensation of thirst is triggered by the hypothalamus in response to increased serum osmolality or decreased EABV to increase water intake. Thirst serves as a protective mechanism against water loss and the development of hypernatraemia.

Hyponatraemia

Definition

- An excess of water in relation to the body's Na^+ stores

- Serum sodium concentration, Na^+ <135 mmol/L

Classification

Severity:
- Mild: 130–134 mmol/L

- Moderate: 125–129 mmol/L

- Severe: <125 mmol/L

Time/duration:
- Acute: <48 hours

- Chronic: ≥48 hours or unknown onset

Symptomatic vs. asymptomatic:
- Asymptomatic: Subtle impairments in mentation and gait, increased risk of falls/fractures

- Symptomatic: Mild-moderate — headache, fatigue, lethargy, nausea/vomiting, dizziness, gait disturbances, forgetfulness, confusion, muscle cramps; Severe — seizures, obtundation, coma, respiratory arrest

Tonicity:
- Hypotonic: Serum osmolality, S_{Osm} < 275 mOsm/kg

- Non-hypotonic: S_{Osm} > 275 mOsm/kg

    — Pseudohyponatraemia: Hyperlipidaemia, Paraproteinaemia

    — Translocational: Hyperglycaemia, Mannitol, Glycine

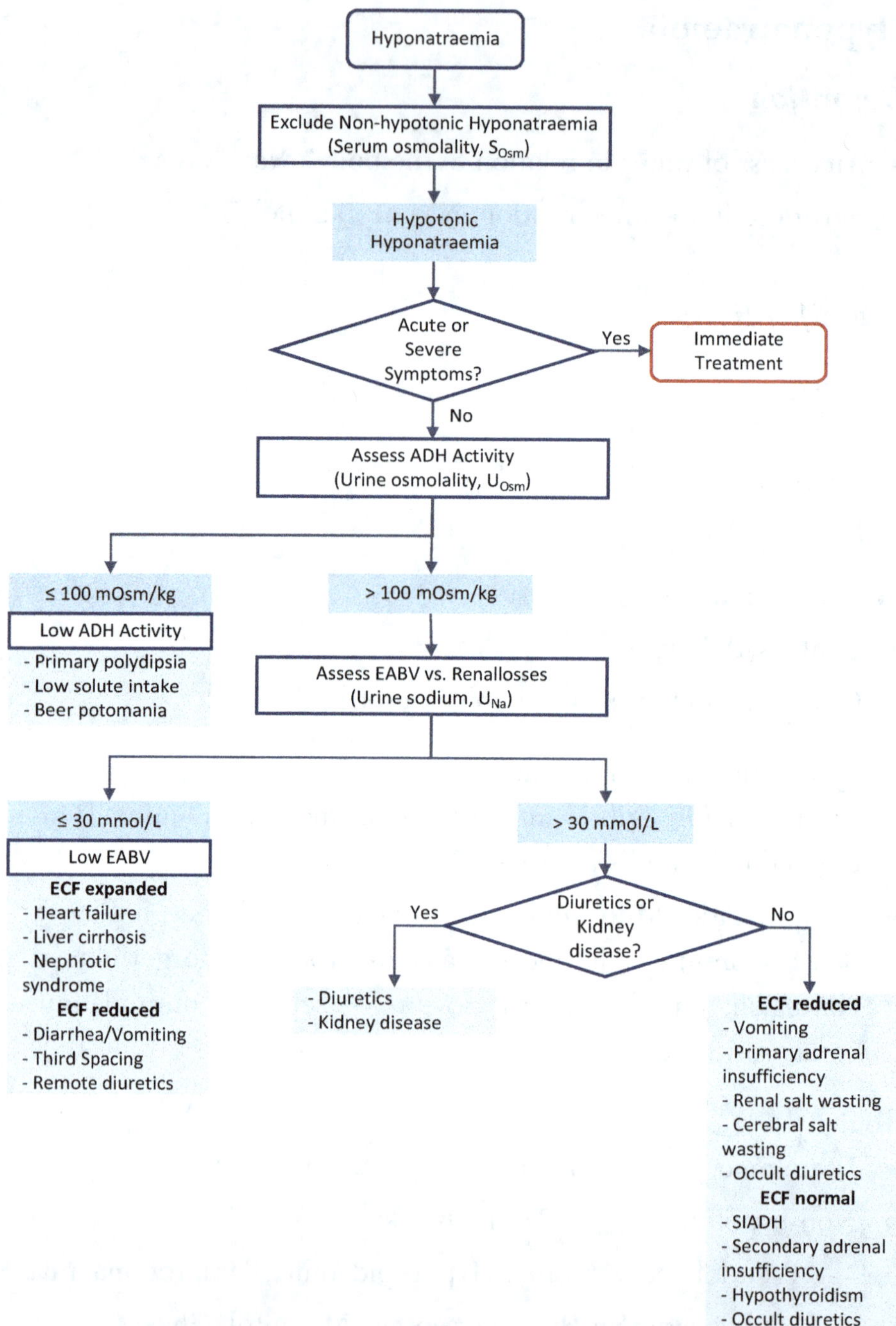

Figure 5.2:   Algorithm for diagnosis of hyponatraemia

Abbreviations: ADH: anti-diuretic hormone, EABV: effective arterial blood volume, ECF: extracellular fluid, SIADH: syndrome of inappropriate anti-diuretic hormone

Source: *Eur J Endocrinol* (2014). ***170***(3): G1–G47. (ESICM, ESE, ERA-EDTA Clinical Practice Guidelines).

Step-by-step approach

1. Exclude non-hypotonic hyponatraemia (serum osmolality, S_{Osm})

S_{Osm} < 275 mOsm/kg: Hypotonic hyponatraemia

S_{Osm} > 275 mOsm/kg: Pseudohyponatraemia, translocational hyponatraemia

Osmolar gap = Measured S_{Osm} – Calculated S_{Osm}; > 10 is suggestive of additional osmolar substance (i.e., translocational hyponatraemia)

Calculated $S_{Osm} = 2 \times [Na] + [Glu] + [Urea]$ (all units in mmol/L)

2. Assess ADH activity (urine osmolality, U_{Osm})

U_{Osm} < 100 mOsm/kg: Low ADH activity (e.g., primary polydipsia, beer potomania, low solute intake)

U_{Osm} ≥ 100 mOsm/kg: Presence of ADH activity (e.g., true hypovolaemia, effective hypovolaemia, SIADH (Table 5.1), hypothyroidism, adrenal insufficiency)

3. Assess effective arterial blood volume (EABV) vs. renal losses (urine sodium, U_{Na})

U_{Na} < 30 mOsm/kg: Low effective arterial blood volume

U_{Na} > 30 mOsm/kg: Elevated Na^+ excretion — rule out diuretic use or kidney disease

4. Assess extracellular fluid status

Table 5.1: Diagnostic Criteria for Syndrome of Inappropriate Antidiuretic Hormone Secretion

- Hypotonic hyponatraemia, serum osmolality (S_{Osm}) < 275 mOsm/kg
- Euvolaemia
- Less than maximally dilute urine: U_{Osm} > 100 mOsm/kg
- Elevated urine sodium excretion with lack of sodium retention: U_{Na} > 30 mmol/L
- Absence of severe kidney disease, cirrhosis, or heart failure
- Absence of alternative causes of euvolaemic hypotonic hyponatraemia with less than maximally dilute urine including but not limited to hypothyroidism, glucocorticoid insufficiency, or diuretic use

Management

Acute or symptomatic hyponatraemia

- Hypertonic saline (3% NaCl) 1–2 mL/kg body weight per hour (typically 50–100 mL)

- Monitor Na^+ every 2 hours, aim to increase in Na^+ by 1 mmol/L per hour (~4–6 mmol/L in the first 6 hours)

Chronic and asymptomatic hyponatraemia

- **Treatment according to underlying cause**

  - Euvolaemic (normal ECF) hyponatraemia: treat underlying cause

  - Hypovolaemic (reduced ECF) hyponatraemia: volume repletion with isotonic saline or balanced crystalloids

  - Hypervolaemic (expanded ECF) hyponatraemia: fluid restriction ± diuretics

  - SIADH: fluid restriction ± increased solute intake (NaCl tabs)

- **Limit increase in Na^+ by 8 mmol/L in any 24-hour period**

  - Monitor Na^+ every 4–6 hours and urine output

- ■ In the event of over-rapid correction, consider re-lowering Na⁺ with electrolyte-free water ± desmopressin (1–2 mcg every 6 hours)
- **Estimation of effects of infusate**
  - ■ $\Delta[\text{Na}] = ([\text{Na}]_{\text{infusate}} + [\text{K}]_{\text{infusate}} - [\text{Na}]_{\text{serum}})/(\text{TBW} + 1)$

Osmotic demyelination syndrome

- Acute demyelination in the setting of osmotic changes associated with rapid correction of hyponatraemia
- Risk factors: [Na] < 105 mmol/L, hypokalaemia, hypophosphataemia, alcoholism, malnutrition, liver disease

Hypernatraemia

Definition

- A deficit of water in relation to the body's Na⁺ stores
- Serum sodium concentration, Na⁺ > 145 mmol/L

Classification

Time/duration:

- ■ Acute: < 48 hours
- ■ Chronic: ≥ 48 hours or unknown onset

Step-by-step approach

1. Assess ADH activity (urine osmolality, U_{Osm})

U_{Osm} < 600 mOsm/kg: Renal concentrating defect

U_{Osm} < 300 mOsm/kg: Pure water loss — Diabetes insipidus (DI)

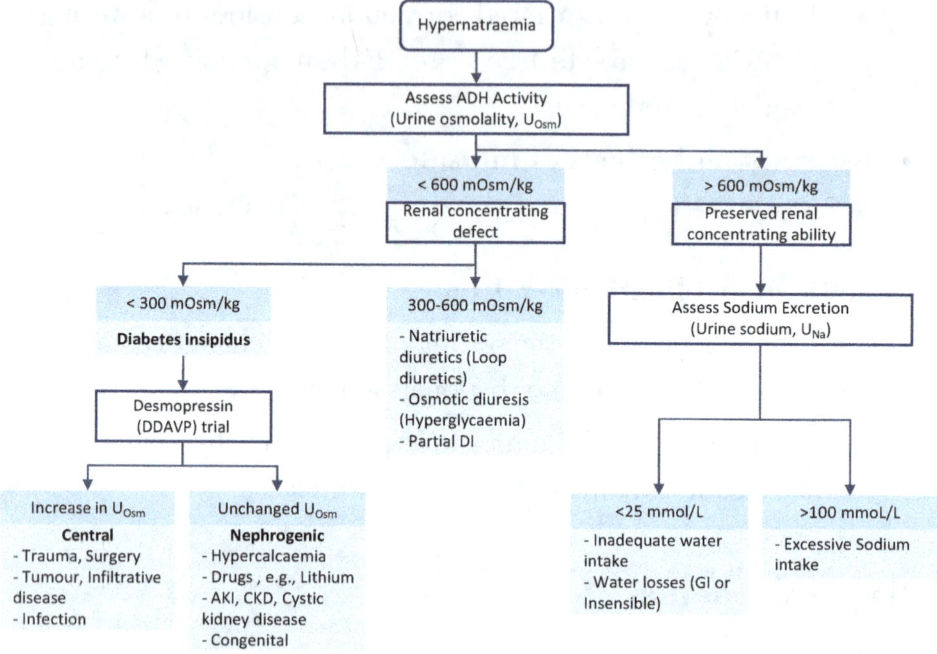

Figure 5.3:   Algorithm for diagnosis of hypernatraemia

U_{Osm} 300–600 mOsm/kg: Driven by natriuretic diuresis or osmotic diuresis — Loop diuretics, hyperglycaemia; partial DI

U_{Osm} > 600 mOsm/kg: Preserved renal concentrating ability

2. If U_{Osm} < 300 mOsm/kg, desmopressin (DDAVP) trial

Differentiate central/neurogenic vs. nephrogenic DI

3. If U_{Osm} > 600 mOsm/kg, assess sodium excretion (urine sodium, U_{Na})

U_{Na} < 25 mmol/L: inadequate water intake, extrarenal hypotonic fluid losses (gastrointestinal or insensible)

U_{Na} > 100 mmol/L: excessive sodium intake

Management

- Address underlying cause – Specific treatment for underlying cause (e.g., correction of electrolyte abnormalities, hyperglycaemia, desmopressin for central DI, stop water/fluid losses, restore access to water)
- Assess free water deficit

  Free water deficit = Total body water $\times$ ([Na] – 140)/140 (all units in mmol/L)

  Will need to account for ongoing free water losses
- Determine rate of correction
  - Acute: Aim for Na^+ decrease by 1 mmol/h
  - Chronic: Limit Na^+ decrease by 10 mmol/24h (~0.5 mmol/h)
  - Estimation of effects of Infusate

    $$\Delta[Na] = ([Na]_{infusate} + [K]_{infusate} - [Na]_{serum})/(\text{Total body water} + 1) \text{ (all units in mmol/L)}$$
- Monitor Na^+ every 4–6 hours and urine output

References

Adrogué HJ and Madias NE (2000). Hypernatremia. *N Engl J Med* **342**(20): 1493–1499.

Adrogué HJ and Madias NE (2000). Hyponatremia. *N Engl J Med* **342**(21): 1581–1589.

Adrogué HJ and Madias NE (2012). The challenge of hyponatremia. *J Am Soc Nephrol* **23**(7): 1140–1148.

Seay NW, Lehrich RW and Greenberg A (2020). Diagnosis and management of disorders of body tonicity-hyponatremia and hypernatremia: Core curriculum 2020. *Am J Kidney Dis* **75**(2): 272–286.

Spasovski G, Vanholder R, Allolio B, *et al.* (2014). Clinical practice guideline on diagnosis and treatment of hyponatraemia. *Eur J Endocrinol* **170**(3): G1–G47. Erratum in: Eur J Endocrinol. 2014 Jul;171(1):X1.

Sterns RH (2015). Disorders of plasma sodium: Causes, consequences, and correction. *N Engl J Med* **372**(1): 55–65.

6 Potassium Disorders

Nigel Fong, Kwek Jia Liang

Potassium Balance

- Total body potassium (K^+) stores are about 55 mmol/kg and distributed mainly intracellularly (98%), with extracellular K^+ (2%) concentration tightly regulated within the narrow range of 3.5–5.0 mmol/L.

- The average daily dietary intake of K^+ ranges between 2500 and 3500 mg/day. About 90% is excreted in the urine while 10% is excreted in the stool and sweat.

- K^+ uptake into the intracellular compartment is stimulated by:
  - insulin (facilitating post-meal uptake of dietary K^+)
  - catecholamines (enabling cellular uptake of K^+ released by exercising the muscles)
  - beta-agonism (e.g., nebulised salbutamol)

- In the kidney, K^+ is freely filtered and almost completely reabsorbed. Regulation of K^+ levels occur in the aldosterone-sensitive distal nephron, hinging on the balance between mineralocorticoid activity and sodium delivery to the tubular lumen of the distal nephron (Figure 6.1).

- In physiologic states, aldosterone activity and distal sodium delivery move in opposite directions such that K^+ homeostasis is unaffected.

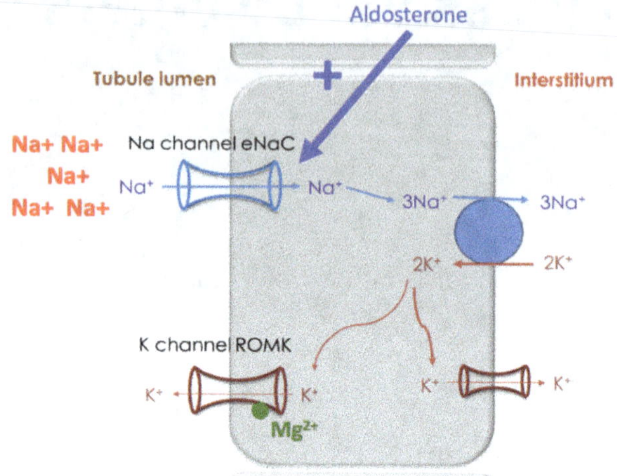

Figure 6.1:   Key Channels involved in potassium homeostasis

- For instance, hypovolaemia stimulates the renin-angiotensin-aldosterone system while simultaneously increasing proximal sodium reabsorption, hence decreasing distal sodium delivery. The increase in aldosterone activity stimulates sodium reabsorption through the epithelial sodium channel (ENaC), which is coupled to increased K^+ secretion through the renal outer medullary potassium (ROMK) channel.

- Conversely, the decrease in distal sodium delivery decreases sodium reabsorption through the ENaC and decreases K^+ secretion through the ROMK channel, which counterbalances the effect of an increase in aldosterone activity.

- Hence, salt and water retention occur without affecting K^+ homeostasis.

- It is only in pathologic states, when aldosterone activity and distal sodium delivery move in parallel, that abnormal K^+ homeostasis occurs.

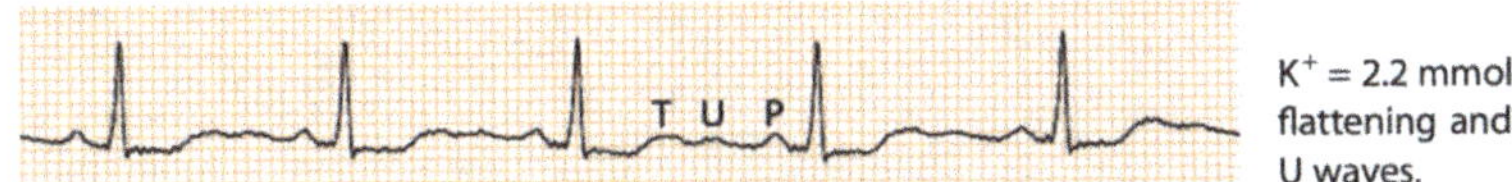

Figure 6.2:   Electrocardiographic Changes of Hypokalaemia

Figure used with permission: Fong N, Algorithms in Differential Diagnosis, 2019.

- An additional factor affecting renal K$^+$ homeostasis is magnesium. The ROMK channel is physiologically inhibited by intracellular Mg^{2+}. In hypomagnesaemia, K$^+$ efflux through the ROMK channel is uninhibited, leading to hypokalaemia.

Hypokalaemia

- Mild hypokalaemia (K$^+$ 3.0–3.5 mmol/L) is common and frequently asymptomatic.

- Severe hypokalaemia may cause cardiac instability (Figure 6.2), gastrointestinal dysmotility, skeletal muscle weakness, and rhabdomyolysis.

- Chronic hypokalaemia may lead to interstitial nephritis and chronic kidney disease.

Approach

- Mechanisms of hypokalaemia include:
  - cellular shifts — for instance in insulin administration, beta adrenergic stimulation, or hypokalaemic periodic paralysis
  - reduced K$^+$ intake
  - gastrointestinal losses such as in diarrhoea, or
  - renal K$^+$ losses

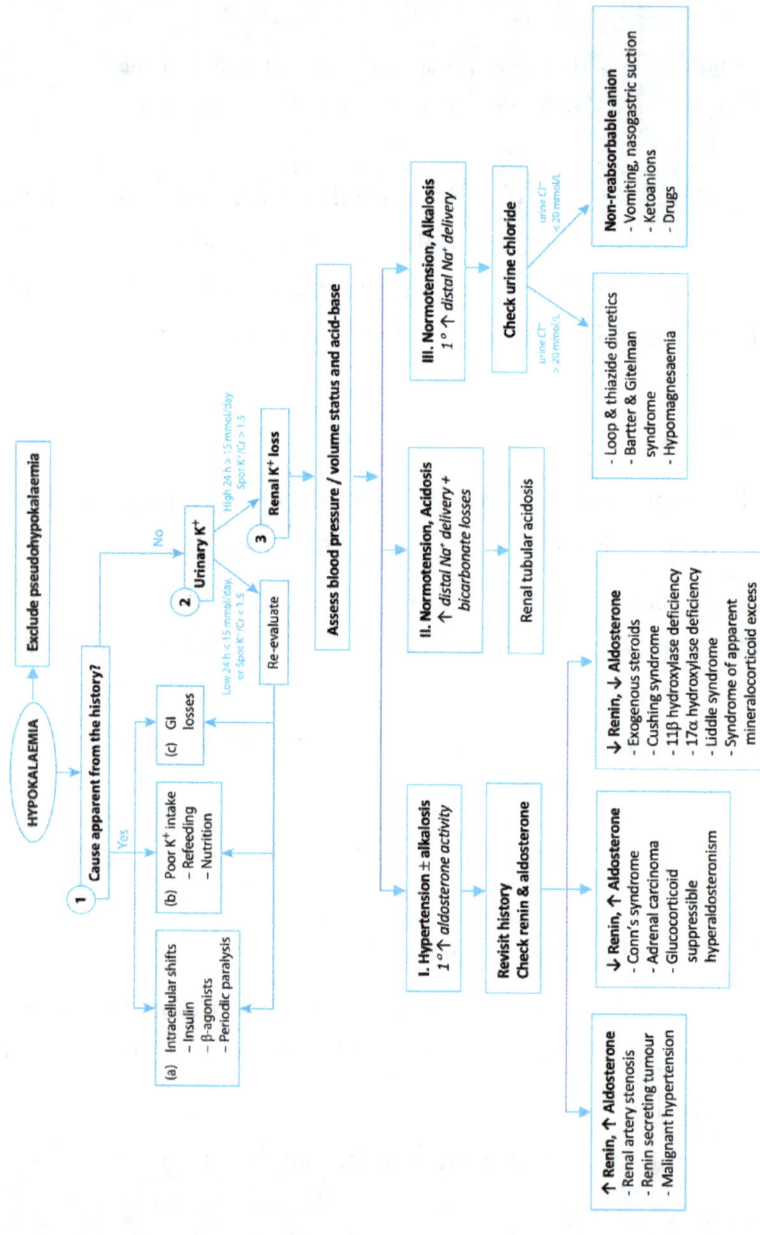

Figure 6.3: Diagnostic approach to hypokalaemia

A stepwise approach to the diagnosis of hypokalaemia (Figure 6.3) can be taken.

1. The first step is to exclude pseudohypokalaemia, as occurs in patients with marked leukocytosis, in whom uptake of K^+ by metabolically active cells may occur in the sample tube following blood collection.
2. Take a careful history for a cause of hypokalaemia as the latter is often apparent from the clinical history — for instance, in a patient with profuse diarrhoea.
3. If a cause is not apparent, proceed with further workup. The first dichotomy is between renal and non-renal K^+ loss, which can be distinguished with a spot urine K^+/creatinine ratio or 24-hour urine K^+ levels. In the setting of hypokalaemia, a spot urine K^+/creatinine ratio of >1.5 or 24-hour urine K^+ secretion of >15 mmol suggests inappropriate renal K^+ wasting.
4. If there is inappropriate renal K^+ wasting, distinguish between these three distinct patterns based on volume and blood pressure, as well as acid/base status.

I. Hypertension and/or volume expansion: This is a primary increase in aldosterone activity that is not in response to hypovolaemia. This increases sodium absorption through the ENaC, leading to hypertension, hypokalaemia, and metabolic alkalosis. The defect lies along the renin-angiotensin-aldosterone axis and can be further distinguished by plasma renin activity and aldosterone levels:

- High Renin, Low Aldosterone — Increase in renin activity, e.g., renal artery stenosis

- Low Renin, High Aldosterone — Increase in aldosterone activity, e.g., Conn's syndrome

- Low Renin, Low Aldosterone — Non-aldosterone stimulation of the ENaC, e.g., steroid excess (exogenous steroids or endogenous Cushing's syndrome), constitutional ENaC activation (Liddle's syndrome)

II. Hypokalaemia with low-normal blood pressure and metabolic acidosis. This is the hallmark of renal tubular acidosis (RTA). RTA arises from impaired bicarbonate reclamation in the proximal tubule (Type II) or impaired H^+ excretion in the distal tubule (Type I). The mechanism of hypokalaemia is increased distal sodium delivery, which accompanies bicarbonate losses. RTA may be associated with drugs, autoimmune disease, or paraprotenaemia. Type II RTA may also manifest as a generalised proximal tubulopathy (Fanconi's syndrome).

III. Hypokalaemia with low-normal blood pressure and metabolic alkalosis. This represents a primary increase in distal sodium delivery. Causes can be distinguished by the urinary chloride level:

- Spot urinary chloride >20 mmol/L: loop diuretics (and its genetic parallel Bartter syndrome), thiazide diuretics (and Gitelman syndrome), or hypomagnesaemia (which both inhibits thick ascending limb sodium absorption and leads to unopposed K^+ efflux through the ROMK channel).

- Spot urinary chloride <20 mmol/L: non-reabsorbable anions such as bicarbonates (in the setting of alkalosis due to vomiting or high nasogastric aspirates), ketoanions, or anionic drugs such as penicillins. This anion would be accompanied by an increase in distal sodium delivery to maintain charge balance.

Management

- Hypokalaemia is treated by correcting the underlying cause along with K^+ replacement.
- The K^+ content of common K^+ replacements is given in Table 6.1.
- Intravenous replacement is recommended where K^+ <2.8 mmol/L or in the presence of ECG changes.
- Tips on correcting potassium:

Table 6.1:   Common Potassium Replacements

Replacement	K content	Notes
IV potassium chloride	10–20 mmol in 100 mL of 5% dextrose	Concentrations >10 mmol/100 mL require infusion through a central venous access
Oral span K tablet	8 mmol per 600 mg tablet	
Oral mist KCl liquid	13.4 mmol per 10 mL solution	
Oral potassium citrate	27.8 mmol per 10 mL solution	Also provides alkali buffer

- Patients with normal kidney function often require considerable replacement as total body K^+ potassium deficits may be quite large — each 0.1 mmol/L decrease in serum K^+ is estimated to reflect a 30–40 mmol decrease in total body K^+ stores.

- Conversely, patients with impaired K^+ excretion (especially patients on dialysis) should receive conservative doses of K^+ as over-replacement can lead to hyperkalaemia.

- If there is hypomagnesaemia, magnesium should be replaced before or alongside K^+. Otherwise, serum K^+ may fail to rise with replacement due to continued K^+ losses through the ROMK channel.

- If there is concomitant hypokalaemia and acidosis, correct K^+ before acidosis as correction of acidosis will lead to K^+ shifts into the intracellular compartment, which risks further falls of serum K^+ levels. In patients with RTA, potassium citrate is ideal to both provide K^+ replacement and correct acidosis.

- Some patients have an underlying etiology of chronic hypokalaemia that cannot be resolved and may require high doses of long-term K^+ replacements. Such patients may benefit from small doses of ENaC blockers (e.g., amiloride 2.5 mg or 5 mg daily) to reduce K^+ efflux through the ROMK channel.

Hyperkalaemia

Definition

- Hyperkalaemia is a serum K^+ of more than 5 mmol/L.

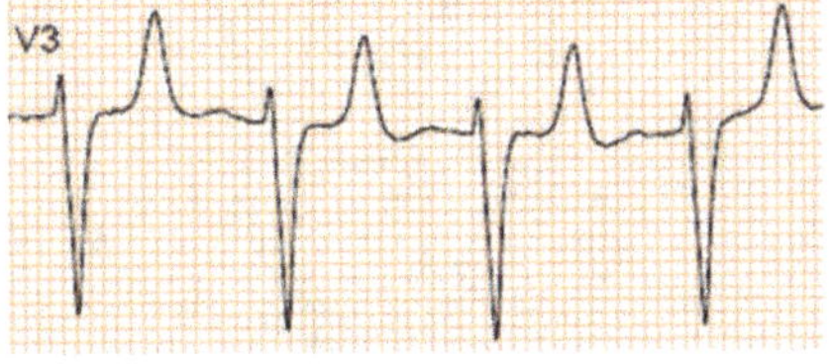

(a) Hyperkalaemia, $K^+ = 7.0$ mmol/L. Recognise the tall tented T waves.

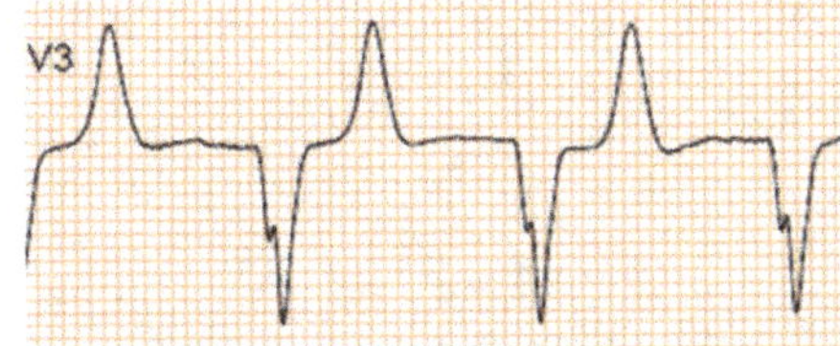

(b) As K^+ rises further to 9.0 mmol/L, the QRS complex widens, a bundle brunch block develops and P waves disappear.

Figure 6.4:   ECG changes in hyperkalaemia

(*Figure used with permission:* Fong N, Algorithms in Differential Diagnosis, 2019.)

- Hyperkalaemia leads to cardiac depolarisation, manifesting as tented T waves, QRS widening, and eventual asystole (Figure 6.4). It can also lead to neuromuscular weakness.

- A rapid rate of rise in K^+ levels is less well tolerated than chronic hyperkalaemia.

Principles

- The kidney has a large capacity to excrete K^+. In fact, in healthy individuals, a high-potassium–low-sodium diet reduces blood pressure and cardiovascular events, with no untoward hyperkalaemia.

- Chronic hyperkalaemia arises in the setting of reduced renal capacity for K^+ excretion, such as in chronic kidney disease or in situations of decreased aldosterone activity or decreased distal sodium delivery (see the preceding chapter on hypokalaemia).

- Superimposed insults may include increased dietary K^+ intake or cellular shifts.

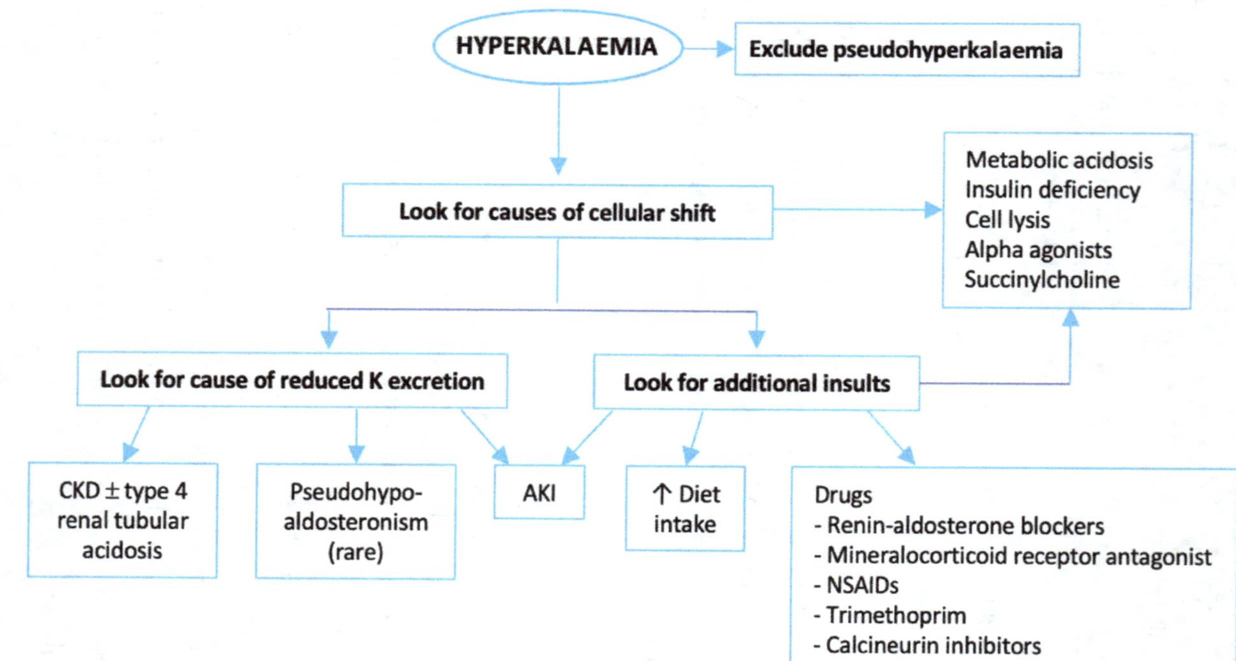

Figure 6.5:   Diagnostic approach to hyperkalaemia

CKD: chronic kidney disease; AKI: acute kidney injury; NSAIDs: non-steroidal anti-inflammatory drugs

(*Figure used with permission:* Fong N, Algorithms in Differential Diagnosis, 2019.)

Step-by-step approach

A stepwise approach to diagnostic workup of hyperkalaemia is as follows:

1. Exclude pseudohyperkalaemia

This occurs when blood is haemolysed during specimen collection (most laboratory systems indicate sample haemolysis) or due to ex-vivo cellular lysis in patients with severe leukocytosis or thrombocytosis.

2. Look for any causes of cellular shift of potassium. These include:

- Metabolic acidosis
- Insulin deficiency, as in diabetic ketoacidosis
- Drugs e.g., alpha agonists (phenylephrine), succinylcholine
- Cell lysis, as occurs in tumour lysis syndrome, massive haemolysis, organ ischaemia, and rhabdomyolysis.

3. Inquire the cause of reduced renal potassium excretion

- Most patients will have acute kidney injury (AKI) or chronic kidney disease (CKD). The risk of hyperkalaemia is inversely proportional to the glomerular filtration rate (GFR) and is typically seen below a GFR of 20–30 mL/min/1.73 m^2.
- However, hyperkalaemia may develop with higher levels of GFR due to Type IV renal tubular acidosis, a hypoaldosteronic state which occurs in diabetic nephropathy, chronic interstitial nephritis, or obstructive uropathy.
- Rarely, hyperkalaemia may occur in patients with normal renal function due to genetic defects in the ENaC, leading to

reduced mineralocorticoid effect (pseudohypoaldosteronism Type I), or in the WNK4 channel (pseudohypoaldosteronism Type II, also known as Gordon syndrome).

4. **Search for additional insults that precipitate hyperkalaemia, especially in CKD patients who previously had stable potassium levels. Such insults may include:**
   - Superimposed AKI or progression of CKD
   - Increased dietary K^+ intake
   - Medications that inhibit aldosterone activity, particularly nonsteroidal anti-inflammatory drugs, calcineurin inhibitors, angiotensin-converting enzyme inhibitors and angiotensin receptor blockers, and mineralocorticoid receptor antagonists
   - Drugs that inhibit renal K^+ secretion, such as trimethoprim

Management

1. **Correct hyperkalaemia emergently if K >6 mmol/L or if there are ECG changes:**
   - Calcium gluconate (10 mL of a 10% solution) to stabilise cardiac myocytes.
   - Insulin (10 units) with dextrose (40 mL) to shift K^+ into cells. This buys temporary reprieve but does not remove K^+ from the body.
   - Potassium binding resins such as sodium polystyrene sulfonate (resonium, 10–15 g q6–8h) or sodium zirconium cyclosilicate (lokelma, 10 g TDS q8h). Sodium zirconium has a more rapid onset than resonium, but may be more costly.

- Dialysis should be undertaken if medical therapy fails or if K^+ is anticipated to rise rapidly as in cases of tumour lysis syndrome, crush injury, or severe oliguric acute kidney injury.

2. Once the patient is stabilised, consider measures to promote normokalaemia:

- Reduce dietary K^+ intake and stop K^+ supplements, if any.

- Avoidance of drugs that predispose to hyperkalaemia.

- Correction of metabolic acidosis — patients with CKD should be given oral sodium bicarbonate supplementation aiming for a serum bicarbonate of >22 mmol/L.

- Chronic loop or thiazide diuretic therapy if indicated (this will also increase K^+ excretion).

References

Gumz ML, Rabinowitz L and Wingo CS (2015). An integrated view of potassium homeostasis. *N Engl J Med* **373**(1): 60–72.

Packham DK, Ramussen HS, Lavin PT, *et al.* (2015) Sodium zirconium cyclosilicate in hyperkalemia. *N Engl J Med* **372**(3): 222–231.

Palmer BF and Clegg DJ (2019). Physiology and pathophysiology of potassium homeostasis: Core curriculum 2019. *Am J Kidney Dis* **74**(5): 682–695.

7 Calcium Disorders

Kog Zheng Xi, Wong Jiunn

Calcium Balance

- Total body calcium (Ca^{2+}) stores are ~1000 g with ~99% in bone, 0.9% intracellular, and 0.1% extracellular.

- Average dietary intake of Ca^{2+} is 500–1000 mg/day – $\frac{2}{3}$ excreted in stools and $\frac{1}{3}$ in urine.

- Extracellular Ca^{2+} is measured as total calcium (45% free/ionised calcium and physiologically active; remaining 10% anion-bound, 45% albumin-bound); systemic acidosis decreases calcium binding to albumin → increasing serum levels while alkalosis has an opposite effect.

- Ca^{2+} is regulated by (i) parathyroid hormone (PTH), (ii) vitamin D; physiologic role of other regulatory hormones such as calcitonin, oestrogens, and prolactin are unclear.

Parathyroid Hormone

- PTH is a protein made from 84 amino acids; initially cleaved from pre-pro PTH → pro PTH → PTH within the parathyroid gland and then secreted/catabolised into *N*-terminal (active) and *C*-terminal fragments (also referred to as "7–84" fragments).

- PTH has several functions as follows:

  - Increases Ca^{2+} reabsorption (and decreased phosphate (PO_4^{3-}) reabsorption) in the distal convoluted tubules. However, in disease states like primary hyperparathyroidism, hypercalciuria can occur as a result of systemic hypercalcaemia.

  - Increases bone resorption (numerous mechanisms)

  - Indirectly increases intestinal absorption of Ca^{2+} by enhancing 1-hydroxylation of 25(OH) vitamin D to 1,25(OH)$_2$ vitamin D in the kidneys

- PTH secretion is regulated by changes in the Ca^{2+} level:

  - Hypocalcaemia (lowering of ionised Ca^{2+} → calcium-sensing receptor [CaSR] inactivation → PTH release), vitamin D deficiency (loss of inhibition), hyperphosphataemia and severe hypomagnesemia → stimulate PTH secretion

  - Hypercalcaemia (inhibitory effect on PTH secretion via CaSR activation), vitamin D excess (inhibitory effect on PTH secretion via vitamin D receptor in parathyroid gland) → inhibit PTH secretion

Vitamin D

- Main sources of vitamin D are dietary (D_2 ergocalciferol) and skin (via conversion of 7 dehydrocholesterol by UV light to D_3 cholecalciferol).

- D_2 and D_3 carried by D-binding protein to the liver and 25-hydroxylated to 25(OH)D.

- 25(OH)D is subsequently 1-hydroxylated by 1-α-hydroxylase in the kidney to 1,25(OH)$_2$,D (calcitriol).

- Vitamin D has several functions:

  - Increases mineralisation and enhances osteoclast activity in the bone

- Increases Ca^{2+} and phosphate (PO_4^{3-}) absorption in the intestines

- Inhibits PTH secretion via vitamin D receptors in the parathyroid gland; vitamin D deficiency $\rightarrow$ PTH secretion $\rightarrow$ enhanced 1-α-hydroxylase activity $\rightarrow$ increased $1,25(OH)_2D$ production

- Vitamin D 1-α-hydroxylase activity is increased with hypocalcaemia, hypophosphatemia, and vitamin D deficiency/PTH secretion.

Hypocalcaemia

Introduction

- Hypocalcaemia can be spurious (due to hypoalbuminaemia) or due to a change in ionised Ca^{2+}. For example, alkalosis increases the binding of calcium to albumin and lowers the serum ionized calcium concentration.

- Ca^{2+} absorption in the gastrointestinal tract (GIT) is a selective process — only 25% total dietary Ca^{2+} is absorbed under normal conditions; calcitriol is the most important regulatory hormone for Ca^{2+} absorption $\rightarrow$ calcitriol binds to vitamin D receptors in the GIT $\rightarrow$ increases active transport of Ca^{2+}; amount of dietary Ca^{2+} intake regulates the proportion of GIT Ca^{2+} absorption

- Calcium reabsorption in the kidney is increased by extracellular volume contraction, hypocalcaemia, PTH, and PTHrP

  - 50–60% in the proximal convoluted tubule

  - 3–10% in the proximal pars recta of the loop of Henle

  - 20–25% in the thick ascending limb of the loop of Henle

  - 5–10% in the distal convoluted tubule

  - <2% in the collecting tubule

  - 1–3% excreted

Table 7.1:   Aetiology of Hypocalcaemia

High Plasma PO4^{3-}	Low Plasma PO4^{3-}	Others
1. Hypoparathyroidism – Post-surgical – Post-radiation – Infiltrative disorders, e.g., amyloidosis – Congenital/hereditary – Autoimmune 2. Pseudohypoparathyroidism 3. Pseudohypoparathyroidism or Albright hereditary osteodystrophy – short neck – round face – short metacarpal – end-organ resistant to PTH 4. AKI or CKD	1. Post-parathyroidectomy or hungry bone syndrome 2. Vitamin D deficiency – malnutrition – malabsorption, e.g., post-gastrectomy, primary biliary cirrhosis, intestinal Ca^{2+} malabsorption – Decreased 25 (OH) D production e.g., liver disease, anticonvulsant – Decreased 1,25 (OH)$_2$ Production e.g., kidney impairment, Type I vitamin D-dependent rickets – Resistance to calcitriol (Type II vitamin D-dependent rickets)	1. Hypomagnesaemia 2. Sequestration – hyperphosphataemia e.g. rhabdomyolysis, tumour lysis syndrome, kidney impairment – acute pancreatitis

Abbreviations: AKI, acute kidney injury; CKD, chronic kidney disease; PTH, parathyroid hormone

Diagnosis

- Symptoms of hypocalcaemia

  - Perioral/peripheral numbness/paraesthesia, muscle cramps/ carpal-pedal spasm/tetany

  - Chvostek's sign — twitching of the facial muscle upon tapping the area innervated by the facial nerve

  - Trousseau's sign — carpopedal spasm during inflation of blood-pressure cuff to above systolic pressure for 3 minutes

- History suggesting possible aetiology

  - Previous thyroid, parathyroid, or neck surgery

  - Previous neck radiation therapy

  - Underlying autoimmune disorders

- History of renal impairment

- History of GI surgery

- History of obstructive jaundice, pruritus

- History of steatorrhea +/– symptoms related to malabsorption of other fat-soluble vitamins (e.g., vitamin A — night blindness, vitamin K — bruising)

- Risk factors — lack of sunlight, low dietary intake of calcium and vitamin D

- Family history

- Investigations

  - Serum calcium, phosphate, albumin

  - Ionised serum calcium

  - Serum magnesium

  - iPTH assay

  - 25(OH) vitamin D levels

Management

- Immediate management of hypocalcaemia

  - Address causes of acute respiratory alkalosis/ hyperventilation — if functional, breathing into paper bag (CO_2 retention) may suffice.

  - Intravenous (IV) calcium gluconate 10% 10 mL infusion administered rapidly over 10 minutes (as opposed to routine infusion over 1 hour) in the event of severe, symptomatic hypocalcaemia followed by additional doses subsequently; calcium gluconate preferred to calcium chloride which can lead to extensive skin necrosis in the event of accidental extravasation.

- Management of chronic hypocalcaemia
  - Post-meal per oral (PO) calcium supplements, administered at least 2 hours away from meals, dose 1–4 g/day
  - Elemental calcium content of calcium carbonate ($CaCO_3$) is 40% whereas elemental calcium content of calcium acetate is 25%
  - Correction of hypomagnesaemia
  - Vitamin D supplementation
  - Consider the use of thiazide diuretics
- Management of hypocalcaemia secondary to hypoparathyroidism
  - Activated vitamin D options include PO/IV calcitriol 0.25–1.5 μg per day or PO/IV 1-α-hydroxycholecalciferol/alfacalcidol 0.25–3.0 μg per day; need to monitor for hypercalcaemia/hypercalciuria → nephrolithiasis/nephrocalcinosis
  - Consider the use of thiazide diuretics to reduce urinary calcium concentration, in conjunction with salt restriction and high fluid intake

Hypercalcaemia

Aetiology of hypercalcaemia

- Primary hyperparathyroidism (55%)
  - Parathyroid adenoma (>80% of cases of primary hyperparathyroidism)
  - Parathyroid hyperplasia (10–15% of cases of primary hyperparathyroidism)
  - Parathyroid adenocarcinoma (<5% of cases of primary hyperparathyroidism)

- Multiple endocrine neoplasia (MEN) syndrome — in particular MEN-1 (parathyroid, anterior pituitary, enteropancreatic, and other endocrine tumours; inactivating germ-line mutations of a tumour suppressor gene with autosomal dominant inheritance) and MEN-2A (parathyroid, thyroid medulla, and adrenal medulla tumours; activating mutations of the *RET* proto-oncogene with autosomal dominant inheritance)
- Malignancy-related (35%)
  - Parathyroid hormone related peptide (PTHrP) — lung, oesophagus, head and neck, renal cell, ovary, bladder
  - Bone metastases → local osteolysis — breast and multiple myeloma
  - Ectopic production of 1,25-dihydroxyvitamin D - lymphoma
- Tertiary hyperparathyroidism (usually in the setting of end-stage renal failure)
- Endocrine disorders — thyrotoxicosis, acromegaly, pheochromocytoma
- Medications
  - Thiazide diuretics
  - Lithium
  - Calcium supplements (milk-alkali syndrome — usually ingestions of large amounts of calcium carbonate, e.g., excessive use of antacids)
  - Vitamin D supplements
  - Vitamin A supplements
- Prolonged immobilisation
- Granulomatous disorders — sarcoidosis

- Genetic disorders
  - Familial hypocalciuric hypercalcaemia (inappropriately low urine calcium excretion in the setting of high-normal serum calcium; inactivating mutations in the gene for calcium sensing receptor (CaSR) with autosomal dominant inheritance)
  - Jansen's metaphyseal chondrodysplasia (rare skeletal dysplasia disorder, "dwarfism", mutations in the PTH receptors with autosomal dominant inheritance)

Diagnosis

- Symptoms of hypercalcaemia ("painful bones, renal stones, abdominal groans, and psychic moans")
  - Musculoskeletal symptoms — generalised myalgia, muscle weakness, bone pain; depending on underlying aetiology — risk of osteoporosis and pathological fractures
  - Renal and urinary symptoms — flank pain, haematuria, nocturia, polyuria, thirst; depending on underlying aetiology — risk of nephrolithiasis and nephrocalcinosis
  - Gastrointestinal symptoms — nausea, constipation, abdominal pain; hypercalcaemia can lead to peptic ulcer disease and pancreatitis
  - Neurological symptoms — headache, altered mentation (confusion, somnolence, and rarely coma)
  - Electrocardiographic signs — in setting of severe hypercalcaemia, prolonged PR interval, short QT interval, widening of QRS complexes, and bradycardia
- History of underlying aetiology
  - Localising symptoms and signs of malignancy

- Constitutional symptoms
- Medication use — thiazide diuretics and lithium
- Family history

- Investigations
  - Serum Ca^{2+}, phosphate, albumin

    Correction of total serum Ca^{2+} measured when there is abnormal low or high serum albumin levels = [(normal serum albumin usually taken as 40 g/L — patient's serum albumin, e.g., 30 g/L) × 0.02] + current measured total serum Ca^{2+}

  - Serum-ionised Ca^{2+}

  - Intact parathyroid hormone (iPTH) assay is a 2nd-generation immunoassay that detects capture antibodies against epitopes located within the C-terminal and detection antibodies directed to amino acid sequences 12–20 within the amino terminal end — assumes that it captures intact PTH 1-84; cross-reactivity with PTH 7-84 fragments that accumulate in patients with CKD → over-estimation of iPTH

    High-normal or high levels of PTH in the setting of hypercalcaemia → primary hyperparathyroidism

  - 25(OH) vitamin D levels

  - 24-hour urine Ca^{2+} and creatinine (paired with serum Ca^{2+} and creatinine) → calculate Ca^{2+} to creatinine clearance (CrCL) ratio to differentiate familial hypocalciuric hypercalcaemia (FHH) from primary hyperparathyroidism

  - Ca^{2+}/CrCL Ratio $= \dfrac{24 \text{ hour urine Ca} \times \text{serum creatinine}}{\text{serum calcium} \times 24 \text{ hour urine creatinine}}$; Ca^{2+}/CrCL ratio <0.01 in ~80% of patients with various forms of FHH whereas Ca^{2+}/CrCL ratio >0.02 in most patients with primary hyperparathyroidism (NOTE: some patients with primary hyperparathyroidism, particularly those with concomitant vitamin D deficiency, may have Ca^{2+}/CrCL ratio <0.01)

- 24-hour urine Ca^{2+} can be used to determine the risk of nephrolithiasis and need for surgical intervention in cases of primary hyperparathyroidism

- Ultrasound or computer tomography scan of the neck (US neck or CT neck to identify parathyroid adenoma) +/– parathyroid scintigraphy in cases of suspected primary hyperparathyroidism

- Consider malignancy screening and parathyroid hormone-related peptides (send-out test) in cases of suspected malignancy-related hypercalcaemia

Management

- Classification of hypercalcaemia
  - Mild — total serum Ca 2.5–3 mmol/L or ionised serum Ca 1.4–2.0 mmol/L
  - Moderate — total serum Ca 3–3.5 mmol/L or ionised serum Ca 2.0–2.5 mmol/L
  - Severe — total serum Ca >3.5 mmol/L or ionised serum Ca >2.5 mmol/L
- Immediate management of severe, symptomatic hypercalcaemia
  - Cessation of causative medications — calcium supplements, vitamin D supplements, thiazide diuretics
  - Strict input-output (IO) charting
  - IV fluids to correct volume depletion, reduce proximal tubule calcium reabsorption, and enhance calcium excretion

- SC or IV inhibitors of osteoclast-mediated bone resorption
  - Subcutaneous (SC) administration of calcitonin, dose 4 units/kg q12 hourly but can be increased to 8 units/ kg q6–12 hourly, limit total duration of therapy to 24–48 hours due to rapid development of tachyphylaxis
  - IV bisphosphonates, options include IV pamidronate 15–90 mg over 1–3 days (diluted in isotonic saline or dextrose and infused over at least 2 hours) or IV zoledronate 4 mg once (diluted in isotonic saline or dextrose and infused over at least 15 minutes) — exercise caution with patients with moderate to severe kidney impairment (CrCL <35 mL/min).

    Contraindications to bisphosphonates (e.g., severe kidney impairment or bisphosphonate allergy)
  - SC denosumab 60–120 mg — no kidney dose adjustment but close monitoring of serum Ca^{2+} is required because denosumab is associated with a higher risk of hypocalcaemia than bisphosphonates
- Consider kidney replacement therapy for patients with:
  - Serum Ca 4.5–5.0 mmol/L and neurologic symptoms who are haemodynamically stable
  - Severe hypercalcaemia along with severe kidney impairment or heart failure (which prevents administration of IV hydration due to risks for fluid overload)

- Management of primary hyperparathyroidism-related hypercalcaemia
  - Avoid high calcium diet >1000 mg/day but maintain moderate calcium intake 800–1000 mg/day and moderate vitamin D intake 400–800 IU/day to maintain a serum 25(OH)D level of at least 20–30 ng/mL

- Avoid medications that can aggravate hypercalcaemia, e.g., thiazide diuretics, lithium, calcium supplementation, vitamin D supplementation (very small risk of exacerbating hypercalcaemia/hypercalciuria — if desired to do so cautiously)
- Avoid volume depletion, prolonged bed rest/immobility
- Calcimimetics, options include PO cinacalcet 25–50 mg/day; common adverse drug reactions include nausea, vomiting, abdominal pain, musculoskeletal pain
- Surgical parathyroidectomy in symptomatic disease (symptomatic hypercalcaemia nephrolithiasis, fractures). It is the definitive care and will decrease risk of nephrolithiasis, improve bone mineral density, reduce risk of fracture, and improve quality of life.

- Management of granulomatous disorder related hypercalcaemia — corticosteroids, options include PO prednisolone 0.5–1.0 mg/kg/day to decrease macrophage synthesis of calcitriol

References

Moe SM (2008). Disorders involving calcium, phosphorus, and magnesium. *Prim Care* **35**(2): 215–237, v–vi.

Turner JJO (2017). Hypercalcaemia: Presentation and management. *Clin Med* **17**(3): 270–273.

Walker MD and Shane E (2022). Hypercalcemia: A review. *J Am Med Assoc* **328**(16): 1624–1636.

8 Magnesium Disorders

Kog Zheng Xi, Wong Jiunn

Magnesium Balance

- Magnesium (Mg^{2+}) is not routinely measured in clinical practice and is called the "forgotten" cation. However, it is the second most common intracellular cation after K^+ and is important in many cellular functions.

- Approximately 21–28 g of Mg^{2+} is contained in the human body with most of it being intracellular (50–60% of total body Mg^{2+} in bone, 30% in muscle, and 10–20% in other tissue). Less than 1% is in extracellular fluid, mostly as free ionised Mg.

- Food containing Mg^{2+} includes vegetables, seafood, and nuts. The recommended daily Mg^{2+} intake is 420 mg for men and 320 mg for women.

- Magnesium (Mg^{2+}) homeostasis is dependent on intestinal absorption and kidney reabsorption of Mg^{2+}:

Intestinal Absorption

- Electrochemically driven paracellular and solvent-driven cellular uptake in the small intestine and uptake through transient receptor potential melastatin cationic channel 6 and 7 (TRPM6 and TRPM7) in the large intestine.

- Mg^{2+} intestinal absorption is dependent on Mg^{2+} intake — increasing when dietary intake of Mg^{2+} is low and decreasing when intake of Mg^{2+} is high.

Kidney Absorption

- The kidney is the main organ maintaining Mg^{2+} balance where volume contraction and hypomagnesaemia stimulate Mg^{2+} absorption.

- 70% of Mg^{2+} is filtered by the glomeruli but most is absorbed by the tubules — proximal tubule (30%), thick ascending loop of Henle (60%), distal convoluted tubule (10%).

Hypomagnesaemia

- Hypomagnesaemia (Table 8.1) is more common than hypermagnesaemia. Magnesium deficiency usually does not result from poor dietary intake alone, although prolonged/severe dietary magnesium restriction <0.5 mmol/day can eventually produce severe/symptomatic magnesium deficiency.

- Hypomagnesaemia can be associated with Hypocalcemia (decreased release of parathyroid hormone and end-organ responsiveness) and hypokalaemia (urinary losses).

Diagnosis

- Symptoms of hypomagnesaemia are usually only present in cases of severe hypomagnesaemia:
  - Neurological — Generalised weakness, neuromuscular hyperexcitability with hyperreflexia, carpopedal spasms, tremors, altered mentation, seizures, rarely tetany

Table 8.1:   Causes of Hypomagnesaemia

Redistribution from Extracellular to Intracellular Fluids	Significant Reduction in Dietary Intake	Reduced Gastrointestinal Absorption	Renal Losses	Drugs
• Insulin treatment • Correction of metabolic acidosis • Hungry bone syndrome post-parathyroidectomy • Catecholamine excess state, e.g., alcohol withdrawal • Acute pancreatitis • Excessive lactation	• Starvation • Chronic alcoholism • Prolonged post-operative state, particularly in patients on nasogastric tube feeding without magnesium supplements	• Chronic diarrhoea with malabsorption and steatorrhea, e.g., celiac disease • Diffuse bowel injury, e.g., inflammatory bowel disease • Primary intestinal hypomagnesaemia with secondary hypocalcaemia • Small bowel resection/bypass surgery • Intestinal/biliary fistula • Use of proton pump inhibitors • Non-Mg^{2+} laxative abuse	• Alcohol-induced tubular dysfunction • Hypercalcaemia • Poorly controlled diabetes • Recovery phase of acute tubular necrosis • Volume expansion • Genetic disorders, e.g., Bartter/Gitelman syndrome, familial hypomagnesaemia with hypercalciuria and nephrocalcinosis, autosomal dominant/recessive isolated hypomagnesaemia • Acute intermittent porphyria associated with inappropriate vasopressin secretion	• Loop and thiazide diuretics • Aminoglycosides • Amphotericin B • Cisplatin • Pentamidine • Cyclosporine

- Cardiovascular — Electrocardiogram (ECG) changes include prolonged QT interval, ST depressions with predisposition to ventricular arrhythmias, and potentiation of digoxin toxicity

- A thorough history may often reveal the underlying aetiology of hypomagnesaemia.

- Investigations:

  - Serum and urine Mg^{2+} — calculate fractional excretion of magnesium $(FE_{Mg}) = \frac{urineMg \times serumCr}{urineCr \times serumMg}$

  - Renal panel

  - Calcium/phosphate

  - Albumin

  - ECG

Management

Immediate management of hypomagnesaemia

IV magnesium sulfate 1–2 g administered as rapid infusion over 15 minutes (alternatively over 1 hour) followed by additional doses subsequently.

Management of chronic hypomagnesaemia

- Dietary modifications — nuts (almonds, cashews, peanuts), rice, cereal, bran flakes, oatmeal, wheat bran, yogurt, spinach, halibut

- Administration of magnesium supplements

- Correct hypocalcaemia

- Consider use of potassium-sparing diuretics (e.g., amiloride, triamterene) in patients with diuretic-induced hypomagnesaemia or renal losses

Hypermagnesaemia

- Hypermagnesaemia (>1.1 mmol/L) is uncommon — symptoms include nausea/vomiting, lethargy, headaches, and flushing.

- Severe hypermagnesaemia (>3.0 mmol/L) is associated with bradycardia, hypotension, paralysis, coma, and ECG changes (e.g., prolonged PR, QRS, and QT interval). Cardiac arrest and asystole may occur.

- Management of hypermagnesaemia involves searching (thence removing) an underlying cause (Table 8.2) and treatment when there are neurological and/or cardiovascular complications:

  - Usually requires admission to the intensive care unit

  - IV calcium gluconate to stabilise neurological and cardiovascular function

  - IV saline

  - IV loop diuretics

  - Haemodialysis if kidney function is impaired or there are severe complications of hypermagnesaemia

Table 8.2:   Causes of Hypermagnesaemia

- Kidney disease
- Magnesium infusion
- Massive oral ingestion
- Magnesium enemas
- Miscellaneous — usually mild hypermagnesaemia
  - primary hyperparathyroidism
  - familial hypocalciuric hypercalcaemia
  - hypercatabolic states (e.g., tumour lysis syndrome)
  - lithium ingestion
  - milk-alkali syndrome
  - adrenal insufficiency

Source: Reddy ST, Soman SS and Yee J (2018). Magnesium balance and measurement. *Adv Chronic Kidney Dis* **25**(3): 224–229.

References

Moe SM (2005). Disorders involving calcium, phosphorus, and magnesium. *Am J Kidney Dis* **45**(1): 213–218.

Pham PC, Pham PA, Pham SV, *et al.* (2014). Hypomagnesemia: A clinical perspective. *Int J Nephrol Renovasc Dis* **7**: 219–230.

Reddy ST, Soman SS and Yee J (2018). Magnesium balance and measurement. *Adv Chronic Kidney Dis* **25**(3): 224–229.

9 Acid-Base Disorders

Ivan Lee, Jason Choo

Introduction

- Acidaemia refers to the concentration of H^+ in the extracellular fluid (ECF) compartment. It is tightly regulated to maintain a normal serum pH of 7.35–7.45 (7.4).

$$pH = -\log[H^+]$$
$$\log[H^+] = -7.4$$
$$[H^+] = 3.98 \times 10^8 \text{ mol/L} \simeq 40 \text{ nmol/L}$$

- Movement between the physiological range of pH 6.8 to 7.8 involves change in $[H^+]$ from 16 nmol/L to 160 nmol/L.

- The body's mechanism to prevent large changes in pH is by buffering. Carbonic acid is the most abundant buffer in the ECF.

$$CO_2 + H_2O \leftrightarrow H_2CO_3 \leftrightarrow H^+ + HCO^{3-}$$

- The equation above demonstrates the ability of the carbonic acid buffer system to maintain acid-base homeostasis. $[HCO^{3-}]$ in the ECF by the kidneys and PCO_2 by alveolar ventilation (15,000 mmol/d!) are controlled separately. The resultant pH can then be expressed by the Henderson–Hasselbalch equation:

$$pH = 6.1 + \frac{\log[HCO^{3-}]}{0.03PCO_2}$$

- Or by the modified equation:

$$[H^+] = 24 \times \frac{PCO_2}{[HCO^{3-}]}$$

- From these two equations, it is immediately appreciated that "acute compensation" when there is a proton load is simply the carbonic acid buffer system at work.

- The kidneys' role in acid-base homeostasis is by net acid excretion (NAE), where:

$$NAE = Volume\ ([NH^{4+}] + [Titratable\ acid] - [HCO^{3-}])$$

- In contrast to the huge capacity of the lungs to remove CO_2, the kidneys are only able to eliminate about 1 mmol/kg/d of H^+.

Step-by-step Approach to Acid-base Disorders

- Identify acidaemia or alkalaemia on arterial blood gases (ABG)
- Corroborate using the modified Henderson equation with serum $[HCO^{3-}]$
  - Testing $[HCO^{3-}]$ involves adding acid to a serum sample and measuring the CO_2 released; it may be overestimated in severe respiratory acidosis (allow for 10% difference between measured $[HCO^{3-}]$ and std HCO^{3-}).
- Identify the primary defect
- Check for appropriate secondary responses
- Identify a mixed disorder (if any)
- Corroborate diagnosis with clinical history and findings

Compensation Formulas

Metabolic acidosis	Winter's formula: Expected $pCO_2 = 1.5 \times [HCO^{3-}] + 8 \pm 2$ Alternatively: Expected $pCO_2 = 40 - (\Delta[HCO^{3-}] \times \mathbf{1.2})$
Metabolic alkalosis	Expected $pCO_2 = 40 + (\Delta[HCO^{3-}] \times \mathbf{0.6 - 0.7})$
Respiratory acidosis	Acute respiratory acidosis: $[HCO^{3-}]$ increased by **0.1 mmol/L** for every 1 mmHg increase in $PaCO_2$
	Chronic respiratory acidosis: $[HCO^{3-}]$ increased by **0.4 mmol/L** for every 1 mmHg increase in $PaCO_2$
Respiratory alkalosis	Acute respiratory alkalosis: $[HCO^{3-}]$ decreased by **0.2 mmol/L** for every 1 mmHg decrease in $PaCO_2$
	Chronic respiratory alkalosis: $[HCO^{3-}]$ increased by **0.5 mmol/L** for every 1 mmHg decrease in $PaCO_2$

Abbreviations: HCO_3, bicarbonate; pCO_2, partial pressure of carbon dioxide

Anion gap

- The aetiology of metabolic acidosis can be classified into either:
  - The addition of protons either by hydrochloric acid or relatively strong acids (proton-donators) or
  - The decrease in the content or concentration of bicarbonate
- The common clinical diagnostic approaches to differentiate the above are through either:

- The commonly used "physiologic approach" or
- The Stewart approach (also known as the strong ion difference)

- The basis of either method is to identify the addition of acid by calculating the difference between cations and anions in equilibrium. The "GambleGram" depicts the "physiologic approach" elegantly:

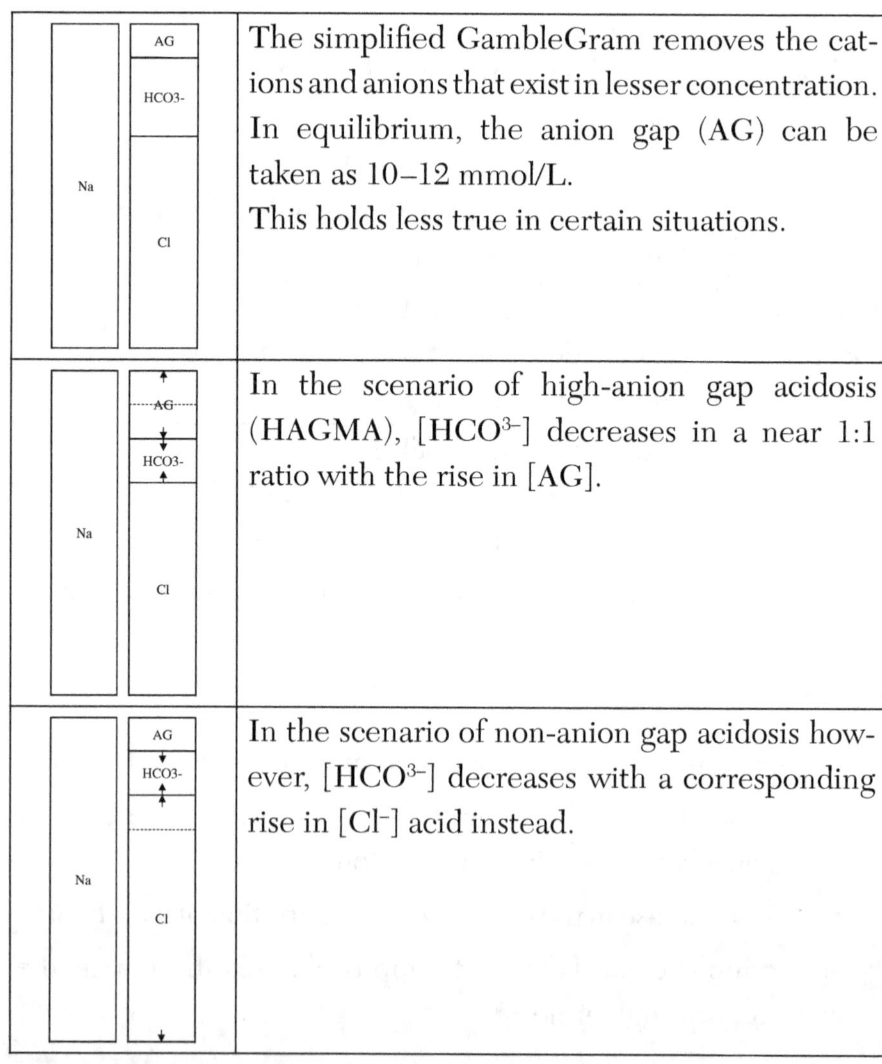

<table>
<tr><td></td><td>The simplified GambleGram removes the cations and anions that exist in lesser concentration.
In equilibrium, the anion gap (AG) can be taken as 10–12 mmol/L.
This holds less true in certain situations.</td></tr>
<tr><td></td><td>In the scenario of high-anion gap acidosis (HAGMA), $[HCO_3^-]$ decreases in a near 1:1 ratio with the rise in [AG].</td></tr>
<tr><td></td><td>In the scenario of non-anion gap acidosis however, $[HCO_3^-]$ decreases with a corresponding rise in $[Cl^-]$ acid instead.</td></tr>
</table>

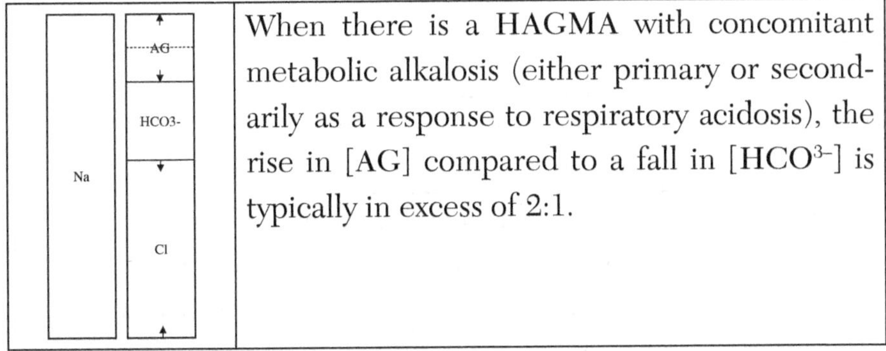

Abbreviations: AG, anion gap; CL, chloride; HCO_3, bicarbonate; Na, sodium

- The major unmeasured anion is albumin, which represents 2.5 mEq/g/L albumin; it must be accounted for in hypoalbuminaemia

$$\text{Corrected AG} = \text{AG} + (40 - \text{sAlb})/4$$
$$\text{Or, expected AG} = 12 - (40 - \text{sAlb})/4$$

- The advantage of the Stewart approach to detect anion gap acidoses over the "physiologic approach" is eliminated by employing the corrected anion gap.

High Anion Gap Acidosis

- Elevated anion gap acidosis occurs either from an endogenous process resulting in increased production of an organic anion or the addition of an exogenous anion.

- The updated GOLD MARK mnemonic can be used to remember the major causes of HAGMAs.

Glycols	Propylene glycol, ethylene glycol, diethylene glycol
5-**O**xoproline	Chronic paracetamol use — typically in malnourished women
L-lactate	Type A: imbalance in oxygen consumption and delivery to metabolically active tissues Type B: unrelated to perfusion or hypoxia (mitochondrial toxins, liver failure, thiamine deficiency, inborn errors of metabolism)
D-lactate	Produced by gastrointestinal bacteria
Methanol	Organic acid formation from metabolism of toxic alcohols
Aspirin	Salicylic acid
Renal failure	Impaired ability to excrete H^+ and NH^{4+}
Ketoacidosis	Diabetic, starvation, alcoholic, keto diet

Low/negative Anion Gap

- The causes of non-anion gap metabolic acidosis are much simpler:
  - Gastrointestinal bicarbonate losses: diarrhoea, fistulas, urinary diversions
  - Acid load: ammonium chloride, hyperalimentation
  - Renal tubular acidosis
- Occasionally, one may encounter an abnormally low anion gap without an acid-base disturbance:

Decreased unmeasured anion	Albumin Paraproteinaemia
Increased chloride	Bromide ingestion Thiocyanate
Increased "unaccounted" cation	Hypercalcaemia Hypermagnesaemia Lithium
Pseudohyperbicarbonataemia	Paraproteinaemia interference with HCO^{3-} assay
Pseudohyponatraemia	Hypertriglyceridemia, severe obstructive jaundice

The utility of the urinary NH4+ excretion

- Given the NAE as expressed in the introduction, urinary H+ is excreted as either titratable acid or NH^{4+}.

- The capacity of the kidney to excrete NH^{4+} is much greater than the capacity to increase titratable acid.

- Urine NH^{4+} excretion is a useful tool to assess the adequacy of the renal response to an acid load or the lack thereof in a pathological state.

  - This can be calculated by the urine anion gap:

$$uAG = uNa + uK - uCl$$

  - The urine anion gap may be falsely low in states where other unmeasured anions may be excreted with NH4+ (e.g., ketoacids, hippuric acid) and hence the following formula may be used:

$$uNH^{4+} = \{uOsmolality - [2\,(uNa + uK) + uUrea + uGlucose]\} / 2$$

- The various permutations that arise are as follows:

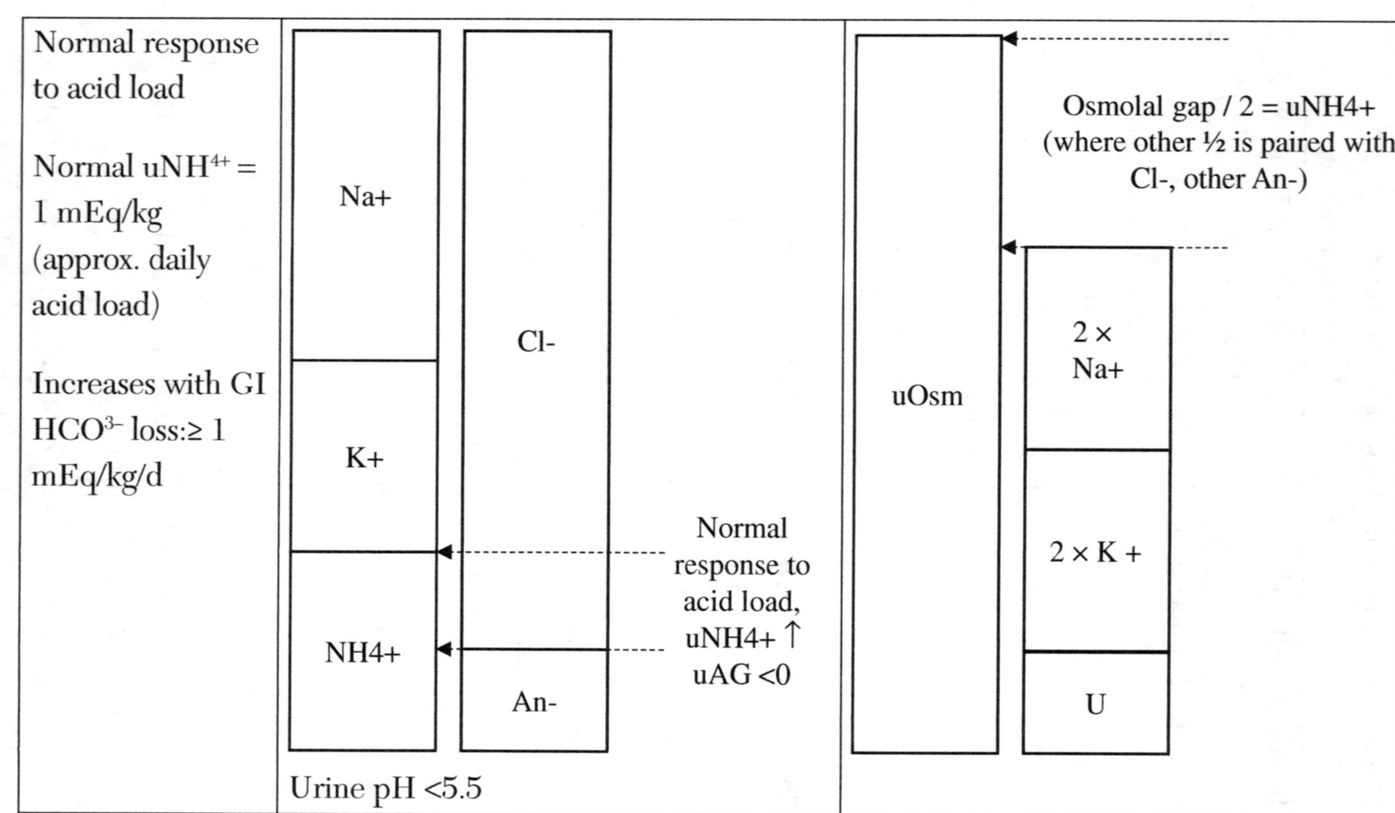

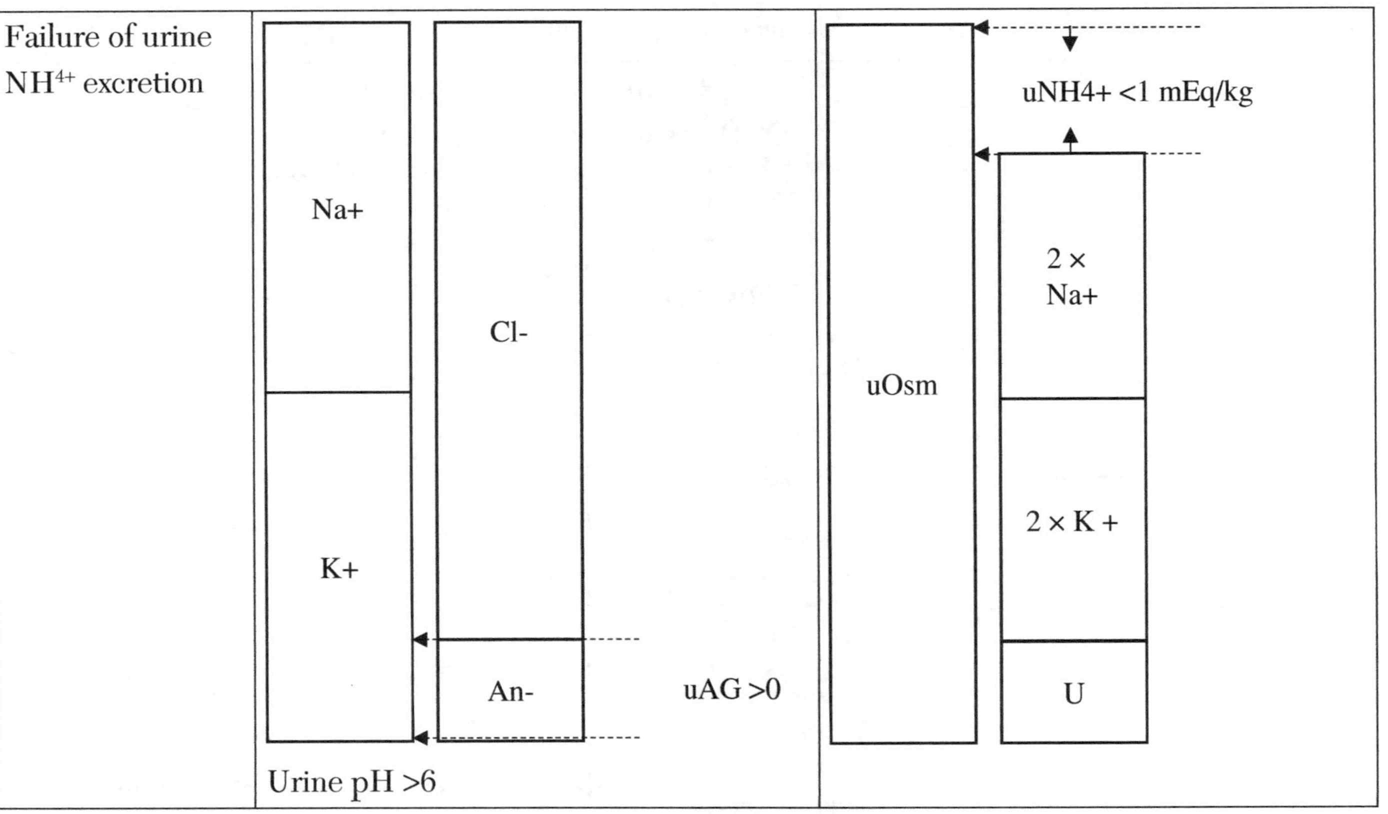
Failure of urine NH4+ excretion
Na+
K+
Cl-
An-
uAG >0
Urine pH >6
uOsm
uNH4+ <1 mEq/kg
2 × Na+
2 × K +
U

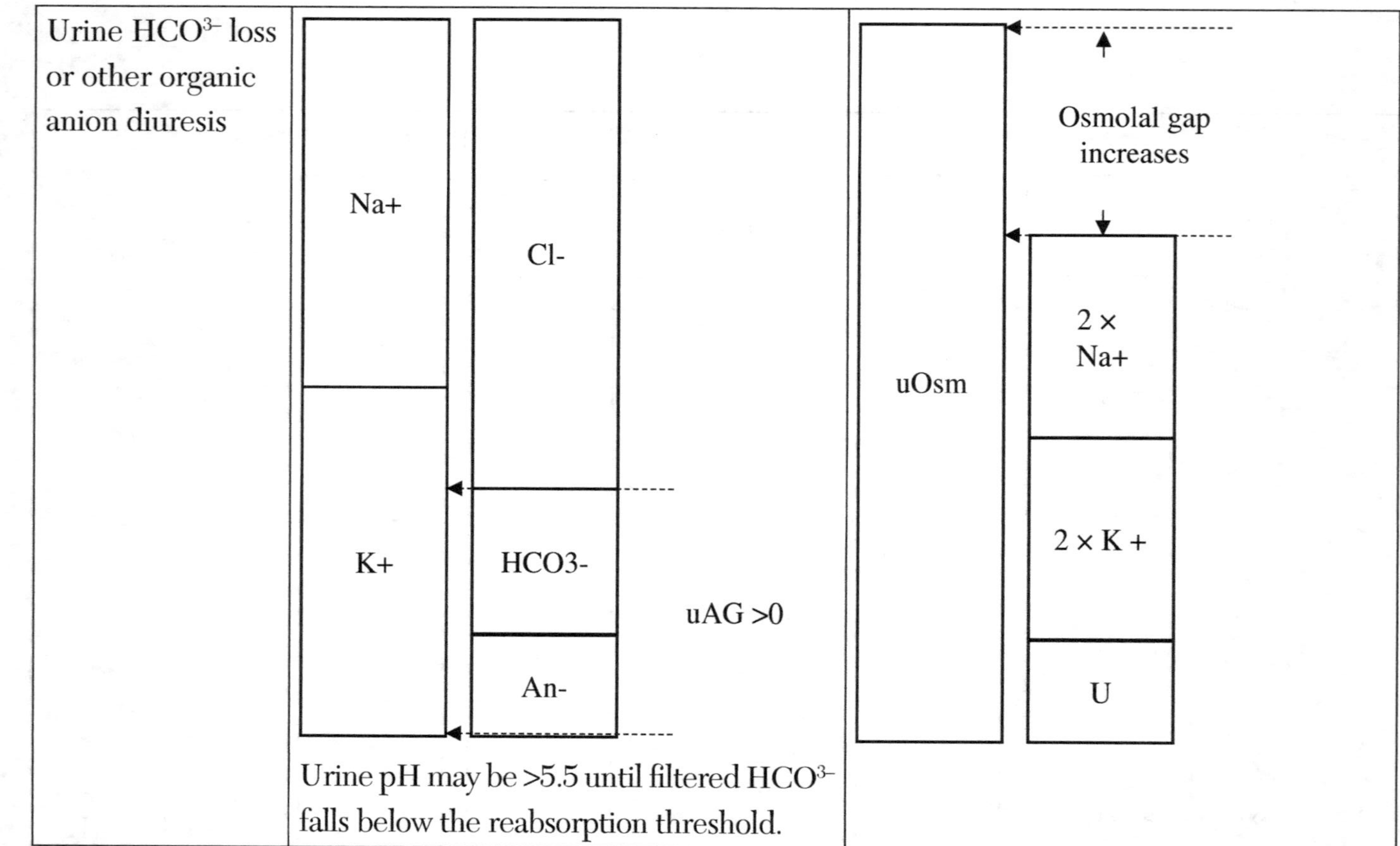

Abbreviation: An, anion; CL, chloride; HCO_3, bicarbonate; K, potassium; Na, sodium, NH4, ammonium; U, urea; uOsm, urine osmolality

Renal tubular acidosis

	Type I RTA (distal)	Type II RTA (proximal)	Type IV RTA
Pathophysiology	Inability to generate a pH gradient between blood and distal tubular fluid	Reduced capacity to reclaim bicarbonate at the proximal tubule	Impaired Na+/K^+-H^+ cation exchange (hypoaldosteronism or resistance)
Serum K^+	Low/normal	Low/normal	High
Urine	upH >5.5 uAG positive uNH^{4+} low	upH may be <5.5 when filtered bicarbonate goes below reclamation threshold uNH^{4+} low uAG positive uOG may be high	upH <5.5 uAG positive uNH^{4+} low
Confirmatory test	Failure to acidify urine with ammonium chloride loading (0.1 g/kg)	FEBi >0.15 with bicarbonate loading (PO 4 mEq/kg or slow infusion of IV $NaHCO_3$)	FEBi high
Other features	Nephrocalcinosis (from hypercalcaemia, hypocitraturia, alkaline urine) Rickets from reduced 1 alpha-hydroxylase activity	Glycosuria Phosphaturia Amino aciduria Rickets, osteomalacia	Bone disease absent

Aetiology	Sporadic	Sporadic	Sporadic
	Inherited	Inherited	Inherited
	Secondary causes:	Secondary causes:	Secondary causes:
	Interstitial nephritis	Sjogren syndrome	Obstructive uropathy
	Sickle cell nephropathy	Wilson disease	Pyelonephritis
	Medullary sponge kidney	Myeloma	Diabetes mellitus
	Lupus nephritis	Cisplatin	Sickle cell nephropathy
	Vesicoureteric reflux	Ifosfamide	Trimethoprim/ sulfamethox-azole
	Amphotericin B	Sodium valproate	ACE inhibitors
	Lithium	Aminoglycoside	Calcineurin inhibitors
	Cisplatin	Heavy metals	
		Primary hyper-parathyroidism	

Abbreviations: ACE, angiotensin-converting enzyme; FEBi, fractional excretion of bicarbonate; H, hydrogen; K, potassium; Na, sodium; $NaHCO_3$, sodium bicarbonate; PO, per oral; RTA, renal tubular acidosis; upH, urine AG, urine anion gap; urine NH_4, urine ammonium; urine OG, urine osmolar gap; urine pH

Metabolic Alkalosis

- Syndrome characterised by high $[HCO^{3-}]$ and low $[H^+]$, involving a sequence of generation and maintenance phases:
  - <u>Generation phase</u>: alkali gain or acid loss — urinary Cl^- may be used to evaluate the aetiological causes.

		Urine [Cl⁻]	Others
Alkali load	Bicarbonate infusion Citrate administration (citrated blood products, extracorporeal circuit anticoagulation) Milk-alkali syndrome	>20	upH high uOG high >200 mOsm
Acid loss	Gastric losses: Vomiting Nasogastric suctioning Chloride-losing diarrhea	<20	uNa may be high upH high uOG high
	Urinary: Diuretic use Bartter, Gitelman syndromes	>20	uCa to differentiate
	Remote diuretics	<20	
	Cystic fibrosis	<20	
EABV expansion with K depletion	Cushing syndrome Renin-angiotensin-aldosterone system activation Syndromes of apparent mineralocorticoid excess Glucocorticoid-remediable aldosteronism Liddle syndrome	>20	Hypertensive

Abbreviations: uCa, urine calcium; uNa, urine sodium; uOG, urine osmolar gap; upH, urine pH

- **Maintenance phase**: from highly conserved or altered mechanisms to preserve volume:

Haemodynamic response — decreased GFR	
Reabsorption of filtered $[HCO_3^-]$	
Hypochloraemia	Impairs excretion of $[HCO_3^-]$ via inactivation of pendrin
Hypokalaemia	Increases ammoniagenesis by increasing glutamine uptake and increasing $[HCO_3^-]$ generation Increases $[HCO_3^-]$ reabsorption at PCT Increases expression of H+ ATPase and H^+/K^+-ATPase at the collecting duct Reduces pendrin expression
Renin-angiotensin-aldosterone system activation	
Elevated PCO_2	Increases $[HCO_3^-]$ reabsorption

Abbreviation: GFR, glomerular filtration rate; H, hydrogen; HCO_3, bicarbonate; K, potassium

- The **recovery phase** from metabolic alkalosis occurs when the generating event is withdrawn or treated and maintaining factors are reversed.

  - Competing comorbidities such as heart failure and lung disease limit volume expansion with NaCl.

  - In severe cases, administration of acid (NH4Cl, HCl, arginine HCl) or acetazolamide may be considered.

  - Treatment with RAAS blockade or K-sparing diuretics may be considered for specific circumstances.

References

Do C, Vasquez PC and Soleimani M (2022). Metabolic alkalosis pathogenesis, diagnosis, and treatment: Core curriculum 2022. *Am J Kidney Dis* **80**(4), 536–551.

Krish P and Jhaveri KD (2012). The case: Hyperbicarbonatemia in a patient with Waldenstrom's macroglobulinemia. The diagnosis: Pseudohyperbicarbonatemia due to paraproteinemia. *Kidney Int* **81**(6): 603–605.

Lerma EV, Sparks MA and Topf JM (2019). XIII: Acid-base and electrolyte disorders. In: *Nephrology Secrets 4th ed.* Elsevier, Philadelphia, PA.

Mehta AN, Emmett JB and Emmett M (2008). GOLD MARK: An anion gap mnemonic for the 21st century. *Lancet* **372**(9642): 892.

Chronic Kidney Disease

10 Diagnostic Approach to Chronic Kidney Disease

Kwek Jia Liang

Introduction

- Chronic kidney disease (CKD) is a global health burden with high economic cost to healthcare systems around the world.

- The estimated global prevalence is around 9.1% in 2017. In Singapore, it is projected that the local prevalence of CKD will increase from 12.2% in 2007 to 24.3% in 2035.

- Most CKD patients are in stage 1–3 (CKD stage 1–2: 5.0%, stage 3: 3.9%, stage 4: 0.16%, stage 5: 0.07%, dialysis: 0.041%, transplant: 0.011%)

Definition

- CKD is defined as abnormalities of kidney structure or function, present for >3 months, and carries implications for health (Table 10.1).

- Staging of CKD is based on a heatmap, using glomerular filtration rate (GFR in mL/min/1.73 m^2) categories and persistent albuminuria (albumin:creatinine ratio or ACR in mg/mmol) categories to determine its severity (Table 10.2).

Table 10.1:　Definition of Chronic Kidney Disease

Either of the following present for >3 months	
Markers of kidney damage	• Albuminuria (ACR ≥3 mg/mmol) • Urine sediment abnormalities • Electrolyte and other abnormalities due to tubular disorders • Abnormalities detected by histology • Structural abnormalities detected by imaging • History of kidney transplantation
Decreased GFR	• GFR <60 mL/min/1.73 m² (GFR categories G3a – G5)

Abbreviations: ACR, albumin: creatinine ratio; GFR, glomerular filtration rate

Table 10.2:　Classification of Chronic Kidney Disease Using GFR and ACR Categories

Glomerular filtration rate categories

Category	GFR (mL/min)	Kidney Function
G1	≥90	Normal and high
G2	60–89	Mild reduction related to normal range for a young adult
G3a	45–59	Mild to moderate reduction
G3b	30–44	Moderate to severe reduction
G4	15–29	Severe reduction
G5	<15	Kidney failure

Albumin: creatinine categories

Category	ACR (mg/mmol)	Albuminuria
A1	<3	Normal to midly increased
A2	3–30	Moderately increased
A3	>30	Severely increased

Abbreviations: ACR, albumin: creatinine ratio; GFR, glomerular filtration rate

Epidemiology

- In 2013, among patients with incident stage 5 CKD in Singapore, diabetic kidney disease was the most common cause (63.5%), followed by hypertension and renovascular disease (15.0%), glomerulonephritis (14.9%), polycystic/other cystic kidney diseases, obstructive uropathy/kidney stone disease, vesicoureteral reflux, chronic pyelonephritis, and unknown causes.

- Risk factors for CKD include:
  - Metabolic diseases (e.g., diabetes mellitus, hypertension, obesity)
  - Cardiovascular disease
  - Genetic or hereditary diseases (polycystic kidney disease, Alport's syndrome)
  - Family history of CKD
  - Smoking
  - Reduced renal mass (solitary kidney, previous nephrectomy)
  - Urinary tract obstruction (renal stones, tumours, strictures)
  - Recurrent urinary tract infection
  - Previous recurrent or severe acute kidney injury
  - Exposure to nephrotoxins (analgesics, aminoglycosides, radiocontrast)

Approach

- The first step to manage CKD is to diagnose it and accurately identify underlying causes.

History

- Medical history of any of the following and its duration:
  - Metabolic diseases (e.g., Type II or long-standing Type I diabetes mellitus), hypertension (long-standing, usually >10 years duration), gout, obesity

- Cardiovascular diseases (e.g., ischaemic heart disease), cerebrovascular disease, peripheral vascular disease
- Organ failure (e.g., heart failure, liver failure)
- Prior recurrent or severe acute kidney injury (especially requiring dialysis support)
- Autoimmune diseases which often affect the kidneys (e.g., systemic lupus erythematosus, Sjogren's syndrome)
- Multiple myeloma or monoclonal gammopathy
- Obstructive uropathy (e.g., kidney stones, strictures)
- Recurrent and complicated urinary tract infection
- Renal or urological anatomical abnormalities (e.g., kidney agenesis, previous nephrectomy, vesicoureteral reflux)
- Cancer treated with chemotherapy, molecular-targeted therapy, immunotherapy, or radiotherapy
- Previous urologic, pelvic, or retroperitoneal surgery
- Viral infection (e.g., hepatitis B, hepatitis C, human immunodeficiency virus; HIV)
- Chronic or recurrent exposure of nephrotoxin, (e.g., analgesics, aristolochic acid) or toxic environmental exposures (e.g., lead)
- Smoking
- Family history of chronic kidney disease, inheritable disease (e.g., polycystic kidney disease, Alport's syndrome), metabolic diseases (e.g., diabetes mellitus, hypertension, cardiovascular disease)

- Symptoms
  - Generally asymptomatic until advanced CKD (stage 4–5) develops where symptoms of uraemia, fluid overload, and other non-specific symptoms may be present.

- Symptoms related to underlying causes, such as:
  - Nephritic-nephrotic syndrome — oliguria, macroscopic haematuria, excessively frothy urine, lower limb oedema
  - Renovascular disease — recently diagnosed hypertension or acute worsening of previously well-controlled hypertension
  - Obstructive uropathy — lower urinary tract symptoms
  - Urinary tract infection (dysuria, fever)
  - Recent or ongoing illness/infection

Physical Examination

- Hypertension (BP >140/90 mmHg)
- Hydration status (overload or dehydrated)
- Presence of oedema and its extent
- Abdominal examination — previous surgical scar, enlarged kidneys, abdominal or renal bruits, palpable bladder
- Complications of CKD — fluid overload (bibasal crepitations, raised jugular venous pressure, peripheral edema), uraemic flap, confusion, lethargy pericardial rub, pleural rub
- For patients with diabetes mellitus, other complications of diabetes mellitus (e.g., retinopathy, neuropathy, peripheral vascular disease)
- For patients with autoimmune diseases, manifestations, and activity of underlying condition (e.g., rash, photosensitivity, arthralgia of small joints)

Investigations

- Renal panel including sodium, potassium, chloride, bicarbonate, urea, creatinine, and estimated GFR (using the Chronic Kidney Disease Epidemiology Collaboration or CKD-EPI equation)

- Urine microscopy, urine phase contrast

- Spot urine albumin or protein — albumin: creatinine ratio (ACR) or protein: creatinine ratio (PCR)

- Ultrasound kidney, ureters, bladder (KUB), ultrasound doppler of renal arteries (if renal artery stenosis is suspected)

- Serum albumin

- Fasting lipid panel

- Fasting glucose, HbA1C

- Complement levels — C3, C4

- Erythrocyte sedimentation rate (ESR)

- Autoimmune screen (if there is suspected underlying autoimmune disease, nephrotic syndrome, or nephritic syndrome):
  - Anti-neutrophil antibody (ANA)
  - Anti-dsDNA antibody
  - Anti-phospholipase A2 receptor antibody (anti-PLA2R)
  - Anti-streptolysin O titer (ASOT)
  - Anti-neutrophil cytoplasmic antibody (ANCA)
  - Anti-glomerular basement membrane antibody (anti-GBM)

- Virology screen for hepatitis B, C and HIV (if chronic viral diseases suspected): Hepatitis B Ag, Hepatitis C screen, HIV screen

- Urine and serum protein electrophoresis if suspected of multiple myeloma or monoclonal gammopathy (e.g., >40 years old,

>1g/day proteinuria), anaemia, hypercalcaemia, bony lesions or no other obvious cause of CKD

- Kidney biopsy (after assessing indications, benefits, and risks of procedure)

Guide for Referral to a Nephrologist

- Refer to the emergency department for the following:
  - Previously unknown estimated GFR <15 mL/min/1.73 m^2 or serum creatinine >500 µmol/L
  - Evidence of acute kidney injury
  - Severe electrolyte disturbances (e.g., serum potassium >6.0 mmol/L)
- Early referral (within 2–6 weeks)
  - Previously unknown estimated GFR of 15–29 mL/min/1.73 m^2
  - Recent rapid decline of eGFR by >30% to 15–29 mL/min/1.73 m^2
  - New onset nephrotic syndrome
  - New onset nephritic syndrome
  - Sustained increase in serum creatinine by >30% from baseline with no apparent cause
- Non-urgent referral
  - Known CKD with estimated GFR <45 mL/min/1.73 m^2, not previously assessed by renal physician and a potential candidate for kidney replacement therapy
  - Sustained increase in serum creatinine by >30% from baseline upon starting RAS blockers

- Sustained decline in estimated GFR by >5 mL/min/1.73 m² in 1 year or >10 mL/min/1.73 m² in 5 years

- Suspected genetic cause of chronic kidney disease (e.g., polycystic kidney disease)

- Significant proteinuria (urine PCR >1g/g or ACR >70 mg/mmol), despite maximally tolerated RAS blockers and optimal blood pressure control

- Significant proteinuria (urine PCR >0.5 g/g or ACR >30mg/mmol) with persistent haematuria

- Uncontrolled hypertension in patient with CKD despite 4 antihypertensive medications

- Uncontrolled hyperkalaemia (serum potassium >5.5 mmol/L) in patients with CKD — Hyperkalaemia should be treated first prior to referring; consider referring to the emergency department in cases with serum potassium >6.0 mmol/L

References

GBD Chronic Kidney Disease Collaboration (2020). Global, regional, and national burden of chronic kidney disease, 1990–2017: A systematic analysis for the Global Burden of Disease Study 2017. *Lancet* **395**(10225): 709–733.

Kidney Disease: Improving Global Outcomes (KDIGO) CKD Work Group (2013). KDIGO clinical practice guideline for the evaluation and management of chronic kidney disease. *Kidney Int **Suppl** 3*: 1–150.

Singapore Renal Registry Annual Registry Report 2012–2013

Wong LY, Liew AST, Weng WT, *et al.* (2018). Projecting the burden of chronic kidney disease in a developed country and its implications on public health. *Int J Nephrol* **2018**: 5196285.

11 Slowing Progression of Chronic Kidney Disease

Kwek Jia Liang

Introduction

- Chronic kidney disease (CKD) is a global health burden with high economic cost to healthcare systems around the world.

- Risk factor-appropriate screening of CKD is important because CKD is asymptomatic in the earlier stages.

- Older adults (45 years or older), especially with risk factors such as diabetes mellitus, hypertension, cardiovascular disease, and family history of chronic kidney disease should be screened for CKD.

- In Singapore, the Ministry of Health (MOH) recommends annual screening for CKD with estimated glomerular filtration rate (eGFR) and urinary albumin assessment in patients with diabetes (five years after diagnosis of type 1 diabetes and during diagnosis for type 2 diabetes) and patients with hypertension.

Approach

- Start with accurately diagnosing the underlying cause of CKD.

- Initiate cause-specific treatments as appropriate in a timely manner.

- Initiate general and non-targeted intervention to slow down progression of CKD.

Treat underlying cause of chronic kidney disease

- Diagnose the underlying cause of CKD accurately through history taking, physical examination, and appropriate investigations.

- Initiate cause-specific treatments as appropriate in a timely manner.

Prevent acute kidney injury

- Acute kidney injury (AKI) is associated with progression of CKD

- Review patient's risk factors for AKI

- Avoid hypotension

- Avoid malignant hypertension

- Avoid obstruction of urinary tract

- Avoid nephrotoxins (e.g., chronic ingestion of non-steroidal anti-inflammatory drugs (NSAIDS) or Cox-2 inhibitors)

Renin-angiotensin System (RAS) Blockade

- Angiotensin-converting enzyme inhibitors (ACEi) and angiotensin-2 receptor antagonists (ARB) are renin-angiotensin system (RAS) blockers.

- They work by decreasing intraglomerular hypertension through efferent arterioles vasodilation.

- ACEi and ARB are first line therapies in patients with albuminuric CKD (Figure 11.1)

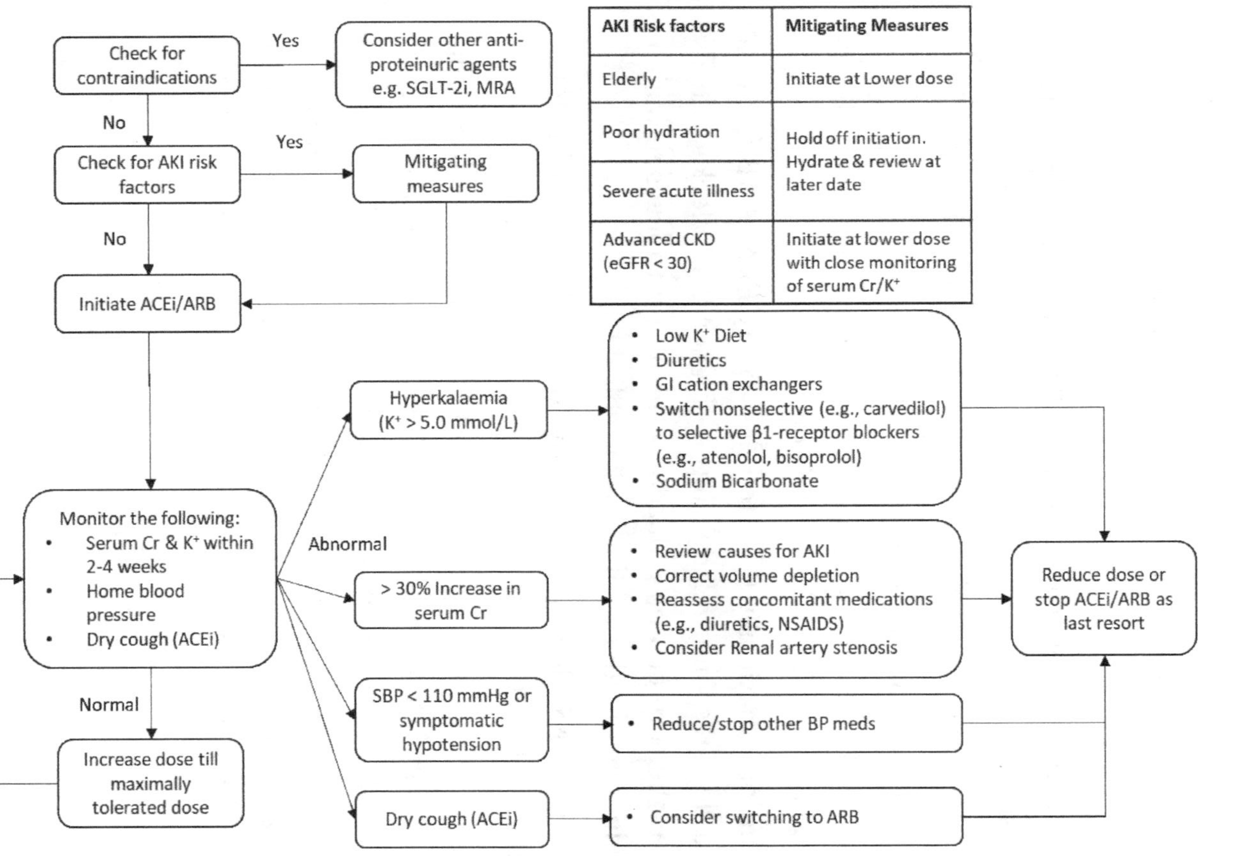

Figure 11.1:   Initiation and optimisation of RAS blockers.

(Adapted from the SingHealth Renal Retardation Programme (SiRRP) Clinical Guide Version 13th March 2022.)

- Review for contraindications to RAS blockers:
  - Bilateral renal artery stenosis
  - Known hypersensitivity to RAS blockers
  - Pregnancy

  There are also relative contraindications to starting RAS blockers such as:
  - Ongoing hyperkalaemia (serum potassium >5.0mmol/L)
  - Acute kidney injury or acute illness

- Start RAS blockers cautiously at a lower dose in elderly patients and patients with GFR <45 mL/min/1.73 m^2.

- Aim for a maximally tolerated dose of ACEi or ARB as there is a dose-response relationship — higher RAS blockade leads to higher proteinuria reduction, which in turn leads to higher reduction of kidney failure risk (Table 11.1).

- Couple RAS blockers with a low sodium diet to enhance the effect of the RAS blockers.

- Use of combination therapy of ACEi with ARB or use of direct renin inhibitors is not recommended because of the lack of proven benefit and increased risk of adverse effects.

- Use of supramaximal dose of RAS blockers has been largely superseded by initiation of other classes of medications that have been found to be effective in slowing down progression of CKD.

Table 11.1:   Dose Reference Guide to Renin-Angiotensin Blockers

Name	Initial Dose	Max Dose	Name	Initial Dose	Max Dose
Losartan	50 mg OD (*25 mg*)	100 mg OD/ 50 mg BD	Enalapril	5 mg OD (*2.5 mg*)	20 mg BD
Irbesartan	150 mg OD (*75 mg*)	300 mg OD	Lisinopril	10 mg OD (*5 mg*)	40 mg OD
Valsartan	80 mg OD (*40 mg*)	320 mg OD	Perindopril Erbumine	4 mg OD (*2 mg*)	8 mg OD
Candesartan	8 mg OD (*4 mg*)	32 mg OD	Perindopril Arginine	5 mg OD (*2.5 mg*)	10 mg OD
Telmisartan	40 mg OD (*20 mg*)	80 mg OD	Ramipril	2.5 mg OD	20 mg OD/ 10 mg BD
Olmesartan	20 mg OD (*10 mg*)	40 mg OD	Captopril	12.5 mg BD (*6.25 mg BD*)	50 mg TDS

**Lower initial dose in ( ) may be considered in the elderly or in patients with CKD 3b and above. Adapted from the SingHealth Renal Retardation Programme (SiRRP) Clinical Guide Version 13th March 2022*

Abbreviations: BD, twice a day; OD, once a day; TDS, three times a day

- Adverse effects of RAS blockers should be managed first before considering discontinuation (Table 11.2).

- Monitor blood pressure, serum creatinine, and potassium within 2–4 weeks of initiating or up-titration of RAS blockers.

- Aim for target blood pressure, serum potassium < 5.5 mmol/L and less than 30% increase in serum creatinine.

Table 11.2:   Management of the Adverse Effects of Renin-Angiotensin Blockers

Adverse Effects	Management
Cr rise ≥30%	• Exclude pre-renal, intrinsic renal, and post-renal causes of AKI (e.g., dehydration, sepsis, nephrotoxic drugs). • Correct volume depletion. • Reassess concomitant medications (e.g., diuretics, NSAIDS). • Stop or reduce ACEi/ARB to previous dose. • Evaluate for underlying renal artery stenosis if no other obvious causes of acute kidney injury (AKI) are found (especially patients with suboptimal blood pressure control).
K^+ >5.0 mmol/L	• Review concurrent drugs (e.g., potassium supplements, potassium-sparing diuretics, beta blockers). • Lower dietary potassium intake. • Consider initiating thiazide diuretic or loop diuretics (eGFR <30 mL/min/1.73 m²) if BP >110/70 mmHg. • Stop or switch from nonselective (e.g., carvedilol) to selective β1-receptor blockers (e.g., atenolol, bisoprolol). • Consider sodium bicarbonate (if metabolic acidosis is present). • Consider GI cation exchangers (e.g., sodium polystyrene sulfonate, sodium zirconium cyclosilicate). • Stop or reduce ACEi/ARB if K^+ ≥5.5 mmol/L persistently despite the above measures.
SBP <110 mmHg or symptomatic hypotension	• Reduce or discontinue other anti-hypertensives.
Persistent dry cough	• Establish temporal relationship between cough and ACEi. • Exclude other causes of chronic cough. • Consider switching from ACEi to ARB.

Adapted from the SingHealth Renal Retardation Programme (SiRRP) Clinical Guide Version 13th March 2022

Abbreviations: ACEI, angiotensin-converting enyzyme inhibitor; ARB, angiotensin receptor blocker; AKI, acute kidney injury; BP, blood pressure; Cr, creatinine; eGFR, estimated glomerular filtration rate; GI, gastrointestinal; K, potassium; NSAIDS, non-steroidal anti-inflammatory drugs; SBP, systolic blood pressure

Sodium-glucose Cotransporter-2 Inhibitor (SGLT-2i)

- Sodium-glucose cotransporter-2 inhibitor (SGLT-2i) has been shown to confer significant reno- and cardio-protective benefits in patients with diabetic or non-diabetic kidney disease (Figure 11.2).

- These benefits are independent of the glucose-lowering effects of SGLT-2i.

- These benefits have been shown in patients with eGFR as low as 20 mL/min/1.73 m^2 (Table 11.3).

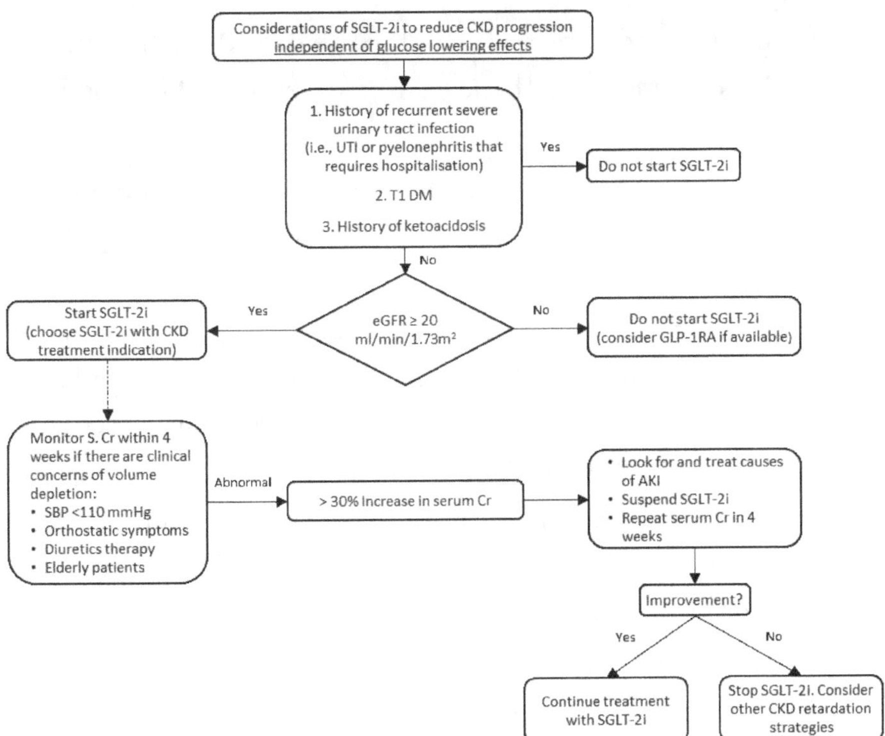

Figure 11.2:   Algorithm for the initiation of SGLT-2i to slow down CKD progression.

(Adapted from the SingHealth Renal Retardation Programme (SiRRP) Clinical Guide Version 13th March 2022.)

Table 11.3: GFR Cut-Offs for the Initiation of SGLT-2i for Non-Glycaemic Indications

SGLT-2i	Dapagliflozin	Empagliflozin	Canagliflozin
	eGFR cut-off (mL/min/1.73 m^2) for initiation		
CKD treatment (Patients with T2DM)	≥25 (10 mg) continue until dialysis	≥20 (10 mg) continue until dialysis	≥30 (100 mg) continue until dialysis
CKD treatment (Patients without T2DM)			No indication

Adapted from the SingHealth Renal Retardation Programme (SiRRP) Clinical Guide Version 13th March 2022

Abbreviations: CKD, chronic kidney disease; eGFR, estimated glomerular filtration rate; SGLT-2i, sodium glucose cotransporter-2 inhibitor; T2DM, type 2 diabetes mellitus

- Precautions need to be taken for the use of SGLT-2i in patients with diabetes mellitus who are at increased risk of diabetic ketoacidosis (Table 11.4).

- Like RAS blockers, an initial increase in serum creatinine up to 30% can be expected and is not an indication to stop if the trend stabilises.

- Majority of patients do not need to have routine monitoring of renal function after initiation of a SGLT-2i. These patients can safely have the next set of blood tests done at subsequent scheduled appointments.

- However, monitoring of serum creatinine and volume status within 4 weeks of initiation of SGLT-2i would be prudent in certain group of patients:

  - Elderly patients

  - Patients at-risk of volume depletion or acute kidney injury (e.g., patients with systolic blood pressure <110 mmHg, signs/symptoms of volume depletion, concurrent diuretics therapy)

Table 11.4:   Precautions for SGLT-2i Use in Patients With Diabetes Mellitus at Increased Risk of Diabetic Ketoacidosis

Patient Groups	What to do
T1DM	Do not use SGLT-2i.
Newly diagnosed T2DM with osmotic symptoms (e.g., polyuria, polydipsia)	Consider SGLT-2i only after 6–12 months of initial treatment with lifestyle modifications and other glucose lowering agent(s).
T2DM patients with HbA1c ≥10% (lower threshold if they exhibit any osmotic symptoms)	Consider insulin therapy. May consider SGLT-2i after glycaemic control improves (HbA1c <10%) and patient has no osmotic symptoms.
Patients with past history of ketoacidosis	Do not use SGLT-2i.

Adapted from the SingHealth Renal Retardation Programme (SiRRP) Clinical Guide Version 13th March 2022

Abbreviations: T1DM, type 1 diabetes mellitus; T2DM, type 2 diabetes mellitus; SGLT-2i, sodium glucose cotransporter-2 inhibitor

Consider decreasing dosages of pre-existing diuretics before commencement of SGT-2i and advise patients about the symptoms of volume depletion and hypotension.

- For patients at-risk for hypoglycaemia or tight glycaemic control, it may be necessary to stop or reduce the dose of a glucose-lowering drug other than metformin to facilitate the addition of an SGLT-2i.

- There is a possibility of an increased risk of urogenital infections associated with SGLT-2i, hence personal hygiene education should be recommended for all patients initiating SGLT-2i.

- Consider withholding SGLT-2i during times of prolonged fasting, surgery, or critical medical illness (when patients may be at greater risk of euglycaemic and hyperglycaemic diabetic ketoacidosis).

- Counsel patients on the risks of rare but severe complications such as euglycaemic diabetic ketoacidosis and Fournier's gangrene.

- SGLT-2i can be continued until patients are initiated on kidney replacement therapy, even if the prevailing eGFR is below the eGFR at which SGLT-2i was commenced.

Mineralocorticoid Receptor Antagonists

- Addition of non-steroidal mineralocorticoid receptor antagonists (MRA) to RAS blockers has been shown to reduce the risk of progression of CKD in patients with diabetic kidney disease.

- Research on similar benefits in patients with non-diabetic kidney disease is ongoing (at the time of publishing of this book).

- Non-steroidal MRAs can be considered in addition to RAS blockers and/or SGLT-2i in patients with persistent albuminuria or proteinuria (Figure 11.3).

- There is less evidence of steroidal MRAs in reducing the risk of progression in CKD and they have more adverse effects, but they may be considered if patients have other concomitant medical conditions (e.g., heart failure, need for further optimisation of blood pressure with close monitoring of adverse effects).

- Finerenone (non-steroidal MRA) dosing (initiation when eGFR at least $\geq$25 mL/min/1.73 m^2)
    - Initiation 20 mg once in the morning (OM) (max 20 mg OM)
    - eGFR $\geq$25 – <60 mL/min/1.73 m^2 – initiation 10 mg OM (max 20 mg OM)

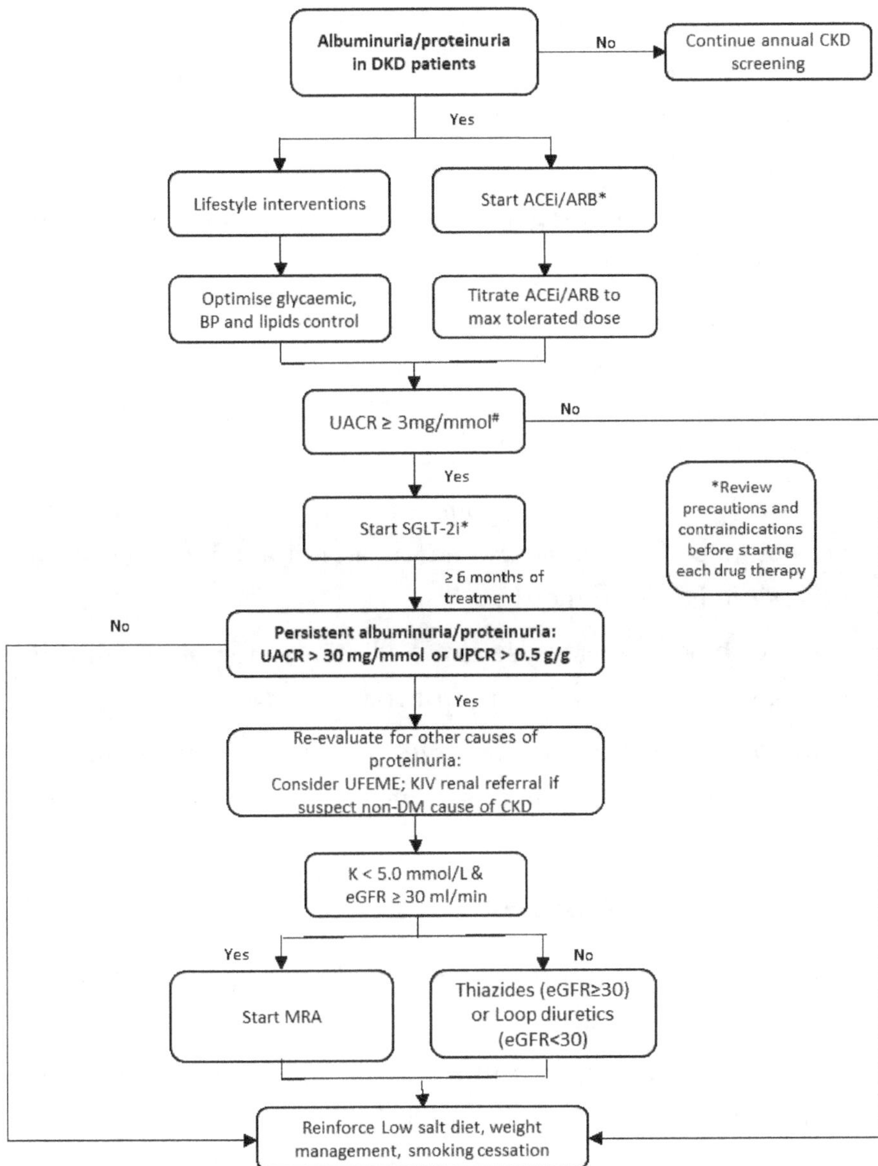

Figure 11.3:   Approach to Persistent Albuminuria/Proteinuria in Patients with DM and CKD

Adapted from the SingHealth Renal Retardation Programme (SiRRP) Clinical Guide Version 13th March 2022

- Spironolactone (steroidal MRA) dosing (initiation when eGFR is at least ≥30 mL/min/1.73 m²)

    - eGFR >50 mL/min/1.73 m² — initiation 12.5 mg OM (max 25 mg BD)

    - eGFR ≥30–50 mL/min/1.73 m² — initiation 12.5 mg OM (max 25 mg OM)

- MRAs have a similar adverse effects profile as RAS blockers (e.g., hyperkalaemia acute kidney injury). Other adverse effects (e.g., hypotension, gynecomastia) are less evident in non-steroidal MRAs compared to steroidal MRAs.

- Research has shown that non-steroidal MRAs increase serum potassium by 0.2 mmol/L, hence avoid initiating it when serum potassium is >4.8 mmol/L.

- Monitor blood pressure, serum creatinine, and potassium within 2–4 weeks of initiating or up-titration of MRAs.

- Aim for blood pressure at target pressure, serum potassium <5.5 mmol/L and less than 30% increase in serum creatinine.

Blood Pressure Control

- Aim for clinic blood pressure <140/90 mmHg in patients with non-albuminuric CKD.

- Aim for clinic blood pressure <130/80 mmHg in patients with albuminuric CKD.

- Home blood pressure measurement is approximately –5/–5 mmHg compared to clinic measurement.

- KDIGO guideline has recommended for systolic blood pressure (SBP) <120 mmHg using standardised office measurement with evidence based mainly from the SPRINT study subgroup analysis of non-DM patients with CKD.

- In the SPRINT CKD sub-group analysis, SBP < 120 mmHg compared to < 140 mmHg reduced primary composite cardiovascular and all-cause mortality outcomes but not composite renal outcomes.

Diabetic Control (In Patients with Diabetes Mellitus)

- Individualised HbA1c target of <6.5% to <8.0%, depending on risk factors:
  - Severity of CKD
  - Presence of macrovascular complications
  - Comorbidities
  - Life expectancy
  - Hypoglycaemia awareness
  - Resources for hypoglycaemia management
  - Propensity of treatment to cause hypoglycaemia
- Lifestyle therapy (weight loss, nutrition, and physical activity)
- First line diabetic treatments are metformin and SGLT-2i

Correction of Acidosis

- Risk of acidosis increases as eGFR decreases to <40 mL/min/1.73 m^2.
- Low to moderate certainty evidence suggests that oral alkali supplementation or reduction in dietary acid intake may slow

the rate of kidney function decline and risk of end-stage kidney disease.

- Aim for serum bicarbonate between 22 and 26 mmol/L, using the lowest dose of sodium bicarbonate or through dietary changes to reduce dietary acid intake.

- Consider initiating sodium bicarbonate tablets if acidosis is not related to other causes or acute kidney injury.

- Start sodium bicarbonate tablet 1 to 2 g/day with monitoring of serum bicarbonate levels. The maximum dose is approximately 4.5 g/day.

- Monitor fluid status, serum potassium and calcium levels, when starting oral sodium bicarboante therapy.

Dietary and Lifestyle Interventions

- Limit sodium intake to <2 g sodium/day (<90 mmol sodium/day or <5 g sodium chloride/day).

- Smoking cessation for current smokers.

- High protein diet (>1.0 g protein/kg body weight/day) may cause harm to patients with CKD.

- Aim for protein intake of 0.6–0.8 g protein/kg body weight/day depending on patient comorbidities and presence of diabetes.

- Plant-based diet has been advocated, though caution is needed for patients prone to hyperkalaemia or at a more advanced stage of CKD.

- Moderate-intensity physical activity (i.e., able to talk but not sing the words of a song, e.g. brisk walking, cycling) for a cumulative duration of at least 150 min per week or to a level compatible with their cardiovascular and physical tolerance.

CKD Monitoring Frequency

- eGFR and urinary albumin: creatinine ratio (ACR) should be monitored (Table 11.5).
- Other investigations may be included for complications of CKD depending on the stage of CKD.

Table 11.5: Recommendations for the Monitoring of Chronic Kidney Disease

Severity of Chronic Kidney Disease	Monitoring Frequency
• eGFR 45 to <60 mL/min/1.73 m² and ACR <3 mg/mmol • eGFR ≥60 mL/min/1.73 m² and ACR 3–30 mg/mmol	12 monthly
• eGFR 30 to <45 mL/min/1.73 m² and ACR <3 mg/mmol • eGFR 45 to <60 mL/min/1.73 m² and ACR 3–30 mg/mmol • eGFR ≥60 mL/min/1.73 m² and ACR >30 mg/mmol	6 monthly
• eGFR 15 to <30 mL/min/1.73 m² and ACR <3 mg/mmol • eGFR 15 to <45 mL/min/1.73 m² and ACR 3–30 mg/mmol • eGFR 30 to <60 mL/min/1.73 m² and ACR >30 mg/mmol	4 monthly
• eGFR <15 mL/min/1.73 m² and any ACR • eGFR 15 to <30 mL/min/1.73 m² and ACR >30 mg/mmol	3 monthly

Abbreviations: ACR, albumin:creatinine ratio; eGFR, estimated glomerular filtration rate

References

Atkins RC, Briganti EM, Lewis JB, *et al.* (2005). Proteinuria reduction and progression to renal failure in patients with type 2 diabetes mellitus and overt nephropathy. *Am J Kidney Dis* **45**(2): 281–287.

Cheung AK, Rahman M, Reboussin DM, *et al.* (2017). Effects of intensive BP control in CKD. *J Am Soc Nephrol* **28**(9): 2812–2823.

Kidney Disease: Improving Global Outcomes (KDIGO) CKD Work Group (2013). KDIGO clinical practice guideline for the evaluation and management of chronic kidney disease. *Kidney Int Suppl* **3**: 1–150.

Kidney Disease: Improving Global Outcomes (KDIGO) Diabetes Work Group (2020). KDIGO 2020 clinical practice guideline for diabetes management in chronic kidney disease. *Kidney Int* **98**(4S): S1–S115.

Navaneethan SD, Shao J, Buysse J, *et al.* (2019). Effects of treatment of metabolic acidosis in CKD: A systematic review and meta-analysis. *Clin J Am Soc Nephrol* **14**(7): 1011–1020.

12 Fluid Overload in Chronic Kidney Disease

Carolyn Tien, Chan Choong Meng

Introduction

- Fluid overload is defined as a clinical state of excess total body sodium and water with expansion of extra cellular fluid.

- This commonly occurs in chronic kidney disease patients especially as their kidney function worsens.

- Diuretics form a cornerstone of management of fluid overload in addition to fluid and salt restriction.

Causes

Renal causes
- Worsening chronic kidney disease
- Acute kidney injury
- Worsening proteinuria/nephrotic syndrome

Precipitating factors
- Fluid indiscretion
- Salt indiscretion
- Non-compliance to diuretics

Other causes
- Cardiac causes such as congestive cardiac failure, acute coronary event, valvular disease
- Liver failure
- Protein-losing enteropathy

Diagnosis

Clinical	• Symptoms — shortness of breath, orthopnoea, paroxysmal nocturnal dyspnoea, lower limb swelling • Signs — lung crepitations, flank/sacral/pedal oedema
Laboratory	• Renal panel • Full blood count • Liver function test • Cardiac enzymes • N-terminal pro brain natriuretic peptide • ± Arterial blood gas • Urine protein:creatinine ratio • Electrocardiogram
Radiological	• Chest X-ray
Adjuncts	• Bio-impedance analysis • Point of care ultrasound (POCUS) — lung fields, inferior vena cava • Transthoracic echocardiogram

Management

- Stabilisation of haemodynamics and oxygen saturation
- If tachypnoeic or drowsy, do arterial blood gas to rule out Type II respiratory failure
- Strict I/O charting and consider the use of an indwelling catheter or urosheath for the initial period
- Fluid restricted to 800 mL/day; low salt diet (<2 g/day)
- Daily weight

Table 12.1:   Diuretic Drugs for Fluid Overload

Diuretic Type		Mode of Action	Use
Proximal tubule	Carbonic anhydrase inhibitor (e.g., acetazolamide)	Block carbonic anhydrase enzyme, indirectly blocking Na/H+ exchanger	Weak diuretic and thus most often used with other diuretics in the treatment of metabolic alkalosis accompanied by oedematous state Generates a hyperchloraemic metabolic acidosis especially with prolonged use
	Osmotic diuretic (e.g., mannitol)	Increases osmotic pressure within lumen of proximal tubule causing water diuresis	Caution for use as there is risk of causing pulmonary oedema during the intravascular hypertonic phase, especially in patients with reduced cardiac output Thus, use mainly or only for cerebral oedema/raised intraocular pressure
Loop diuretics (e.g., furosemide, bumetanide) *Bumetanide 1 mg = furosemide 40 mg		Inhibit Na-K-2Cl transporter in the thick ascending limb in the loop of Henle, causing reduced reabsorption of Na and dilute urine formation with net fluid loss	Onset of action • IV 5 minutes, PO 30–60 minutes Duration of action • IV 2 hours, PO 4–6 hours Oral dose has to be doubled compared to IV as oral bioavailability is only 50% for furosemide Dosing: • Moderate CKD (stage 3–4): Furosemide 80 mg, bumetanide 2–3 mg • Severe CKD (stage 5): Furosemide 160–240 mg, bumetanide 8–10 mg Caution as there is risk of ototoxicity if dose is given rapidly or the daily total dose >1 g

(Continued)

Table 12.1: (*Continued*)

Diuretic Type	Mode of Action	Use
Thiazide diuretics (e.g., hydrochlorothiazide, indapamide, metolazone)	Inhibit Na-Cl co-transporter in distal convoluted tubules	Hydrochlorothiazide is often ineffective in patients with advanced renal impairment (eGFR <30 mL/min) Instead, thiazides are often used as combination therapy for sequential blockade with loop diuretic for more effective diuresis (e.g., metolazone)
Collecting Duct	Epithelial sodium channel antagonist (e.g., amiloride)	Inhibit Na reabsorption by blocking apical epithelial sodium channel	Considered as weak diuretics and often needs to be used with other diuretics to augment diuresis Monitor K closely as there is risk of hyperkalaemia especially in CKD patients
	Aldosterone antagonist (e.g., spironolactone)	Competitive antagonist of aldosterone causing natriuresis and K retention	Used as first line for certain conditions • Spironolactone in liver cirrhosis with ascites • Amiloride in the treatment of Liddle syndrome

- Administer diuretic therapy (Table 12.1)

- Ensure adequate bolus dosing of **IV** furosemide based on kidney function (often higher doses needed in patients with reduced eGFR).

- Consider continuous furosemide infusion 10–30 mg/hour if there is a poor response to bolus dosing.

- Consider co-administration of **IV** albumin if hypoalbuminaemic.

- Addition of sequential blockade with thiazide such as metolazone 5–20 mg om.

- Trend the kidney function and monitor for side effects of diuretic therapy such as hypokalaemia, hyponatraemia, hyperuricaemia, hypercalcaemia, or hypocalcaemia.

- If there is poor urine output response to diuretic therapy, worsening fluid overload, and kidney function, consider initiating kidney replacement therapy.

References

Kitsios GD, Mascari P, Ettunsi R, *et al.* (2014). Co-administration of furosemide with albumin for overcoming diuretic resistance in patients with hypoalbuminemia: A meta-analysis. *J Crit Care* **29**(2): 253–259.

Ng KT and Yap JLL (2018). Continuous infusion vs. intermittent bolus injection of furosemide in acute decompensated heart failure: Systematic review and meta-analysis of randomised controlled trials. *Anaesthesia* **73**(2): 238–247.

13 Anaemia of Chronic Kidney Disease

Carolyn Tien, Chan Choong Meng

Introduction

- Anaemia is a common problem among patients with chronic kidney disease (CKD) and has many causes (Table 13.1 and Figure 13.1).

- It is diagnosed in males when haemoglobin (Hb) level <13 g/dL and for females when Hb <12 g/dL.

Table 13.1: Causes of Anaemia in Chronic Kidney Disease

Inadequate production	• Erythropoietin deficiency in CKD • Iron deficiency • Folate/B12 deficiency • Bone marrow issues such as haematological malignancies • Pure red cell aplasia
Increased losses	• Blood loss, e.g., gastrointestinal bleeding, loss of blood from dialysis circuit clotting • Haemolysis
Others	• Poorly controlled hyperparathyroidism • Use of angiotensin-converting enzyme or angiotensin receptor blockers • Chronic inflammation/infection

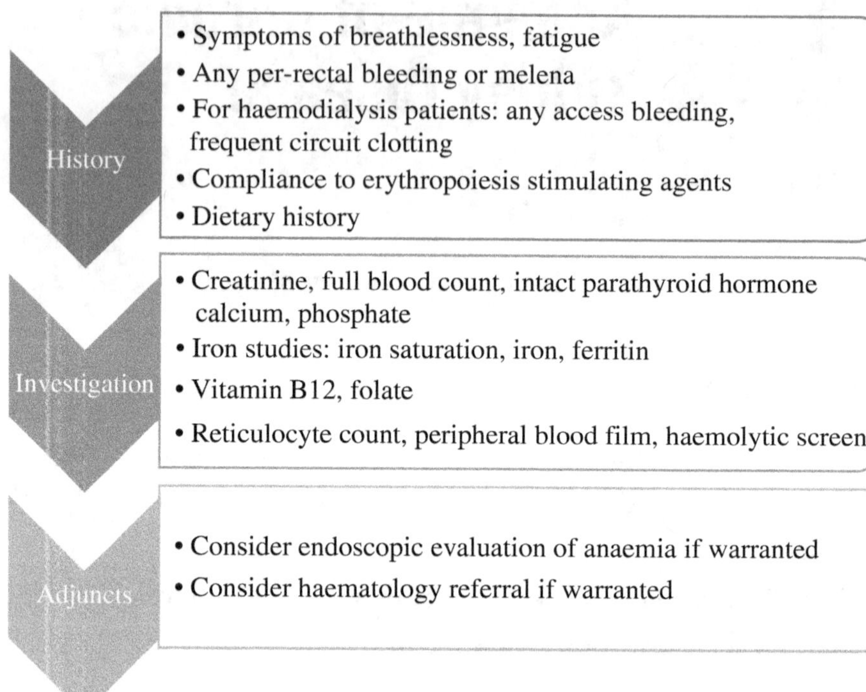

Figure 13.1:   Approach to anaemia in patients with chronic kidney disease

Management

- Ensure adequate iron stores (Table 13.2).
- Initiation of erythropoiesis-stimulating agents (Table 13.3).

Table 13.2:   Iron Replacement Therapy in Chronic Kidney Disease

Indications to replace with IV iron* *For CKD non dialysis patients, a 1–3-month trial of oral iron therapy can be given as an alternative to IV iron	For adult CKD patients with anaemia not on iron or ESA therapy with a. TSAT <30% and ferritin <500 ng/mL b. Desire to increase Hb level without starting ESA For adult CKD patients on ESA who are not receiving iron with a. TSAT <30% and ferritin <500 ng/mL b. Desire to increase Hb level OR a decrease in ESA dose is desired	
Types of iron replacement	Oral	Ferrous fumarate: 200 mg – 65 mg of elemental Fe (33%) Iron polymaltose: 1 mL – 50 mg of elemental Fe Ferrous gluconate (Sangobion): 250 mg = 29.2 mg of elemental Fe (11.5%)
	Intravenous	Iron sucrose (venofer) 100 mg Ferric carboxymaltose (ferinject) 500–1000 mg Ferric derisomaltose (monofer) 500–1000 mg
How to replace	In haemodialysis patients, IV iron can be given across dialysis, e.g.: • IV venofer 100 mg/week for 5–10 doses as loading followed by maintenance thereafter monthly or • IV monofer 500 mg once every 2 weeks for 2 doses as loading followed by maintenance of 500 mg once a month In PD or CKD patients, IV iron will require IV access and can be given as a once-dose loading of either ferinject or monofer followed by PO iron	

(Continued)

Table 13.2:   (Continued)

Monitoring	During IV iron infusion:
	• Monitor for hypotension, dyspnoea, anaphylaxis
	• Do not administer when patients have active systemic infection
	Check iron stores (TSAT and ferritin) 3 monthly

Abbreviations: CKD, chronic kidney disease; ESA, erythropoiesis-stimulating agent; Fe, iron; Hb, haemoglobin; IV, intravenous; PD, peritoneal dialysis; PO, per os/oral; TSAT, transferrin saturation.

Table 13.3:   Erythropoiesis-stimulating Agents in Chronic Kidney Disease

Indications to start ESA	For adult CKD ND patients with Hb >10 g/dL
	– do NOT start ESA
	For adult CKD ND patients with Hb <10 g/dL
	– decision to start ESA depends on:
	• rate of fall of Hb
	• prior response to IV iron
	• risk of needing a transfusion
	• risks related to ESA
	• presence of symptoms due to anaemia
	For adult CKD dialysis patients
	– start ESA when Hb is between 9 to 10 g/dL
Types of ESA and dosing	Erythropoietin, e.g., recormon (epoetin beta), eprex (epoetin alfa)
	– SC or IV 20–50 IU/kg 3 times per week
	Darbepoetin-alfa
	– SC or IV route: 0.45 µg/kg once weekly or
	– SC 0.75 µg/kg once every 2 weeks
	Mircera
	– SC or IV 0.6 µg/kg once every 2 weeks or
	– SC or IV 1.2 µg/kg once a month
How to give ESA	SC route in PD or CKD ND patients
	• SC erythropoietin is 20% more potent than IV for the same dose

Table 13.3:   (*Continued*)

	• To note, the SC route for eprex is contraindicated due to its strong association with antibody-mediated pure red cell aplasia (PRCA), but the SC route for recormon is acceptable IV route preferred in HD patients as it can be given during HD Caution on risk for hypertension, increased risk of thromboembolic event, and PRCA. To also use with caution in patients with active malignancy or history of malignancy and history of stroke due to risk of tumour progression/thromboembolic complications
Monitoring (Table 13.4)	Consider monitoring Hb monthly for HD/PD patients and 3 monthly for CKD ND patients Target Hb 10–11.5 g/dL and avoid >13 g/dL Aim to rise Hb by 1–2 g/dL per month Titrate ESA dose adjustment in steps of 25% and not more than 50% at once, e.g., EPO 4000 u once a week increase to once every 5 days (50% increase) or decrease to 4000 U per 10 days (25% decrease) Interval of dose adjustment should not be shorter than 4 weeks as the ESA effect takes time to set in Consider ESA hyporesponsiveness if: • Initial phase: No increase in Hb from baseline after first month of appropriate weight-based dosing of ESA • Maintenance phase: After stable doses of ESA, now requiring 2 increases in ESA doses up to 50% beyond the dose at which they had been stable to maintain a stable Hb concentration

Abbreviations: CKD ND, chronic kidney disease non-dialysis; ESA, erythropoiesis-stimulating agent; Hb, haemoglobin; HD, haemodialysis; IU, international units; IV, intravenous; kg, kilograms; PD, peritoneal dialysis; PRCA, pure red cell aplasia; SC, subcutaneous.

Table 13.4:   Monitoring of Anaemia in Chronic Kidney Disease

CKD without anaemia	Stage 3	Annually
	Stage 4–5 non-dialysis	Twice a year
	Stage 5 on dialysis	Every 3 months
CKD with anaemia not on ESA	Stage 3–5 non-dialysis	Every 3 months
	Stage 5 on dialysis	Monthly
CKD with anaemia on ESA	Initiation phase	Monthly
	Maintenance phase	CKD ND — 3 monthly CKD dialysis — Monthly

Abbreviations: CKD, chronic kidney disease; ESA, erythropoiesis-stimulating agent

Reference

Locatelli F, Nissenson AR, Barrett BJ, *et al.* (2008). Clinical practice guidelines for anemia in chronic kidney disease: Problems and solutions. A position statement from Kidney Disease: Improving Global Outcomes (KDIGO). *Kidney Int* **74**(10): 1237–1240.

14 Hypertension in Chronic Kidney Disease

Liew Zhong Hong, Wong Kok Seng

Introduction

- Hypertension (HTN) is very common among patients with chronic kidney disease (CKD) and its frequency increases as glomerular filtration rate (GFR) falls. More than 80% of patients with stage 4–5 CKD have HTN.

- It is important to control HTN in CKD as it can reduce proteinuria, retard the progression of CKD, and reduce the risk of cardiovascular morbidity and mortality.

- The pathophysiology of HTN in CKD is complex, mediated by multiple factors such as:

  - Increase in sympathetic tone (vasoconstriction)

  - Activation of the renin-angiotensin-aldosterone system (salt and water retention)

  - Increased salt sensitivity

  - Endothelial dysfunction

  - Increased arterial stiffness

Measurement of Blood Pressure

- Blood pressure (BP) should be measured at every clinic visit for patients with CKD, but the measurement should be standardised as follows:

  - The patient should be rested quietly for 5 minutes prior to BP measurement using a validated and calibrated device (e.g., oscillometric or manual BP device).

  - Caffeine and exercise should be avoided for 30 minutes prior to BP measurement.

  - The cuff should be placed on the arm at the level of the atrium with the correct cuff size (the bladder of the cuff should encircle 80% of the arm).

  - The patient should sit with feet flat on the ground and back supported by the chair.

  - At least 2 readings should be obtained to classify hypertension (Table 14.1).

Table 14.1:   Classification of Hypertension According to ACC/AHA 2017 Guidelines on High Blood Pressure

BP Category	SBP (mmHg)		DBP (mmHg)
Normal	<120	and	<80
Elevated	120–129	and	<80
Hypertension			
Stage 1	130–139	or	80–89
Stage 2	≥140	or	≥90

Abbreviations: ACC, American College of Cardiology; AHA, American Heart Association; DBP, diastolic blood pressure; SBP, systolic blood pressure

Note:
- BP should be based on an average of ≥2 careful readings obtained on ≥2 occasions
- Individuals with SBP and DBP in 2 categories should be designated to the higher BP category.

- Out-of-clinic BP readings correlate more strongly with kidney and cardiovascular outcomes than office readings. There are several reasons why home BP measurements with validated devices should be encouraged:
  - To detect nocturnal hypertension and systolic BP variability, which is frequent and associated with an increased risk of cardiovascular events.
  - To establish the degree of control of BP — resistant HTN is common among patients with CKD. On the other hand, white coat HTN may lead to excessive anti-hypertensive treatment, causing hypotension at home.

Evaluation of Hypertension in Chronic Kidney Disease

- Though HTN is very common among patients with CKD, secondary causes should be evaluated for when:
  - The onset of hypertension occurred before puberty and preceded the development of CKD
  - There is sudden worsening of BP in a patient with previously controlled HTN
  - There is severe or malignant HTN that is out of proportion to the severity of CKD
  - HTN is resistant to treatment

Target Blood Pressure in Chronic Kidney Disease

- Various guidelines have recommended different target BP for patients with CKD (Table 14.2).
- In general, blood pressure should be lowered to less than 140/80 mmHg and eventually less than 130/80 mmHg espe-

Table 14.2:   Recommended Target Blood Pressure for Chronic Kidney Disease According to Various Guidelines

Guidelines	Target Blood Pressure (mmHg)
European Society of Cardiology (ESC) and European Society of Hypertension (ESH) 2018 guidelines	Systolic BP < 130–140 Diastolic BP < 70–80
American College of Cardiology (ACC) and American Heart Association (AHA) 2017 guidelines	Systolic BP < 130 Diastolic BP < 80
Kidney Disease Improving Global Outcomes (KDIGO) 2012 guidelines	Without albuminuria, systolic BP < 140 and diastolic BP < 90 With albuminuria, systolic BP < 130 and diastolic BP < 80
NICE 2019	Systolic BP < 130 Diastolic BP < 80
Hypertension Canada 2020	Systolic BP < 120 for severe CKD

Abbreviations: BP, blood pressure; CKD, chronic kidney disease

cially in younger and/or proteinuric patients. Nevertheless, blood pressure targets should be individualised to the patient's condition, tolerance to anti-hypertensive treatments, and interactions with other treatments.

Non-pharmacological Management of Hypertension in Chronic Kidney Disease

- Reduce dietary salt intake to less than 2 g/day — the DASH (Dietary Approaches to Stop Hypertension) diet may not be appropriate in patients with CKD due to the risk of hyperkalaemia when eating more fruits and vegetables as recommended by the DASH diet.

- Limit intake of alcohol to no more than 2 drinks a day in men or 1 drink a day in women.

- Stop smoking

- Moderate-intensity physical activity for ≥150 minutes per week, if tolerated

- Lose weight, if overweight or obese

Pharmacological Management of Hypertension in Chronic Kidney Disease

- Drug therapy for HTN should be individualised to the patient's condition and concurrent therapies. However, multiple anti-hypertensive drugs are frequently needed, and polypharmacy increases the risk of adverse effects, drug interactions, non-adherence, and drug costs.

- During initiation and titration of anti-hypertensive therapy, patients should be:

  - advised to record home BP measurements which can be reviewed at the next clinic visit — the technique of measuring BP at home should be reviewed.

  - reviewed 2 to 4 times per week if BP is poorly controlled to titrate doses or start additional anti-hypertensive agents (after 1–2 adjustments of initial anti-hypertensive drugs). Patients with severe asymptomatic HTN (e.g., systolic BP ≥180 mmHg and/or diastolic BP ≥110 mmHg) should be reviewed earlier (e.g., 1 week after initiation of anti-hypertensive drug treatment).

  - checked for non-adherence to lifestyle modifications and anti-hypertensive drugs.

- Nocturnal dosing of anti-hypertensive medications has been shown to achieve better BP control and reduce the incidence of cardiovascular events than morning dosing.

- Renin-angiotensin system (RAS) blockers such as angiotensin-converting enzyme inhibitors (ACEi) and the angiotensin II-receptor blocker (ARB) are the first-line anti-hypertensive drugs of choice to treat HTN in patients with CKD. They reduce both the kidney and cardiovascular risks in CKD. In addition, they reduce proteinuria independent of their effect on BP. However, they can cause:

  - Hyperkalaemia, which can be mitigated by dietary restrictions, diuretics, correction of metabolic acidosis, adjustment of medications that cause hyperkalaemia, and the use of potassium binders such as sodium zirconium cyclosilicate (Lokelma®) or polystyrene sulfonate (Resonium®).

  - Reversible decline in GFR (generally less than 30%) at the start of therapy which by itself is not an indication to discontinue RAS blockers.

Combination therapy with ACEi and ARB are no longer recommended as they have been shown to increase the risk of adverse effects without improvement in the progression of CKD or cardiovascular events.

There is insufficient evidence to support routine discontinuation of ACEi and ARB in progressive CKD — generally, ACEi and ARB should only be discontinued if there are adverse effects or contradictions have emerged.

- Calcium channel blockers (CCB) are often added to RAS blockers if BP remains uncontrolled or they are acceptable initial agents when CKD is not associated with proteinuria.

A combination of CCBs and RAS blockers has been shown to reduce the progression of kidney disease and cardiovascular events. CCB may be added first if the patient is not yet suitable for RAS blockers (e.g., hyperkalaemia). Non-dihydropyridine CCBs (e.g., diltiazem) are better than dihydropyridine CCBs (e.g., amlodipine) in reducing proteinuria but are associated with significant interactions with other drugs. The most common side effect of CCB is peripheral oedema.

- Diuretics can be prescribed when there is fluid overload or as an additional anti-hypertensive drug after RAS blockers and CCB have been prescribed. Loop diuretics are the preferred diuretics in CKD but can be combined with thiazide diuretics for synergistic effect. Higher doses of diuretics are required as the GFR declines. Diuretics should generally be avoided in polycystic kidney disease due to accelerated cyst growth.

- Beta blockers are useful when there is coronary artery disease or cardiac failure. Otherwise, they are added only if blood pressure remains uncontrolled despite RAS blockers, CCBs, and diuretics. Beta blockers that are hepatically excreted and with vasodilatory properties (e.g., carvedilol) are preferred.

- Aldosterone antagonists (e.g., spironolactone, finerenone) can also be considered as they can lower BP and proteinuria and may retard the progression of CKD. They are an alternative to beta blockers as a fourth anti-hypertensive agent but are associated with a risk of hyperkalaemia. They are also beneficial in patients with left ventricular dysfunction.

- Other anti-hypertensive drugs such as ∝-adrenoceptor antagonists (e.g., prazosin) and vasodilators (e.g., hydralazine) have not been shown to reduce cardiovascular events or progression of CKD, but they may be added when HTN is poorly controlled.

- Sodium-glucose cotransporter 2 (SGLT2) inhibitors are often prescribed in eligible patients to retard the progression of CKD. However, they can also reduce BP but the effect is modest.

References

Boffa RJ, Constanti M, Floyd CN and Wierzbicki AS (2019). Hypertension in adults: Summary of updated NICE guidance. *Br Med J* **367**: l5310.

Hermida RC, Ayala DE, Mojón A and Fernández JR (2011). Bedtime dosing of antihypertensive medications reduces cardiovascular risk in CKD. *J Am Soc Nephrol* **22**(12): 2313–2321.

Kidney Disease: Improving Global Outcomes (KDIGO) Blood Pressure Work Group (2021). KDIGO 2021 clinical practice guideline for the management of blood pressure in chronic kidney disease. *Kidney Int* **99**(3S): S1–S87.

Rabi DM, McBrien KA, Sapir-Pichhadze R, *et al.* (2020). Hypertension Canada's 2020 comprehensive guidelines for the prevention, diagnosis, risk assessment, and treatment of hypertension in adults and children. *Can J Cardiol* **36**(5): 596–624.

Whelton PK and Carey RM (2017). The 2017 clinical practice guideline for high blood pressure. *J Am Med Assoc* **318**(21): 2073–2074.

Williams B, Mancia G, Spiering W, *et al.* (2018). 2018 ESC/ESH Guidelines for the management of arterial hypertension: The Task Force for the management of arterial hypertension of the European Society of Cardiology and the European Society of Hypertension. *J Hypertens* **36**(10): 1953–2041.

15 Kidney Mineral Bone Disease

Wong Jiunn

Introduction

- Chronic Kidney Disease-Mineral Bone Disorder (CKD-MBD) is a systemic disorder of mineral and bone metabolism due to CKD, manifested by either one of a combination of:

  - Abnormalities of calcium, phosphate, PTH, or vitamin D metabolism

  - Abnormalities in bone turnovers, mineralisation, volume, linear growth, or strength

  - Vascular or other soft tissue calcification

- Hyperparathyroidism is the primary presentation of CKD-MBD but differs from primary hyperparathyroidism in that hyperparathyroidism due to CKD-MBD is usually secondary to reduction of the kidney's ability to excrete phosphate.

- As the glomerular filtration rate (GFR) declines, the kidney's ability to excrete phosphate is progressively impaired and hyperphosphataemia develops (Figure 15.1). To maintain a normal phosphate level, the kidney adapts by increasing fibroblast growth factor 23 (FGF-23) secretion. FGF-23 stimulates urinary excretion of phosphate and together with impaired kidney function, also inhibits the hydroxylation of 25 vitamin D to its active form 1,25 vitamin D. This causes vitamin D deficiency,

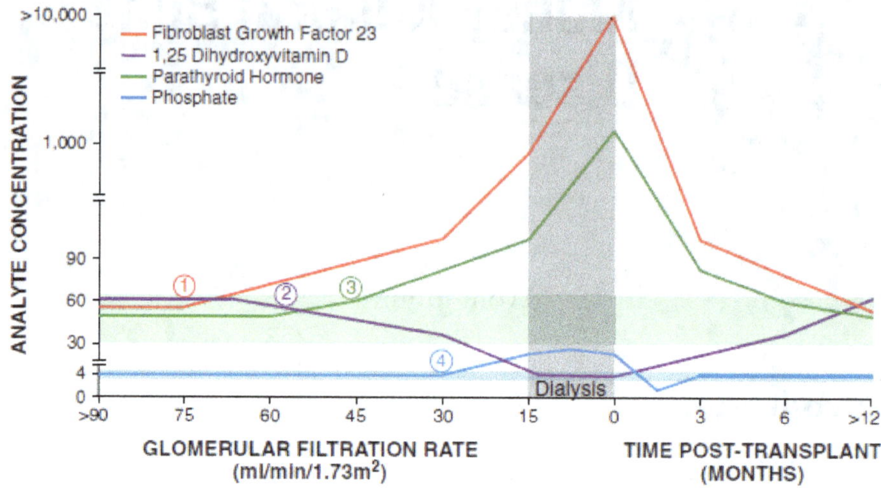

Figure 15.1:   Phosphate Metabolism with Declining Kidney Function

Source: Wolf M (2010). Forging forward with 10 burning questions on FGF23 in kidney disease. *J Am Soc Nephrol* **21**(9): 1427–1435.

which is associated with reduced absorption of phosphate from the kidneys and gastrointestinal tract.

- These changes subsequently lead to a reduction in serum calcium and stimulate serum parathyroid hormone (PTH) levels to rise. PTH increases serum calcium levels through bone resorption as well as increased reabsorption by the kidney and gastrointestinal tract.

- As kidney function deteriorates further, this adaptive mechanism is overwhelmed and the parathyroid glands become autonomous, leading to tertiary hyperparathyroidism (Table 15.1).

- Secondary and tertiary hyperparathyroidism would subsequently lead to the other 2 manifestations of CKD-MBD — abnormalities in bone turnovers, mineralisation, volume, linear growth, or strength, as well as vascular or other soft tissue calcification.

Table 15.1: Biochemical Differences Between Primary, Secondary, and Tertiary Hyperparathyroidism

Biochemical Parameter	Primary Hyperparathyroidism	Secondary Hyperparathyroidism	Tertiary Hyperparathyroidism
Calcium	↑	↓	↑
Phosphate	↓	↑	↑
iPTH	↑	↑	↑

Abbreviation: iPTH, ionised parathyroid hormone

Management of Chronic Kidney Disease Mineral Bone Disease

Control phosphate

- The main treatment strategy for preventing and treating hyperparathyroidism due to CKD-MBD is mainly to reduce phosphate load to the kidney.

- This can be achieved via the following

  - Restriction of phosphate in diet

  - Phosphate binders

  - Phosphate transport inhibitor

  - Optimising dialysis

- The main strategies in early CKD, even prior to evidence of hyperphosphataemia, is to restrict phosphate in the diet. Phosphate from dietary sources is absorbed in the gastrointestinal tract to varying degrees — plant based phosphate (20–40%), animal-based phosphate (30–80%), and inorganic phosphate from food additives (90–100%).

- However, it is important to avoid malnutrition while restricting dietary phosphate — the Kidney Dialysis Outcomes Quality

Table 15.2:   Types of Phosphate Binders Available in Singapore

Phosphate Binders	Dosage	Content	Potential Advantages	Potential Disadvantages
Calcium acetate*	667 mg Total elemental calcium intake should not exceed 2 g/day (dietary 500 mg + elemental Ca in phosphate binder 1500 mg)	Contains 25% elemental Ca /tab (160 mg)	Effective Less calcium absorption	Potential for hypercalcaemia Gastrointestinal side effects More costly than calcium carbonate
Calcium carbonate*	625 mg, 1250 mg Total elemental calcium intake should not exceed 2 g/day (dietary 500 mg + elemental Ca in phosphate binder 1500 mg)	Contains 40% elemental Ca (250 mg or 500 mg /tab)	Effective Inexpensive	Potential for hypercalcaemia Gastrointestinal side effects
Sevelamer	800 mg–1600 mg TDS with meals		Effective No calcium/metal Not absorbed Reduce low density lipoprotein level Slow progression of vascular calcification	Cost Metabolic acidosis May require calcium supplement in the presence of hypocalcaemia Gastrointestinal side effects
Lanthanum	500 mg–1 g TDS with meals or immediately after meals		Effective Non-calcium binder Chewable Slow progression of vascular calcification	Cost Potential for accumulation due to gastrointestinal absorption Long term clinical consequences unknown Gastrointestinal side effects
Sucroferric oxyhydroxide (velphoro)	500 mg TDS	500 mg of iron (minimally adsorbed)	Effective Non-calcium binder Easy to chew Slow progression of vascular calcification	Cost Gastrointestinal side effect

Abbreviations: Ca, calcium; TDS, three times a day

Table 15.3:   Practical Tips in the Use of Phosphate Binders

- The phosphate-binding properties of calcium acetate and calcium carbonate are largely similar. However, the choice of one over the other may depend on their calcium content, which differs (calcium acetate and calcium carbonate has 325 and 500 mg of elemental calcium, respectively).

- Non-calcium-based phosphate binders such as sevelamer, lanthanum, and velphoro are preferred in CKD patients with vascular calcification, low PTH, or adynamic bone disease. However, they are more costly.

- Adherence to phosphate binders can be challenging for patients. The best phosphate binder is the one that the patient is taking.

- Dialysis may eventually be indicated to control phosphate when dietary restriction and phosphate binders become inadequate to control phosphate in advanced CKD.

- Phosphate transport inhibitors (e.g., tenapanor) block sodium phosphate co-transported in the GI tract but is not available for clinical use at the time of writing.

Initiative (KDOQI) guidelines recommend a dietary phosphate/protein ratio of 12–16 mg phosphorus/g of protein.

- As GFR continues to decline, dietary phosphate restriction alone would not be sufficient to prevent hyperphosphataemia and phosphate binders would be required (Tables 15.2 and 15.3). Phosphate binders need to be taken with food so that it can mix and bind the phosphate in the diet.

- Chewing/crushing for certain types of phosphate binders may increase surface area and improve binding capacity.

Avoid calcium loading

- Corrected total calcium should be maintained within the normal range for the lab used, preferably toward the lower end (2.1 to 2.37 mmol/L). However, the serum calcium level may not be truly reflective of the total body calcium level.

- Dialysate calcium of 1.25 mmol/L should be used in most patients on dialysis unless serum calcium levels are low or after parathyroidectomy.

- Calcium-based phosphate binders should be avoided in patients who are hypercalcaemic or show significant evidence of vascular calcification.

Vitamin D and PTH

- Serum calcium, phosphate, and vitamin D levels should be measured in patients with stage 3, 4, and 5 CKD who have elevated iPTH levels. Any abnormalities found should be corrected.

- For stage 3 and 4 CKD stage patients, treat vitamin D insufficiency or deficiency if the vitamin 25(OH)D level is <30 ng/mL (Table 15.4).

Table 15.4:   Recommended Supplementation for Vitamin D Deficiency/ Insufficiency in Patients with Stage 3 and 4 Chronic Kidney Disease

Serum 25(OH)D (ng/mL) (nmol/L)	Definition	Ergocalciferol Dose	Duration	Comment
<5 [12]	Severe vitamin D deficiency	50,000 IU/wk orally × 12 weeks, then monthly 500,000 IU as single IM dose	6 months	Measure 25 (OH) D levels after 6 months
5–15 [12–37]	Mild vitamin D deficiency	50,000 IU/wk orally × 4 weeks then 50,000 IU/ month orally	6 months	Measure 25 (OH) D levels after 6 months
16–30 [40–75]	Vitamin D insufficiency	50,000 IU/month orally	6 months	

Source: National Kidney Foundation (2003). K/DOQI clinical practice guidelines for bone metabolism and disease in chronic kidney disease. *Am J Kidney Dis* **42**(4 Suppl 3): S1–S201.

- Alphacalcidiol and vitamin D analogs are not routinely recommended for adult patients with CKD G3a–G5 (GFR <60 mL/min/1.73 m²) who are not on dialysis. However, it is reasonable to use alphacalcidol and vitamin D analogs for patients with CKD G4–G5 (GFR <30 mL/min/1.73 m²) who have severe and progressive hyperparathyroidism.

- In patients with CKD G5D (on dialysis) requiring PTH-lowering therapy, calcimimetics, alphacalcidol/vitamin D analogs, or a combination of calcimimetics with alphacalcidol/vitamin D analogs can be used.

- Alphacalcidol l or other vitamin D sterols should be reduced or stopped when there is hypercalcaemia and hyperphosphataemia.

- Pulse therapy of alphacalcidol and vitamin D analogs (e.g., 2–3 doses per week) is preferred, especially in the presence of hypercalcaemia and hyperphosphataemia.

    - Usual starting doses are 0.25–0.5 μg 3 times/week (start at no higher than 1 μg 3 times/week).

    - Up to 3 μg 3 times per week can be used but with risk of worsening vascular calcification.

    - Intravenous therapy for dialysis patients improves compliance and possibly reduces intestinal absorption of calcium and phosphate.

    - Monitoring with adjustment of doses is required to avoid hypercalcaemia. Serum calcium and phosphate level should be monitored during therapy with vitamin D.

- Vitamin D should be avoided in patients with low iPTH level.

- Alternatives to alphacalcidiol and vitamin D analogs are calcimimetic agents (e.g., cinacalcet and etelcalcitide). They increase the sensitivity of the Ca-sensing receptor in parathyroid cells to activation by extracellular Ca, thereby downregulating PTH levels and consequently lowering serum Ca and phosphorus. A limiting factor to their widespread use is high prescribing cost.

Parathyroidectomy

- Under conditions of persistent hyperphosphataemia, hypocal-caemia, and vitamin D deficiency, calcium sensing and vitamin D receptors in the parathyroid gland are downregulated. Eventually, the parathyroid glands would develop into adenomas which are no longer responsive to medical therapy.

- Parathyroidectomy would be the treatment of choice in the following clinical situations:

  - Clinical complications — Calciphylaxis, bone pain, fractures, intractable pruritis not responding to medical therapy

  - Radiological complications — Progressive metastatic calcification, brown tumours, bone resorption, rugger-jersey spine, pepper pot skull, chondrocalcinosis

  - Biochemical — Hypercalcaemia with or without concurrent vitamin D therapy; the latter may be necessary to control secondary hyperparathyroidism

- Two major types of parathyroidectomies are performed around the world — subtotal parathyroidectomy and total parathyroidectomy with deltoid implants

- Some of the major risks associated with surgeries are:

- Local complication — bleeding, infection, haematoma, recurrent laryngeal nerve injury (causing weakness or paralysis of the vocal cords)
- Hungry bone syndrome
- Hypoparathyroidism with prolonged severe hypocalcaemia
- Recurrent hyperparathyroidism with deltoid implant or subtotal parathyroidectomy

References

Kidney Disease: Improving Global Outcomes (KDIGO) CKD-MBD Work Group (2009). KDIGO clinical practice guideline for the diagnosis, evaluation, prevention, and treatment of Chronic Kidney Disease-Mineral and Bone Disorder (CKD-MBD). *Kidney international. Supplement* (113): S1–S130.

Martin KJ and González EA (2007). Metabolic bone disease in chronic kidney disease. *Journal of the American Society of Nephrology: JASN* **18**(3): 875–885.

National Kidney Foundation (2003). K/DOQI clinical practice guidelines for bone metabolism and disease in chronic kidney disease. *American journal of kidney diseases: The official journal of the National Kidney Foundation* **42**(4 Suppl 3): S1–S201.

Wagner CA (2020). Coming out of the PiTs-novel strategies for controlling intestinal phosphate absorption in patients with CKD. *Kidney international* **98**(2): 273–275.

Wolf M (2010). Forging forward with 10 burning questions on FGF23 in kidney disease. *Journal of the American Society of Nephrology: JASN* **21**(9): 1427–1435.

16 Parathyroidectomy

Wong Jiunn

Introduction

- Parathyroidectomy remains an important treatment option for patients with severe hyperparathyroidism that is refractory to medical therapy. Even though calcimimetics have significantly reduced the number of parathyroidectomies done worldwide, many patients still undergo this procedure.

- There is currently no consensus on the threshold parathyroid hormone (PTH) level for a parathyroidectomy to be performed. The type of parathyroidectomy and the management after a parathyroidectomy also vary significantly across centres.

- Parathyroid hormone (PTH) level may not be a good predictor of parathyroid-mediated high turnover disease — most parathyroid hormone level assays are 2nd-generation assays that detect PTH fragments which accumulate in end-stage kidney disease.

- Alternative bone turnover markers such as bone-specific alkaline phosphatase (ALP) may improve the prediction of bone turnover when interpreted together with the PTH level.

Total Parathyroidectomy vs. Subtotal Parathyroidectomy vs. Total Parathyroidectomy with Auto Implantation

- Parathyroidectomy can be total with or without auto-implantation or subtotal.

- All 3 surgical techniques have been demonstrated to improve quality of life in patients with severe hyperparathyroidism.

- Improvement in symptoms is usually seen early — within a month post parathyroidectomy and may persist for up to 1 year following surgery.

- Systematic reviews have also shown that parathyroidectomy is associated with better cardiovascular as well as overall mortality.

- The rate of recurrence has been documented to be higher in patients who underwent subtotal parathyroidectomy vs. total parathyroidectomy with auto implantation or in those who underwent total parathyroidectomy without auto implantation.

- The choice of surgical technique should be determined based on the patient profile. However, in Singapore where dialysis survival is high and the waiting time for a transplant may be more than a decade, total parathyroidectomy with auto implantation is preferred over subtotal parathyroidectomy. Total parathyroidectomy without auto implantation is avoided because of concerns with permanent hypoparathyroidism.

Hungry Bone Syndrome

- Hungry bone syndrome is a state of profound and often prolonged hypocalcaemia associated with hypophosphataemia and hypomagnesaemia occurring after parathyroidectomy.

- There is no consensus on the diagnostic criteria and the incidence of hungry bone syndrome varies widely in the literature.

- The severity of hungry bone syndrome is proportionate to the extent of parathyroid-mediated high turnover bone disease.

- PTH increases both bone formation as well as resorption. The mechanism of hungry bone syndrome is postulated to be due to acute reversal of parathyroid hormone-mediated bone resorption to maintain serum calcium concentration. Sudden reduction in PTH following parathyroidectomy causes an imbalance between osteoblast and osteoclast activities. A sudden decrease in osteoclastic activity with continued osteoblast activity drives the influx of calcium and phosphate into bones.

- Multiple risk factors for hungry bone syndrome have been identified, but none are well validated. Some of the risk factors reported in the literature include:

  - Old age
  - Size of the gland removed
  - Pre-operative PTH level
  - Pre-operative ALP level
  - Vitamin D deficiency

Treatment of hungry bone syndrome

- There is insufficient data-driven evidence on the best means to treat, minimise, or prevent this complication.

- Treatment is aimed at replacing severe calcium deficit with high dose of calcium as well as vitamin D supplements.

- KDIGO in 2005 recommends that oral calcium should be initiated as soon as the patient is allowed to take orally, and a calcium gluconate infusion should be initiated at a rate of 1 to 2 mg elemental calcium per kg bodyweight per hour when ionic calcium falls below <0.9 mmol/L (corrected total serum calcium of 1.80 mmol/L).

- Phosphate replacement should be avoided in patients with hungry bone syndrome since phosphate can combine with calcium to further reduce plasma calcium concentration.

- Magnesium levels should be checked and replaced accordingly, as hypomagnesaemia can contribute to refractory hypocalcaemia by potentially further diminishing PTH secretion and inducing PTH resistance.

- Pre-operative administration of bisphosphonates has been postulated to prevent severe hungry bone syndrome, but this remains to be proven.

- Most centres have developed protocols for dialysis patients who undergo parathyroidectomy. The protocol at the Singapore General Hospital (SGH) was developed with the following considerations:

  - ALP level is a better surrogate marker of bone turnover than PTH as the assay used in SGH remains a 2nd-generation assay which detects PTH fragments that accumulate in patients with end-stage kidney disease.

  - Intravenous calcium replacement is given prophylactically rather than waiting for hypocalcaemia to occur.

  - The amount of intravenous calcium replacement is determined by the pre-operative ALP level and titrated according to patients' calcium level.

References

Apetrii M, Goldsmith D, Nistor I, *et al.* (2017). Impact of surgical parathyroid-ectomy on chronic kidney disease-mineral and bone disorder (CKD-MBD): A systematic review and meta-analysis. *PLoS One* **12**(11): e0187025.

Filho WA, van der Plas WY, Brescia MDG, *et al.* (2018). Quality of life after surgery in secondary hyperparathyroidism, comparing subtotal parathyroid-ectomy with total parathyroidectomy with immediate parathyroid autograft: Prospective randomized trial. *Surgery* **164**(5): 978–985.

See A, Lim AEL, Wong J, *et al.* (2019). The effect of parathyroidectomy on patients' symptoms in tertiary hyperparathyroidism. *Head Neck* **41**(8): 2748–2755.

17 Hypertensive Emergencies

Liew Zhong Hong, Wong Kok Seng

Introduction

- Hypertensive crisis is a collective term for hypertensive emergencies and urgencies (Table 17.1) — 1 to 2% of patients with hypertension (HTN) will suffer a hypertensive crisis in their lifetime.

Hypertensive Urgencies

- Hypertensive urgency is the most common type of hypertensive crisis.

- It is usually asymptomatic, or a mild headache may be reported.

- Hypertensive urgency can be treated by intensification, resumption of pre-existing antihypertensive drugs, or initiation of antihypertensive therapy in the treatment naïve.

- Patients do not require referral to the emergency department or hospitalisation.

- Blood pressure (BP) can be slowly reduced over 24–48 hours, aiming for ≤25% reduction within the first 24 hours.

- Patients should be followed-up within a week to ensure BP is controlled.

Table 17.1:   Definitions of Hypertensive Emergencies and Urgencies

Hypertensive emergency	Severe elevations of BP (≥180/120 mmHg) associated with new or worsening target organ damage (**BARKH** acronym) ■ **B**rain – Hypertensive encephalopathy – Intracranial or subarachnoid haemorrhage – Acute cerebral infarction ■ **A**rteries – Aortic dissection – Eclampsia ■ **R**etina – Hypertensive retinopathy ■ **K**idney – Acute kidney failure – Thrombotic microangiopathy ■ **H**eart – Acute myocardial infarction – Acute left ventricular failure/acute pulmonary oedema – Myocardial ischaemia (e.g., angina pectoris or infarction)
Hypertensive urgency	Severe elevations of BP (≥180/120 mmHg) in otherwise stable patients without acute or impending change in target organ damage or dysfunction.

Abbreviation: BP, blood pressure

Hypertensive Emergencies

- Hypertensive emergencies are potentially lethal with a 1-year mortality rate >79%.

- Risk factors for hypertensive emergencies include:

  - Males

  - Older age

  - Black

  - Non-adherence to treatment

  - Lack of insurance or a primary care doctor

- Unlike hypertensive urgency, hypertensive emergencies require admission to a high dependency or intensive care unit for continuous BP monitoring, frequent neurological and kidney function assessment, and the administration of intravenous (IV) antihypertensive drugs.

Evaluation of hypertensive emergencies

- The most common presentation of hypertensive emergencies are cerebral infarction, hypertensive encephalopathy, and pulmonary oedema.

- Determine:
  - Symptoms and signs of specific target end-organ damage (Table 17.2) including doing a fundoscopy to detect papilledema and retinopathy — arteriolar spasm, retinal

Table 17.2:   Symptoms and Signs of Hypertensive Emergencies

Organ System	Symptoms	Signs
Neurological	Visual disturbances, dizziness, headache, seizures, change in mental state, dysphagia, loss of sensation, paraesthesia, loss of movement, nausea/vomiting (sign of raised intracranial pressure)	Carotid bruit, focal neurological signs
Cardiac	Chest pain, dyspnoea, diaphoresis, orthopnoea, paroxysmal nocturnal dyspnoea, palpitations, back pain (sign of aortic dissection)	Jugular venous distension, murmurs, friction rub, additional heart sound, lateral displacement of the apex beat, lung crepitations, differences in BP between arms (sign of aortic dissection), peripheral oedema
Kidney	Reduced urine output	Renal bruit

Abbreviation: BP, blood pressure

oedema, retinal haemorrhages, retinal exudates (cotton-wool spots), engorged retinal veins

- History of HTN — duration, level of control or recent worsening, anti-hypertensive drug therapy — adherence, change in doses or type of drugs
- Conditions associated with HTN, e.g., endocrinopathies, chronic kidney disease (CKD), etc.

Use of drugs that can elevate BP

  - Non-steroidal anti-inflammatory drugs (NSAIDs)
  - Oral contraceptives
  - Sympathomimetics
  - Glucocorticoids
  - Mineralocorticoids
  - Calcineurin inhibitors
  - Erythropoietin
  - Vascular endothelial growth factor inhibitors
  - Illicit drugs (e.g., cocaine)
  - Herbal supplements
  - Drug or food interactions with monoamine oxidase inhibitors
- Lifestyle — excessive dietary salt intake, alcohol consumption, obesity
- The date of last menstrual period for pregnancy status

- Laboratory examination
  - Renal panel
  - Full blood count (FBC)
  - Peripheral blood film
  - Lactate dehydrogenase (LDH)
  - Haptoglobin

- Urine full and microscopic examination (UFEME)
- Chest X-ray (CXR)
- Electrocardiogram (ECG)
- Other investigations depending on presentation and clinical findings, such as:
    - Cardiac enzymes
    - Brain natriuretic peptide
    - Toxicology screen
    - CT or magnetic resonance imaging MRI of the brain
    - CT chest or aortogram
    - Echocardiogram
    - Tests for specific causes of secondary hypertension

Management of hypertensive emergencies

- Treatment should not be delayed while performing diagnostic tests.
- The choice of drug, desired BP target, and the time course to achieve the target BP depends on target organ involvement, comorbidities, drug pharmacology, and contraindications (Table 17.3).
- The US Joint National Committee on Prevention, Detection, Evaluation and Treatment of High Blood Pressure recommends that the initial goal of therapy in hypertensive emergencies is to reduce the mean arterial BP (MAP) by no more than 25% (within minutes to 1 hour), then, if stable, to 160/100–110 mmHg within the next 2–6 hours. If the initial level of reduced BP is well tolerated, further gradual reductions toward a normal BP (<130/80 or 140/90 mmHg) can be targeted over the next 24 to 48 hours.

Table 17.3: Hypertensive Emergencies and Preferred Choice of Antihypertensive Drugs at the Singapore General Hospital

Condition	Preferred Treatment	Comment
Cerebral infarction	IV labetalol or IV nitroprusside	If patient is for thrombolytic therapy, aim for BP < 185/110 mmHg otherwise withhold antihypertensive treatment unless SBP > 220 mmHg or DBP > 120 mmHg
Intracerebral haemorrhage	IV labetalol or IV esmolol	If there is raised intracranial pressure (ICP), aim for SBP < 180 mmHg (MAP < 130 mmHg) for the first 24 hours but if there is no raised ICP, aim for SBP < 160 mmHg (MAP < 110 mmHg)
Subarachnoid haemorrhage	IV labetalol or IV esmolol	Aim for SBP < 160 mmHg until the aneurysm is treated or cerebral vasospasm occurs
Hypertensive encephalopathy	IV labetalol or IV esmolol or IV nitroprusside	Aim for 20–25% reduction in MAP Avoid hydralazine
Aortic dissection	IV labetalol or IV esmolol with or without IV nitroprusside or IV glyceryl trinitrate	Aim for SBP < 120 mmHg within 20 minutes and maintain <110 mmHg if tolerated. Beta blockers should precede vasodilator administration to prevent reflex tachycardia and worsen shear stress on the intimal flap. However, avoid beta blocker if there is aortic regurgitation or cardiac tamponade.
Myocardial ischaemia or infarction	IV esmolol + IV glyceryl trinitrate IV labetalol + IV glyceryl trinitrate	Aim for BP < 160/100 mmHg — thrombolytics are contraindicated if BP > 185/100 mmHg
Left ventricular failure	IV glyceryl trinitrate or IV nitroprusside Both with IV diuretics	Beta blockers are contraindicated

Table 17.3:   (*Continued*)

Condition	Preferred Treatment	Comment
Acute kidney failure	IV labetalol or IV glyceryl trinitrate	IV nitroprusside is contraindicated
Pre-eclampsia or eclampsia	IV labetalol or IV hydralazine	IV nitroprusside is contraindicated

Abbreviations: IV, intravenous; BP, blood pressure; SBP, systolic blood pressure; DBP, diastolic blood pressure; MAP, mean arterial pressure

Table 17.4:   Intravenous Antihypertensive Drugs for Treatment of Hypertensive Emergencies Available at the Singapore General Hospital

Class	Drugs	Usual Dose Range	Comments
Alpha and nonselective beta receptor antagonist	Labetalol	Initial IV slow bolus 0.3–1.0 mg/kg/dose (maximum 20 mg) every 10 mins or Initial IV infusion 0.4–1.0 mg/kg/hr up to 3 mg/kg/hr. Adjust rate up to total cumulative dose of 300 mg. This dose can be repeated every 4–6 hrs.	Contraindicated in • Reactive airway disease • Second- or third-degree heart block • Bradycardia It may worsen heart failure but is useful for hyperadrenergic symptoms.
$Beta_1$ receptor selective antagonist	Esmolol	Loading bolus dose 500–1000 mcg/kg/min over 1 min followed by a 50 mcg/kg/min infusion. For additional dosing, the bolus dose is repeated and the infusion increased in 50 mcg/kg/min increments as needed to a maximum of 200 mcg/kg/min.	Contraindicated in • Concurrent beta blocker therapy • Bradycardia • Decompensated heart failure Monitor for bradycardia May worsen heart failure Higher doses may block $beta_2$ receptors and worsen reactive airway disease

(*Continued*)

Table 17.4:   (*Continued*)

Class	Drugs	Usual Dose Range	Comments
Nitric oxide dependent vasodilator	Glyceryl trinitrate	Initial 5 mcg/min; increase in increments of 5 mcg/min every 3–5 min to a maximum of 20 mcg/min	Use only in patients with acute coronary syndrome or acute pulmonary oedema. Do not use in volume depleted patients.
Nitric oxide dependent vasodilator	Sodium nitroprusside	Initial 0.3–0.5 mcg/kg/min; increase in increments of 0.5 mcg/kg/min to achieve BP target; maximum dose 10 mcg/kg/min; duration of treatment as short as possible. For infusion rates $\geq$4–10 mcg/kg/min or duration >30 mins, thiosulphate can be coadministered to prevent cyanide toxicity	Intra-arterial BP monitoring recommended to prevent "overshoot". Lower dosing adjustment required for the elderly. Tachyphylaxis common with extended use. Cyanide toxicity with prolonged use can result in irreversible neurological changes and cardiac arrest.
Direct vasodilator	Hydralazine	Initial 10 mg via slow IV infusion (maximum initial dose 20 mg); repeat every 4–6 hrs as needed.	BP begins to decrease within 10–30 mins and the fall lasts 2–4 hrs. Unpredictability of response and prolonged duration of action do not make hydralazine a desirable first-line agent for acute treatment in most patients.

Abbreviations: IV, intravenous; mg, milligrams; kg, kilograms; mcg, micrograms; hrs, hours; min, minutes; BP, blood pressure

- However, there are specific conditions which require more rapid lowering of SBP to <140 mmHg in the first hour of treatment, such as:
    - Aortic dissection
    - Severe preeclampsia or eclampsia

- ▪ Pheochromocytoma with hypertensive crisis
- Continuous infusion of short-acting anti-hypertensive drugs is preferred (Table 17.4). Once the BP is stabilised and the risk of end-organ damage has subsided, IV antihypertensive drugs can be titrated downwards, followed by conversion to oral antihypertensive drugs.

References

Rossi GP, Rossitto G, Maifredini C, *et al.* (2021). Management of hypertensive emergencies: A practical approach. *Blood Press* **30**(4): 208–219.

Unger T, Borghi C, Charchar F, *et al.* (2020). 2020 International Society of Hypertension global hypertension practice guidelines. *Hypertension* **75**(6): 1334–1357.

Whelton PK, Carey RM, Aronow WS, *et al.* (2018). 2017 ACC/AHA/AAPA/ABC/ACPM/AGS/APhA/ASH/ASPC/NMA/PCNA guideline for the prevention, detection, evaluation, and management of high blood pressure in adults: A report of the American College of Cardiology/American Heart Association Task Force on clinical practice guidelines. *Hypertension* **71**(6): e13–e115.

18 Renovascular Hypertension

Riece Koniman, Tan Chieh Suai

Introduction

- Renovascular hypertension (HTN) is defined as systemic HTN caused by compromised blood supply to the kidneys, usually due to renal artery stenosis (RAS).

- Renovascular HTN is the most common (75%) cause of secondary HTN (Table 18.1).

- The 2 most common causes of renovascular HTN are atherosclerosis and fibromuscular dysplasia (FMD) (Table 18.2).

Table 18.1: Causes of the Syndrome of Renovascular Hypertension

Unilateral Disease	Bilateral Disease
• Atherosclerotic RAS	• Stenosis to a solitary functioning kidney
• Fibromuscular dysplasia	• Bilateral RAS
• Renal artery aneurysm	• Aortic coarctation
• Arterial embolus	• Systemic vasculitis (e.g., Takayasu's polyarteritis)
• Arteriovenous fistula (congenital/ traumatic)	• Atheroembolic disease
• Segmental arterial occlusion (post-traumatic)	• Vascular occlusion due to endovascular aortic stent graft
• Extrinsic compression of renal artery (e.g., pheochromocytoma)	
• Renal compression (e.g., metastatic tumour)	

Abbreviation: RAS, renal artery stenosis

Table 18.2:   Atherosclerotic Renal Artery Stenosis vs. Fibromuscular Dysplasia

	Atherosclerotic RAS (ARAS)	Fibromuscular Dysplasia (FMD)
Cause of renovascular hypertension	90%	10%
Pathogenesis	Atherosclerosis	Medial fibroplasia
Prevalence	10–15% aged over 50 years, increasing to 50–60% in older patients with atherosclerosis elsewhere	1–3%
Age at onset	Older >50 years	Younger <40 years
Gender	Male > Female	Female > Male
Prevalence	High	Low
Location of renal artery stenosis	Ostial or proximal	Middle or distal Multiple segments of stenosis, giving rise to the string of beads appearance
Extrarenal involvement	Atherosclerosis can affect other arterial beds	FMD can affect other arterial beds
Progression to end-stage kidney disease	Common — With 5 years — 51% will progress, 8–16% will occlude, and 17% will become bilateral renal artery stenosis	Unusual — progression is not well-defined
Effective intervention	Angioplasty + stent	Angioplasty
Cure of hypertension	Unlikely	Normotension in most patients (e.g., 74% at 1 year)

Abbreviation: RAS, renal artery stenosis

- RAS can lead to ischaemic nephropathy, which is defined as a reduction in glomerular filtration rate (GFR) and a loss of renal parenchyma caused by haemodynamically significant RAS (stenosis that reduces the vessel diameter by 60%).

- According to the Goldblatt model of RAS:

  - Unilateral RAS causes reduction in the affected kidney perfusion pressure, activation of the renal angiotensin-aldosterone system (RAAS), suppression of renin release, and pressure natriuresis from the contralateral kidney.

  - Bilateral RAS or RAS of a single functioning kidney is similar but because there is no other normal functioning kidney, activation of the RAAS causes impaired sodium excretion and volume-dependent HTN.

The Goldblatt model assumes the kidneys are normal and have a normal RAAS response — this may apply for patients with FMD but not with ARAS where there are other causes of HTN. As a result, HTN may not improve with revascularisation in patients with atherosclerotic RAS (ARAS).

Clinical Clues that Suggest Renovascular Hypertension

- Young onset HTN without a family history
- New onset of severe HTN or acute worsening of blood pressure (BP) or HTN over a previously stable baseline
- Drug-resistant HTN — HTN despite treatment with >3 drugs of different classes at optimal doses
- Acute kidney injury (AKI) after starting an angiotensin-converting enzyme inhibitor (ACEI) or angiotensin receptor blocker (ARB)
- Severe HTN and/or kidney impairment in patients with diffuse atherosclerosis
- Recurrent episodes of acute pulmonary oedema

- Systolic-diastolic abdominal bruit on one side of the abdomen
- Renal asymmetry (>1.5 cm) on imaging

Screening and Diagnostic Tests

- Routine work-up is not specific — urine microscopy is unremarkable, proteinuria is absent or mild, serum creatinine may or may not be elevated. Biochemical tests like plasma renin concentrations lack specificity.

- Imaging (Table 18.3) for renovascular HTN should be performed for patients with clinical suspicion and who are likely to benefit from revascularisation.

Table 18.3:   Screening Tests for Renal Artery Stenosis

	US Doppler	**CTA**	**MRA**
Advantages	• Inexpensive • Non-invasive • No radiation • No contrast • Easier to perform serially to monitor for recurrent RAS	• Non-invasive • More sensitive and specific than the US doppler	• Non-invasive • No radiation
Disadvantages	• Time consuming • Technically difficult to perform • Results are operator-dependent • Obesity and bowel gas may impair quality of images	• More expensive • Involves radiation • Requires contrast, so there is risk of contrast-induced nephropathy • Distal RAS like those by FMD is more difficult to visualise	• Most expensive • Requires contrast, so there is risk of nephrogenic systemic fibrosis in patients with low GFR

Abbreviations: US, ultrasound; CTA, computed tomography angiogram; MRA, magnetic resonance angiogram; RAS, renal artery stenosis; FMD, fibromuscular dysplasia; GFR, glomerular filtrate rate

- An ultrasound (US) doppler is usually the first-line imaging modality because it is the cheapest and does not involve contrast agents — duplex criteria for RAS >60% include:

  - Renal artery peak systolic velocity (PSV) >200 cm/s

  - Ratio of PSV in renal artery to PSV in aorta (renal/aortic ratio) >3.5

  Resistive index (RI = [PSV – end diastolic velocity]/PSV) >80 may indicate irreversible kidney damage and hence a lower likelihood of benefit from revascularisation.

- For computed tomography angiogram (CTA) or magnetic resonance angiography (MRA), a stenosis >75% or a 50% stenosis with post-stenotic dilatation suggests a haemodynamically significant stenosis.

- Catheter angiography is the gold standard test to confirm the diagnosis of RAS, but it is invasive and involves contrast exposure.

Management

Medical therapy

- Medical therapy should be offered to all with renovascular HTN.

- Anti-hypertensive drugs:

  - Frequently multiple drug regimens

  - ACEI/ARB should be tried first but must be monitored carefully for acute kidney injury

  - If BP cannot be controlled with ACEI/ARB, other agents like thiazide diuretics, long-acting calcium channel blockers, mineralocorticoid receptor antagonists, or beta blockers may be added as necessary

- Statin to control hyperlipidaemia
- Antiplatelet agent (e.g., low dose aspirin)
- Weight loss
- Smoking cessation
- Medical treatment should be monitored closely for:
  - Impaired kidney function with ACEI/ARB
  - Progression of stenosis and vascular occlusion
  - Normalisation of systemic arterial pressure which may result in renal hypoperfusion and ischaemic renal atrophy

Percutaneous revascularisation

- Several studies (DRASTIC, STAR, ASTRAL, CORAL) on the revascularisation of ARAS reported no difference in renal function as well as cardiovascular and mortality outcomes when revascularisation was compared to medical therapy while reduction of BP was only modest. However, these studies were limited by methodological problems. Nevertheless, this suggests that routine revascularisation is not warranted for all patients.
- Only a select group of patients may benefit from revascularisation:
  - Short duration of HTN (duration <1 years)
  - Drug-resistant HTN
  - Intolerance to medical therapy
  - Progressive kidney impairment
  - Bilateral RAS with progressive loss of renal functional mass

- Single native kidney or transplanted kidney with RAS

- Flash pulmonary oedema

- If revascularisation proceeds, a haemodynamically significant stenosis needs to be confirmed prior to balloon angioplasty ± stent which is defined as:

  - 70% lumen occlusion

  - Mean gradient >10 mmHg across the lesion

  - Fractional flow reserve <0.8 before revascularisation

- FMD is treated with angioplasty alone while ARAS is treated with angioplasty and stent placement because primary patency is better maintained with lesser frequency of restenosis.

- There is a 3–5% complication rate (e.g., atheroemboli, dissection, renal artery rupture, thrombosis) and 13–39% restenosis rate.

Surgical Revascularisation

- Surgical revascularisation is reserved for a select group of patients with one or more of the following conditions:

  - Multiple small renal arteries

  - Early primary branching of the main renal artery

  - Require aortic reconstruction near renal arteries for other indications

  - Have had failed renal artery stenting procedures

  - Repeated in-stent restenosis

  - Complex FMD that extends into segmental arteries and with macroaneurysms

- Surgical revascularisation does not confer better outcomes than medical therapy or angioplasty with stenting. Surgical options include:
  - Aortorenal bypass
  - Extra-anatomical bypass
  - Unilateral nephrectomy
  - Extracorporeal microvascular reconstruction
  - Endarterectomy or atherectomy

References

Bhalla V, Textor SC, Beckman JA, *et al.* (2022). Revascularization for renovascular disease: A scientific statement from the American Heart Association. *Hypertension* **79**(8): e128–e143.

Safian RD (2021). Renal artery stenosis. *Prog Cardiovasc Dis* **65**: 60–70.

19 Autosomal Dominant Polycystic Kidney Disease

Alvin Tng, Kwek Jia Liang

Introduction

- Autosomal dominant polycystic kidney disease (ADPKD) is the most common hereditary kidney disease in Singapore.

    - Majority of cases are associated with autosomal dominant inheritance of a defect in PKD1, encoding polycystin-1 (85%) or PKD2 gene, encoding polycystin-2 (15%) — 50% of children of an affected individual will inherit the defect.

- PKD1 is more common than PKD2 — PKD1 patients become symptomatic earlier (between the ages of 30 and 50) and progress faster than PKD2.

- 10–20% have disease because of a de novo gene defect.

- Mutations impair ciliary function and lead to disruption of intracellular signalling pathways (including cyclic adenosine monophosphate (cAMP)-activated ones). This promotes fluid secretion from the renal tubular epithelial cells and proliferation of cyst epithelial cells. As a result, cysts grow and compress blood vessels, causing renal ischaemia and fibrosis. There is also activation of the renin-angiotensin-aldosterone (RAAS) system, leading to increased systemic vascular resistance and sodium retention.

- Patients may maintain normal function for decades due to compensatory hyperfiltration — kidney function deteriorates, typically after the fourth decade of life and 50% will have end-stage kidney disease (ESKD) by the age of 60.

Clinical Manifestations

Renal

- Hypertension (HTN)
- Haematuria
- Proteinuria
- Impairment of kidney function
- Flank pain due to kidney enlargement/cysts, haemorrhage, infection, calculi, tumour
- Kidney stone, typically uric acid, or calcium oxalate
- Infection — cyst, urinary tract infection (UTI)
- Kidney cell carcinoma
- Palpable kidneys
- Effects of compression by enlarging kidney or cysts — inferior vena cava (hypotension, thromboembolism, hepatic venous outflow obstruction), gastric outlet obstruction (by right kidney cysts)

Extra-renal

- Polycystic liver disease
- Cysts in other organs — pancreas, spleen, epididymis, thyroid, subarachnoid, seminal vesicle
- Intracranial aneurysms (in up to 40%) — cause intracranial haemorrhage and death in 8–11%

- Valvular heart disease — commonly mitral valve prolapse, aortic regurgitation
- Other aneurysms — thoracic, iliac, aorta, coronary artery
- Other vascular diseases — intracranial arterial dissection and dolichoectasia, megadolichobasilar artery
- Colonic diverticula
- Abdominal hernia

Screening for Intra-cranial Aneurysms

- Screening can be performed with either CT angiography (CTA) or MR angiography (MRA) and is indicated for high-risk patients:
    - Headache and other neurological symptoms
    - Previous intracranial haemorrhage
    - Positive family history of intracranial haemorrhage, intracranial aneurysm, or unexplained stroke
    - High risk occupation, in which loss of consciousness would pose a risk to the patient and others
    - Prior to surgery that is likely to be associated with haemodynamic instability and hypertension
- For patients with initially negative radiographic studies, repeat screening every 5 years for those with a family history of cerebrovascular accidents or intracranial haemorrhage.
- For patients with intracranial aneurysms that do not need surgery, perform surveillance yearly with CTA or MRA for 2 years and then once every 2 years if the aneurysm is clinically and radiographically stable.

Diagnosis

- Diagnosis is usually made by family history and age-specific kidney imaging criteria (see below) while gene testing is reserved only for special situations (e.g., a young person wanting to be a kidney donor to a family member with ADPKD).

- ADPKD should be suspected in the following:
    - Enlargement of the kidneys or liver on physical examination
    - Hypertension in young individuals (<35 years)
    - Family history
    - Multiple bilateral kidney cysts where other causes are excluded
    - Cysts in other organs (e.g., liver)
    - Intracranial aneurysm

- Ultrasound (US) is commonly used to make the diagnosis of ADPKD using an age-specific US criteria (Table 19.1) when there is an affected first-degree relative (see below). The positive predictive value is 100% if the gene defect is PKD1- or PKD2-related but the sensitivity of US decreases with non-PKD1 gene defects.

Table 19.1: Age-Specific US Diagnostic Criteria for Autosomal Dominant Polycystic Kidney Disease

Age (years)	US Criteria for those with an Affected First-degree Relative	Sensitivity According to Genotype		
		PKD1	PKD2	Unknown
15–30	≥3 cysts unilaterally or bilaterally	94.3	69.5	81.7
30–39	≥3 cysts unilaterally or bilaterally	96.6	94.9	95.5
40–59	≥2 cysts unilaterally or bilaterally	92.6	88.8	90

Abbreviations: US, ultrasound; PKD; polycystin gene
Note: In patients ≥60 years, ≥4 cysts in each kidney confirms the diagnosis of ADPKD.

Table 19.2:   Indications for Gene Testing

1. Equivocal or atypical renal imaging techniques
2. Sporadic PKD with no family history
3. Early and severe PKD
4. PKD with syndromic features
5. Reproductive counselling
6. Potential living kidney donor

Abbreviation: PKD, polycystic kidney disease

- For patients without a family history of ADPKD, diagnosis by ultrasound is made if there are 10 or more cysts (≥ 5 mm) in each kidney, especially if the kidneys are enlarged or liver cysts are present.

- CT or MRI is more sensitive than US and useful:

  - if US is equivocal

  - if there is a suspicious cyst or mass

  - to calculate height-adjusted total kidney volume (htTKV) to evaluate risk of progression and need for disease-modifying treatment

  - to exclude cysts in the potential kidney donor of a related and affected kidney transplant recipient

- For patients 40 years and younger with a positive family history of ADPKD, > 10 renal cysts in total on CT or MRI scan have a sensitivity and specificity of 100% for making a diagnosis of ADPKD while < 5 renal cysts in total can exclude ADPKD.

- Gene testing can be considered for special indications (Table 19.2) for PKD1 and PKD2, but is not commonly performed due to high costs and mutations are only detected in 41–63% of cases.

Screening of Asymptomatic Individuals Suspected to be at Risk of ADPKD

- Pre-symptomatic screening is not currently recommended for at-risk children.

- However, the potential benefits of pre-symptomatic screening (usually with a US) for at-risk adults usually outweigh the risks though adults should ensure they have adequate insurance coverage prior to screening.

Monitoring of ADPKD

- Height-adjusted total kidney volume (HtTKV) should be measured using CT or MRI for initial evaluation.

- The Consortium for Radiologic Imaging Studies in Polycystic Kidney Disease (CRISP) group suggested that TKV is an early and accurate measure of individual cystic burden and likely growth rate trajectory when the estimated glomerular filtration rate (eGFR) > 60 mL/min/1.73 m^2.

- The Mayo imaging classification system (Table 19.3) is a prediction model to identify rapid progressors among ADPKD patients. An online calculator is available to determine the Mayo imaging classification system by inputting kidney dimensions, height and age. Serum creatinine, gender and race are additional variables to age and the Mayo classification to predict future eGFR.

- Repeated measurement of HtTKV in asymptomatic patients without intervention to slow disease progression is not recommended.

- However, HtTKV could be remeasured once every 3–5 years and compared with baseline HtTKV in patients on tolvaptan to ensure efficacy.

Table 19.3:   The Mayo Imaging Classification System

Mayo Class	Estimated TKV Annual Percentage Increase	Estimated Slope of Change in eGFR (mL/min/1.73 m^2)		Risk for eGFR Decline
		Male	Female	
1A	<1.5%	–0.23	0.03	Low risk
1B	1.5–3.0%	–1.33	–1.13	Intermediate risk
1C	3.0–4.5%	–2.63	–2.43	High risk
1D	4.5–6.0%	–3.48	–3.29	High risk
1E	>6.0%	–4.78	–4.58	High risk

Abbreviations: TKV, total kidney volume; GFR, glomerular filtration rate

- However, the eGFR and proteinuria/albuminuria should be measured to monitor ADPKD progression.

Management

- Diet, metabolic, and lifestyle modification (so refer to a dietician):
  - Adequate hydration to aim for first morning urine osmolality of ≤280 mOsm/kg except in patients who have a eGFR of <30, are hyponatraemic, or are on diuretics
  - Reduce sodium (≤3 g/day), protein (≤1 g/kg/day), and phosphate intake (≤800 mg/day)
  - Aim for normal body mass index (BMI)
  - Treat hyperlipidaemia with statin or ezetimibe
  - Maintain serum sodium bicarbonate ≥ 22 mmol/L — can prescribe sodium bicarbonate
  - Aim for normal serum uric acid level
  - Avoid caffeine and smoking
  - Regular exercise

- Treat HTN:
  - HTN is due to intrarenal activation of the renin angiotensin-aldosterone system secondary to the growth of cysts and endothelial dysfunction.
  - Control of HTN prevents left ventricular hypertrophy, reduces albuminuria, and slows down growth of kidney cysts.
  - First-line anti-hypertensive drugs include angiotensin-converting enzyme inhibitors (ACEI) and angiotensin receptor blockers (ARB).
  - Aim for blood pressure (BP) < 130/80 mmHg — aim lower ≤ 110/75 mmHg for those aged 18–50 with an eGFR of >60 mL/min/1.73 m² and Mayo Clinic class 1C-1E or with intracranial aneurysms.
- Treat complications (Table 19.4).
- Nephrectomy is indicated only for:
  - Recurrent infection
  - Massive kidney volume leading to impaired quality of life, anorexia, nutritional deficiency, severe intractable pain
  - Recurrent nephrolithiasis

Disease-Modifying Drugs to Reduce Disease Progression

- Arginine vasopressin stimulates adenyl cyclase to produce cAMP, which stimulates cyst formation and growth. Tolvaptan (Jinarc) is a PO vasopressin V2-receptor antagonist which decreases cAMP levels and thence slows the rate of cyst growth. It is metabolised by the CYP3A4 system.

Table 19.4: Treatment of Complications

Complications	Management
Flank pain	Pharmacological (avoid NSAIDs) first, but if pain is intractable — cyst decompression, aspiration and sclerosis, renal artery embolisation, laparoscopic or surgical cyst fenestration, kidney denervation, nephrectomy
Cyst haemorrhage or gross haematuria	Bed rest, analgesics, hydration, blood transfusion, segmental arterial embolisation, nephrectomy
Cyst infections	Cyst penetrating antibiotics (preferentially cyst-penetrating lipid soluble antibiotics) based on individual characteristics and bacterial resistance risk profiles.
Stones	Hydration, analgesia, potassium citrate, extracorporeal shockwave lithotripsy, percutaneous nephrostolithotomy
Intracranial aneurysms	Surgical clipping as surgically indicated

Abbreviation: NSAIDS, non-steroidal anti-inflammatory drugs

- The other effects of V2-receptor antagonism are:
  - Increased free water excretion, resulting in net body fluid loss
  - Increased serum Na^+
  - Decreased urine osmolality
- Two of the largest phase III multi-centre randomised controlled trials (TEMPO 3:4 and REPRISE) showed that tolvaptan reduced decline in kidney function (Table 19.5).
- Other benefits from these trials and other studies have shown that tolvaptan can prolong the time to ESKD by 6.5 years, increase life expectancy by 2.5 years, and reduce BP (slightly), pain, haematuria, stone, and UTI.

Table 19.5:   Efficacy of Tolvaptan on a Decline in the eGFR of Patients with ADPKD

Parameter	TEMPO 3:4	REPRISE
Therapy investigated	Tolvaptan vs. placebo	Tolvaptan vs. placebo
Number of patients	1445	1370
Age (years)	18–50	18–65
Baseline eGFR (mL/min/1.73 m^2)	>60	25–65
Efficacy on decline in renal function (therapy vs. placebo)	–2.72 vs. –3.70 mL/min/1.73 m^2	–2.34 vs. –3.61 mL/min/1.73 m^2
Discontinuation (therapy vs. placebo)	23 vs. 14%	9.5 vs. 2.2%
Adverse effects	Aquaresis (100%) Hepatic injury (4.9%)	Aquaresis (100%) Hepatic injury (5.6%)

Abbreviations: TEMPO, Tolvaptan Efficacy and Safety in Management of Autosomal Dominant Polycystic Kidney Disease and its Outcome; REPRISE, Replicating Evidence of Preserved Renal Function: an Investigation of Tolvaptan Safety and Efficacy in ADPKD.

- Tolvaptan is approved to slow kidney function decline in adults at risk of rapidly progressive ADPKD.

- At the time of writing, prescribing tolvaptan is restricted to physicians who have completed a risk management training programme required by the Singapore's Health Sciences Authority and Otsuka Pharmaceuticals. However, some general prescribing considerations are presented in Table 19.6.

- The operational and regulatory processes of prescribing, monitoring, and maintenance therapy are complicated and beyond the scope of this book.

Table 19.6:   Prescribing Considerations for Tolvaptan for Autosomal Dominant Polycystic Kidney Disease

Area	Prescribing Considerations
Indication	To slow the progression of cyst development and renal insufficiency in adults with ADPKD and CKD stage 1–3 with rapidly progressing disease. It should be combined with basic renal protective measures (see under "Management").
Contraindications	Pregnancy, lactation, uncorrected hypernatraemia, history of significant liver injury not due to polycystic liver disease, hypovolaemia, inability to sense or respond to thirst, urinary tract obstruction
Decision analysis in prescribing	Confirm diagnosis of ADPKD and determine the Mayo class (see Table 19.4) — recommend tolvaptan if the Mayo class is IC, 1D, or 1E + eGFR $\geq$ 25 mL/min + age 18–55 years). Patients must be informed of risks and benefits of tolvaptan.
Dosing	Initial dose is 45 mg in the morning and 15 mg in the afternoon (8 hours after morning dose) and adjust in 15 mg increments every 1–2 weeks if tolerated or until the urine osmolality is $\leq$280 mOsm/kg (to 60/30 or 90/30 mg)
Adverse effects	Polyuria, pollakiuria (frequent, abnormal urination during the day), thirst, fatigue, uric acid elevations (rarely gout), idiosyncratic liver injury, possible drug interaction (CYP3A inhibitor)
Mandatory monitoring	Liver panel before starting and after 2 and 4 weeks, then monthly for 18 months and once every 3 months thereafter
Drug interactions	Avoid or lower dose with concurrent use of CYP3A inhibitors

Abbreviations: ADPKD, autosomal dominant polycystic kidney disease; CKD, chronic kidney disease; eGFR; estimated glomerular filtration rate

Poor Prognostic Factors

- Male gender

- Diagnosis before age 30 years

- First episode of haematuria before age 30 years

- Onset of hypertension before age 35 years

- Hyperlipidaemia

- High BMI

- GFR decline rate $\geq$ 2.5 mL/min/year

- High urine sodium excretion

- Lower kidney blood flow

- Lower serum high-density lipoprotein cholesterol

- Large total kidney volume

- HtTKV growth rate of $\geq$5% per year

- Mayo imaging class 1C, 1D, or 1E

- Presence of truncating PKD1 variant

End-stage Kidney Disease in ADPKD

- Kidney transplantation (KT) is preferred over haemodialysis (HD) or peritoneal dialysis (PD). Survival outcomes are similar to or better than non-ADPKD KT recipients.

- Nephrectomy may be needed before KT to free up space for implantation of the new kidney — thence pre-emptive KT may not be possible. However, simultaneous nephrectomy and KT have been performed in some centres.

- Polycystic kidneys *in-situ* after KT may shrink due to fibrosis or calcineurin inhibitors or mTOR-based regimens.

- A higher frequency of intracranial haemorrhage, post-transplant diabetes mellitus (PTDM), erythrocytosis, and diverticular complications have been observed in KT recipients with ADPKD.

- PD is not a contraindication in ADPKD patients but may not be suitable for those with massive kidneys, abdominal hernias, or previous episodes of diverticular disease.

Family Planning

- ADPKD patients planning a family should receive genetic counselling and preimplantation genetic testing before pregnancy.

References

Alam A and Perrone RD (2010). Management of ESRD in patients with autosomal dominant polycystic kidney disease. *Adv Chronic Kidney Dis* **17**(2): 164–172.

Chapman AB, Devuyst O, Eckardt KU, *et al.* (2015). Autosomal-dominant polycystic kidney disease (ADPKD): executive summary from a Kidney Disease: Improving Global Outcomes (KDIGO) Controversies Conference. *Kidney Int* **88**(1): 17–27.

Chebib FT, Perrone RD, Chapman AB, *et al.* (2018). A practical guide for treatment of rapidly progressive ADPKD with tolvaptan. *J Am Soc Nephrol* **29**(10): 2458–2470.

Grantham JJ, Torres VE, Chapman AB, *et al.* (2006). Volume progression in polycystic kidney disease. *N Engl J Med* **354**(20): 2122–2130.

Halvorson CR, Bremmer MS and Jacobs SC (2010). Polycystic kidney disease: inheritance, pathophysiology, prognosis, and treatment. *Int J Nephrol Renovasc Dis* **3**: 69–83.

Raina R, Houry A, Rath P, *et al.* (2022). Clinical utility and tolerability of tolvaptan in the treatment of autosomal dominant polycystic kidney disease (ADPKD). *Drug Healthc Patient Saf* **14**: 147–159.

Torres VE, Chapman AB, Devuyst O, *et al.* (2012). Tolvaptan in patients with autosomal dominant polycystic kidney disease. *N Engl J Med* **367**(25): 2407–2418.

Torres VE, Chapman AB, Devuyst O, *et al.* (2017). Tolvaptan in later-stage autosomal dominant polycystic kidney disease. *N Engl J Med* **377**(20): 1930–1942.

Torres VE, Grantham JJ, Chapman AB, *et al.* (2011). Potentially modifiable factors affecting the progression of autosomal dominant polycystic kidney disease. *Clin J Am Soc Nephrol* **6**(3): 640–647.

Chapter

20 Tubulointerstitial Nephritis

Terence Kee

Introduction

- Tubulointerstitial nephritis (TIN) is an inflammatory nephropathy characterised by an inflammatory infiltrate in the tubules/interstitium, which can cause either an acute (acute tubulointerstitial nephritis or ATIN) or slower (chronic tubulointerstitial nephritis or CTIN) decline in kidney function.

- The trigger for inflammation can be immunological processes (e.g., drug-induced ATIN), infections (e.g., BK virus-associated nephropathy), abnormal accumulation of metabolic end-products (e.g., urate nephropathy), toxicity (e.g., lead nephropathy), or genetic factors (e.g., autosomal dominant tubulointerstitial kidney disease).

- Incidence of TIN is generally 1–5% and the causes vary according to the patient's age, geography, drug exposures, family history, and specific disease states (Table 20.1).

- In general, drug-induced TIN is most common, followed by autoimmune and infective interstitial nephritis.

- As TIN is defined by histopathological features, a definitive diagnosis of TIN is by kidney biopsy.

Table 20.1:   Causes of Interstitial Nephritis

Acute Interstitial Nephritis	
Medications (71–90%)	• Antibiotics • NSAIDS • Proton pump inhibitors • Checkpoint inhibitors • Others
Autoimmune factors (5–20%)	• Sarcoidosis • Sjogren • Tubulointerstitial nephritis and uveitis (TINU) syndrome • IgG4-related disease • ANCA vasculitis • Systemic lupus erythematosus
Infections (4–17%)	• Viruses: cytomegalovirus, Epstein–Barr virus, hantavirus, human immunodeficiency virus, polyomavirus • Bacteria: brucella, campylobacter, escherichia coli, legionella, salmonella, streptococcus, staphylococcus, yersina, leptospira, syphilis, diphtheria • Others: tuberculosis, toxoplasmosis, mycoplasma
Chronic Tubulointerstitial Nephritis	
Genetic	• Autosomal dominant tubulointerstitial kidney disease • Family nephronophthisis • Cystinosis • Karyomegalic interstitial nephritis
Metabolic	• Hypokalaemia (hypokalaemic chronic interstitial nephritis or kaliopenic nephropathy) • Hyperoxaluria (oxalate nephropathy) • Hyperuricaemia/hyperuricosuria (uric acid nephropathy)
Endemic nephritis	• Itai-Itai disease (Japan) • Balkan endemic nephropathy (Sebria, Bulgaria, Croatia, Romania, Bosnia) • Meso-american nephropathy (Nicaragua, El Savador, Costa Rica) • Sri Lanka CKDu (Sri Lanka) • Uddanam nephropathy (India CKDu) (India)
Others	• Radiation nephropathy

Abbreviations: NSAIDS, non-steroidal anti-inflammatory drugs; ANCA, anti-neutrophilic cytoplasmic antibodies; CKDu, chronic kidney disease of unknown origin

Diagnosis of Tubulointerstitial Nephritis

- Most affected patients will present with an asymptomatic elevation of the serum creatinine, and TIN should always be part of
  the differential diagnosis when evaluating acute kidney injury
  (AKI) or chronic kidney disease (CKD).

- If symptomatic, patients with TIN may present with symptoms
  and signs of AKI or advanced CKD — a classic triad of fever,
  skin rash, and eosinophilia has been associated with ATIN, but
  this occurs only in 10% of cases.

- In addition, if TIN is associated with systemic conditions (e.g.,
  autoimmune diseases), then patients may have symptoms and
  signs of the systemic conditions.

- There are no laboratory tests that can help confirm the diagnosis of TIN, but they may raise the suspicion of TIN as a cause of
  AKI or CKD (Table 20.2).

- TIN is confirmed with a kidney biopsy where there is tubular
  cell injury/necrosis and inflammation which:
    - is frequently consisting of lymphocytes, macrophages,
      plasma cells, and less frequently eosinophils, mast cells,
      and neutrophils
    - is only observed in the interstitium (interstitial nephritis)
      or extends into the tubular compartment (TIN)
    - is most commonly occurring in the cortex but also can occur
      at the corticomedullary junction (drug-induced TIN) or
      medulla (polyomavirus nephropathy, bacterial pyelonephritis)
    - with interstitial oedema suggests active TIN while
      interstitial fibrosis and tubular atrophy suggest active on
      chronic TIN
        - may be associated with other non-specific histopathological
          features such as non-necrotising interstitial granulomas,

Table 20.2:   Laboratory and Radiological Investigations for Tubulointerstitial Nephritis

Tests	Finding
Serum creatinine	Elevated
Electrolyte abnormalities	May be present due to tubular damage (e.g., a high FENa of >1%)
FBC	Eosinophilia may be present in 20–25% of cases, especially antibiotic-associated ATIN
CRP	Elevated but not specific
ESR	Elevated but not specific
Urinalysis	Urinalysis abnormalities such as pyuria, haematuria, proteinuria, and casts may be present but up to 20% of patients may have normal urinalysis. Eosinophiluria ($\geq$1% of urinary WBC) may be detected but is not sensitive or specific enough to diagnose TIN.
Proteinuria	Variable severity of proteinuria may be observed — nephrotic range proteinuria may be seen if there is concurrent glomerulonephritis or drug-induced minimal change or membranous nephropathy.
Ultrasound/CT	No diagnostic features on imaging but may reveal bilateral kidney enlargement and diffuse cortical hyper-echogenicity due to oedema and tubulointerstitial inflammation.
Other diagnostic tests	[67]Gallium scintigraphy and PET-CT would demonstrate uptake of [67]gallium or FDG in the kidneys. MRI would show heterogeneous striated enhancement of the cortex and restricted water diffusion on DW-MRI. None of these tests are diagnostic but may help provide supplementary information, especially for patients who are unable to undergo kidney biopsy to confirm the diagnosis.

Abbreviations: ATIN, acute tubulointerstitial nephritis; CRP, C-reactive protein; CT, computed tomography; DW, diffusion weighted: ESR, erythrocyte sedimentation rate; FBC, full blood count; FDG, fluorodeoxyglucose; FENa, fractional excretion of sodium; MRI, magnetic resonance imaging; PET, positron emission tomography

extra-tubular Tamm–Horsfall protein (THP), giant cells, and tubulovenous herniation (rupture of tubules into veins resulting in venous thrombi containing inflammatory cells and THP)

- As the most common cause of interstitial nephritis is exposure to an inciting drug, a thorough review of the medication history is important (Table 20.3), but the culprit drug may be difficult

Table 20.3: Causes of Drug-Induced Tubulointerstitial Nephritis

Drug Class		Drugs Known to Cause Acute Tubulointerstitial Nephritis
Antibiotics	Penicillins	Amoxicillin, ampicillin, aztreonam, benzylpenicillin, cloxacillin, methicillin, nafcillin, oxacillin, piperacillin/tazobactam
	Fluoroquinolones	Ciprofloxacin, levofloxacin, moxifloxacin, norfloxacin
	Cephalosporins	Cefazolin, cefotaxime, cefoxitin, cefuroxime, ceftriaxone, cephalexin
	Sulfonamides	Trimethoprim-sulfamethoxazole
	Macrolides	Azithromycin, clarithromycin, erythromycin, telithromycin
	Others	Cefepime, chloroamphenicol, clindamycin, colistin, doxycycline, ethambutol, gentamicin, griseofulvin, imipenem, isoniazide, linezolid, nitrofurantoin, polymyxin B, quinine, rifampicin, teicoplanin, vancomycin
Anti-retrovirals	Abacavir, acyclovir, atazanavir, foscarnet, indinavir	
Non-steroidal anti-inflammatory drugs	COX2 inhibitors	Celecoxib, rofecoxib
	Others	Aceclofenac, diclofenac, fenoprofen, flurbiprofen, ibuprofen, indomethacin, ketoprofen, meloxicam, naproxen, phenylbutazone

(Continued)

Table 20.3: (*Continued*)

Drug Class		Drugs Known to Cause Acute Tubulointerstitial Nephritis
5-aminosalicylates		Basalazine, mesalazine, olsalazine, sulfasalazine
Gastric secretion inhibitors	Proton pump inhibitors	Esomeprazole, lansoprazole, omeprazole, pantoprazole, rabeprazole
	H2 antagonists	Cimetidine, famotidine, ranitidine
Anticancer drugs	Immune checkpoint inhibitors	Atezolizumab, ipilimumab, nivolumab, pembrolizumab
	Tyrosine kinase inhibitors	Sorafenib, sunitinib
	Others	Adriamycin, alendronate, azathioprine, bacillus Calmette-Guerin, bevacizumab, bortezomib, platinum-based (e.g., cisplatin), gemcitabine, interleukin-2, ifosfamide, lenalidomide, methotrexate, pemetrexed, vemurafenib
Diuretics	Thiazides	Hydrochlorothiazide, indapamide, metolazone
	Loop of Henle diuretics	Furosemide, torasemide
	Potassium sparing	Amiloride, triamterene
Antihypertensives	Angiotensin-converting enzyme inhibitors	Captopril, lisinopril
	Angiotensin receptor antagonists	Candesartan, losartan
	Calcium channel antagonists	Amlodipine, nifedipine
Anticonvulsants		Carbamazepine, diazepam, lamotrigine, levetiracetam, phenobarbital, phenytoin, valproate
Other drugs		Allopurinol atorvastatin, carbimazole, chlorpropamide, exenatide, febuxostat, flecainide, gemfibrozil, leflunomide, metamizole, propranolol, propylthiouracil, risedronate, sildenafil, lithium salt

Source: Atta MG and Perazella MA (2022). *Tubulointerstitial Nephritis. 1st ed.* (p. 51). Springer, Cham.

to determine due to polypharmacy and the observation that TIN can develop from a few days to months after the exposure of the offending drug (the exact time depends on the type of drug).

- If drugs are not implicated, further investigations are guided by the suspicion of other causes (Table 20.4).

- Persistent ATIN, if left untreated, can progress to CTIN but there are other causes of CTIN that generally present as CKD (Table 20.5).

- Diagnosis of CTIN is often based on history and physical examination — specific diagnostic tests may be applicable for

Table 20.4: Investigations for a Suspected Systemic Cause of Tubulointerstitial Nephritis

Investigation	Suspected Cause of Tubulointerstitial Nephritis
Chest X-ray	Sarcoidosis, tuberculosis
Serum calcium level	Sarcoidosis (hypercalcaemia)
24-hour urinary calcium	Sarcoidosis (hypercalciuria)
TB-SPOT test	Tuberculosis
C3, C4 level	Systemic lupus erythematosus, IgG4-related disease
Autoantibodies	Systemic lupus erythematosus (ANA, anti-dsDNA), Sjogren's syndrome (anti-Ro/SSA and anti-LA/SSb, Rh F, ANCA-associated vasculitides (anti-PR3 and MPO-ANCA)
IgG4	IgG4-related disease
Microbiological	Specific test guided by clinical suspicion — HBsAg, anti-HBs, anti-HCV, HIV Ag-Ab serologies, and HBV/HCV/HIV nucleic acid testing should be performed in anticipation of immunosuppressive therapy

Abbreviations: ANCA, anti-neutrophil cytoplasmic antibody; ANA, anti-nuclear antibody; C3, complement C3; C4, complement C4; dsDNA,double-stranded deoxyribonucleic acid; HBsAg, hepatitis B surface antigen; HCV, hepatitis C virus; HIV, human immunodeficiency virus; MPO, myeloperoxidase; PR3, proteinase-3; RhF, rheumatoid factor; TB, tuberculosis

Table 20.5:   Types of Chronic Tubulointerstitial Nephritis

Types of Chronic Tubulointerstitial Nephritis	Pathogenesis	Clinical Presentation
Autosomal dominant tubulointerstitial kidney disease (ADTKD)	• Due to mutations encoding uromodulin (ADTKD-UMOD), hepatocyte nuclear factor-1β (ADTKD-HNF1β), renin (ADTKD-REN), mucin-1 (ADTKD-MUC1), and SEC61 (ADTKD-SEC61A1) • These mutations affect multifunctional proteins (UMOD, MUC-1), transcription factors (HNF1β), angiotensinogen protease (REN), and protein transporter (SEC61) • ADTKD-UMOD, MUC1 and REN are considered protein storage disorders as they are characterised by intracellular accumulation of abnormal proteins (e.g., uromodulin, mucin-1, renin)	• Positive family history of CKD — autosomal dominant inheritance • Early-onset hyperuricaemia or gout • Hypokalaemia and hypomagnesaemia (ADTKD-HNF1β) or acidosis and hyperkalaemia (ADTKD-REN) • Urinary concentration defect ± polydipsia-polyuria, enuresis or nocturia in children • Lack of significant HTN in the early stages • Onset in childhood common for ADTKD-REN, HNF1β and SEC61A1 • Progressive CKD, ESKD occurs after age 30 • Bland urine sediment • No or mild proteinuria • Normal or small-sized kidneys ± cysts • HNF1β mutations can also be associated with congenital anomalies of the kidney, urinary tract, genitals, neuro-developmental problems, endocrinopathies, and digestive problems
Familial nephronophthisis (NPHP)	• Mutations in nephrocystin genes that are involved in ciliary function (ciliopathy) • Histologically characterised by corticomedullary cysts	• Autosomal recessive inheritance • Most common form is juvenile nephronophthisis which present with ESKD at a mean age of 13 years • Typically present with urinary concentration defect (polyuria, polydipsia), enuresis, short stature, severe anaemia, CKD, ESKD • 15–20% also have extra-renal manifestations (e.g., eye, liver, heart, CNS, bones)

Karyomegalic interstitial nephritis (KIN)	• Mutation of Fanconi anaemia-associated nuclease 1 (FAN1) gene which facilitates repair of DNA crosslinks • Biopsy will show enlarged, hyperchromatic, and dysplastic nuclei in renal tubular epithelial cells (tubular karyomegaly)	• Autosomal recessive inheritance • CKD • Recurrent upper respiratory tract infections • Abnormal liver function • Linked to hereditary colorectal cancer, microcephaly, and bone marrow failure
Cystinosis	• Mutations in the cystinosin (CTNS) gene, a lysosomal H^+/cystine symporter which leads to lysosomal cystine accumulation • Cystine crystals can be seen on phase contrast microscopy and EM of kidney tissue sample	• Autosomal recessive inheritance • The most common presentation is infantile cystinosis, presenting with growth retardation, rickets, Fanconi's syndrome, CKD progressing to ESKD around age 10 years • Extra-renal manifestations include corneal crystals, hepatomegaly, endocrinopathies, myopathy, and increased intracranial pressure
Hypokalaemic chronic interstitial nephritis	• Associated with conditions causing chronic hypokalaemia — eating disorders, hyperaldosteronism, Bartter and Gittelman syndromes, herbs • Hypokalaemia leads to increased $NH4^+$ in the medullary interstitium and trigger complement-mediated damage	• CKD • Hypokalaemia • High aldosterone and variable renin levels • Tubular proteinuria (albuminuria is infrequent) • Medullary renal cysts

(*Continued*)

Table 20.5:   (*Continued*)

Types of Chronic Tubulointerstitial Nephritis	Pathogenesis	Clinical Presentation
Oxalate nephropathy	• May be primary (genetic defect leading to increased production of oxalate) or secondary (fat malabsorption, e.g., after bariatric surgery, high dietary oxalate, medications (ascorbic acid, orlistat), juicing drinks, ethylene glycol) • Excessive urinary oxalate leads to binding with calcium, forming calcium oxalate crystals (causing inflammation), calcium oxalate stones, and nephrocalcinosis • Calcium oxalate crystals may be seen in the tubules and interstitium on biopsy	• CKD • Haematuria • Proteinuria • Urinary calcium oxalate crystals • High serum and urinary oxalate levels • Nephrolithiasis
Uric acid nephropathy	• May be primary (UMOD mutation) or secondary (high dietary intake of purines, diuretics, high cell turnover states, e.g., tumour lysis) • Uric acid induces inflammation through crystal dependent and independent mechanisms • Uric acid can be seen as needle-like crystals and micro-tophi in the tubules and medulla	• CKD • Gout • Hyperuricaemia • Bland urine sediment • Proteinuria • Uric acid nephrolithiasis • Medullary cysts

Heavy metal toxicity (e.g., arsenic, cadmium, chromium, lead, mercury, uranium)	• Due to prolonged exposure, largely in occupational settings (e.g., mining) • Heavy metals cause tubular damage from reactive oxygen species or interruption of normal metabolic processes	• Positive exposure history • CKD • Fanconi's syndrome • Extra-renal manifestations depending on type of heavy metal exposure • Elevated blood and/or urine levels of heavy metal
Plants, mushrooms, herbal medications	• Classic example is aristolochic acid (AA) nephropathy which includes Balkan endemic nephropathy (BEN) and Chinese herb nephropathy (CHN) • Involves DNA damage by AA	• Positive exposure history • CKD • Disproportionate anaemia • HTN is often absent • Tubular dysfunction • Pyuria • Proteinuria • Urothelial cancers
Radiation nephropathy	• Ionising radiation can induce oxygen radicals which damage DNA	• Occurs in patients receiving radiation for cancer treatment or exposed to radiation in other settings (e.g., occupational, nuclear plant accidents/war) • Develops 3–12 months after radiation exposure • Disproportionate anaemia and HTN
Endemic nephritis/chronic kidney disease of unknown origin/chronic interstitial nephritis in agricultural communities	• A type of CKD that mainly affects marginalised agricultural communities in specific areas of the world	• CKD affecting otherwise healthy young to middle-aged persons living in agricultural areas in Meso-America, Sri Lanka, and India

Abbreviations: Abbreviations: CKD, chronic kidney disease; CNS, central nervous system; DM, diabetes mellitus; DNA, deoxyribonucleic acid; ESKD, end-stage kidney disease; HTN, hypertension; TIN, tubulointerstitial nephritis

With modifications from Atta MG and Perazella MA (2022). *Tubulointerstitial Nephritis. 1st ed.* (p. 51). Springer, Cham.

Table 20.6:   Endemic Nephritis or Chronic Kidney Disease of Unknown Origin

Chronic Kidney Disease of Unknown Origin (CKDu)	Endemic Areas	Aetiology Confirmed	Risk Factors
Itai-Itai disease	Japan	Cadmium	Water — crops, mining pollution
Balkan endemic nephropathy (BEN)	Serbia Bulgaria Croatia Romania Bosnia	Aristocholic acid	Wheat
Meso-American nephropathy (MEN)	Nicaragua El Salvador Costa Rica	Unexplained	Sugarcane, heat stress, agrochemical exposure, heavy metals exposure, genetic predisposition, alcohol "LIJA" consumption
Sri Lanka CKDu	Sri Lanka	Unexplained	Agricultural work, heat stress, agrochemical exposure, heavy metals exposure, genetic predisposition, alcohol/betel/tobacco consumption
India CKDu (Uddanam nephropathy)	India	Unexplained	Agricultural workers, heat stress, agrochemical exposure, heavy metals, genetic predisposition

Source: Atta MG and Perazella MA (2022). *Tubulointerstitial Nephritis. 1st ed.* (p. 14). Springer, Cham.

certain CTIN, such as genetic testing for genetic CTIN, slit-lamp corneal examination, and cystine levels (cytinosis). Some CTIN are restricted to geographical regions (Table 20.6).

Management of Acute Tubulointerstitial Nephritis

- For drug-induced ATIN, management should include:
  - Discontinuation of the offending drug.

- Providing dialysis as indicated — this may also be required to reduce the risk of bleeding in uraemic patients needing biopsy.

- Kidney biopsy to confirm the diagnosis and determine the extent of chronic damage (unless there are contraindications) — patients with >50% interstitial fibrosis and tubular atrophy (IFTA) may not benefit from corticosteroid therapy.

- Among patients with non-severe ATIN (not requiring dialysis), observation for recovery of kidney function for 7–10 days following discontinuation of the offending drug may be appropriate. Otherwise, if kidney function does not improve or is severe enough to require dialysis, PO or IV corticosteroids can be used to treat drug-induced ATIN as there are no differences in efficacy between these routes of administration (Table 20.7).

- Factors that are associated with a poor response to corticosteroids include:
  - severe chronic damage on biopsy (e.g., >50% IFTA)
  - severity of kidney dysfunction
  - timing of corticosteroid therapy (e.g., starting >1–2 weeks of stopping the causative drug)

- For patients who do not respond well to corticosteroids after 8 to 12 weeks, reassessment is required before continuing further immunosuppression, such as:
  - Reconsidering diagnosis especially if biopsy was not performed
  - Considering if there are other offending drugs that may require discontinuation
  - Excluding other causes of persistent kidney dysfunction

Table 20.7:   Corticosteroid Treatment Regimens for Acute Tubulointerstitial Nephritis from Randomised Controlled Trials

Study	n	Corticosteroid Regimen	Outcome
Ramachandran *et al.*	29	Group 1: PO Prednisolone 1 mg/kg for 3 weeks followed by rapid tapering over subsequent 3 weeks or Group 2: IV Methylprednisolone 30 mg/kg (maximum 1 g) for 3 days then PO Prednisolone 1 mg/kg for 2 weeks, tapered over 3 weeks	Complete remission was achieved in 50% of Group 1 and 61% of Group 2 (no statistically significant differences between groups) Partial remission was achieved in 50% of Group 1 and 39% of Group 2 (no statistically significant differences between groups)
Chowdry *et al.*	31	Group A: PO Prednisolone 1 mg/kg for 2 weeks Group B: IV Methylprednisolone 30 mg/kg (maximum 1 g) for 3 days then PO Prednisolone 1 mg/kg for 2 weeks, tapered over 2 weeks	Complete remission was achieved in 56.2% of Group A and 60% of Group B (no statistical difference between groups) Partial remission was achieved in 41.93% of Group A and 43.7% of Group B (no statistical difference between groups)

Note: Complete remission defined as improvement in eGFR to $\geq$60 mL/min/1.73 m^2; partial remission defined as improvement in eGFR but <60 mL/min/1.73 m^2.

- – Futility of treatment because of established IFTA
- For those who are steroid-resistant, one can consider a switch to MMF at a dose of 1–2 g/day and taper according to response.

- Appropriate anti-microbial and anti-ulcer prophylaxis should be provided in patients receiving corticosteroids.

- For TIN due to other causes, treatment is directed towards the specific cause of the interstitial nephritis.

Management of Chronic Tubulointerstitial Nephritis

- Management of CTIN is through addressing CKD and specific complications (Table 20.8).

Table 20.8: Specific Treatments for Chronic Tubulointerstitial Nephritis

Chronic Tubulointerstitial Nephritis	Specific Treatment
Autosomal dominant tubulointerstitial kidney disease, familial nephronophthisis, karyomegalic interstitial nephritis	• No specific therapies available
Cystinosis	• PO cysteamine therapy
Hypokalaemic chronic interstitial nephritis	• Potassium supplementation, potassium-sparing diuretics
Oxalate nephropathy	• Restrict dietary oxalate and fat intake • Increased fluid and calcium intake • Potassium citrate • Pyridoxine • Restoration of bowel continuity in secondary causes related to bariatric surgery • For primary oxaluria Type I — SC lumarsiran (reduce oxalate synthesis), combined liver-kidney transplantation for primary hyperoxaluria
Uric acid nephropathy	• Urine alkalinisation • Allopurinol or febuxostat

(Continued)

Table 20.8:   *(Continued)*

Chronic Tubulointerstitial Nephritis	Specific Treatment
Heavy metal toxicity	• Stop exposure to offending heavy metal • Chelation therapy
Aristolochic acid nephropathy	• Stop exposure to aristolochic acid • Corticosteroids — 1 mg/kg × 4 weeks then taper to maintenance dose of 0.15 mg/kg if rapid deterioration with GFR >20 mL/min/1.73 m²; stop treatment if no stabilisation of kidney function after 6 months • Screen for cancer of the urinary tract — cystoscopy, CT/MRI

Abbreviations: PO, per oral; GFR, glomerular filtration rate; CT, computed tomography; MRI, magnetic resonance imaging

Prognosis

- Complete and partial kidney recovery is experienced in approximately 50% and 40%, respectively. End-stage kidney disease (ESKD) is observed in approximately 10%.

- Risk factors for a poor prognosis include:

  - Baseline patient characteristics — older age, female, hypertension

  - Clinical presentation — haematuria, severe proteinuria, recurrent ATIN

  - Histological features — significant glomerulosclerosis and interstitial fibrosis/tubular atrophy (IFTA), granulomas

References

Atta MG and Perazella MA (2022). *Tubulointerstitial Nephritis 1st ed*. Springer, Cham.

Chowdry AM, Azad H, Mir I, *et al.* (2018). Drug-induced acute interstitial nephritis: Prospective randomized trial comparing oral steroids and high-dose intravenous pulse steroid therapy in guiding the treatment of this condition. *Saudi J Kidney Dis Transpl* **29**(3): 598–607.

Ramachandran R, Kumar K, Nada R, *et al.* (2015). Drug-induced acute interstitial nephritis: A clinicopathological study and comparative trial of steroid regimens. *Indian J Nephrol* **25**(5): 281–286.

Tan Chee Wooi, Terence Kee

Introduction

- Contrast-induced nephropathy has been historically used to describe the onset of acute kidney injury (AKI) following intravenous or intra-arterial administration of iodinated contrast media or contrast agents. However, it is increasingly recognised that AKI following contrast exposure may occur simultaneously in the presence of other factors that can cause AKI (e.g., dehydration) and hence contrast exposure may not be the only implicating factor.

- As a result, AKI following exposure to contrast agents may now be defined as a sudden decrease in kidney function within 48 hours following an intravenous or intra-arterial administration of iodinated contrast medium. It can be further defined as contrast-induced AKI (CI-AKI), which is where exposure of contrast is causally related to the AKI or contrast-associated AKI (CA-AKI), which is where exposure of contrast occurs together with other risk factors for AKI. As a result, CA-AKI is more common than CI-AKI.

Table 21.1:   KDIGO Definition of AKI Following Contrast Exposure

1. Absolute increase in sCr ≥26.4 μmol/L
2. Relative increase in sCr ≥50% (≥1.5 × baseline)
3. Urinary volume <0.5 mL/kg/hr for ≥6 hr

Abbreviations: sCr, serum creatinine; μmol/L, micromole per litre; mL, millilitres; kg, kilogram; hr, hour

Diagnosis

- CA-AKI or CI-AKI can be diagnosed if any one of the KDIGO-defined criteria occurs within 48 hours after intravascular administration of contrast media (Table 21.1).

- The elevation in serum creatinine levels peaks by 3 to 5 days and usually returns to baseline by 7 to 10 days.

- Urine microscopy may show granular casts and tubular epithelial cells, and the fractional excretion of sodium (FeNa) is usually low.

- It is important to exclude other causes of AKI following exposure to iodinated contrast media (e.g., atheroemboli released during angiography).

Nephrotoxicity of Iodinated Contrast Media

- The pathogenicity of iodinated contrast media may involve several mechanisms such as:

    - Direct cytotoxicity on tubular epithelial and endothelial cells

    - Enhances generation of reactive oxygen species, causing oxidative stress

    - Kidney hypoxia through renal vasoconstriction

- Iodinated contrast media vary in their potential for nephrotoxicity according to their:

  - Osmolality (number of particles in a solution for a given concentration of iodine in the contrast media) — high osmolality iodinated contrast media is associated with a higher frequency of CA-AKI.

  - Volume — small doses (<70 mL) are less frequently associated with CA-AKI than higher doses. Several equations have been developed to determine the threshold dose of contrast media that will be associated with CA-AKI.

  - Route — the intra-arterial route is associated with a higher risk of CA-AKI than the intravenous route, but this may be related to the fact that doses of contrast administered by the intra-arterial route is much higher (first-pass effect).

Risk Factors

- As there is no definitive treatment for CI-AKI, it is important to prevent it by identifying patients at risk for CI-AKI (Table 21.2). Risk factors can be patient- and procedure-related.

- The most important risk factor for CA-AKI and CI-AKI is kidney dysfunction, and the degree of kidney dysfunction affects the risk of CI-AKI associated with a certain volume of contrast media. Guidelines advise that the dose of contrast media should be limited to threshold ratios of contrast dose to kidney function, for example:

  - Contrast media dose (grams of iodine)/absolute eGFR (mL/min) <1.1

Table 21.2:   Risk Factors for Acute Kidney Injury Following Contrast Exposure

Patient-related Risk Factors	Procedure-related Risk Factors
• Older age	• Route of administration — intra-arterial
• Female	• Type of procedure — catheter-based
• Kidney dysfunction especially GFR <45 mL/min/1.73 m²	• Type of contrast — high osmolality
• DM	• Volume of contrast — higher volume
• Cardiovascular disease including HTN	• Repeated contrast media administration within 24–72 hrs
• Reduced intravascular volume	
■ Dehydration	
■ Blood loss	
■ Congestive heart failure	
■ Liver cirrhosis	
■ Nephrotic syndrome	
• Malignancy	
• Anaemia	
• Hyperuricaemia	
• Nephrotoxic medications	
■ Diuretics	
■ NSAIDs	
■ Aminoglycosides	
■ Amphotericin B	
■ Antiviral drugs (e.g., acyclovir)	
■ Cyclosporine	
■ Cisplatin	

Abbreviations: GFR, glomerular filtration rate; DM, diabetes mellitus; HTN, hypertension; NSAIDs, non-steroidal anti-inflammatory drugs; hrs, hours

- ■ Contrast media volume (mL)/eGFR mL/min/1.73 m² <3.0

- ■ Contrast volume/creatinine clearance <2.44

- In order to estimate the risk for CI-AKI, the Mehran score is the gold standard and most validated scoring system for

Table 21.3: Mehran Scoring System to Predict Risk for Contrast-Induced Acute Kidney Injury Following Percutaneous Coronary Intervention

Variable		Point
Hypotension	No	0
	Yes	5
Intra-aortic balloon pump	No	0
	Yes	5
Congestive heart failure	No	0
	Yes	5
Age >75 years	No	0
	Yes	4
Anaemia	No	0
	Yes	3
Diabetes	No	0
	Yes	3
Contrast media volume		1 point per 100 mL contrast
eGFR, mL/min/1.73 m^2	≥60	0
	40 to <60	2
	20 to <40	4
	<20	6

Mehran Risk Score	Risk of CI-AKI	Risk of CI-AKI Requiring Dialysis
≤5	7.5%	0.04%
6 to 10	14%	0.12%
11 to 15	26.1%	1.09%
≥16	57.3%	12.6%

Abbreviations: eGFR, estimated glomerular filtration rate; CI-AKI, contrast-induced acute kidney injury

predicting CI-AKI after percutaneous coronary intervention (intra-arterial contrast administration) (Table 21.3). Unfortunately, it has not been validated for patients receiving intravenous contrast administration.

Prevention of CA-AKI and CI-AKI

- There is no specific treatment for CA-AKI and CI-AKI and minimising the risks is the cornerstone of management (Table 21.4).

Table 21.4:   Minimising the Risks of Contrast-Induced Acute Kidney Injury

Risk Stratification	Identify Risk Factors
Indication	• Review the indication of contrasted imaging and explore alternate imaging modalities and interventions — risks and benefits of different options need to be weighed and discussed with the patient.
Communication	• Proper counselling and education prior to contrast exposure.
Hydration	• Hydration is the mainstay of preventing CI-AKI — it improves the patient's volume status, dilutes contrast media, and increases kidney blood flow as well as tubular urine flow, which will reduce retention of contrast media and toxicity in the tubular lumen. • Intravenous fluid hydration (0.9% sodium chloride preferred — isotonic bicarbonate does not provide additional benefits). • Oral hydration is not recommended. • IV hydration is tailored to the patient's volume status, urine output, and comorbidities (e.g. fixed 500 mL or 1–3 mL/kg/hr) • IV hydration should be started at least 1–4 hours before and continue to 3–12 hours post-contrast exposure. • IV hydration may be considered for patients on HD or PD who have signficant residual kidney function to preserve the latter. • Fluid overload should be avoided when hydrating the patient.
N-acetylcysteine (NAC)	• There is no strong evidence or consensus to support the routine use of IV or PO NAC to reduce the risk of CI-AKI.

Table 21.4: (*Continued*)

Risk Stratification	Identify Risk Factors
Adjust medications	• Stop nephrotoxic drugs (e.g., NSAIDs). • Diuretics may need to be withheld in order for sufficient hydration to occur. • Stop metformin temporarily as it increases risk of lactic acidosis if CI-AKI occurs — it can be restarted if kidney function is stable 48 hours after contrast exposure. • There is no recommendation in the guidelines about the stopping or reducing of ACEI/ARB but this may be reasonable considering that hyperkaaemia may be exacerbated if CI-AKI should occur. • Statins should be continued as they may be beneficial in reducing CI-AKI.
Contrast agents	• Use low-osmolar or iso-osmolar contrast media • Minimise volume of contrast media • Limit maximum contrast volume • Consider interval of contrast administration (multiple doses within 24–72 hours increase risk of CI-AKI)
Prophylactic HD	• Not recommended as it has not been shown to reduce the incidence of CI-AKI • In patients already on HD, extra HD or change in HD schedule in relation to contrast administration is also not recommended unless there is fluid overload
Monitoring	• Monitor renal function closely especially among high risk patients

Abbreviations: ACEI, angiotensin-converting enzyme inhibition; ARB, angiotensin receptor blockers; CI-AKI, contrast-induced acute kidney injury; HD, haemodialysis; IV, intravenous; NAC, N-acetylcysteine; NSAIDs, non-steroidal anti-inflammatory drugs; PD, peritoneal dialysis

References

Cho E and Ko GJ (2022). The pathophysiology and the management of radio-contrast-induced nephropathy. *Diagnostics* **12**(1): 180.

Mehdi A, Taliercio JJ and Nakhoul G. (2020). Contrast media in patients with kidney disease: An update. *Clevel Clin J Med* **87**(11): 683–694.

22 Urinary Tract Infections in the Non-Transplant Setting

Jasmine Chung

Introduction

- Urinary tract infections (UTIs) are common infections encountered by every specialty both in the hospital as well as in the community.

- The spectrum of disease is broad, ranging from asymptomatic bacteriuria (ASB) to cystitis to pyelonephritis, and in the most extreme of cases, the infection may potentially be life-threatening.

- Because UTIs are so common, it is very easy to treat "every UTI" with a course of antibiotics and stop there. However, there are opportunities for improved care if we put things in context. ASB does not usually warrant treatment. When UTIs are too frequent, complications develop, or if they occur in patients from special populations, our approach must be adjusted accordingly (Figure 22.1).

- For the non-kidney transplant patients, they may have:

  - Underlying structural/renal tract problems, such as reflux nephropathy, polycystic kidney disease, obstructive lesions (e.g., strictures, benign prostatic hypertrophy)

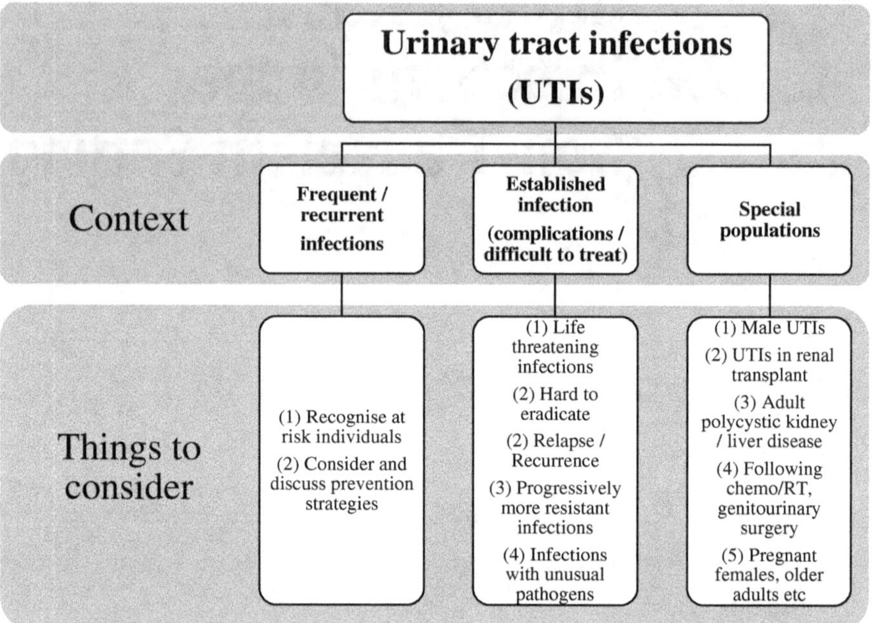

Figure 22.1:   Approach to Managing Patients with Urinary Tract Infections — Putting Things in Context

- Chronic kidney disease (CKD) — recurrent UTI in this case may result in progression of the CKD or a severe UTI may tip the patient over and dialysis may be required

- Renal stone disease

- Foreign body *in situ* (e.g., genitourinary stents *in situ*)

- Neurogenic bladder

- In working up the patient for UTIs, the following factors are important:

  - **Host characteristic** (e.g., gender, comorbidities, underlying genitourinary structural abnormalities, pregnancy)

  - **Risk factors/precipitating event** (e.g., lifestyle, sexual behaviour, recent surgery, genitourinary instrumentation)

- **Syndrome**

  It is important to assess the severity of the infection and determine if it is a lower UTI (e.g., cystitis) or upper UTI (e.g., pyelonephritis where the patient may be systematically unwell and the infection could be life-threatening).

- **Bug/offending pathogen**

  UTIs are usually caused by uropathogens such as gram-negative pathogens (faecal flora) or gram-positive organisms such as *Staphylococcus saprophyticus* and *Streptococcus agalactiae* (otherwise known as Gp B *Strep*). If an unusual pathogen is isolated from the urine cultures, further workup is warranted. For example, in the case of *Staphylococcus aureus* being isolated from the urine, a more sinister process needs to be excluded (e.g., a bacteraemia, which was an antecedent event, and infective endocarditis has to be excluded). For unusual pathogens isolated (e.g., *Mycobacterium* species, *Actinomyces* species), we have to consider the pathophysiology behind the UTI, assess for predisposing factors, and address the underlying cause.

Definitions

- There are 2 very important entities to consider in evaluating and managing patients with suspected UTI. The first is ASB and the latter is clinically symptomatic UTI. The former often does not warrant treatment except during pregnancy, prior to invasive urological procedures with mucosal trauma, or within the first month following kidney transplantation (older publications recommend up to 3 months).

- ASB is defined as the presence of 1 or more species of bacteria growing in the urine at specified quantitative counts ($\geq 10^5$ colony-forming units [CFU]/mL or $\geq 10^8$ CFU/L), irrespective of the presence of pyuria and in the absence of signs or symptoms attributable to UTI. ASB is a common finding in some healthy females and in many women or men with abnormalities of the genitourinary tract that impair voiding.

- For clinical purposes, patients with UTIs must have a compatible clinical syndrome (lower tract symptoms are characterised by dysuria, frequency, urgency, and/or suprapubic pain, while patients with upper tract symptoms may experience fever, flank pain, and costoverterbral tenderness and may also be systemically unwell), evidence of urinary tract inflammation (e.g., documented pyuria), ± uropathogen isolated from their urine cultures. In patients who have been pretreated with antibiotics prior to collection of urine specimen, urine cultures are likely to return positive.

- For the purposes of healthcare surveillance and clinical research, there are existing definitions of UTIs proposed but they are not universally accepted definitions, and may vary between the published guidelines. Nonetheless, it is still important to appreciate the various definitions used as this would have implications for healthcare communication and patient care.

- One useful framework is the UTI classification based on the European Association of Urology (EAU) urological infections guidelines (Table 22.1).

Table 22.1: Common Terminology Used in the Evaluation and Management of Urinary Tract Infections

	Definitions
Uncomplicated UTI	Acute, sporadic, or recurrent lower (uncomplicated cystitis) and/or upper (uncomplicated pyelonephritis) UTI, limited to non-pregnant women with no known relevant anatomical and functional abnormalities within the urinary tract or comorbidities.
Complicated UTI	UTIs in a patient with an increased chance of a complicated course; e.g., all men, pregnant women, patients with relevant anatomical or functional abnormalities of the urinary tract, indwelling urinary catheters, renal diseases, and/or with other concomitant immunocompromising diseases (e.g., diabetes).
Recurrent UTI	Recurrences of uncomplicated and/or complicated UTIs, with a frequency of at least 3 UTIs/year or 2 UTIs in the last 6 months.
CAUTI	CAUTIs refers to UTIs occurring in a person whose urinary tract is currently catheterised or has had a catheter in place within the past 48 hours.
Urosepsis	Urosepsis is defined as life-threatening organ dysfunction caused by a dysregulated host response to infection originating from the urinary tract and/or male genital organs.

Abbreviations: UTI, urinary tract infections; CAUTIs, catheter associated urinary tract infections

Diagnosis

- The diagnosis of UTI is based on history, clinical examination, and/or urine examination.

- The indication and type of urine examination depends on the clinical diagnosis. In general, we should only be performing a urine examination if an infection is suspected and we plan to treat it (Table 22.2).

Table 22.2: Indications for Urine Examination Based on Clinical Diagnosis

Diagnosis	Implications for Testing
ASB	Targeted testing — We should only screen for ASB in pregnant women, patients undergoing urological procedures with mucosal trauma, and kidney transplant recipients within the first month of transplant surgery.
Acute uncomplicated UTI (cystitis)	The diagnosis can be made on focused history alone. In the community setting, urine dipstick may be useful in patients presenting with atypical symptoms. Urine cultures are not routine. Patients often respond to antibiotics based on guideline recommendations.
Acute pyelonephritis	Urine cultures recommended.
Non-resolving UTI	Urine cultures recommended.
UTI recurring within 2–4 weeks upon completion of therapy	Urine cultures recommended.
Complicated UTI	Urine cultures recommended.

Modalities of Urine Examination for the Assessment of Urinary Tract Infections

Urine dipstick

- Point of care testing with the dipstick urinalysis is widely used in the community setting; the presence of leukocyte esterase and/or nitrites in a midstream urine specimen (MSU) supports the diagnosis of a UTI.

- The leukocyte esterase is 75–96% sensitive and 94–98% specific for detecting uropathogens at 10^5 CFU per mL of urine.

- The sensitivity of urine nitrite tests is 35–85% sensitive and 95% specific; the reduced sensitivity of urine nitrate can be explained by the fact that some uropathogens such as *Entero-coccus spp.*, *S. saprophyticus* and *Acinetobacter* are non-ni-trate-reducing.

- The urine dipstick is useful in evaluating patients presenting with atypical symptoms. In patients with a low pretest proba-bility for a UTI, a negative urine dipstick for leukocyte esterase and nitrite is a good rule-out test. In contrast, a positive dip-stick for leukocyte esterase and nitrite increases the likelihood of a UTI.

Urine microscopy

Urine microscopy has to be interpreted in context (Table 22.3).

Urine cultures

- Urine cultures are important in patients who may be at risk of developing severe infections (e.g., pyelonephritis, com-plicated UTIs) and those with non-resolving or recurrent infections. The burden of antimicrobial resistance is high, and appropriately collected urine cultures (prior to antibiotic administration) are important for culture-directed therapy for optimal outcomes.

- Ideally, the urine specimens should be sent to the microbi-ology laboratory soon after collection for processing. If urine cultures cannot be sent immediately (this usually happens

Table 22.3:   Interpretation of Urine Microscopy

	Findings in Urinary Tract Infections	Caveats
Urinary RBC (normal range: ≤3 RBC/hpf)	Haematuria may be present	May be due to UTI, but one has to consider other non-infectious causes.
Urinary WBC (normal range: 2–5 WBC/hpf)	>10/hpf	It has to be interpreted in light of clinical symptoms. Pyuria in the absence of clinical symptoms is not indicative of UTI. Absence of pyuria and bacteriuria may indicate colonisation rather than infection, or a contaminated urine specimen. Sterile pyuria could be due to infection with atypical organisms (e.g., *Chlamydia*, *Ureaplasma urealyticum*, tuberculosis) or other non-infective causes.
Urinary EC (normal range: 1–5 EC/hpf)	—	>5 EC/hpf suggests a contaminated urine specimen.

Abbreviations: UTI, urinary tract infections; RBC, red blood cell; WBC, white blood cell; EC, epithelial cell; hpf, high power field

after office hours), the specimen should then be stored in a refrigerator at 4°C. This is because bacteria will continue to proliferate in the warm medium of freshly voided urine and may lead to increased bacterial counts and affect the interpretation of urine culture results.

- The colony count should also be considered when interpreting urine culture results.(Table 22.4).

Table 22.4: Interpreting Urine Cultures Based on Colony Count Criteria

Classification of UTI	Laboratory Investigation of Urine/Evidence for Bacteria in Terms of CFU/mL
ASB	10^5 CFU/mL of uropathogen
Acute simple cystitis in a female	>10 WBC/hpf >10^3 CFU/mL of uropathogen
Acute pyelonephritis	>10 WBC/hpf >10^4 CFU/mL of uropathogen

Abbreviations: ASB, asymptomatic bacteriuria; CFU, colony forming unit; WBC, white blood cell; hpf, high power field

Microbiology

- For most cases of UTIs, it is usually a monomicrobial infection. Community-acquired UTIs are commonly caused by drug-susceptible gram-negative uropathogens such as *E. coli, Klebsiella spp, Proteus spp.*, or some gram-positive uropathogens such as *Staphylococcus saprophyticus* and *Group B Streptococcus*. UTIs occurring in patients with recent receipt of antibiotics or healthcare exposures may be caused by more resistant pathogens such as Amp C and extended spectrum beta-lactamases (ESBL) carrying *Enterobacterales*. They may also be caused by common nosocomial pathogens such as *Pseudomonas aeruginosa* and *Enterococcus spp*, which may also be drug-resistant strains.

- If more than one pathogen is isolated in the urine culture, it is either a contaminant or a true polymicrobial infection indicative of a fistula developing in the genitourinary system, or it could be a urine specimen collected from an existing nephrostomy tube.

UTIs in Special Populations

UTIs in males

- UTIs in males are uncommon due to longer urethral length, drier periurethral environment, and antibacterial resistance in prostatic fluid. Risk factors include insertive anal intercourse and lack of circumcision. In this group of patients, we have to be vigilant for the prostatitis or upper urinary tract infection. In addition, urological abnormalities and other medical conditions such as poorly controlled diabetes mellitus or immunocompromising conditions have to be excluded.

UTIs in older adults

- Older adults often present with non-specific symptoms and it may be challenging to diagnose a true UTI in this population (i.e., the patient may have another medical condition, infective or otherwise, while having concomitant ASB). A thorough evaluation, appropriate workup, and review of the medication list is recommended prior to starting empiric antibiotics for UTI. Treatment of ASB in the elderly often results in overuse of antibiotics which is a driver for antimicrobial resistance.

Catheter-associated UTIs

- The use of urinary catheters is common in the healthcare setting. In patients with indwelling urinary catheters or those with intermittent catheterisation, it is again important to distinguish between catheter-associated ASB (CAASB) and catheter-associated UTI (CAUTI).

- Patients with CAASB are asymptomatic, and those with CAUTI must have a compatible clinical syndrome. In clinical practice, the diagnosis of CAUTI is often overcalled and antibiotics are overprescribed.

- As a general rule of thumb, routine urine cultures in asymptomatic catheterised patients is not recommended. In catheterised patients, the presence of pyuria or malodorous urine does not distinguish between CAASB from CAUTI.

- CAASB does not require treatment. In contrast, CAUTI is a common cause of nosocomial infection and treatment is warranted. In patients with CAUTIs, the urine specimen should be obtained for culture prior to initiation of antimicrobial therapy. If the catheter is still indicated, it should be replaced (especially if it has been in place for >2 weeks at the onset of CAUTI) and urine cultures should be obtained from the freshly placed catheter. Conversely, if the catheter can be discontinued, then a midstream urine specimen should be obtained. Obtaining urine cultures for culture-directed therapy is important as CAUTIs are usually caused by more drug-resistant pathogens.

- In general, a 7-day course of treatment should suffice; however, a longer course of treatment (~10–14 days) may be recommended for those with delayed responses and the catheter should be replaced if it is still required.

- Regarding CAUTIs, prevention is better than cure. Indwelling catheters should be placed only if there is a clear indication to do so. Adherence to infection prevention practices (e.g., CAUTI bundle) is recommended. The CAUTI bundle includes clear documentation of indication for the catheter, insertion of the catheter under aseptic technique by trained staff, maintaining perineal hygiene, maintaining a closed system to ensure sterility, placing the urinary bag below the bladder but above the floor, ensuring unobstructed urinary flow, and daily review of the ongoing indication of the urinary catheter. Indwelling catheters should be removed promptly when no longer required.

UTIs in diabetic patients on sodium glucose co-transporter-2 (SGLT2) inhibitors

- SGLT2 inhibitors (SGLT2i) are beneficial for diabetic patients with cardiorenal comorbidities as they improve cardiorenal outcomes. SGLT2i work by blocking glucose reabsorption in the proximal tubules. While this improves diabetic control, it results in significant glycosuria, and this may explain the increased risk of UTIs and genitourinary yeast infections. However, the numbers needed to treat to improve cardiorenal outcomes are much smaller than the numbers needed to harm regarding UTI and genitourinary yeast infections risk.

- Nevertheless, some caution must be exercised in patients on SGLT2i. Vigilance is prudent, and patients should be counseled to make sure that they are well hydrated, avoid holding their bladder, and maintain good personal (including perineal) hygiene. If UTIs develop, patients with mild and uncomplicated infections can be managed expectantly and continue the use of SGLT2i. For those with recurrent UTIs, severe UTIs (e.g., emphysematous pyelonephritis), or life-threatening complications, we may have to consider modification of therapy.

Management of UTIs

- Management depends on whether it is a lower UTI (cystitis) or upper UTI (pyelonephritis), and whether it is simple (uncomplicated) or complicated.

Acute uncomplicated cystitis

- Acute uncomplicated cystitis (usually occurs in the community setting in otherwise healthy individuals) responds very well to oral antibiotics of which there are a few options. Augmentin, oral cephalosporins, ciprofloxacin, co-trimoxazole, nitrofurantoin, and fosfomycin are possible options.

- In the hospital setting, cystitis among inpatients (with more complex medical conditions and frequent healthcare attendances) may run a more tenuous course and with infections caused by more drug-resistant pathogens. In such settings, the choice of empiric therapy is guided by local antibiogram, and urine cultures collected prior to antibiotic therapy will help further refine antibiotic selection especially if the infection is non-resolving.

Mild to moderate uncomplicated pyelonephritis

- Mild to moderate uncomplicated pyelonephritis may be treated with a course of oral ciprofloxacin (for 7 days) or co-trimoxazole (for 14 days). For complicated pyelonephritis, septic patients may have to be attended to emergently. Appropriate imaging may be required to exclude abscesses and to look for urinary obstruction. A longer course of antibiotics until resolution of the infection may be required.

Complicated urinary tract infections

- In the evaluation and management of complicated UTIs:

  - The severity of the infection determines the pace of our medical interventions and the locus of care.

  - The underlying urological abnormality has to be addressed (e.g., urinary obstruction relieved and structural abnormalities corrected where possible, sizeable abscesses may have to be drained).

  - Antimicrobials should be culture-directed where possible for optimal outcomes. Patients with prior urological procedures, urinary catheterisation, recent receipt of antibiotics, and recent hospitalisation often have UTIs with more drug-resistant organisms, and patients may require admission for IV antibiotics.

  - Principles of antibiotic selection are illustrated (Tables 22.5 and 22.6). Of note, oral fosfomycin and nitrofurantoin are not recommended for upper UTIs and in patients with renal impairment. Although oral fosfomycin is available for the treatment of simple cystitis, it is not recommended as first line where it must be preserved in the armamentarium for use in the treatment of multi-drug resistant infections (this is administered intravenously for the latter indication, mainly for systemic infections).

Recurrent UTIs

- Risk factors for recurrent UTIs in young pre-menopausal women include sexual intercourse, use of spermicide, a new sexual partner, a mother with a history of UTI, and history of childhood UTI.

Table 22.5:   Commonly Used Oral Antibiotics for the Treatment of Acute Uncomplicated Cystitis — Caveats to Consider

	Nitrofurantoin	Fosfomycin	Bactrim	Fluoroquinolones	β-lactams
Mechanism of action	Targets bacterial ribosomes/inhibits protein synthesis; bactericidal for UTI	Inhibits bacterial wall synthesis; bactericidal activity	Interferes with bacterial folic acid synthesis; bactericidal activity in combination	Direct inhibitors of bacteria DNA synthesis; bactericidal activity	Inhibitors of cell wall synthesis; bactericidal activity
Uncomplicated UTI	✓	✓	✓	✓	✓
Complicated UTI	X	X (off-label use)	✓	✓	✓
Renal impairment	CrCl >30 mL	—	Not recommended for CrCl <15 mL/min	Dose adjustment	Dose adjustment
Advantages	Efficacious in uncomplicated UTI for community acquired infections	Once daily dosing	Oral agent; good bioavailability	Oral agent; good bioavailability	Different agents
Disadvantages	Retroperitoneal fibrosis, pulmonary fibrosis in patients on long term	Decreased efficacy compared to other first-line agents	Hyperkalaemia AKI SJS/TENS High baseline resistance rates	High baseline resistance	Broad spectrum agents only available in IV form
Baseline resistance rates	—	—	High	High	Amp C/ESBL rates in the hospital not low

Abbreviations: UTI, urinary tract infection; CrCl, creatinine clearance; X; not to use; AKI, acute kidney injury; SJS, Steven-Johnson syndrome; TENS, toxic epidermal necrolysis; DNA, deoxyribonucleic acid; ESBL, extended spectrum beta-lactamase; IV, intravenous

Table 22.6:   Additional Considerations When Selecting Antibiotics for the Treatment of UTI — Bug Drug Match

	Gram-positive (e.g., *Enterococcus*, *S. aureus*, *Streptococcal spp.*)	Gram-negative (no *Pseudomonas aeruginosa*)	Gram-negative (*Pseudomonas aeruginosa*)
β-lactams			
Penicillin (amoxicillin/augmentin/ tazocin)	+/− (for sensitive strains)	+/− (for sensitive strains)	+ (tazocin)
Monobactam (aztreonam)	−	+	+
Cephalosporin (cefazolin, cefuroxime, ceftriaxone, cefepime, ceftazidime)	+ (cefazolin/cefuroxime for MSSA; ceftazidime has very little gram-positive cover)	+	+ (cefepime/ceftazidime)
Carbapenem (ertapenem, meropenem, imipenem, doripenem)	+ (apart from imipenem, its activity is not ideal for *Enterococcus*)	+ (useful for more resistant organisms, e.g., Amp C/ESBL)	+ (only meropenem, imipenem, doripenem)
Aminoglycosides (gentamicin, amikacin)	− (usually used for synergism for complicated infections)	+	+
Fluoroquinolone* (ciprofloxacin, levofloxacin)	−	+	+
Bactrim	+ (for MRSA/MSSA)	+	−

Abbreviations: MSSA, methicillin sensitive Staphylococcus Aureus; MRSA, methicillin resistant Staphylococcus Aureus; ESBL, extended spectrum beta-lactamase

*Baseline fluoroquinolone resistance rates in our local hospitals are high at approximately 30–40%. A local antibiogram has to be taken into consideration when selecting fluoroquinolones for the empiric treatment of UTIs. It is advisable to perform culture-directed therapy.

- In post-menopausal and elderly women, the risk factors are slightly different. They include history of UTI prior to menopause, urinary incontinence, atrophic vaginitis due to oestrogen deficiency, cystocoele, increased post-void urine volume, urine catheterisation, and poor functional status/clinical deterioration in the elderly patient.

- Apart from treating the acute episode of UTI, we have to also address the underlying risk factors with non-antimicrobial strategies including behavioural modifications (e.g., adequate hydration, timely emptying of the bladder, wiping from front to back following defecation), topical oestrogen for atrophic vaginitis, as well as addressing urinary retention (intermittent self-catheterisation may be necessary in select cases).

- There may be evidence to suggest that D-mannose or probiotics may be useful. The role of cranberry products and methamine hippurate is less clear.

- The use of antibiotic prophylaxis for the prevention of UTI is controversial. Some meta-analyses have shown antibiotic prophylaxis to be effective in the prevention of UTIs, but the optimal duration is not known and UTIs recur once prophylaxis is discontinued. Antibiotic prophylaxis is a driver for antimicrobial resistance, and this strategy is not likely to be beneficial for patients given the high resistance rates in the Asian region. Having said that, post-coital prophylaxis is likely to be beneficial in pregnant women with a history of frequent UTI prior to the onset of pregnancy.

Test of cure

- This is not necessary for uncomplicated cystitis, pyelonephritis, and patients who have appropriate responses to therapy. However, follow-up cultures may be required:

    - if patients are not responding to therapy,

    - in patients with recurrent/difficult-to-treat UTIs, especially those with anatomic/functional abnormalities of the genitourinary tract, or

    - in the case of unexplained abnormal urinalysis findings

Candida in the urine

- Candida isolated from urine cultures could reflect one of a few possibilities:

    - In asymptomatic patients, it could be a contaminated urine specimen or, very commonly, reflect bladder colonisation (which is the case for many hospitalised patients with a urinary catheter *in situ*). For these cases, patients are expectantly managed. For candiduria occurring in the kidney transplant recipient in the early post-transplant period, there is a risk of fungal arteritis and graft loss, so treatment is recommended. If fluconazole is used, drug-drug interactions with the calcineurin inhibitors must be monitored. If amphotericin is used, then we have to be vigilant for nephrotoxicity.

    - In symptomatic patients who are at-risk hosts (e.g., patients with poorly controlled diabetes or those with urinary tract abnormalities), this may be a significant infection and a fungal ball may develop. Ultrasound of the genitourinary system is recommended and cystoscopy may be indicated for the removal of the fungal ball.

- Candiduria may be indicative of a systemic candida infection (e.g., candidaemia), and this has to be correlated with the other clinical signs, symptoms, and investigations.

Specific Complicated UTIs

- For the renal unit, it is also important to be aware of a few specific infections.

Emphysematous pyelonephritis

- Emphysematous pyelonephritis is a form of acute severe necrotising infection of the renal parenchyma and surrounding tissue characterised by radiological evidence of gas in the renal parenchyma, collecting system, or perinephric tissue.
- Risk factors for development of emphysematous pyelonephritis include:
  - poorly controlled diabetes mellitus
  - urinary tract obstruction
  - history of drug abuse
  - neurogenic bladder
  - alcoholism, and
  - anatomical abnormality of the genitourinary system
- The reported incidence is higher in females, and it is also more common in Asians.
- Patients present with clinical signs and symptoms of pyelonephritis, and crepitus may be present in the costovertebral or

scrotal region. Approximately 50% of patients are bacteraemic. Septic complications may be present and are associated with poorer prognosis. However, emphysematous pyelonephritis is a radiological diagnosis.

- If there is extensive emphysematous pyelonephritis with extension of the gas into the perinephric/para-renal space, or if it occurs in bilateral kidneys (or in a solitary kidney for that matter), nephrectomy may be required. Timely referral to the urologist is indicated.

Infections in patients with polycystic kidney disease

- In patients with autosomal dominant polycystic kidney disease, approximately 30–50% will have UTIs in their lifetime, and they are also at risk of cyst infections. Cyst infections develop because of ascending UTI or as a result of haematogenous spread. It may be difficult to differentiate these cyst infections between cyst rupture or haemorrhage. Of those who develop cyst infections, approximately 10% of cases are hospitalised. Even if these patients go on to receive a kidney transplant, the native kidneys can still get infected post-transplant.

- The diagnosis of a definite cyst infection is based on evidence for neutrophilic debris on aspiration of cyst fluid and/or identification of an offending pathogen; however, this may not always be possible. Cyst fluid aspiration is associated with bleeding risks, cyst rupture, and contamination of adjacent cysts.

- There may be clues from clinical examination to suggest this — patients usually complain of fever and abdominal pain (usually a focal area of tenderness on palpation), inflammatory markers are elevated (usually C-reactive protein >50 mg/L), and there is no radiological evidence for cyst bleeding nor is there alternative cause of fever identified. Therefore, blood cultures are also recommended as part of the workup.

- In general, it is hard to obtain a microbiological diagnosis of cyst infections. Because the cysts are separate from the collecting system, the yield of urine cultures to obtain a microbiological diagnosis is low. Imaging of the cysts (either by ultrasound, CT, or MRI) may reveal evidence of enhanced wall thickening and/or perilesional inflammation. FDG-PET CT is more specific as infected cysts may light up and it allows us to identify pyocysts for drainage if indicated.

- Treatment is usually with prolonged courses of antibiotics (until source control is achieved) ± drainage of the pyocyst either percutaneously or surgically. Recurrent cyst infections are not uncommon.

References

Bonkat G, Bartoletti R, Bruyère F, *et al.* EAU guidelines on urological infections 2022. https://d56bochluxqnz.cloudfront.net/documents/full-guideline/EAU-Guidelines-on-Urological-Infections-2022.pdf

Goldman JD and Julian K (2019). Urinary tract infections in solid organ transplant recipients: Guidelines from the American Society of Transplantation Infectious Diseases Community of Practice. *Clin Transplant* **33**(9): e13507.

Hooton TM, Bradley SF, Cardenas DD, *et al.* (2010). Diagnosis, prevention, and treatment of catheter-associated urinary tract infection in adults: 2009 International clinical practice guidelines from the Infectious Diseases Society of America. *Clin Infect Dis* **50**(5): 625–663.

Kranz J, Schmidt S, Lebert C, *et al.* (2018). The 2017 update of the German clinical guideline on epidemiology, diagnostics, therapy, prevention, and management of uncomplicated urinary tract infections in adult patients: Part 1. *Urol Int* **100**(3): 263–270.

Nicolle LE, Gupta K, Bradley SF, *et al.* (2019). Clinical practice guideline for the management of asymptomatic bacteriuria: 2019 update by the Infectious Diseases Society of America. *Clin Infect Dis* **68**(10): e83–e110.

Rowe TA and Juthani-Mehta M (2014). Diagnosis and management of urinary tract infection in older adults. *Infect Dis Clin North Am* **28**(1):75–89.

Tan CW and Chlebicki MP (2016). Urinary tract infections in adults. *Singapore Med J* **57**(9): 485–490.

23 Assessment of Patients With Advanced Chronic Kidney Disease for Dialysis or Transplant

Liew Ian Tatt

Introduction

- In 2020, the Singapore renal registry reported 2,079 patients newly diagnosed with Stage V chronic kidney disease (CKD) with a median age of 68.6 years at the time of diagnosis. In addition, there were 1,378 patients started on definitive dialysis or transplant for end-stage kidney disease (ESKD).

- The most common aetiology of ESKD in Singapore is diabetic kidney disease.

- ESKD education should be emphasised to patients with irreversible deterioration of glomerular filtration rate (< 20 mL/min/1.73 m^2) that is expected to decline further. Patients should have the following options offered as treatment for ESKD:

    1. Kidney supportive care (KSC)/nondialytic kidney management strategies

    2. Kidney transplantation (KT)

    3. Peritoneal dialysis (PD)

    4. Haemodialysis (HD)

- Choice of kidney replacement therapy (KRT) or KSC must be individualised to the patient and considered holistically, such as:

  - Medical aspects

    - If KRT is medically possible or if there are medical contraindications to KRT (e.g., other life-limiting diseases)

    - If KRT is anticipated to prolong and improve the patient's life

  - The patient's goals of care

  - The patient's understanding of ESKD as well as expectations of KRT and KSC

  - The socioeconomic background of the patient

- Effective preparation for KRT requires time and the input of multiple stakeholders including the patient's caregivers, medical, nursing, pharmacy, dieticians, social workers and in some cases psychological support. A multidisciplinary clinic such as a low clearance clinic can be a tool to consolidating input.

Timing of Initiation of KRT

- Patients with CKD should undergo assessment of their risk for progression to ESKD. There are various tools for such risk stratification including Tangri's kidney failure risk calculator which has been validated in Singapore. The need for timely preparations for dialysis is paramount.

- Indications for dialysis initiation may be recalled via the acronym, A-E-(I)-O-U:

  A — Acidosis

E — Electrolyte abnormality, particularly refractory hyperkalaemia, hypocalcaemia, and hyperphosphataemia

I — Intoxication

O — Fluid overload nonresponsive to diuretic control

U — Uraemia

Self-evidently, the "I" would be an uncommon cause for initiation on chronic dialysis.

- Initiation on chronic dialysis also considers:
  - Subtle signs of uraemia, including pruritus, lethargy, discomfort, nausea, and protein-energy wasting
  - Recurrent/uncontrollable fluid overload
  - Impending therapies that require optimisation (e.g., initiation of dialysis for a patient with Stage V CKD with upcoming coronary bypass surgery)
  - GFR of less than 7 mL/min/1.73 m^2

- Whilst KRT may be delayed if the patient is asymptomatic for advanced CKD, consideration of KRT initiation should be made in symptomatic patients or in asymptomatic patients with extremely low GFR (eGFR of <7 mL/min/1.73 m^2 is usually poorly tolerated). The landmark IDEAL study randomised patients to dialysis initiated at a GFR of 10–14 mL/min/1.73 m^2 ("early") or 5–7 mL/min/1.73 m^2 ("late"). The mean eGFR at the start of dialysis was 9 mL/min/1.73 m^2 in the early dialysis arm compared to 7.2 mL/min/1.73 m^2 in the late dialysis arm. The late dialysis arm was commenced on dialysis on an average of 5.6 months after the early dialysis arm. There were no significant difference in mortality or clinical outcomes at a median of 3.5 years of follow-up between the early and late initiation of dialysis.

Kidney Transplantation

- If suitable for KRT, efforts should be made for a KT as the preferred modality as KT offers a greater survival advantage and quality of life over dialysis modalities.

- Graft outcomes are superior in patients who have received a living donor KT (compared to deceased donor KT) and for recipients of a pre-emptive KT (compared to KT after chronic dialysis has been initiated). The best outcomes are therefore seen in patients who have received a preemptive living donor KT.

- Optimal timing for pre-emptive KT is unclear but may be considered when GFR <20 mL/min/1.73 m² and renal function has showed progressive deterioration over the last 6–12 months.

- Because of the need for general anaesthesia, major intra-abdominal surgery, and lifelong immunosuppression therapy, KT candidates are subject to significant scrutiny. This includes a thorough cardiorespiratory assessment for operative fitness as well as contraindication to immunosuppression including infective, malignant, and metabolic derangements.

- Because of the scarcity of deceased donor kidneys, there are additional criteria imposed nationally as to the eligibility of proposed candidates for deceased donor KT. The goal of distribution is an egalitarian one — allografts are allocated to the patients who are anticipated to benefit the greatest or have the longest graft survival to maximise the use of this scarce national resource.

Peritoneal Dialysis

- PD has several advantages over in-centre HD. This includes improved survival in the first 2 years of initiation of KRT due to the preservation of residual kidney function, a home-based dialysis modality, lower rates of anaemia, greater cost-savings, and possibly better quality of life. For these reasons, Singapore has adopted a PD-preferred approach when advocating for KRT.

- The only absolute contraindication to PD is failure of peritoneal membranes. Relative contraindications to PD have been surmounted by PD centres using various modifications of PD techniques (Table 23.1).

Haemodialysis

- In Singapore, >70% of patients on KRT are on HD with in-centre HD being the main form of administration (Figure 23.1).

- All patients should be evaluated for permanent vascular access creation in the form of an arteriovenous fistula (AVF) or an arteriovenous graft (AVG). Timely creation of vascular access should be prioritised for patients to initiate dialysis on a functioning vascular access instead of a dialysis catheter. Rates of primary failure (non-function) of an AVF/AVG are increased in elderly, diabetic, and female patients. In such patients, consideration

Table 23.1: Methods of Circumventing Relative Contraindications in PD

Relative Contraindication	Methods of Overcoming Relative Contraindications
Unable to self-care/self-perform PD	Assisted PD
Obesity	Advanced PD catheter placement techniques including substernal exits
Polycystic kidney disease	Automated PD with low fill volumes
Adhesions from previous surgeries	Adhesiolysis during PD catheter insertion
Unplanned/urgent dialysis initiation	Insertion of PD catheter with urgent-start PD

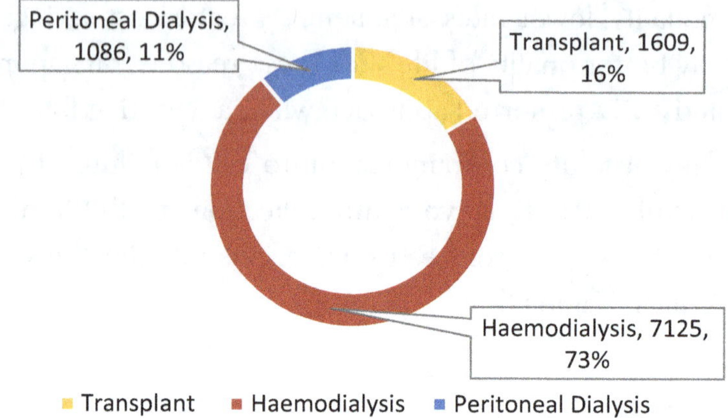

Figure 23.1:   Prevalent Treated ESKD Population by Kidney Replacement Therapy
Source: Singapore Renal Registry 2020.

should be made for PD or earlier access creation to allow time for adequate maturation, modification, or repeat surgery in case of primary failure.

- HD catheters carry risks of catheter malfunction, vessel thrombosis, central vein stenosis, and infections. Long-term tunneled dialysis catheters may be considered in patients with an anticipated limited lifespan who are still considering haemodialysis (e.g., frail, elderly patients who may not benefit from a permanent vascular access).

- Logistical issues to be considered for HD are transport and mobility of the patients. Patients need to travel or be transported to their dialysis centre thrice weekly. In addition, patients should have sufficient mobility to be transferred for weighing and remain seated in a dialysis chair for 4 hours for dialysis. Candidates for HD also need to be compliant to administration of HD which includes needling of the AVF/AVG and tolerating the duration of dialysis. Patients with dementia or specific needle phobias may face difficulties with this.

- Patients on HD have risk of exposure to blood-borne viruses including hepatitis B and C. Candidates for HD who are sero-negative for hepatitis B surface antibody should be immunised. Because of poor serological response to standard vaccinations in advanced CKD, enhanced doses of vaccines are required to achieve seroconversion. An example of an enhanced vaccination regime in advanced CKD is intramuscular administration of 40 mcg Engenrix-B® at months 0, 1, 2, and 6.

Reference

Cooper BA, Branley P, Bulfone L, *et al.* (2010). A randomized, controlled trial of early versus late initiation of dialysis. *N Engl J Med* **363**(7): 609–619.

Glomerulonephritis

24 Nephrotic Syndrome

Irene Mok

Introduction

- Nephrotic syndrome (NS) is a clinical syndrome (Table 24.1) with an incidence in the adult general population reported to be 3 new cases per 100,000.

- Potentially serious complications can occur if NS is left undiagnosed and untreated (Table 24.2).

Causes

- Most causes of NS are caused by primary glomerular disease but can also be secondary to systemic diseases (Table 24.3).

- In Singapore, the 3 most common glomerulonephritis are IgA nephropathy (27%), focal segmental glomerulosclerosis (25%), and minimal change disease (20%) (Table 24.4). These may cause NS but the more common causes of NS in adults are focal segmental glomerulosclerosis, membranous nephropathy, minimal change disease, and diabetic nephropathy.

- NS needs to be differentiated from other oedematous conditions like liver cirrhosis and cardiac failure.

Table 24.1: Definition of Nephrotic Syndrome

Features of Nephrotic Syndrome	Pathophysiology
Severe proteinuria: 24-hr UTP 3–3.5 g/day Urine protein: creatinine ratio 300–350 mg/mmol	• Increased glomerular permeability due to alterations in the charge- and size-selective barriers of the glomerular basement membranes
Hypoalbuminaemia serum albumin <30 g/L	• Urinary losses of protein
Hyperlipidaemia, lipiduria*	• Increased synthesis of lipoproteins • Reduce lipoprotein lipase activity
Oedema	• Underfill mechanism — Hypoalbuminaemia reduces plasma oncotic pressure and results in shift of fluid from capillaries to extracellular tissue. This activates the renin-angiotensin system to retain sodium and increases intravascular blood volume. • Overfill mechanism — Elevated blood volume occurs due to salt and water retention mediated by activation of the epithelial sodium channel (ENaC). As a result, the intravascular blood volume increases and the low plasma oncotic pressure facilitates shift of fluid into the extracellular space, causing oedema.

*Oval fat bodies may be seen in the urine which are sloughed tubular epithelial cells filled with lipid droplets.

Evaluation of Nephrotic Syndrome

History

• Screen for symptoms, causes, and complications of NS (Table 24.5).

Table 24.2: Complications of Nephrotic Syndrome

Complication	Pathophysiology
Acute kidney injury	• Hypovolaemia • Intrarenal oedema with tubular compression • Acute tubular necrosis • Rapid progression of primary kidney disease • Renal vein thrombosis • Raised intra-abdominal pressure due to tense ascites • Use of ACEI/ARB • Drug-induced tubulointerstitial nephritis
Thromboembolism	• Increased hepatic synthesis of procoagulant proteins • Urinary loss of anticoagulants (e.g., antithrombin III) • Increased platelet activation and aggregation • Reduced fibrinolysis (low plasminogen levels) • Haemoconcentration with thrombocytosis • Accelerated atherosclerosis due to hyperlipidaemia
Increased risk of infection	• Loss of IgG and complements in the urine • Skin breaks from oedematous skin • Impaired phagocytic and lymphocytic function • Immunosuppressive treatments
Loss of lean body mass	• Increased urine protein losses
Vitamin D deficiency	• Urinary losses of vitamin D-binding proteins

Abbreviations: ACEI, angiotensin-converting enzyme inhibitor; ARB, angiotensin receptor blocker

Table 24.3: Causes of Nephrotic Syndrome

Primary Glomerulopathies	Secondary Glomerulopathies

• Minimal change disease (MCD)
• Focal segmental glomerulosclerosis (FSGS)
• Membranous nephropathy (MN)
• IgA nephropathy (IgAN)
• Membranoproliferative GN (MPGN)
	• Systemic diseases
	  – Diabetes Mellitus
	  – SLE (Lupus nephritis)
	  – Amyloidosis
	• Infections
	  – Mycoplasma
	  – Syphilis

(Continued)

Table 24.3:   (Continued)

Primary Glomerulopathies	Secondary Glomerulopathies
	– HBV
	– HCV
	– HIV
	– Acute post-streptococcal GN
	– Malaria
	– Schistosomiasis
	– Filariasis
	– Toxoplasmosis
	• Malignancies
	– Breast
	– Lung
	– Gastrointestinal tract
	– Myeloma
	– Lymphoma
	• Drugs
	– Gold
	– NSAIDs
	– Penicillamine
	– Bisphosphonates
	– Antibiotics
	– Tamoxifen
	– Captopril
	– Lithium
	– Interferon alpha
	– Heroin
	• Congenital causes
	– Alport's syndrome
	– Congenital nephrotic syndrome of the Finnish type
	– Pierson's syndrome
	– Nail-patella syndrome
	– Denys-Drash syndrome
	• Secondary FSGS
	– Obesity
	– Reflux nephropathy

Abbreviations: HBV, hepatitis B virus; HCV, hepatitis C virus; HIV, human immunodeficiency virus; GN, glomerulonephritis; NSAIDs, non-steroidal anti-inflammatory drugs; SLE, systemic lupus erythematosus

Table 24.4:   Spectrum of Primary Glomerulonephritis Over 4 Decades in Singapore

Histology	1st Decade (1978–1988)	2nd Decade (1988–1998)	3rd Decade (1998–2008)	4th Decade (2008–2018)
Minimal change disease	9%	13%	19%	20%
Focal global sclerosis	6%	12%	4%	1%
Mesangial proliferative GN	32%	17%	7%	4%
IgA nephropathy	42%	45%	40%	27%
Focal segmental glomerulo-sclerosis	5%	6%	15%	25%
Membranous GN	3%	6%	11%	15%
Crescenteric GN	1%	1%	1%	3%

Abbreviation: GN, glomerulonephritis

Table 24.5:   Medical History Evaluation for Nephrotic Syndrome

History	Specific
Symptoms of nephrotic syndrome	• Weight gain • Oedema — periorbital, peripheral • Abdominal discomfort and distension — ascites • Dyspnoea — pleural effusion • Frothy urine • Macroscopic haematuria with upper respiratory tract infection (synpharyngitic haematuria of IgA nephropathy) • Diarrhoea (due to gut oedema)

(*Continued*)

Table 24.5:   (*Continued*)

History	Specific
Symptoms of complications	• Skin blistering from oedema • Infective symptoms • Flank pain and haematuria (renal vein thrombosis) • Painful swelling in one leg (DVT) • Chest pain and dyspnoea (PE)
Symptoms of secondary causes	• Infective symptoms (e.g., cellulitis, tonsillitis, URTI, GE) • Symptoms of malignancy (e.g., weight loss, lumps, change in bowel habits) • Symptoms of rheumatological diseases (e.g. Butterfly rash, oral ulcers, alopecia, arthralgia, SLE)
Exclude urinary tract infection	• Dysuria • Frequency • Urgency • Haematuria • Fever
Past medical history	• DM; level of control and complications • Hearing loss (e.g., Alport's syndrome)
Medication history	• Prescribed medications • Over the counter medications • Traditional remedies • Substance abuse
Family history	• Kidney diseases (e.g., nephrotic syndrome, haematuria)

Abbreviations: DM, diabetes mellitus; DVT, deep venous thrombosis; GE, gastroenteritis; PE, pulmonary embolism; SLE, systemic lupus erythematosus; URTI, upper respiratory tract infection

Physical examination

• Blood pressure — hypertension may be present

• Proteinuria — frothy urine

• Oedema — periorbital, lower limb, genital, abdominal wall, ascites

- Hypoalbuminaemia — muehrcke lines (transverse white linear bands parallel to nail lanular)
- Pleuritic chest pain, tachypnea, tachycardia — pulmonary embolism
- Tachycardia — pulmonary embolism
- Dyspnoea — pleural effusion
- Hyperlipidaemia — eruptive xanthomata, xanthelasma
- Oropharyngeal examination — examine dental hygiene, tonsillar enlargement
- Skin — rashes suggestive of vasculitis or tubulointerstitial nephritis
- Heart sounds — murmurs for infective endocarditis
- Chest examination — dull percussion note, reduced air entry suggestive of pleural effusion
- Abdominal examination — organomegaly, masses
- Lymph nodes — lymphadenopathy
- Digital examination — prostatomegaly, rectal masses
- Pelvic examination in females — masses
- Breast and axilla in females — masses

Table 24.6:   Laboratory Evaluation of Nephrotic Syndrome

Area of Evaluation	Laboratory Tests	Possible Findings
Confirmation of diagnosis	24-hour urine total protein or urine protein: creatinine ratio	Nephrotic range proteinuria
	Liver panel	Hypoalbuminaemia
	Fasting lipid panel	Hyperlipidaemia
	UFEME	Haematuria, pyuria
	Urine phase contrast	Dysmorphic RBC suggesting GN

(*Continued*)

Table 24.6: *(Continued)*

Area of Evaluation	Laboratory Tests	Possible Findings
Determining cause	Autoimmune screen – ANA – anti-dsDNA – ANCA – anti-GBM Ab – anti-PLA2R – ASOT – C3 – C4	Positive tests suggest possible cause though a kidney biopsy is performed prior to a decision on immunosuppressive therapy. Tissue obtained from kidney biopsy should be sent for light microscopy, immunofluorescence, electron microscopy examination.
	Infection screen – HBsAg, anti-HBs, anti-HBc Ab – Anti-HCV – HIV Ag-Ab screen – Nucleic acid test for HBV, HCV, HIV Malignancy screen – CTAP – FOB – PSA (males) – Mammogram (females) – Cervical smear (females) – Urine immunoelectrophoresis (myeloma panel) Fasting glucose HbA1C Cryoglobulins Kidney biopsy	
Excluding complications	Electrolytes	Pseudo hyponatraemia due to hyperlipidaemia
	Chest X-ray	Pleural effusion
	US doppler kidneys	Renal vein thrombosis
	US doppler lower limbs	Deep venous thrombosis

Table 24.6:   (*Continued*)

Area of Evaluation	Laboratory Tests	Possible Findings
Exclude infection	Blood C/S Urine C/S Swab for respiratory viruses as indicated	Infection should be treated first before immuno-suppression is started.
Others	PT/aPTT GXM	Preparation for kidney biopsy.

Abbreviations: ART, antigen rapid test; ANA, anti-nuclear antibody; dsDNA, double stranded DNA; ANCA, anti-neutrophil cytoplasmic antibody; ASOT, anti-streptolysin O titre; C, complement; C/S; culture and sensitivity; CTAP, computed tomography of abdomen and pelvis; FOB, faecal occult blood; GBM, glomerular basement membrane; GN, glomerulonephritis; GXM, group and crossmatch; HbA1C: haemoglobin A1C; HBsAg, hepatitis B surface antigen; anti-HBc Ab; anti-hepatitis B core antibody; HCV, hepatitis C virus; HIV, human immunodeficiency virus; UFEME, urine full examination and microscopy; GN, glomerulonephritis; PCR, polymerase chain reaction; PL2R; phospholipase A2 receptor; PSA, prostate specific antigen; PT/aPTT, prothrombin time/ activated partial thromboplastin time; RBC, red blood cells; US, ultrasound

Table 24.7:   Management of Nephrotic Syndrome

Symptom or Complication	Treatments
Oedema	• Restrict salt intake (<3 g/day) • Restrict fluid intake • Loop diuretics — may need IV at high doses (furosemide 80–120 mg) due to gut oedema • ±PO thiazides (e.g., metolazone or ±PO amiloride if there is an inadequate response to loop diuretics) • ±IV albumin to improve diuresis — improves diuretic delivery to tubule, expands plasma volume but evidence for benefit remains scant • Monitor I/O and daily weight • Aim for net negative fluid balance — 0.5–1 L/day
Proteinuria	• PO ACEI or ARB, titrated to maximal dose tolerated • Aim for 50% reduction of proteinuria • Immunosuppressive therapy for primary causes of nephrotic syndrome

(Continued)

Table 24.7: (*Continued*)

Symptom or Complication	Treatments
Hypoalbuminaemia	• Protein intake 0.8 g/kg/day + amount in urinary losses
Blood pressure	• Target blood pressure 125–130/75–80 mmHg — PO ACEI or ARB are preferred agents since they treat proteinuria too
Acute kidney injury	• Require close monitoring and may need a period of kidney replacement therapy while awaiting effect of specific immunosuppressive therapies to take place
Hyperlipidaemia	• Restrict dietary fat intake • Statin therapy
Thromboembolism	• Prophylactic anticoagulation, e.g., low molecular weight heparin or warfarin should be considered in severe NS and those at higher risk for thrombosis. • Some patients may not be suitable for anticoagulation and aspirin can be considered as an alternative. • Risk stratification scores and tools, e.g., GN tools (https://www.med.unc.edu/gntools/), Imperial College prophylaxis regimen* are available for certain conditions to estimate benefits relative to risks.
Infections	• Antimicrobial prophylaxis when immunosuppressive therapies are given (e.g., TMP-SMX for PCP prophylaxis) • Monitor for specific infections (e.g., CMV) • Ensure appropriate vaccination

*Imperial College prophylaxis regimen — serum albumin > 30g/L: No thromboembolism prophylaxis; serum albumin 20–30 g/L: Daily aspirin; serum albumin < 20g/L: anticoagulate.

Abbreviations: ACEI, angiotensin-converting enzyme inhibitor; ARB, angiotensin receptor blocker; GN, glomerulonephritis; I/O, input and output; IV, intravenous; PCP, pneumocystis pneumonia; PO, per oral; TMP-SMX, trimethoprim-sulfamethoxazole.

Laboratory investigation

• Laboratory evaluation is aimed to determine the diagnosis, cause of NS, and presence of complications (Table 24.6).

Management

- The principles of management of NS include controlling oedema, reducing proteinuria, treating complications, and addressing the underlying cause of NS (Table 24.7).

References

Hedin E, Bijelić V, Barrowman N, *et al.* (2022). Furosemide and albumin for the treatment of nephrotic edema: A systematic review. *Pediatr Nephrol* **37**(8): 1747–1757.

Orth SR and Ritz E (1998) The nephrotic syndrome. *N Engl J Med* **338**(17): 1202–1211.

Woo KT, Chan CM, Lim C, *et al.* (2019). A global evolutionary trend of the frequency of primary glomerulonephritis over the past four decades. *Kidney Dis* **5**(4): 247–258.

25 Nephritic Syndrome and Rapidly Progressive Glomerulonephritis

Irene Mok, Jason Choo

Introduction

- The presence of haematuria, proteinuria, hypertension, oedema, and varying degrees of kidney dysfunction encompasses the clinical criteria for diagnosing nephritic syndrome.

- This syndromic presentation indicates the presence of kidney injury (glomerular inflammation) and can be variable in its onset of presentation.

- Various causes, such as infections, autoimmune diseases, and drugs, can secondarily cause nephritic syndrome. There is evidence of potential genetic or epigenetic predispositions in affected patients. If undiagnosed and untreated, nephritic syndrome frequently leads to progressive kidney dysfunction, chronic kidney disease (CKD), and end-stage kidney disease (ESKD).

- Rapidly progressive glomerulonephritis (RPGN) refers to the clinical and histopathological triad of:

  - Rapid onset of kidney dysfunction over days and weeks (typically within 3 months) progressing to ESKD.

  - Nephritic urinalysis characterised by glomerular red blood cells (RBC) or presence of dysmorphic RBC in the urine phase contrast, RBC casts, and varying degrees of proteinuria. Haematuria can be gross or microscopic.

■ Kidney histopathology showing crescentic glomerulo-nephritis (GN) characterised by extra capillary proliferation of parietal epithelium or infiltration of inflammatory cells of at least two cell layers thick covering a third or more of the glomerular circumference in more than 50% of glomeruli. Biopsies with 30–50% of crescents can also be considered to have crescentic GN. The presence of crescents signifies severe kidney injury.

Aetiology

• Nephritic syndrome is a common presentation of most proliferative GN (Table 25.1). Causes include lupus nephritis, acute

Table 25.1: Common Glomerular Diseases Presenting as Nephritic Syndrome

Primary Glomerulonephritis	Secondary Glomerulonephritis

• Immunoglobulin A nephropathy
• Membranoproliferative glomerulonephritis
	• Lupus nephritis
	• Infections (PIGN, IRGN)
	  – Acute poststreptococcal glomerulonephritis
	  – Bacterial endocarditis
	  – Abscess
	  – Shunt
	  – HBV
	  – HCV
	  – HIV
	  – Malaria

Abbreviations: HBV, hepatitis B virus; HCV, hepatitis C virus; HIV, human immunodeficiency virus; IRGN, infection-related glomerulonephritis; PIGN, post-infectious glomerulonephritis

Table 25.2: Common Glomerular Diseases Presenting as Rapidly Progressive Glomerulonephritis

Disease	Associations
Goodpasture syndrome (anti-GBM disease)	Pulmonary involvement Anti-glomerular basement membrane AB
Vasculitis (pauci-immune or AAV) Granulomatosis with polyangiitis Microscopic polyangiitis	Pulmonary involvement Cytoplasmic ANCA — anti-PR3 AB Multisystem or renal involvement, perinuclear ANCA — anti-MPO AB
Immune complex disease Systemic lupus erythematosus	Multisystem involvement, ANA, anti-DS DNA AB, low complement C3, C4
IgA nephropathy or IgAV PIGN, IRGN Endocarditis	Characteristic rash in IgAV, normal complement levels Signs of infection (e.g., skin, URTI) Elevated anti-streptolysin O antibody titre New cardiac murmur, positive blood cultures, low C3

Abbreviations: AAV, anti-neutrophil cytoplasmic antibody associated vasculitis; ANA, anti-nuclear antibody; ANCA, anti-neutrophil cytoplasmic antibody; AB, antibodies; anti-DS DNA, anti-double stranded deoxyribonucleic acid; GBM, glomerular basement membrane; IgAV, IgA vasculitis; MPO, myeloperoxidase; PR3, proteinase 3; URTI, upper respiratory tract infection

proliferative GN (postinfectious (PIGN), infection related (IRGN), immunoglobulin A nephropathy (IgA nephropathy), or the earlier presentation of crescentic/rapidly progressive GN (RPGN) (Table 25.2).

- IRGN may occur in association with certain infections, such as bacterial infections (e.g., meningococcaemia, staphylococcal endocarditis, pneumococcal pneumonia), viral infections (mainly hepatitis B, hepatitis C, mumps, human immunodeficiency virus (HIV) infection, varicella, and EBV causing infectious mononucleosis), and parasitic infections (malaria and toxoplasmosis).

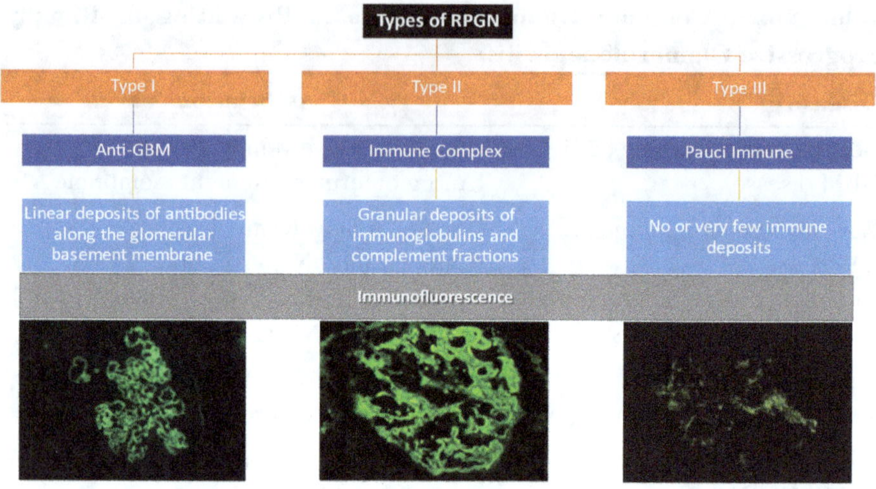

Figure 25.1:   Types of Rapidly Progressive Glomerulonephritis

Abbreviation: RPGN, rapidly progressive glomerulonephritis

- In systemic lupus erythematosus (SLE), patients with focal or diffuse proliferative GN usually present with nephritic syndrome.

- The three main classes of RPGN (Figure 25.1) differentiated by their histopathological and immune complex deposition characteristics include:

  - Anti-GBM disease
    - Linear deposits of antibodies along the glomerular basement membrane (GBM)
    - Kidney limited, lung limited, or kidney and lung involvement (Goodpasture disease)
  - Immune complex glomerulonephritis
    - Granular deposits of immunoglobulins and complement fractions
    - Includes PIGN, IRGN, lupus nephritis, IgA nephropathy, IgA vasculitis, or cryoglobulinaemia

Diagnostic approach principles

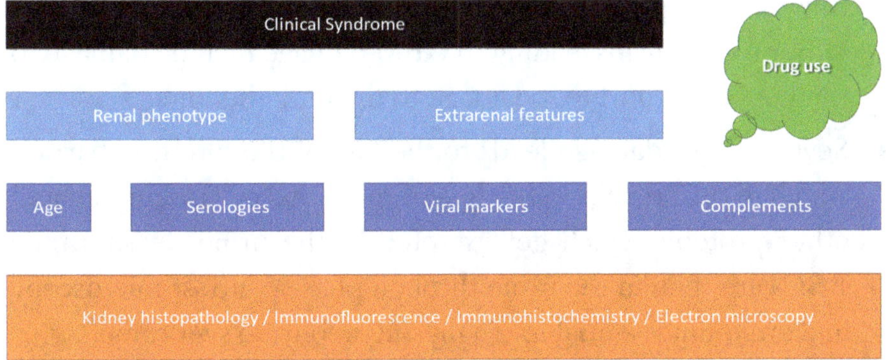

Figure 25.2:   Diagnostic Approach to Rapidly Progressive Glomerulonephritis.

- ■ Pauci-immune GN
  - – None or very few immune deposits
  - – Granulomatous polyangiitis, microscopic polyangiitis, or eosinophilic granulomatous polyangiitis)
  - – Further categorisation is based on anti-myeloperoxidase (MPO) or anti-proteinase-3 antibody positivity
- The other differential diagnoses of patients who present with features of acute kidney injury and active urinary sediment (nephritic urinalysis) include acute thrombotic microangiopathy, atheroembolic kidney disease, acute tubular necrosis, and acute tubulointerstitial nephritis accompanying milder forms of glomerulonephritis.

Pathophysiology

- The underlying pathophysiology of nephritic syndrome depends mainly on the diagnosis. Disruption of GBM ultimately occurs from either direct damage of the glomerular basement membrane or through deposition of immune complexes in the mesangial, subepithelial, or subendothelial space, thus activating the inflammatory milieu within the glomeruli. Other mechanisms leading to GBM damage include damage to the podocytes or direct damage to the endothelium.

- Severe GBM damage leads to the loss of the filtration barrier, which in turn results in the loss of red blood cells, albumin, and other proteins which get excreted in the urine. Dysmorphic RBCs are seen in the urine through phase contrast microscopy and are quintessential to diagnosing nephritic syndrome.

- Crescentic GN signifies severe glomerular damage where there is destruction of the glomeruli with infiltration of inflammatory cells, local cells, and deposition of fibrin. Unopposed immune activation would quickly lead to permanent glomerular damage.

Clinical Suspicion of RPGN

- The first step to managing RPGN patients is appropriate early pickup and diagnosis. Certain types of RPGN are more frequent in certain age groups than others (Table 25.3). Early diagnosis of the cause of the RPGN will allow for early treatment and a better prognosis and outcome (Figure 25.1).

- A high index of suspicion is necessary for patients who present with brown or pinkish-colored urine, gross or significant microscopic haematuria (urine dipstick or microscopy) with constitutional symptoms (e.g., low-grade temperature, general unwellness, fatigue, swelling, out of the ordinary hypertension), and/or a raised serum creatinine when the baseline was normal or lower (no easy explanation). Proteinuria is typically in the non-nephrotic (<3.5 g/day) range.

Table 25.3: Causes of Rapidly Progressive Glomerulonephritis by Age

Immunopathologic Category	All Ages(%)	Age 1–20(%)	Age 21–60(%)	Age > 60(%)
Anti-GBM disease	15	12	15	15
Immune complex GN	24	45	35	6
Pauci-immune GN	60	42	48	79
All other glomerular diseases with 50% or more crescents such as thrombotic microangiopathy, diabetic glomerulosclerosis, and monoclonal immunoglobulin deposition disease	1	0	3	0

Source: Jennette JC (2003). Rapidly progressive crescentic glomerulonephritis. *Kidney Int* **63**(3): 1164–1177.

Abbreviations: GBM, glomerular basement membrane, GN, glomerulonephritis

- When in doubt, an early follow-up of the patient with a repeat serum creatinine, urine microscopy, and urine protein quantification can help prevent missing out on an RPGN diagnosis.

- The clinical symptoms can have a very variable course, with some patients having an insidious progression (e.g., anti MPO-AAV) or a more marked fulminant course (typically with features of crescentic GN).

- Other clinical signs and symptoms include:
    - Recent infection of the upper respiratory tract or elsewhere
    - Ulcers, rashes, purpura, swollen joints
    - Lung symptoms (e.g., dyspnoea, haemoptysis)
    - Pallor
    - New heart murmur

Evaluation

Urinalysis

- Microscopic haematuria is defined as the presence of ≥3 RBCs per high-power field on urinary microscopy of a fresh sample of unspun urine. It is important to:

  - exclude concomitant urinary tract infections, trauma, or menstruation (women)

  - repeat urinalysis at least 48 hours after the last strenuous exercise (exercise-induced haematuria or myoglobinuria)

Urine phase contrast

- Routine evaluation of urine sediment for erythrocyte morphology and the presence of RBC casts and/or acanthocytes is indicated in all forms of glomerular disease.

- Flow-assisted cell-sorting techniques can greatly aid automated analyses of haematuria. In patients with GN, the RBCs are commonly (50–80%) misshapen (dysmorphic) and small (microcytic). The presence of casts containing RBCs or the presence of acanthocytes (>5% of all RBCs) usually indicates an inflammatory glomerular disease. It is essential to distinguish between patients with glomerular haematuria versus haematuria of urological origin. Those with predominantly isomorphic or mixed isomorphic and dysmorphic haematuria should be evaluated for urological disease (especially for patients older than 40 years old or with risk factors for urological cancer, e.g., smoking, chronic cystitis, previous cyclophosphamide use, occupational exposure of benzene/amine dyes).

- Complete urological evaluation is performed to exclude stones, infections, and upper and lower urinary tract tumours. Modalities of evaluation include:

  - Urine cytology

  - Ultrasound of kidneys and bladder (KUB)

  - Non-contrast computed tomography (CT) KUB or CT urogram/intravenous pyelography (contrast-enhanced imaging increases sensitivity and specificity for detection of kidney masses, urinary tract calculi, and pelvicalyceal and ureteric transitional cell cancers, but proceed with caution in patients with kidney dysfunction)

  - Cystoscopy examination of the bladder

- Proteinuria should be quantified with urine protein: creatinine ratio (UPCR) or 24-hour collection of urinary total protein (24-hr UTP). The proteinuria is usually sub-nephrotic in range (less than 3.5 g/day), but some can have nephrotic range proteinuria. A 24-hour UTP may be necessary if concomitant nephrotic syndrome is suspected.

- Renal function should be assessed by measuring plasma creatinine and calculating the estimated GFR.

- Other serological tests (Figure 25.3) should be performed as follows:

  - Serum complement levels (C3, C4) — complement levels are low in diseases in which there is an activation of the inflammatory cascade resulting in deposition of immune complexes in the glomerulus

  - Anti-streptolysin O antibody titres (ASOT) indicate a recent streptococcal infection

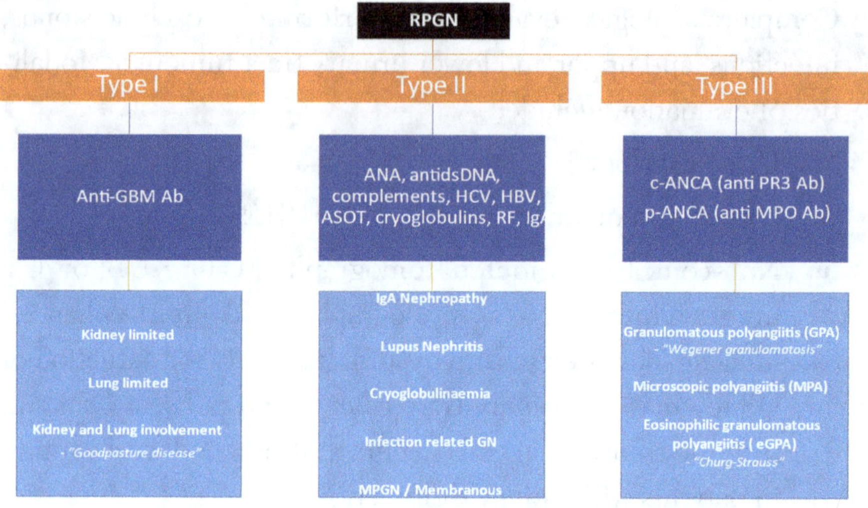

Figure 25.3: Serological Evaluation of Rapidly Progressive Glomerulonephritis

- Anti-neutrophil cytoplasmic antibody — anti-myeloperoxidase (MPO) or anti-proteinase-(PR3) antibodies are evaluated

- Anti-nuclear antibodies (ANA) — to rule out autoimmune disorders

- Anti-double-stranded deoxyribonucleic acid (dsDNA) antibodies

- Anti-GBM antibodies

- Hepatitis B surface antigen and hepatitis B and C antibodies — to rule out hepatitis B and C infection

- Serum protein electrophoresis and serum immunofixation — to identify plasma cell disorders and levels of monoclonal proteins

- Rheumatoid factor — to screen for cryoglobulinaemia in suspected patients

- Kidney biopsy is recommended for definitive diagnosis, prognostication, and ruling out other causes.

Management

Treatment approach principles

- Manage acute symptoms
- Assess kidney function and possible outcomes (natural history, age, sex, ethnicity, genetic background)
- Kidney biopsy
- Prevent and manage complications (e.g., BP, proteinuria, lipid, oedema, coagulation, infection)
- Adjunctive therapies
- Active or disease specific therapies — immunosuppression with or without plasmapheresis
- Other considerations (e.g., pregnancy issues, costs)

General supportive treatment

- Hypertension is very common in GN; it is virtually universal as chronic GN progresses toward CKD/ESKD and is the key modifiable factor in preserving kidney function. As in other CKD, the aim of blood pressure (BP) control is not only to protect against the cardiovascular risks of hypertension, but also to delay progression of the kidney disease.

- In the Modification of Diet in Renal Disease (MDRD) study, patients with proteinuria (>1 g/day) had a better outcome if their BP was reduced to 125/75 mm Hg. The Kidney Disease: Improving Global Outcomes (KDIGO) CKD guidelines recommends a

BP target below 130/80 mm Hg in proteinuric patients, but the SPRINT trial and some specific GN studies suggest that a systolic BP target in the 120 s range may be more effective in certain patient groups.

- ACE inhibitors and ARBs as first-choice therapy is well documented in clinical studies. Additional antihypertensive therapy should be further titrated if target BP cannot be achieved.

- Sodium and water overload is an integral part of the pathogenetic process, and diuretics with dietary sodium restriction are usually an essential part of the treatment.

- Lifestyle modification (salt restriction, weight normalisation, regular exercise, and smoking cessation) is a necessary part of therapy. In situations whereby inflammation is so severe, leading to kidney failure, kidney replacement therapy may be required.

Disease-specific therapies

- Patients should be counselled on intensive immunosuppressive strategies as part of a shared decision-making process considering age, underlying comorbidities, functional status, and the prognosis of the underlying condition with or without immunosuppressive therapy at the time.

- Older nonspecific agents such as corticosteroids and alkylating agents (cyclophosphamide) remain the mainstays of treatment and can result in early dampening of immune and inflammatory activation at multiple levels.

- Other immunosuppressive agents, such as mycophenolate mofetil and rituximab, may be used depending on the nephritic cause. Novel agents that modify inflammatory states in autoimmune conditions (e.g., spleen tyrosine kinase inhibitors) or B cell immunity (e.g., inhibitors of B cell activation factor) are currently under study for efficacy in these acute conditions.

- The benefits of immunosuppression must be weighed against the risks of infections (activations of latent infections or opportunistic infections). Patients at high risk for complications should be appropriately monitored, with risks mitigated by prophylaxis and vaccinations if the patient consents to immunosuppressive therapy.

Reference

Jennette JC (2003). Rapidly progressive crescentic glomerulonephritis. *Kidney Int* **63**(3): 1164–1177.

26 Principles of Immunosuppression in Glomerular Diseases

Tan Hui Zhuan

Introduction

- The immune system can cause kidney damage through various mechanisms, leading to acute kidney injury, chronic kidney disease, and kidney failure.
- These mechanisms can be:
  - direct via targeting specific antigens in the kidneys
  - indirect via systemic dysfunction of the immune system with inadvertent damage to the kidneys
- Immunosuppression is frequently employed to dampen these immune and inflammatory responses, thus allowing for rapid and effective disease control. However, therapy-related adverse events and comorbidities may develop during treatment, often leading to reduced quality of life or life expectancy. Hence, a nuanced, disease-specific approach is required to balance the need for disease control while avoiding excessive harm.
- Personalised risk-benefit assessment should be performed during initial therapeutic decision making, together with appropriate patient counselling. The timing, intensity, and duration of immunosuppression should be based on:

- natural history of the disease
- disease trajectory, including markers of disease activity
- presence of advanced kidney disease, including eGFR at diagnosis and histologic evidence of chronicity
- presence of extra-renal disease in systemic autoimmune diseases
- patient-related variables, such as age and comorbidities

- Immunosuppressive therapy should not be initiated, or should be withdrawn, if or when the risks of immunosuppressive therapy are deemed to outweigh the benefits. Immunosuppression in special populations such as pregnant women, cancer patients, and the elderly will require a nuanced approach and enhanced surveillance of adverse effects. Multidisciplinary team involvement (where appropriate) is necessary.

Evaluation Prior to Immunosuppression Therapies

- As immunosuppressive therapies are potentially toxic, a thorough screening of the patient for suitability to receive immunosuppression should be performed (Table 26.1).

Adjunctive Therapies

Anticoagulation

- Consider prophylactic anticoagulation in nephrotic syndrome (especially membranous nephropathy), if not otherwise contraindicated by high bleeding risk, if there is:
  - Albumin <20–25 g/dL and
  - Other risk factors including but not limited to:

Table 26.1:   Screening for Immunosuppression

Domain	Screening Tests
Infection	• HBsAg • Anti-HBs Ab • Anti-HBc total Ab • Anti-HCV Ab • HIV Ag-Ab screen • HBV, HCV, HIV NAT • VDRL • CXR • Screen for tuberculosis history of exposure
Cancer	• Age-appropriate cancer screening
Metabolic	• Fasting glucose • Lipid

Abbreviations: Ab, antibody; Ag, antigen; CXR, chest X-ray; HBc, hepatitis B core antigen; HBsAg, hepatitis B surface antigen; HCV, hepatitis C; HIV, human immunodeficiency virus; NAT, nucleic acid testing; VDRL, venereal disease research laboratory test

- Transient high-risk event (e.g., prolonged flight)
- BMI >35 kg/m^2
- Heart failure NYHA class III or IV
- Recent orthopedic/abdominal/pelvic surgery
- Prolonged immobilsiation

Consider using www.med.unc.edu/gntools for idiopathic/PLA2R-membranous nephropathy to guide on anticoagulation

Anti-microbial surveillance and prophylaxis

- Screen for tuberculosis, hepatitis B, hepatitis C, HIV, and syphilis as clinically appropriate prior to starting immunosuppressive therapies.
- Prescribe antimicrobial prophylaxis as indicated (Table 26.2).

Table 26.2:   Suggested Antimicrobial Prophylaxis for Glomerulonephritis Treatments

Infection	Immunosuppression	Drug and Dose	Duration of Prophylaxis
Pneumocystis carinii	PRED (>0.5 mg/kg/day), CYC, RITUX or MMF or dual immunosuppression with PRED (>20 mg/day) and a second agent	PO TMP-SMX adjusted to kidney function PO Atovaquone Nebulised pentamidine	Continue until 6–12 weeks after discontinuation of CYC/MMF
Cytomegalovirus	CMV IgG positive serostatus and any 2 of the following: MP, CYC, MMF, RITUX, PLEX, eGFR <15 mL/min or on dialysis, age ≥60 years, absolute lymphocyte count <0.6 × 10^9/L	Monitoring with CMV PCR and treatment if CMV DNA is detected CMV PCR ≥1000 copies/mL — start treatment for CMV CMV PCR <1000 copies/mL — review for symptoms of CMV disease and repeat CMV PCR, FBC, LFT Suggested antimicrobial prophylaxis for glomerulonephritis within 3–5 days CMV PCR ≥1000 copies/mL — start treatment for CMV CMV DNA <1000 copies/mL but increasing during escalation of immunosuppression — start treatment for CMV CMV PCR <1000 and stable with reduction of immunosuppression — continue weekly monitoring	Monitoring and CMV DNA-triggered treatment for the initial 3 to 6 months of induction therapy
Hepatitis B	HBc total antibody positive, HBsAg negative, and HBV DNA negative	PO Entecavir adjusted to kidney function	Continue while on immunosuppression

Abbreviations: CMV, cytomegalovirus; CYC, cyclophosphamide; DNA, deoxyribonucleic acid; FBC, full blood count; HBc, hepatitis core antigen; HBsAg, hepatitis surface antigen; HBV, hepatitis B virus; LFT, liver function test; MMF, mycophenolate mofetil; MP, methylprednisolone; PCR, polymerase chain reaction; PLEX, plasmapheresis; PO, per oral; PRED, prednisolone; RITUX, rituximab; TMP-SMX, trimethoprim-sulfamethoxazole

Vaccinations

- Influenza, pneumococcal, and COVID-19 vaccinations are encouraged for standard immunosuppression.
- Meningococcal vaccination is encouraged for complement inhibitor therapies.
- Live vaccinations are contraindicated for immunocompromised hosts.
- Timing of vaccinations should consider current disease activity and level of immunosuppression (e.g., administer vaccines when dose of prednisolone is less than 20 mg/day or more than 6 months from last dose of rituximab).

Gastroprotection

- Omeprazole 20 mg daily or twice a day if daily dose of prednisolone is 10 mg or more.

Bone protection

- If on steroids (any dose), aim calcium intake 1–1.2 g/day and vitamin D intake 600–800 IU/day. Consider monitoring bone mineral density every 1–2 years for long-term prednisolone therapy.

27 Common Glomerulonephritis and Their Treatment

Cynthia Lim, Jason Choo

The immunosuppressant (IS) regimens suggested are adapted from KDIGO Clinical Practice Guidelines on Glomerular Diseases 2021.

This document only serves as a guide; therapy should be individualised for each patient according to disease and patient profile, treatment goals, and shared decision-making after discussing indication, benefits, risks, and alternatives.

Table 27.1:   Types of Glomerulonephritis

GN	Epidemiology	Pathogenesis	Presentation	Evaluation	Kidney Biopsy
Minimal change disease (MCD)	Most common cause of NS in children with a peak incidence in children aged 2–4 years. Accounts for up to 20% of NS in adults.	Most patients have primary or idiopathic MCD. Secondary MCD may be due to allergies, drugs, malignancies, and/or vaccinations. There is immune dysfunction, especially of the T-cells which contributes to podocyte injury and dysfunction (podocytopathy).	Typically abrupt onset of "full-blown" NS. BP is usually normal. AKI occurs in 30%.	Kidney biopsy is required to make a diagnosis. Exclude secondary causes.	**LM** No or minimal glomerular abnormalities. **EM** Diffuse effacement of podocyte foot processes.
Primary focal segmental glomerulosclerosis (FSGS)	Accounts for up to 35% of NS in adults.	May be primary or secondary to other causes.	Acute/subacute onset of NS.	Kidney biopsy is required to make a diagnosis and will identify	**LM** Segmental mesangial sclerosis involving <50% of all glomeruli.

Primary FSGS is a podocytopathy caused by unknown circulating permeability factors. Secondary FSGS is due to reduced nephron mass and glomerular hyperfiltration injury.	Hypertension occurs in 30–40%. AKI occurs in 20–25%. Compared to primary FSGS, secondary FSGS is associated with lesser degree of oedema and low albumin levels.	different histological subtypes of FSGS that have distinct clinical phenotypes; for example, collapsing FSGS has the worst prognosis while tip lesion has the best prognosis. Perihilar FSGS is usually a secondary FSGS. Exclude secondary and genetic causes (e.g., viral infections, drugs, familial FSGS)	There are 5 variants: Collapsing FSGS: collapse of tuft, podocyte hyperplasia Cellular FSGS: endocapillary proliferation, podocyte hyperplasia Tip lesion: sclerosis or adhesion at proximal tubule pole Perihilar variant: sclerosis and hyalinosis at vascular pole FSGS not otherwise specified (NOS): segmental sclerosis

(*Continued*)

Table 27.1: (*Continued*)

GN	Epidemiology	Pathogenesis	Presentation	Evaluation	Kidney Biopsy
					EM Podocyte foot processes effacement is diffuse in primary FSGS but is less extensive in secondary FSGS.
PLA2R membranous nephropathy (MN) (Previously known as "primary" or "idiopathic" MN)	One of the most common cause of NS in adults (30% of NS) Median age of onset in the 50s, but can occur at any age	Immune complex-mediated GN due to auto-Ab against podocyte antigens (e.g., M-type phospholipase A2 receptor 1 (PLA2R), thrombospondin Type I domain containing protein 7A (THSD7A)).	Insidious onset +/− microscopic haematuria Renal function usually normal or near-normal at presentation If AKI is diagnosed, need to exclude	MN can be also secondary to other diseases medications which needs to be excluded during evaluation Anti-PLA2R Ab are found in 70% of patients with primary MN and is useful in monitoring disease activity.	**LM** Diffuse thickening of GBM; subepithelial "spikes" on silver methenamine stain **IF** Granular deposition of IgG and complement in glomeruli **EM** Subepithelial electron dense deposits. Presence

		There is a dysregulated immune system that leads to complement activation and subsequent podocyte injury.	bilateral renal vein thrombosis, pre-renal causes, or superimposed RPGN Secondary MN can be caused by autoimmune diseases, infections, malignancies, and medications	Presence of anti-PLA2R Ab before or after KT predicts recurrence of MN. • Several other antigens or biomarkers have also been identified in MN but their role in diagnosis and monitoring remains uncertain.	of tubule-reticular inclusions or mesangial/ subendothelial deposits suggests a secondary cause
IgA nephropathy	Most common GN among Asians	Multi-hit pathogenesis with formation of circulating immune complexes	Highly variable clinical presentations: – Asymptomatic haematuria and/or proteinuria	Consider secondary causes: IgA vasculitis, chronic liver disease, celiac disease, infections	**LM** Mesangial ± endocapillary hypercellularity ± crescents (MEST-C)

(*Continued*)

Table 27.1:   (*Continued*)

GN	Epidemiology	Pathogenesis	Presentation	Evaluation	Kidney Biopsy
		(galactose-deficient-IgA1 IgG or anti-gliadin IgA) and alternative ± lectin pathway complement activation	– Gross haematuria – NS – RPGN	(IgA-dominant infection-related GN), connective tissue disease, psoriasis	**IF** IgA ± C3 **EM** Electron dense deposits in the mesangial and paramesangial areas The Oxford (MEST-C) classification system is widely used to identify lesions of prognostic value: Mesangial hypercellularity (M1: present, M0: absent) Endocapillary hypercellularity (E1)

					Segmental sclerosis (S1)
					Tubular atrophy of 3 levels of severity (T0, T1, T2)
					Crescents (C0, C1, C2)
Lupus nephritis	Lupus nephritis occurs in about 30–60% of patients with SLE with variable prevalence — lowest in caucasians and highest in asians.	Multisystem autoimmune disorder	Kidney presentations vary, ranging from asymptomatic microscopic haematuria to NS or nephrotic-nephritic syndrome with or without progressive kidney dysfunction.	Indications for kidney biopsy in patients with SLE: – glomerular haematuria – cellular casts – 24-hr UTP >0.5 g/24 hrs (or spot UPCR >0.5 g/g) – unexplained persistent decline in eGFR. Kidney biopsies are necessary to detect presence	Histopathological diagnosis (International Society of Nephrology/ Renal Pathology Society (ISN/RPS) classification) **Class I** Minimal mesangial LN **Class II** Mesangial proliferative LN **Class III** Focal proliferative LN ± Class V

(*Continued*)

Table 27.1:   (*Continued*)

GN	Epidemiology	Pathogenesis	Presentation	Evaluation	Kidney Biopsy
			Diagnosis of SLE can predate or be diagnosed at time of diagnosis of lupus nephritis.	of concomitant TMA (rule out antiphospholipid syndrome) or exclude acute interstitial nephritis or secondary FSGS.	**<u>Class IV</u>** Diffuse proliferative LN ± Class V **<u>Class V</u>** Membranous LN **<u>Class VI</u>** Advanced sclerosing LN Severe lupus nephritis denotes presence of – >15% crescents – glomerular capillary necrosis – persistent or relapsing disease despite effective immunosuppression (e.g., CYC)

					– proliferative LN features – raised serum creatinine at time of induction therapy
Renal-limited ANCA Associated Vasculitis	Usually in older adults especially 60–70 yr Classification by clinical disease: 1. Granulomatosis with polyangiitis (GPA) associated with anti-PR3 or cANCA 2. Microscopic polyangiitis (MPA) associated with anti-MPO or pANCA;	Necrotising vasculitis ± granulomatous inflammation mediated by circulating ANCAs and alternative complement pathway activation — pauci-immune necrotising ± crescentic GN ± interstitial nephritis	Usually present as RPGN or nephritic syndrome, although may sometimes have a subacute presentation with constitutional symptoms such as fever or weight loss	Assess for extra-renal involvement: upper airway (rhinitis, sinusitis, otitis media, nasal perforation, saddle nose), respiratory tract (alveolar haemorrhage, cavitation, nodules, fibrosis, asthma), eosinophilia, neuropathy, constitutional	Pauci-immune necrotising and/ or crescentic glomerulonephritis

(Continued)

Table 27.1:   (*Continued*)

GN	Epidemiology	Pathogenesis	Presentation	Evaluation	Kidney Biopsy
	3. Eosinophilic GPA (EGPA) or according to ANCA-specificity — PR3-ANCA disease or MPO-ANCA disease Evaluation:			symptoms (fatigue, weight loss, fever). Consider secondary causes: chronic infections, malignancies, thyroid disease, drugs (silica exposure, hydralazine, cocaine, anti-thyroid meds, anti-TNF agents)	
Anti-GBM Disease	Rare, can occur at all ages but typically bimodal distribution Evaluation Management:	Caused by pathogenic autoantibodies against NC1 domain of α3 chain of Type IV collagen.	Usually presents as RPGN — AKI with active urinary sediment, subnephrotic-range proteinuria	Serology: ○ Positive anti-GBM Ab (ELISA) ○ ANCA present in 1/3 of patients	Kidney biopsy: ○ LM: crescentic GN ○ IF: classically linear IgG along GBM

| Exact trigger for antibody production unknown, but smoking and hydrocarbon inhalation implicated. | Extra-renal disease esp pulmonary: clinical exam, SPO2, CXR, Bronchoalveolar lavage, DLCO in selected cases |

Abbreviations: Ab, antibodies; AKI, acute kidney injury; eGFR, estimated glomerular filtration rate; cANCA, cytoplasmic anti-neutrophil cytoplasmic antibodies; EM, electron microscopy; GN, glomerulonephritis; hr; hour IF, immunofluorescence; KT, kidney transplantation; LM, light microscopy; MPO, myeloperoxidase; NS, nephrotic syndrome; pANCA, perinuclear anti-neutrophil cytoplasmic antibodies; PLA2R, phospholipase A2 receptor 1; PR3, proteinase-3; RPGN, rapidly progressive glomerulonephritis; SLE, systemic lupus erythematosus; TMA, thrombotic microangiopathy; TNF, tumour necrosis factor; UTP, urine total protein; UPCR, urine protein: creatinine ratio

Table 27.2:　Immunosuppressive Therapies for Glomerulonephritis

GN	Initial Immunosuppressive Therapy	Prognosis	Special Situations
Minimal change disease (MCD)	**First line:** • PO PRED 0.8–1 mg/kg/d (max 60 mg) or 2 mg/kg/EOD (max 120 mg) • Target 4–16 wks of high-dose as tolerated with subsequent tapering over 6 mths if CR/PR achieved **Steroid minimisation option:** PO PRED 0.5 mg/kg with PO CsA 3–5 mg/kg/d × 6–12 mths (C0: 100–175 ng/mL) or PO TAC 0.05–0.1 mg/kg/d × 6–12 mths (C0: 5–10 ng/mL) or PO CYC 2 mg/kg/d × 2–3 mths	• Spontaneous remission uncommon in adults. • Most adult MCD are SSNS. • 30–40% are FR/SDNS. • Long-term kidney survival excellent in SSNS but poor in SRNS. • The greater the relapse-free interval, the better the prognosis.	**Frequently relapsing/ steroid-dependant:** PO CYC 2 mg/kg/d × 8–12 wks or PO CsA 3–5 mg/kg/d (C0: 100–150 ng/mL) for 6 mths then taper; total duration 1–2 yrs or PO TAC 0.05–0.1 mg/kg/d (C0: 4–7 ng/mL) for 6 mths then taper; total duration 1–2 yrs or PO MMF 0.75–1 g BD for 6 mths then taper; total duration 1–2 yrs or IV RTX 375 mg/m² weekly × 1–4 doses or 1 g 2-weekly × 2 doses

| Primary focal segmental glomerulosclerosis with nephrotic syndrome | **First line:**
• PO PRED 0.8–1 mg/kg/d (max 60 mg) or 2 mg/kg/EOD (max 120 mg)
• Target 4–16 wks of high-dose as tolerated with subsequent tapering over 6 mths if CR/PR achieved

Steroid minimisation option:
PO PRED 0.5 mg/kg/d and CsA 3–5 mg/kg/d
(C0: 100–175 ng/mL)
or
TAC 0.05–0.1 mg/kg/d
(C0: 5–10 ng/mL)
Treat × 12 mths then taper over 6–12 mths | • Usually progressive CKD if untreated/no remission: 2/3 progress to ESRD within 10–15 years
• Poor prognostic factors:
– Older age
– Male gender
– African-American
– Severe proteinuria
– Low GFR
– HTN at presentation
– Histological variants (e.g., collapsing FSGS)
– Severity of interstitial fibrosis
– Genetic forms of FSGS
– Therapy response (remission) is the best single clinical indicator of eventual outcome | **Steroid resistant:**
PO PRED 0.5 mg/kg/d and PO CsA 3–5 mg/kg/d (C0: 100–150 ng/mL)
or
PO TAC 0.05–0.1 mg/kg/d (C0: 5–10 ng/mL)
Aim high-dose for 6 mths then taper
CR/PR: aim to complete total 12–24 mths
• No response: treat ≥ 6 mths before deeming CNI resistant; reconsider secondary causes

Relapse:
Steroid sensitive: re-induce with PO PRED
Steroid resistant: re-induce with CNI
Frequent relapse/steroid-dependent: treat as per MCD |

(*Continued*)

Table 27.2: *(Continued)*

GN	Initial Immunosuppressive Therapy	Prognosis	Special Situations
PLA2R membranous nephropathy	Consider immunosuppression if at high risk for developing progressive kidney failure, as determined by both clinical and immunologic parameters: – eGFR < 60 mL/min – UPCR > 8 g/d for 6 mths – ±PLA2R > 150 RU/mL – complications of NS **Treatment regimens:** CsA 3.5 mg/kg/d (C0 125–200 ng/mL) or TAC 0.05–0.1 mg/kg/d (C0 4–7 ng/mL) ± PO PRED 0.5 mg/kg/d or IV RTX 1 g on D1 and D15 or IV RTX 375 mg/m² weekly for 2–4 doses	Traditionally the rule of thirds — a third undergo spontaneous remission, a third has persistent proteinuria, and another third progresses to ESKD	Monitor PLA2R at 3–6 mths for serologic remission **Refractory:** Consider change of regimen **Relapse:** • Consider repeating initial induction if there was good response/remission ± maintenance • Consider lifetime cumulative CYC dose

Consider maintenance fixed-
  dosing every 6 mths × 2 yrs or
  dose according to PLA2R levels

or

Continuous:

PO PRED 0.5 mg/kg/d + PO CYC
  1.5 mg/kg/d × 3–4 mths

or

Cyclical (Ponticelli):

IV MP 1 g × 3 d (at mth 1, 3, 5)
  then

PO PRED 0.5 mg/kg/d × 28 d +
  PO CYC 2.5 mg/kg/d (at mth 2,
  4, 6)

or

PO MMF 0.75–1 g BD for 6 mths
  then taper, total duration 1–2 yrs
with PO PRED 0.5 mg/kg/d

| IgA nephropathy (IgAN) | Optimise SBP < 120 mmHg
Maximal tolerated ACEi/ARB
±SGLT2i
±omega3-FA
Smoking cessation | The IgAN International prediction tool predicts at the time of kidney biopsy the risk of worsening kidney function over 5–7 years; | **IgAN with light microscopy and clinical presentation consistent with MCD**: treat as per minimal change disease. |

(Continued)

Table 27.2:   (Continued)

GN	Initial Immunosuppressive Therapy	Prognosis	Special Situations
	First line: PO PRED 0.5–1 mg/kg/d × 2 mths then taper, total duration 6 mths **Second line**: PO PRED 0.5 mg/kg/d + MMF 750 mg BD × 6–12 mths	can be used in adults of all ethnicities with primary IgAN. The tool is available on the web for use.	**Crescentic IgAN with RPGN**: IV pulse steroids and cyclophosphamide
Lupus nephritis	**Active Class III/IV ± V Induction:** PO PRED 0.8–1 mg/kg/d × 4–8 wks then taper or IV MP 250–500 mg/d × 3 d then PO PRED 0.3–0.5 mg/kg/d (max 60 mg/d) × 2 wks then taper and IV CYC 500 mg every 2 wks × 6 doses or PO CYC 1–1.5 mg/kg/d (max 150 mg) × 4 mths or MMF 2–3 g/d × 9–12 mths then taper	In general, patients with Class III/IV ± V histological diagnosis necessitates treatment with immunosuppression. Appropriate induction treatment doses should be followed by stabilisation or improvement in eGFR and reduction in proteinuria by 3 mths with further improvement up to 6 or 12 mths targeting for	**Active Class III/IV ± V Refractory**: – Check compliance – Switch from CYC to MMF or vice versa OR add IV rituximab 1 g D1 and D15 **Relapse:** repeat same or alternate induction (consider lifetime cumulative CYC dose)

Consider

Combination MMF + CNI
for mixed Class III/IV + V

Adjunct: HCQ

Maintenance:

Taper to lowest dose to sustain
  remission × 2–3 yrs

MMF 1–2 g/d

or

AZA 1.5–2 mg/kg/d

±

low-dose PO PRED 3–5 mg/d

**Isolated Class V lupus nephritis
  with proteinuria > 3 g/d**

Induction:

PO PRED 0.5–1 mg/kg/d × 4–8
  wks then taper and

MMF 2–3 g/d × 9–12 mths then
  taper

or

PO CsA 3–5 mg/kg/d
(trough 125–200 ng/mL)

complete remission
(proteinuria < 0.5 g/d with
return to baseline serum
creatinine and preferable
inactive urinary sediment)
and overall controlled
extrarenal disease activity.
Patient adherence to
immunosuppressive
treatment regimen is
essential for sustenance of
remission in this chronic
disease.

Lupus podocytopathy

Class I/II with nephrotic
syndrome: treat as per
MCD, maintain with MMF/
AZA/CyA/FK.

(*Continued*)

Table 27.2:   (Continued)

GN	Initial Immunosuppressive Therapy	Prognosis	Special Situations
	or PO TAC 0.05–0.1 mg/kg/d (trough 4–7 ng/mL) **Adjunct:** HCQ **Maintenance:** Taper to lowest dose to sustain remission × 2–3 yrs PO MMF 0.5–1.5 g/d or PO CsA 1–2 mg/kg/d or PO TAC 0.02–0.04 mg/kg/d		
Renal-limited ANCA associated vasculitis	**Induction:** IV CYC 15 mg/kg at 0, 2, 4 wks then every 3 wks or IV CYC 500 mg every 2 wks × 3 mths or PO CYC 2 mg/kg/d × 3–4 mths	If untreated — organ/life-threatening in 70–80% Remission in 60–80% when treated with immunosuppression	Stop immunosuppression after 3 mths if still dialysis-dependent and there is no extrarenal indication.

or
IV RTX 375 mg/m^2 weekly × 4
   doses or 1 g on D1 and D15
All with
IV MP 500 mg × 3 d then PO
   PRED as per PEXIVAS reduced
   dose:

<u>≤50 kg:</u>
50 mg × 7 d then 25 mg × 7 d then
   taper to 6–10 mg/d by 3 mths
   and 5 mg/d by 6 mths

<u>50–75 kg:</u>
60 mg × 7 d then 30 mg × 7 d then
   taper to 6–10 mg/d by 3 mths
   and 5 mg/d by 6 mths

<u>>75 kg:</u>
75 mg × 7 d then 40 mg × 7 d then
   taper to 6–10 mg/d by 3 mths
   and 5 mg/d by 6 mths

<u>Adjunct:</u>
Consider PLEX if SCr >
   300 μmol/L, or concomitant
   anti-GBM.

<u>Maintenance:</u>
PO PRED 5–7.5 mg/d and
RTX 0.5–1 g every 6/12
or
AZA 1–2 mg/kg/d
or
MMF 0.5–1.5 g/d
Total duration 2–4 yrs

<u>Relapsing disease:</u>
Re-induce preferably with
   RTX + PRED regimen.

<u>Refractory disease:</u>
Switch from CYC to RTX or
   vice versa. Consider PLEX.

(Continued)

Table 27.2:   *(Continued)*

GN	Initial Immunosuppressive Therapy	Prognosis	Special Situations
Anti-GBM disease	Percentage of crescents on initial kidney biopsy and pre-intervention kidney function guide treatment strategy and predict outcome. Immunosuppression and PLEX recommended in most patients. Organ supportive care for severe disease Daily PLEX (40–50 mL/kg ideal body weight) until anti-GBM Ab undetectable and PO CYC 2 mg/kg/d × 2–3 mths and IV MP 500 mg × 3 d then PO PRED 0.8–1 mg/kg/d then taper	Generally a monophasic disease. Relapses are rare unless dual positive for ANCA	No immunosuppression if dialysis-dependent, 100% crescents, and no alveolar haemorrhage. No maintenance therapy unless concomitant ANCA positive.

Abbreviations: Ab, antibody; ANCA, anti-neutrophil cytoplasmic antibody; BD, twice a day; CNI, calcineurin inhibitor; C0, trough concentration drug level; CR, complete remission; CsA, cyclosporine; CYC, cyclophosphamide; d, days; eGFR, estimated glomerular filtration rate; EOD, every other day; ESKD, end-stage kidney disease; FR/SDNS, frequent relapsing/steroid dependent nephrotic syndrome; GBM, glomerular basement membrane; GFR, glomerular filtration rate; HTN, hypertension; IV, intravenous; MMF, mycophenolate mofetil; mth, month; MP, methylprednisolone; NS, nephrotic syndrome; PLEX, plasma exchange; PO, per oral; PR, partial remission; PRED, prednisolone; SRNS, steroid resistant nephrotic syndrome; RTX, rituximab; SSNS, steroid sensitive nephrotic syndrome; TAC, tacrolimus; UPCR, urine protein: creatinine ratio; wks, weeks; yrs, years

Haemodialysis

28 Concepts and Modalities of Haemodialysis

Phang Chee Chin, Sheryl Gan

Introduction

- Haemodialysis (HD) is a medical treatment using an artificial semipermeable membrane called a dialyser membrane to remove uraemic toxins, certain electrolytes and fluid in patients with end-stage kidney disease (ESKD) (Figure 28.1).

- During HD treatment, the patient's blood is drawn via an "access" (arteriovenous fistula/graft, dialysis catheter) and pumped through a haemodialyser machine where fresh dialysate from the machine enters in a counter-current flow separated by the dialyser membrane.

- This process allows excess uraemic toxins and fluid to be filtered out from the patient's blood into the dialysate. The used dialysate containing uraemic toxins and fluid leaves the dialyser membrane and is washed down the drain while the treated blood returns to the patient.

- Dialysate is a solution of pure water with a concentration of electrolytes similar to that found in extracellular fluid with the exception of the buffer bicarbonate and potassium concentration.

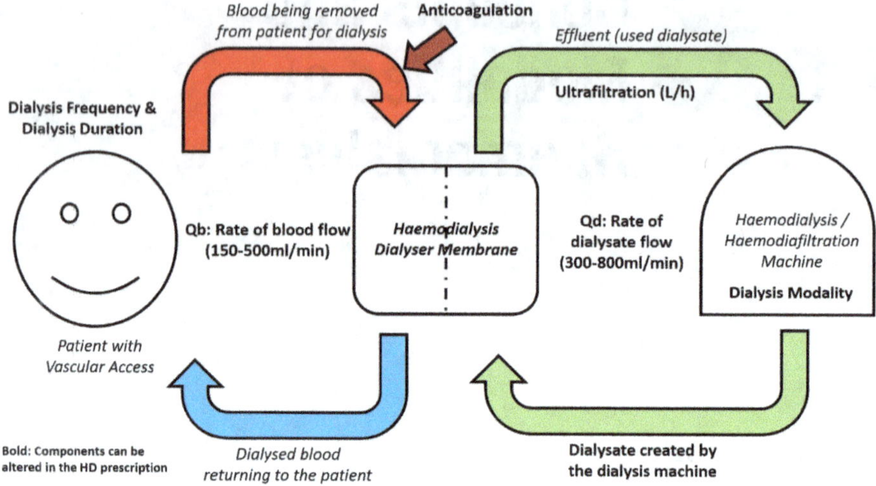

Figure 28.1:　Concept of Haemodialysis

- During HD treatment, uraemic toxins are removed from the patient's blood to the dialysate compartment through the dialyser membrane by diffusion and/or convection.

  Diffusion (Figure 28.2) — a process where solute moves from the high-concentration compartment (patients' blood)

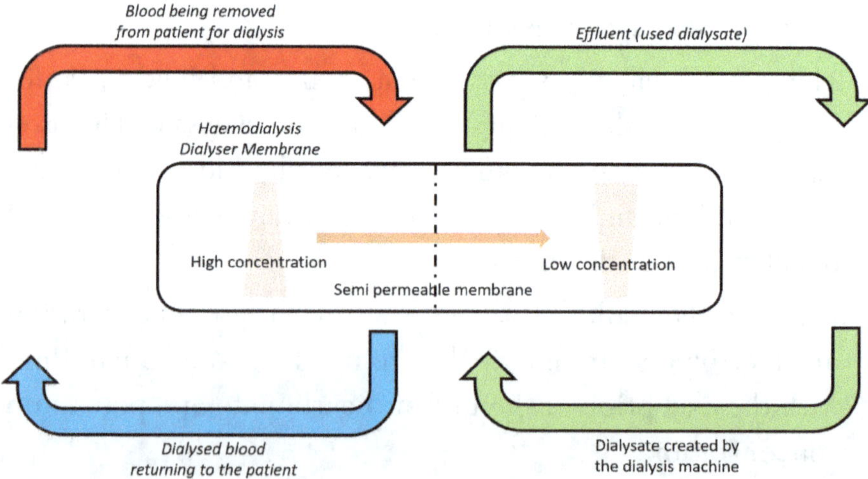

Figure 28.2:　Diffusion

to the low-concentration compartment (dialysate) across the dialyser membrane.

Convection (Figure 28.3) — a process where solute passes through the dialyser membrane due to solvent drag. This fluid movement (ultrafiltration) is achieved by applying a hydrostatic transmembrane pressure gradient. Adsorption of larger molecular weight proteins onto the dialyser membranes occurs at varying degrees in dialysis therapies due to blood exposure to the surface of the dialyser membranes.

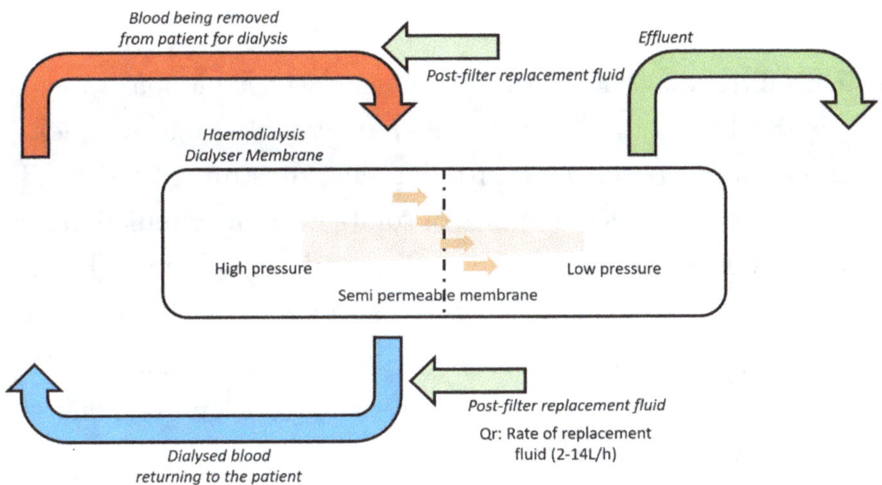

Figure 28.3:   Convection

- The primary mode of solute removal by HD is diffusion. In haemodiafiltration (HDF), a combination of diffusion and convection enhances solute removal. Convection allows a higher degree of removal of middle molecular weight solutes.

Table 28.1: Modalities of Haemodialysis

	Iso-UF	HD	HDF	SLED
Principle	Ultrafiltration	Diffusion	Convection + diffusion	Diffusion
Indications	Removal of fluid	Stable patients	Hypotension Myocardial infarction Cerebrovascular accident Chronic HDF may be provided in stable patients at community-based HD centres	

Abbreviations: HD, haemodialysis; HDF, haemodiafiltration; Iso-UF, isolated ultrafiltration; SLED, slow low-efficiency dialysis

- Ultrafiltration (UF) is the process by which plasma water is removed from the blood circulation across the dialyser membrane in response to a transmembrane pressure gradient. UF leads to the net mass removal of solute from the circulation but no change in the concentration of solute in the plasma. The solute concentration in the UF is the same as that in the plasma.

- HD can be performed in a few ways: in-centre HD, home HD, and nocturnal HD. In-centre HD is usually done at a dialysis facility 3 times a week.

- There are different HD modalities commonly prescribed (Table 28.1).

Conventional HD

Conventional HD is the most common modality performed in ESKD patients who are otherwise stable on maintenance HD. The typical blood flow (Qb) for conventional HD ranges from 200–400 mL/min, and dialysate flow (Qd) 500–800 mL/min. The dialysis duration ranges from 3.5 to 5 hours per session, with a minimum of 3 times a week necessary in ESKD patients with no residual renal function.

Sustained Low-efficiency Dialysis

Sustained low-efficiency dialysis (SLED) is performed in patients with:

- haemodynamic instability,
- acute coronary syndrome,
- acute gastrointestinal bleeding, and/or
- acute cerebrovascular accident without midline shift.

SLED may also be used in newly initiated patients to reduce the risk of dialysis disequilibrium syndrome.

During SLED treatment, lower blood and dialysate flow rates provide better haemodynamic stability by reducing the small solute clearance and associated changes in osmolality. The duration of SLED is typically 6 to 12 hours, but some centres commonly perform this over 4 hours due to various logistical concerns. As SLED is associated with reduced efficiency in solute clearance, patients may require more frequent sessions to achieve adequate solute clearance and fluid removal. Hence, it is crucial to monitor adequacies of solute clearance when patients require multiple sessions of SLED therapy.

Isolated UF

During isolated UF, no dialysate fluid is required. It is performed in patients who require additional fluid removal without the need for solute clearance.

Sequential HD

Sequential HD combines isolated UF and HD/SLED therapy, typically performed in the first HD session, to prevent dialysis disequilibrium syndrome while allowing time for UF in patients with fluid overload.

Haemodiafiltration (HDF)

Haemodiafiltration utilises both diffusive and convective clearance during dialysis treatment. Compared to conventional HD, which predominantly uses diffusive clearance, convective clearance provides more middle-molecular weight solute clearance. During haemodiafiltration, a sterile replacement fluid is infused into the patient's blood circuit to maintain the fluid balance. The replacement fluid can be infused either before the blood enters the dialyser (prefilter) or after the dialyser (postfilter).

References

Himmelfarb J and Ikizler TA (2010). Hemodialysis. *N Engl J Med* **363**(19): 1833–1845.

Lang T, Zawada AM, Theis L, *et al.* (2023). Hemodiafiltration: Technical and medical insights. *Bioeng* **10**(2): 145.

Thajudeen B, Issa D and Roy-Chaudhury P (2023). Advances in hemodialysis therapy. *Fac Rev* **12**: 12.

29 Initiation and Prescription of Haemodialysis

Phang Chee Chin, Liu Peiyun

Indication of Dialysis Initiation

- The decision to start haemodialysis (HD) in patients with chronic kidney disease should be based on the presence of uraemic signs and symptoms, the trajectory of the decline of estimated glomerular filtration rate (eGFR), and the absolute eGFR.

Guidelines	Recommendations
2014 Canadian Society of Nephrology	• Asymptomatic patients when the eGFR declines to below 6 mL/min/1.73 m^2 or • When symptoms occur
2011 European Guidelines	• When eGFR < 15 mL/min/1.73 m^2 and symptomatic • Most patients will be symptomatic and need to start dialysis with eGFR in the range of 6 to 9 mL/min/1.73 m^2
2015 KDOQI	• No specific kidney function was recommended • Timing of initiation should be based on uraemic symptoms, evidence of protein-energy wasting, and the ability to manage metabolic abnormalities and volume overload medically

- Absolute indications to initiate HD:
    - Uraemic pericarditis
    - Uraemic pleuritis
    - Uraemic encephalopathy
- Other common indications:
    - Declining nutritional status
    - Volume overload refractory to medical therapy or difficult to manage with medical therapy (e.g., worsening uraemia)
    - Fatigue and malaise
    - Mild cognitive impairment
    - Refractory acidosis, hyperkalaemia, and hyperphosphataemia

Haemodialysis Prescription

- When prescribing HD (Table 29.1), consider the goals of therapy, volume of fluid needed to be removed, extent of solute clearance, residual kidney function, timing of dialysis, and logistical concerns.
- Care should be taken to prevent dialysis disequilibrium syndrome when initiating HD for the first time in a uraemic patient.
- The HD prescription should specify the following:
    - **<u>Virology</u>**

        As part of infection control measures in the haemodialysis centre, all chronic HD patients are required to be screened for hepatitis B and C as well as HIV at regular time intervals (Table 29.2). The results of these screening tests determine the allocation of HD machines to patients at the HD centre.

Table 29.1:   Summary of Common Dialysis Prescriptions

	Isolated Ultrafiltration	Intermittent Haemodialysis	Haemodiafiltration	Sustained Low-Efficiency Dialysis
Access	Vascular catheter/AVF/AVG			
Time (hrs)	3.5–5.0			
Blood flow rate (mL/min)	150–500	200–500	150–500	150
Dialysate flow rate (mL/min)	Not applicable	500–800	300–800	300
Replacement fluid rate (L/h)	Not applicable	Not applicable	2.0 to ~12 (given prefilter or post-filter)	Not applicable
Anticoagulation	Heparin or heparin free (no heparin given)			
Dialysate Sodium	Fixed 138–140 mmol/L Fixed vs. modelling			
Dialysate Temperature	35–37 °C			
Dialyser Membrane	Low flux	Low or high flux	High flux	Low or high flux
Ultrafiltration	UF not more than 10 mL/hr/kg or > 5% of predialysis weight over 4 hrs			

Abbreviations: AVF, arteriovenous fistula; AVG, arteriovenous graft; UF, ultrafiltration

Table 29.2:   Screening for Blood Borne Diseases at the Renal Dialysis Centre in Singapore (Adopted from the National Infection Prevention and Control Guideline for Outpatient Dialysis Centres 2020)

Predialysis Status	Before Admission	3 Monthly	6 Monthly
All patients	• Anti-HBs • HBsAg • Anti-HBc (Total) • Anti-HCV • HIV Ag-Ab • HBV DNA (if Anti-HBc total positive) • ALT	ALT	

a) HBV-susceptible as defined by
  – HBsAg, anti-HBs, and anti-HBc (total) negative
  – HBsAg, anti-HBs negative, and anti-HBc (total) positive but HBV DNA negative
b) HBC-immune as defined by
  – Anti-HBs positive (>10 mIU/mL)
  – HbsAg negative
  – anti-HBc (total) positive or negative
  – Anti-HBs >100
			• HBsAg
			• Anti-HBs

Anti-HCV negative		Anti-HCV	
Anti-HIV negative			HIV Ag-Ab

Abbreviations: Ab, antibody; HBsAg, hepatitis B surface antigen; HBc, hepatitis B core antigen; ALT, alanine aminotransferase; HCV, hepatitis C virus; HIV; human immunodeficiency virus

- **<u>Blood flow rate (Qb)</u>**

  The blood flow rate is measured in millilitres per minute. The higher the flow, the better the clearance. The commonly prescribed blood flow rate in chronic conventional HD ranges between 250 and 400 mL/min, depending on the clearance and the type of access. Not all fistula or catheters can sustain high flow. Patients initiated on HD for the first time or those at high risk of disequilibrium syndrome should undergo HD at a lower Qb (150–200 mL/min) to reduce the risk of disequilibrium syndrome. The Qb can be gradually increased over the first three sessions.

- **<u>Dialysate flow rate (Qd)</u>**

  The rate of the dialysate fluid flow is known as the Qd, measured in millilitres per minute. The dialysate fluid flows counter-current to the blood flow within the dialyser so as to optimise the concentration gradient between the blood and dialysate compartment. Increasing dialysate flow rate improves clearance but its impact is less effective than the change in blood flow rate (Qb). The typical Qb prescribed in conventional HD ranges from 500 to 800 mL/min.

- **<u>Duration</u>**

  Time on dialysis can range from 2.5 hours for short, frequent dialysis schedules to 6–8 hours for patients on nocturnal dialysis. Increasing the time on dialysis is one of the crucial factors in increasing the efficiency of dialysis. In conventional HD, the dialysis time is typically between 3.5 and 5 hours.

- **<u>Anticoagulation</u>**

  Anticoagulation is prescribed to prevent extracorporeal blood clotting during HD. The dose depends on the patient's weight. Anticoagulation-free HD is recommended in patients with:

- active bleeding
- intracranial haemorrhage
- recent major surgeries or procedures
- severe thrombocytopenia
- coagulation factor VII or VIII deficiency.

No additional anticoagulation is required during HD for patients already on systemic anticoagulation, such as warfarin, enoxaparin, or apixaban. Heparin is contraindicated for patients with a history of heparin-induced thrombocytopenia (HIT), especially HIT Type II. It is important to indicate not to prime or coat the dialysis circuit tubings with heparin or heparin-lock at the end of HD.

- **<u>Dialyser</u>**

The dialyser acts as the "artificial kidney" and filters out excessive uraemic toxins and fluid during HD treatments. Dialysers differ in size depending on the blood volume that will go through them. A bigger-sized dialyser provides better clearance. The type of solutes removed during HD also depends on the dialyser membrane pore size and other characteristics. Most dialysis units use high-flux dialysers to improve the clearance of middle-sized molecules. The term "flux" refers to the permeability of the membrane in the dialyser.

<u>Low flux</u>

Allows removal of smaller-sized molecules like urea and creatinine. They are used in HD and isolated ultrafiltration.

<u>High flux</u>

Allows removal of small and middle-sized molecules but prevents the accidental removal of protein from the blood. They are used in HD and haemodiafiltration (HDF).

- ### <u>Ultrafiltration/dry weight</u>

  Dry weight (DW) is defined as the lowest tolerated post-dialysis weight that can be achieved where there are minimal signs or symptoms of hypovolaemia or hypervolaemia. DW is achieved through a gradual change in post-dialysis weight after each HD session. DW will need to be adjusted when a patient is overloaded with fluids, gains or loses weight, or undergoes amputation of a limb.

  In chronic HD, ultrafiltration (UF) volume is determined by the prescribed DW. However, specific UF volume is ordered in patients who are haemodynamically unstable or unable to be weighed. Assessing a patient's fluid and haemodynamic status is crucial when ordering a specific UF volume. A UF rate of more than 5% of predialysis weight or > 10–13 mL/kg/hr increases the risk of hypotension and mortality.

Dialysis Disequilibrium Syndrome

- Dialysis disequilibrium syndrome (DDS) is characterised by a range of neurological symptoms that affect patients, mainly when they are first initiated on dialysis. Symptoms of DDS are primarily due to movement of water into the brain (causing cerebral oedema), triggered by a change in osmotic gradient between the blood and brain compartment when urea is rapidly removed from the blood during HD.

- Risk factors:
  - First HD treatment
  - Markedly elevated blood urea nitrogen concentration
  - Elderly or children
  - Concomitant hypernatraemia, hyponatraemia, or hyperglycaemia
  - Pre-existing neurologic abnormalities or cerebral oedema
  - Conditions associated with increased permeability of the blood-brain barrier (e.g., meningitis, vasculitis, thrombotic thrombocytopenic purpura or haemolytic uraemic syndrome)
- Common symptoms of DDS include headache, nausea, blurring of vision, and restlessness, which can progress into somnolence, confusion, and disorientation. Mild symptoms are usually self-limited. In severe cases, patients can develop seizures, stupor, and coma. Generally, symptoms cluster occurs at the beginning of the dialysis, but some can happen towards the end.
- DDS is a clinical diagnosis of exclusion (Table 29.3) as there are no specific diagnostic tests. DDS is suspected in patients with typical symptoms during the first HD treatment. Patients with mild self-limited symptoms typical of DDS may be managed

Table 29.3:   Differential Diagnosis of Dialysis Disequilibrium Syndrome

1. Hypo or hyperglycaemia
2. Hypo or hypernatraemia
3. Hypo or hypercalcaemia
4. Uraemia encephalopathy
5. Cerebrovascular accidents or other intracranial processes

expectantly but more severe symptoms require an extensive evaluation.

- The management of DDS should primarily be based on preventative measures to reduce the development of cerebral oedema. The urea reduction rate during the first session of HD treatment should be lower to attenuate the change in plasma osmolality and osmotic gradient at the end of HD. This can be achieved by decreasing the HD time, Qb, Qd, and using a less efficient (smaller) dialyser. A short HD session of 2 hours with a lower Qb rate and a urea reduction ratio goal of 0.4 as an initial prescription is recommended for patients at risk for DDS.

References

Flythe JE, Assimon MM and Wang L (2017). Ultrafiltration rate scaling in hemodialysis patients. *Semin Dial* **30**(3): 282–283.

National Kidney Foundation (2015). KDOQI clinical practice guideline for hemodialysis adequacy: 2015 update. *Am J Kidney Dis* **66**(5): 884–930.

Nesrallah GE, Mustafa RA, Clark WF, *et al.* (2014). Canadian Society of Nephrology 2014 clinical practice guideline for timing the initiation of chronic dialysis. *Canadian Med Assoc J* **186**(2): 112–117.

Patel N, Dalal P and Panesar M (2008). Dialysis disequilibrium syndrome: A narrative review. *Semin Dial* **21**(5): 493–498.

Saha M and Allon M (2017). Diagnosis, treatment, and prevention of hemodialysis emergencies. *Clin J Am Soc Nephrol* **12**(2): 357–369.

Saran R, Bragg-Gresham JL, Levin NW, *et al.* (2006). Longer treatment time and slower ultrafiltration in hemodialysis: Associations with reduced mortality in the DOPPS. *Kidney Int* **69**(7): 1222–1228.

Tattersall J, Dekker F, Heimbürger O, *et al.* (2011). When to start dialysis: Updated guidance following publication of the Initiating Dialysis Early and Late (IDEAL) study. *Nephrol Dial Transplant* **26**(7): 2082–2086.

Zepeda-Orozco D and Quigley R (2012). Dialysis disequilibrium syndrome. *Pediatr Nephrol* **27**(12): 2205–2211.

Sheryl Gan, Liu Peiyun

30 Assessment of Adequacy of Haemodialysis

Chapter

Introduction

- Dialysis adequacy encompasses a broad range of measures and indicators that can be personalised to the dialysis patient to optimise care, achieve optimal quality of life and survival, and reduce the risk of cardiovascular complications.

- These measures would include patient-reported outcome matrices in addition to clinical and dialysis-related indicators.

- Dialysis adequacy is a multi-faceted concept not achieved through the delivery of dialysis dose alone (Figure 30.1).

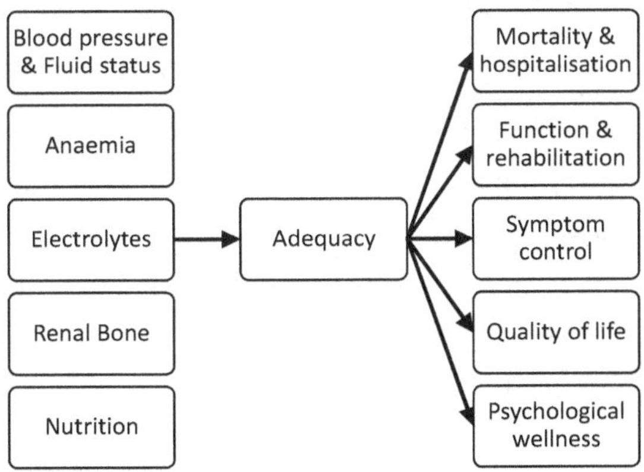

Figure 30.1:   Factors Affecting Dialysis Adequacy

327

Dialysis Dose

- Numerous indicators need to be considered to assess the adequacy of dialysis.

- Currently, urea is utilised as a convenient surrogate marker of dialysis dose for a particular HD session (Table 30.1).

- The delivered dose of HD should be measured at regular intervals 1–3 monthly.

- Patients who may require a higher dialysis dose are as follows:
  - Pregnancy
  - Females attempting to conceive
  - Patients requiring dialysis to remove dialysable poisons or toxins
  - Acutely ill patients with high catabolic output or high obligate fluid intake

Approach to Inadequate Haemodialysis

- A multi-pronged approach is required to address the presence of dialysis inadequacy.

- Table 30.2 specifies the considerations when the measured delivered dialysis dose is low.

- Table 30.3 specifies the measures that can be taken to increase the dialysis dose.

Table 30.1:   Indicators for Adequacy of Haemodialysis

Measure	How it is Done	Targets
Single pool Kt/V (spKt/V)	Mathematical formula with the following components • Sample urea pre and post HD* • Duration of dialysis • Ultrafiltration volume • Weight post patient post HD	3 times a week HD • Target 1.4 per session • Minimum delivered 1.2–1.4 per session
Equilibrated Kt/V (eKt/V)	Mathematical formula using the spKt/V.	3 times a week HD • Target 1.4 per session • Minimum delivered 1.2 per session
Standard Kt/V (stdKt/V)	Mathematical formula with the following components • spKt/V • Number of HD sessions a week • Duration of dialysis	For other HD frequencies apart from 3 times a week • Target 2.3 per week • Minimum delivered 2.1
Urea reduction ratio	• Sample urea pre and post HD* Less accurate as it does not account for: • Contraction in the extracellular volume • Urea generation during HD	3 times a week HD • Target 70% per session • Minimum delivered 65% per session
Online Kt/V	Measurement done on the HD machine Exact methods vary according to the HD machine.	As above, depending on frequency of dialysis.

Abbreviations: KT/V, "K" is dialyser urea clearance, "T" is total dialysis session time, and "V" is volume of distribution of urea; HD, haemodialysis

*All sampling of pre and post HD urea should follow current guidelines. For example, sampling of post HD urea should utilise one of the following methods:

1) Stop dialysate flow method
2) Slow flow method
3) Simplified slow flow method

Table 30.2: Factors Contributing to Inadequate Haemodialysis

Concern	Explanation	Solution
Patient is given their prescribed HD dose	There are numerous reasons why a prescribed dose may not be achieved. Some of the reasons may be chronic or recurrent issues.	Review reasons for why the prescribed HD dose is not achieved and address the concerns accordingly.
Malfunction vascular access	A malfunction vascular access may limit the achieved HD blood flow rate.	Address the vascular access malfunction.
Improper technique in AVF/G cannulation	HD needles sited too close to each other may result in recirculation and reduce clearance.	Review utilised needle size and cannulation technique.
HD circuit clotting	This may reduce the achieved HD time or the effectiveness of the HD membrane due to clot formation in the HD membrane fibres.	Review HD anticoagulation dose
Loss of RKF	The recommended RKF to allow for less than 3 times a week dialysis is urea clearance >2 mL/min.	Preventative measures should be considered to preserve RKF prior to the lost. Consider measuring urea clearance regularly when on less than 3 times a week HD.
Sampling errors in the calculation of Kt/V		Review practices and consider repeating the test.

Abbreviations: HD, haemodialysis; AVF, arteriovenous fistula; AVG, arteriovenous graft; RKF, residual kidney function; KT/V, "K" is dialyser urea clearance, "T" is total dialysis session time, and "V" is volume of distribution of urea

Table 30.3:   Interventions to Improve Adequacy of Haemodialysis

Measure	Considerations
Increasing blood flow rate	• Good vascular access • Review gauge of blood needle used (Table 30.4)
Increasing the dialysate flow rate	• Requires an adequate blood flow Most dialyser membranes may not significantly improve clearance if the blood flow rate is <50% of the dialysate flow rate
Increasing membrane surface area	• Requires an adequate blood flow Most dialyser membranes may not demonstrate a significant improvement in clearance with larger surface areas if the achieved blood flow rate is low

Converting to haemodiafiltration	• Requires the available expertise and infrastructure in addition to shared decision-making with the patient
	• To achieve a high replacement fluid rate (thus higher dose), patients should preferentially be able to
	  i. Have anticoagulation during HD
	  ii. Achieve higher blood flow rates

Increasing HD duration
Increasing HD frequency
	• Requires shared decision-making with the patient
	• Need to review the HD centre's available expertise and infrastructure
	• Consider intensive HD modalities depending on availability
	  i. Nocturnal HD
	  ii. Home HD
	  iii. Short daily HD

Abbreviation: HD; haemodialysis

Table 30.4:   Recommended Needle Size and Associated Blood Flow Rates

Needle Size (G)	Blood Flow (mL/min)
17	<300
16	300–350
15	350–450
14	>450

References

Hemodialysis Adequacy 2006 Work Group (2006). Clinical practice guidelines for hemodialysis adequacy, update 2006. *Am J Kidney Dis* **48**(Suppl 1): S2–S90.

Kerr P, Perkovic V, Petrie J, *et al.* (2005). The CARI guidelines. Dialysis adequacy (HD) guidelines. *Nephrology* **10**(Suppl 4): S61–S80.

Kerr PG, Toussaint ND, Kidney Health Australia, *et al.* (2013). KHA-CARI guideline: Dialysis adequacy (haemodialysis): dialysis membranes. *Nephrology* **18**(7): 485–488.

National Kidney Foundation (2015). KDOQI clinical practice guideline for hemodialysis adequacy: 2015 update. *American J Kidney Dis* **66**(5): 884–930.

Tattersall J, Martin-Malo A, Pedrini L, *et al.* (2007). EBPG guideline on dialysis strategies. *Nephrol Dial Transplant* **22**(Suppl 2): ii5–ii21.

31 Fluid Overload in Haemodialysis Patients

Phang Chee Chin, Lina Choong

Introduction

- Fluid overload is a common complication in patients with end-stage kidney disease (ESKD). It is associated with:
  - Hypertension (HTN) — fluid overload is the most common cause of HTN in HD patients
  - An increased risk of hospitalisation
  - Higher all-cause and cardiovascular mortality
  - Increased arterial stiffness, dilatation of cardiac chambers, and cardiac dysfunction
  - Chronic inflammation
- Fluid overload develops in HD patients because the cumulative fluid intake during interdialytic periods exceeds fluid losses via bodily losses (e.g., urine, stool, respiration, sweat) and ultrafiltration (UF) during HD.
- Common causes of fluid overload in patients on HD include:
  - Non-adherence to dietary salt and fluid restrictions
  - Missed HD sessions

- Cumulative fluid overload due to incomplete HD sessions (e.g., UF was repeatedly discontinued due to recurrent episodes of intradialytic hypotension (IDH))
- Dry weight has not been adjusted to recent weight loss
- Cardiac failure

Non-adherence to dietary intake and HD sessions or incomplete HD sessions can lead to high interdialytic weight gain (IDWG).

- High IDWG can trigger a vicious cycle where a high UF rate and volume to treat high IDWG can lead to IDH prompting discontinuation of UF and saline infusions. This leads to further expansion of fluid volume, hypertension, and addition of antihypertensive drugs. The latter may further increase the risk of IDH in subsequent HD. IDH also causes myocardial stunning which, if recurrent, can lead to myocardial fibrosis and cardiac dysfunction, another risk factor for fluid overload.

Diagnosis of Fluid Overload

- The mainstay of assessing fluid overload is a thorough clinical assessment but this can be challenging at times — clinical assessment may be inaccurate, leading to inappropriate intervention and consequential hypervolaemia or hypovolaemia (Figure 31.1).
- Some technologies and biomarkers have been evaluated to provide a more objective assessment of fluid volume status among HD patients (Table 31.1). For example, lung ultrasound has been shown to be superior to clinical assessment in detecting and monitoring fluid overload in HD patients.

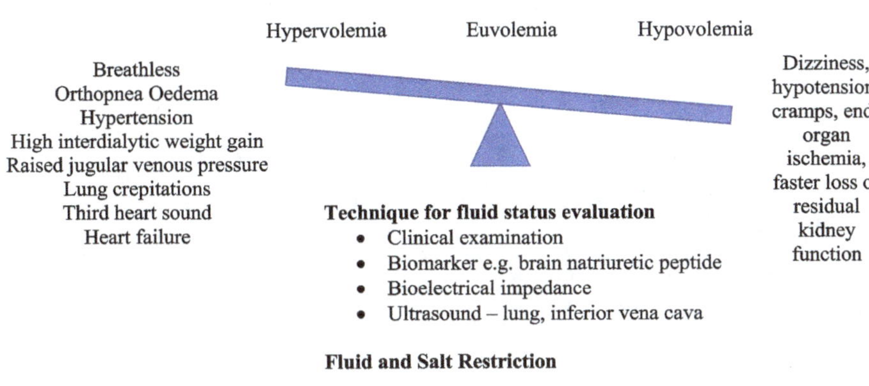

Figure 31.1: Assessment and Management of Fluid Overload in Patients on Haemodialysis

Management of Fluid Overload

• Management of volume overload in patients on HD is often challenging, involving many factors and requiring a multidisciplinary approach that includes nurses, dieticians, psychologists, and social workers.

• IDH, muscle cramps, nausea, and vomiting often constrain UF volumes. Cessation of UF, hypertonic sodium infusion, increasing dialysate sodium concentration, and early termination of IDH as the results of these complications may further impact the volume management of HD patients.

• General approaches to managing fluid overload in haemodialysis patients include:

  ▪ Excluding medical causes (e.g., cardiac failure)

  ▪ Ensuring adherence to salt and fluid dietary restrictions

Table 31.1:   Assessment of Fluid Volume Status in Patients on Haemodialysis

Tool	Methodology	Body Fluid Compartment Evaluated	Advantages	Disadvantages
Clinical	History • Dyspnoea • Orthopnoea • Salt and fluid intake • Control of BP • Changes in BW • IDWG • Adherence to HD sessions • Episodes of IDH with discontinuation of UF Physical examination • Raised JVP • Jugular venous distension • High BP • Third heart sound • Lung crepitations • Reduced air entry (pleural effusion) • Ascites • Oedema	• Total body water • Extracellular water • Intravascular fluid volume	• Inexpensive • Non-invasive • Easy to apply • Readily available	• Historical information may not be forthcoming • Non-standardised • Observer-dependent • Not specific

Chest X-ray	• Dilated upper lobe vessels • Cardiomegaly • Interstitial oedema • Enlarged pulmonary artery • Pleural effusion • Alveolar oedema • Prominent superior vena cava • Kerley B lines	• Extracellular water • Intravascular volume	• Inexpensive • Non-invasive • Readily available	• Involves radiation • Not available at a HD centre • May not be specific (e.g., effusion may be infective)
Bioelectrical impedance	• Determines body's resistance (measure total body water) and reactance (measure body cell mass) by measuring an electric current passing through the body from distant electrodes on the body's surface	• Total body water • Extracellular water • Intracellular water	• Relatively inexpensive • Non-invasive • Easy to apply • Reproducible	• Interpretation is of limited value in some patients (e.g., pacemakers, morbidly obese, intra-abdominal fluid) • Also may require manpower, is time consuming, and may not be widely available • Some studies on bioimpedance-guided fluid removal report reduction in episodes of acute fluid overload, cardiovascular events, HTN, and IDH but no impact on mortality

(Continued)

Table 31.1:   (*Continued*)

Tool	Methodology	Body Fluid Compartment Evaluated	Advantages	Disadvantages
Echo-cardiography	• Assess for echocardiographic parameters of fluid overload (e.g., dilatation of heart chambers like the D-sign (interventricular septal flattening due to right ventricular dilatation), pericardial effusion)	• Only assess intravascular volume	• Non-invasive • Can assess cardiac function and pathology	• Expensive • Requires well trained and proficient staff • Time consuming • Point of care echo-cardiography is not readily available at HD centres
Lung ultrasound	• Assess excessive interstitial lung water which is seen as thickened subpleural interlobular septa (B-lines)	• Only assess interstitial lung water	• Non-invasive • Inexpensive • Easy to apply • Has been shown to improve fluid and BP control	• Observer-dependent • Requires training • Not readily available • Not specific — B-lines can also be due to pulmonary fibrosis • Lung ultrasound-guided treatments have been shown to improve HTN and LVH in HD patients

Inferior vena cava diameter	• Assess diameter and collapsibility of the inferior vena cava during a respiratory cycle	• Only assess intravascular volume	• Non-invasive • Inexpensive • Long-established method	• Operator-dependent • Requires training • Not readily available • May be difficult to perform in patients with obesity or excessive bowel gas • Measurements may be affected by respiration, obesity, right heart function, and intrathoracic or abdominal pressure changes
B-type natriuretic peptide	• Hormone secreted by the heart in response to stretching	• Only assess intravascular volume	• Non-dialysable	• Not readily available • Not specific since levels are elevated in end-stage kidney failure • "Normal" levels in HD patients unknown • Expensive • Mainly used for research

(Continued)

Table 31.1:   (Continued)

Tool	Methodology	Body Fluid Compartment Evaluated	Advantages	Disadvantages
Relative blood volume monitoring	• An online blood volume sensor provide real-time measurement of haematocrit which can estimate changes in plasma volume	• Only assess intravascular volume	• Non-invasive • Real-time monitoring • Reproducible • Useful to identify a critical fluid volume under which intradialytic hypotension will occur	• Only for intradialytic assessment • Not readily available • Low accuracy and reproducibility • Requires expert interpretation • Data is conflicting on whether intradialytic blood volume monitoring is beneficial or not

Modified from Loutradis C, Sarafidis PA, Ferro CJ, *et al.* (2021). Volume overload in haemodialysis: diagnosis, cardiovascular consequences, and management. *Nephrol Dial Transplant* **36**(12): 2182–2193.

Abbreviations: BP, blood pressure; BW, body weight; BNP, brain natriuretic peptide; DW, dry weight; HD, haemodialysis; HTN, hypertension; IDH, intradialytic hypotension; IDWG, interdialytic weight gain; JVP, jugular venous pressure; LVH, left ventricular hypertrophy; UF, ultrafiltration

- Starting loop diuretics in those with residual kidney function
- Reviewing and adjusting dry weight
- Increasing HD duration or frequency to avoid high UF ratae, especially in patients with high interdialytic weight gain

References

Flythe JE, Chang TI, Gallagher MP, *et al.* (2020). Blood pressure and volume management in dialysis: Conclusions from a Kidney Disease: Improving Global Outcomes (KDIGO) Controversies Conference. *Kidney Int* **97**(5): 861–876.

Loutradis C, Sarafidis PA, Ferro CJ, *et al.* (2021). Volume overload in hemodialysis: Diagnosis, cardiovascular consequences, and management. *Nephrol Dial Transplant* **36**(12): 2182–2193.

32 Hypertension in Haemodialysis Patients

Phang Chee Chin, Lina Choong

Introduction

- Hypertension (HTN) is common in dialysis patients, with an estimated prevalence of over 50–85% of haemodialysis (HD) patients. The reported prevalence varies widely because of differences in the definition of HTN and blood pressure monitoring methods.

- Fluid overload is one of the most important risk factors for HTN among HD patients and is the main reason why HTN is most common among patients newly initiated on HD.

- The National Kidney Foundation Kidney Disease Outcomes Quality Initiative guidelines suggest that pre-HD and post-HD blood pressure (BP) should be <140/90 and <130/80 mmHg, respectively. However, these parameters have not been consistently associated with the risks of poor cardiovascular outcomes such as stroke, cardiovascular and all-cause mortality. Instead, inter-dialytic BP is better associated with cardiovascular risks and death.

Diagnosis and Monitoring

- Diagnosis and monitoring of BP in HD patients is challenging due to the variability in BP from ultrafiltration that occurs during HD. In addition, other factors affect the accuracy of BP measurements at the HD centre, such as inadequate time to rest or position properly prior to BP measurement, vascular abnormalities, and current BP machines not having been validated for use in HD patients.

- There are different methods of BP monitoring in HD patients (Table 32.1). However, the current gold standard method in diagnosing and monitoring HTN is ambulatory BP monitoring (ABPM) over a 44-hours interdialytic period.

- A 44-hours interdialytic ABP has been shown to predict risk for mortality in patients on chronic HD. However, this is not routinely available and an acceptable alternative is home BP monitoring.

Pathogenesis

- Hypertension in HD patients is a complex interplay of fluid overload, vasoconstrictive neurohormonal mechanisms, endothelial dysfunction, and comorbid conditions (Figure 32.1).

Management

- Targets for BP control among HD patients remain unclear — there are no large-scale randomised clinical trials to address BP targets in this patient population. As a result, treatment of HTN needs to be individualised to the patient's condition.

Table 32.1:   Methods of Blood Pressure Monitoring in Haemodialysis Patients

Blood Pressure Monitoring	Considerations	Diagnosis
Pre- and post-dialysis BP measurement	• Important for assessing patients' haemodynamic stability before and after HD • However, it does not correlate well with ABPM; predialysis BP is often overestimated, while post-dialysis often underestimates BP readings	• Not recommended for HTN diagnosis or titration of antihypertensive medication
Ambulatory BP monitoring (ABPM)	• The gold standard for diagnosing HTN • Correlates better with LVH and all-cause mortality • Not practical for the day-to-day management of HTN	• An average BP ≥ 130/80 mmHg over 24-hr monitoring during a mid-week day free of HD — better if it is extended to 44 hrs, covering a whole mid-week dialysis interval
Home BP measurements	• A practical and efficient way to diagnose HTN and day-to-day management of BP • Correlates with ABPM and outcomes • Recommended to check home BP readings twice a day for 4 days after the midweek dialysis treatment	• An average BP ≥ 135/85 mmHg for measurements collected in the morning and the evening over 6 non-dialysis days (covering a period of 2 weeks)

Abbreviations: ABPM, ambulatory blood pressure monitoring; BP, blood pressure; HRS, hours; HTN, hypertension; LVH, left ventricular hypertrophy; HD, haemodialysis

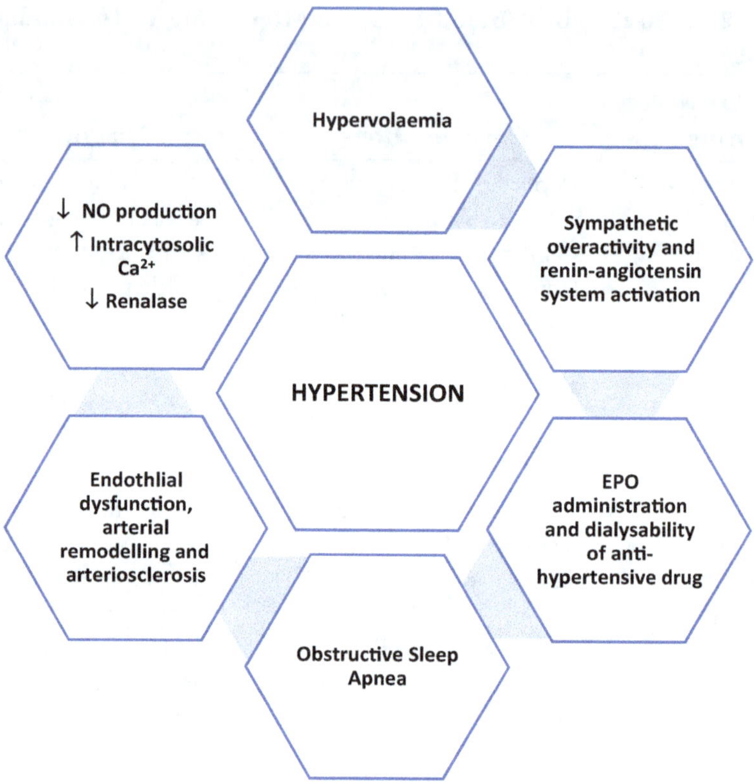

Figure 32.1: Factors Contributing to Hypertension in Patients on Haemodialysis

- HTN in HD patients involve non-pharmacological/haemodialysis-related (Table 32.2) and pharmacological interventions (Table 32.3).

Pharmacological treatment

- Most patients on HD will require antihypertensive therapy despite achieving optimal dry weight.

- The optimal antihypertensive regimen in patients on HD is unknown. Few classes of antihypertensive drugs have been studied specifically in patients on chronic HD.

Table 32.2: Nonpharmacological Treatment for Hypertension in Haemodialysis Patients

Nonpharmacological Treatment	Explanations	Approaches

Volume management	• Fluid overload is the most common cause of HTN in patients on HD
	• The DRIP (**D**ry-weight **R**eduction **I**n hypertensive haemodialysis **Pa**tients) trial showed that reduction of DW in HD patients with HTN resulted in decreased systolic and diastolic BP
		• Optimise and maintain proper volume status:
		  – avoid high IDWG
		  – set an appropriate DW
		• Regular clinical assessment for fluid overload — jugular venous distension, lung crepitations, peripheral oedema, chest X-ray
		• Other tools — bioimpedance analysis, relative plasma volume, measurement of inferior cava diameter, and bedside lung ultrasound may provide additional information to help determine the appropriate DW

Dietary salt restriction	• Salt consumption stimulates thirst and water drinking, leading to volume expansion • High salt intake is associated with high pre-dialysis systolic BP and cardiovascular death • Low salt intake is associated with improved BP control	• The recommended daily dietary sodium intake should not exceed 1.5 g of sodium or 4 g of sodium chloride

(Continued)

Table 32.2:   (*Continued*)

Nonpharmacological Treatment	Explanations	Approaches

Individualise dialysate sodium	High sodium dialysis improves haemodynamic stability and reduces muscle cramps but is associated with thirst, significantly higher IDWG, and BP.
	
	The DISO (Dialysate Individualised Sodium) trial showed that individualised dialysate sodium concentration based on serum sodium was associated with lower IDWG, lower BP, and less intradialytic HTN
		• Avoid high sodium dialysis.
		• Consider matching dialysate sodium to patients' average predialysis serum sodium level.
		• Potential risks with lower dialysate sodium
		  – IDH
		  – cramps
		• Individualise dialysate sodium, considering the patient's haemodynamic status, IDWG, and BP control.

Dialysis duration and frequency	Short dialysis sessions with high UF rates increase the risk of cramps and IDH, limiting optimal removal of fluid More prolonged or frequent dialysis reduces the need for a high UF rate	• Increasing dialysis duration or frequency (intensive dialysis).

Abbreviations: BP, blood pressure; DW, dry weight; HD, haemodialysis; HTN, hypertension; IDWG, inter-dialytic weight gain; IDH, intradialytic hypotension; UF, ultrafiltration

- The choice of antihypertensive drugs will have to be individualised to the patient's needs and conditions — beta and calcium channel blockers (CCB) are often prescribed. Consideration should also be taken on whether they are dialysable or not (Table 32.3).

  - Loop diuretics may be beneficial in patients with residual kidney function as increased urine output can reduce inter-dialytic weight gain which contributes to HTN.

  - Beta blockers have been observed to be associated with a lower risk of new heart failure and cardiovascular/all-cause mortality. They are beneficial in patients with a history

Table 32.3: Antihypertensive Medications and Extent of Drugs Removal with Haemodialysis

Drug	Percent Dialysability	Drug	Percent Dialysability
Angiotensin-converting enzyme inhibitors		**Angiotenin receptor blockers**	
		Losartan	Not dialysable
Ramipril	20–30	Candesartan	Not dialysable
Enalapril	35–50	Telmisartan	Not dialysable
Lisinopril	50	Valsartan	Not dialysable
Perindopril	50	Irbesartan	Not dialysable
Beta blockers		**Calcium channel blockers**	
Carvedilol	Not dialysable		
Bisoprolol	Not dialysable	Amlodipine	Not dialysable
Atenolol	50–75	Nifedipine	Low
Metoprolol	High	Verapamil	Low
Alpha blockers		**Centrally acting sympathomimetic drugs**	
Terazosin	Not dialysable		
Prazosin	Not dialysable		
Doxazosin	Not dialysable	Methyldopa	60
Hydralazine	Not dialysable		

of coronary artery disease and systolic dysfunction. Beta blockers reduce sympathetic overactivity and may prevent ventricular arrhythmias or sudden death. Bisoprolol and carvedilol are preferred since they are not dialysable.

- Calcium channel blockers such as amlodipine have been associated with lower mortality among hypertensive patients on HD. They have no or little dialysability.

- Angiotensin-converting enzyme (ACE) inhibitors and angiotensin receptor blockers (ARB) are beneficial in patients with heart failure and post-myocardial infarction. They also help to preserve residual kidney function and reduce left ventricular mass. However, their impact on mortality remains unclear. ARBs are preferred over ACE inhibitors since they are not dialysable.

- Mineralocorticoid receptor antagonists (e.g., spironolactone) are associated with lower cardiovascular and all-cause mortality, but systematic reviews and meta-analyses have not shown them to have any significant impact on BP control in patients on dialysis.

- Other classes of antihypertensive drugs (e.g., α_1-blockers) and centrally acting sympathomimetics are less frequently used.

Resistant Hypertension

- Some patients may be resistant to non-pharmacological measures and antihypertensive drug therapy. In such patients, it is important to exclude non-adherence, other medical conditions that can cause HTN, and use of drugs that can increase BP (e.g., calcineurin inhibitors, non-steroidal anti-inflammatory drugs).

Intradialytic Hypertension

- In most patients, BP will fall during HD and IDH may even occur. However, some patients may develop paradoxical HTN in the latter part of a HD session where most fluids have already been removed.

- Some factors that may contribute to intradialytic HTN include sympathetic overactivity in response to hypovolaemia, dialysis removal of antihypertensive drugs, improvements in haematocrit, and hypoxia.

- Administration of antihypertensive drugs or isotonic saline in the case of hypovolaemia may be used to treat intradialytic hypertension.

References

Agarwal R, Flynn J, Pogue V, *et al.* (2014). Assessment and management of hypertension in patients on dialysis. *J Am Soc Nephrol* **25**(8), 1630–1646.

Bansal N, Artinian NT, Bakris G, *et al.* (2023). Hypertension in patients treated with in-center maintenance hemodialysis: Current evidence and future opportunities: A scientific statement from the American Heart Association. *Hypertension* **80**(6): e112–e122.

Chen KT, Kang YN, Lin YC, *et al.* (2021). Efficacy and safety of mineralocorticoid receptor antagonists in kidney failure patients treated with dialysis: A systematic review and meta-analysis. *Clin J Am Soc Nephrol* **16**(6): 916–925.

Denker MG and Cohen DL (2015). Antihypertensive medications in end-stage renal disease. *Semin Dial* **28**(4): 330–336.

Rahman M, Dixit A, Donley V, *et al.* (1999). Factors associated with inadequate blood pressure control in hypertensive hemodialysis patients. *Am J Kidney Dis* **33**(3): 498–506.

Sarafidis PA, Persu A, Agarwal R, *et al.* (2017). Hypertension in dialysis patients: A consensus document by the European Renal and Cardiovascular Medicine (EURECA-m) working group of the European Renal Association-European

Dialysis and Transplant Association (ERA-EDTA) and the Hypertension and the Kidney working group of the European Society of Hypertension (ESH). *Nephrol Dial Transplant* **32**(4): 620–640.

Zucchelli P, Santoro A and Zuccala A (1988). Genesis and control of hypertension in hemodialysis patients. *Semin Nephrol* **8**(2): 163–168.

Chapter

33 Intradialytic Hypotension

Liu Peiyun, Sheryl Gan

Introduction

- Intradialytic hypotension (IDH) is a serious and frequent complication of haemodialysis (HD) which has been associated with disabling symptoms, end-organ ischaemia and mortality.

- Blood pressure (BP) falls in most patients during HD and there is no accepted "safe" BP range for chronic HD patients.

- In the literature, intradialytic hypotension (IDH) has been defined in many ways, such as

  - Type of BP parameter used (e.g., decrease in systolic BP (SBP) or mean blood pressure or nadir SBP)

  - An intradialytic SBP value below a specific nadir value

  - SBP drop accompanied by symptoms or need for interventions

- The National Kidney Foundation's Kidney Dialysis Outcomes Quality Initiative guidelines defines IDH as either a decrease in SBP $\geq$20 mmHg or mean BP $\geq$10 mmHg, leading to symptoms (cramping, headache, light headedness, vomiting, or chest pain) and need for interventions (e.g., reduction in ultrafiltration (UF) or administration of fluids).

- The prevalence of IDH differs widely (15–50%) due to variations in patients' characteristics (Table 33.1) and criteria used to define IDH.

353

Table 33.1:   Risk Factors for Intradialytic Hypotension

• Female	• Ischaemic heart disease
• Age >65 years	• Arrhythmias
• Pre-dialysis systolic blood pressure <100 mmHg	• Vascular calcification
• High body mass index	• Autonomic dysfunction
• Severe anaemia	• Poor nutritional status
• High interdialytic weight gain	• Hypoalbuminaemia
• Diabetes mellitus	

Pathophysiology of Intradialytic Hypotension

- IDH occurs because there is a decrease in effective arterial blood volume, leading to reduced cardiac filling and hence cardiac output that is insufficient to maintain BP.

- Increase in heart rate, cardiac contractility, and vascular resistance to the splanchnic and cutaneous beds (shunting blood to the central circulation) occur during hypotension but are impaired in IDH. These mechanisms may be dysfunctional due to patient and haemodialysis factors (Table 33.2).

Clinical Features of Intradialytic Hypotension

- IDH may cause light headedness, headache, nausea/vomiting, cramps, and post-dialysis fatigue in patients, which can be distressing and affect their quality of life.

Complications of Intradialytic Hypotension

- The nadir SBP during HD is prognostically important. An intradialytic nadir SBP <90 mmHg in patients with pre-dialysis

Table 33.2: Pathophysiological Factors Leading to Intradialytic Hypotension

Patient-related Factors	Haemodialysis-related Factors

• Medical complications
  – Cardiac failure with reduced contractility
  – Myocardial infarction
  – Pericardial effusion
  – Arrhythmias
  – Sepsis
• Anti-hypertensive medications
• Cardiac autonomic dysfunction — blunted sympathetic activity, reduced baroreceptor sensitivity
• Intradialytic meals, causing splanchnic vasodilatation and sequestration of blood in the splanchnic vasculature
	• Haemodialysis-related complications
	  – Haemolysis
	  – Air embolism
	  – Dialyser or tubing reaction
	• High UF rates (>10–13 mL/kg/hr) — removal of plasma fluid from the intravascular compartment outpaces the rate of plasma refilling from the interstitial and intracellular compartments.
	• Rapid clearance of waste products during HD may lead to transient reduction in plasma osmolality, shifting water from the extracellular to intracellular space.
	• Heightened Bezold-Jarisch Reflex (BJR), which refers to the triad of bradycardia, hypotension, and vasodilation when cardiac receptors are activated in response to hypovolaemia.
	• Dialysate fluid issues
	  – acetate buffer
	  – low sodium, calcium
	  – low magnesium
	• Thermal stress during HD — increase in core body temperature (due to complement activation) leads to vasodilatation of the skin vasculature and shifting of blood from the central to the skin circulation

SBP <160 mmHg or an intradialytic nadir SBP <100 mmHg in patients with pre-dialysis SBP ≥160 mmHg is strongly associated with mortality.

- Premature termination of HD sessions due to hypotension and symptoms will also contribute to inadequate dialysis and cumulative fluid overload.

Cardiovascular events and mortality

- IDH has been associated with reduction in myocardial perfusion and myocardial stunning (transient regional wall motion abnormalities of the myocardium due to ischaemia). Myocardial stunning is associated with cardiovascular events and mortality. Furthermore, repeated myocardial stunning can eventually lead to irreversible myocardial fibrosis, which reduces cardiac systolic function. As a result, heart failure develops and is predictive of increased cardiovascular mortality.

- IDH is also associated with an increased risk for myocardial infarction, hospitalisation for heart failure, fluid overload, as well as cardiovascular and all-cause mortality.

Cerebral ischaemia

- Intradialytic cerebral ischaemia, defined as a 15% decline in baseline cerebral oxygen saturation, is linked to low mean arterial pressure and occurs in about 25% of HD sessions.

- Repeated episodes of IDH-induced cerebral ischaemia is associated with ischaemic white matter changes and frontal lobe atrophy on brain imaging. Elderly patients experiencing IDH are at risk for dementia — patients experiencing ≥7 episodes of IDH in 90 days have the highest 5-year risk of new-onset dementia.

Other organ ischaemia

- Mesenteric ischaemia and liver ischaemia are less common ischaemic complications of IDH.

Loss of residual kidney function

- IDH has been associated with loss of residual kidney function (RKF), which is much more pronounced in HD than in peritoneal dialysis patients, especially in the first 3 months of dialysis initiation.

- Hence, IDH should be avoided in patients who are newly initiated on HD as these patients have higher RKF.

Vascular access thrombosis

- Patients with the highest quartile of IDH (SBP decline of 44 mmHg) experience a two-fold higher risk of developing thrombosis of an arteriovenous fistula as compared to the lowest quartile of IDH (SBP decline of 26 mmHg).

- However, IDH has not been shown to be associated with AVG thrombosis.

Management

Acute management

- Consider the Trendelenburg position (where the feet are raised higher than the head) to improve venous return to the heart.

- Stop UF on the HD machine.

- Administer oxygen therapy.

- If BP does not improve with the above measures, consider infusion of 250–500 mL of isotonic saline.

- Exclude complications relating to HD and other acute medical conditions (Table 33.2).

- Consider lowering blood and dialysate flow rates to reduce rate of change in plasma osmolality and osmotic gradients between plasma and intracellular compartments.

Prevention

- After excluding medical complications that can cause IDH, IDH can be prevented by adjustment of the HD prescription (Table 33.3), optimisation of patient condition (Table 33.4), and the use of biofeedback technologies (Table 33.5).

- Pharmacological agents (Table 33.6) should only be used if non-pharmacological measures fail to reduce the frequency of IDH.

Table 33.3:   Haemodialysis Prescription Factors to Reduce the Risk of Intradialytic Hypotension

Haemodialysis Prescription Factor	Adjustments to Prevent Intradialytic Hypotension
Avoid high UFR >10–13 mL/hr/kg	• Increase frequency of dialysis sessions per week • Increase duration of HD treatments
Cool dialysate	• Reduce temperature of the dialysate (35–36 °C) below the core body temperature to induce vasoconstriction and activate the sympathetic nervous system • Patients may not tolerate the cold sensations • The KDOQI and EBPG guidelines recommend the use of cool dialysate in patients with frequent IDH
Increase dialysate calcium concentration to 1.5 mmol/L	• Increase cardiac contractility, but high dialysate calcium concentration can lead to possible positive calcium balance and vascular calcification
Higher dialysate magnesium concentration	• Avoid low magnesium 0.25 mmol/L dialysate • High dialysate Mg may reduce intradialytic hypotension and risk for arrhythmias

Table 33.3: (*Continued*)

Haemodialysis Prescription Factor	Adjustments to Prevent Intradialytic Hypotension
Dialysate sodium modelling	• Removal of uraemic toxins reduces extracellular fluid osmolarity, resulting in a shift of extracellular fluid into cells • In sodium modelling, dialysate sodium concentration is high in the beginning of the dialysis session to maintain osmotic gradient and plasma refill. Dialysate sodium is then gradually decreased during treatment as uraemic toxins are cleared from plasma. • However, higher dialysate sodium in sodium modelling can result in thirst and volume expansion and increases BP. It may also be associated with higher all-cause and cardiovascular mortality. Thence, KDOQI and EBPG guidelines do not recommend sodium modelling
Isolated UF or sequential dialysis	• Removal of fluid isotonic to plasma, resulting in minimal change to plasma osmolality and potentially reducing IDH • Risk of inadequate clearance since time for solute clearance is reduced
Ultrafiltration profiling	• Provide higher UFR early in HD when interstitial space is larger and plasma refilling is higher • As treatment proceeds, interstitial space decreases in size, refilling rates decline, and UFR is reduced • Limited evidence for its efficacy
Haemodiafiltration	• Improved haemodynamics with convective therapy — alternative to cool dialysis • Treatment is more expensive
Switch to PD	• Requires assessment of potential barriers and patient's desire to perform self-care • Patient would have to undergo another surgery and training

Abbreviations: EBPG, European Best Practice Guidelines; UFR, ultrafiltration rate; KDOQI, Kidney Dialysis Outcomes Quality Initiative

Table 33.4: Patient Factors to Reduce the Risk of Intradialytic Hypotension

Patient Related Factors	Adjustments to Reduce Intradialytic Hypotension
Minimise inter-dialytic weight gain	• Restrict dietary intake of sodium • Loop diuretics for patients with residual kidney function • Preservation of residual kidney function by avoiding nephrotoxic agents

Set an optimal dry weight	• Regular clinical assessment is the mainstay but there are several newer methods to assess dry weight:
	  – Bioelectrical impedance spectroscopy (BIS): measures fluid status by measuring body resistance to electrical currents. Evidence remains insufficient to justify routine use for intradialytic volume management, and the interpretation of results is complicated in elderly and malnourished patients. BIS cannot be performed in patients with cardiac devices, metal implants and pregnancy.
	  – Lung ultrasonography: detect lung congestion using B line score
	  – Inferior vena cava measurement but significant intra and inter-observer variability and difficult to interpret in patients with heart failure and tricuspid regurgitation
	• The challenges of these novel tests are their costs, need for training to use them, and time required to perform them

Evaluate for underlying cardiac disease	• Optimise cardiovascular status (e.g., cardiac intervention)
Optimise nutrition	• Prevent protein energy wasting • Consider avoiding food intake during or just before dialysis if patient has recurrent IDH to avoid redistribution of blood from the central to the splanchnic circulation (controversial)

Table 33.4: (*Continued*)

Patient Related Factors	Adjustments to Reduce Intradialytic Hypotension
Optimise haemoglobin level	• Anaemia is a risk factor for IDH • Evaluate anaemia and consider increasing dose of erythropoietin stimulating agents, administration of iron, or blood transfusion
Intradialytic exercise	• Increase cardiac output and venous return
Intermittent pneumatic compression of the lower limbs	• Improves venous tone

Table 33.5: **Biofeedback Technologies to Prevent Intradialytic Hypotension**

Biofeedback Mechanisms	Description
Blood volume monitoring (BVM)	• Optical sensing device placed at the arterial end of the dialyser • Plasma refilling is estimated from relative blood volume changes calculated from changes in the haematocrit • Ultrafiltration rate and conductivity are adjusted accordingly after the information is processed by software • Evidence is conflicting on whether BVM can predict intradialytic hypotension
Temperature biofeedback	• Temperature at the arterial and venous lines of the extra-corporeal circuit is measured • Dialysate temperature is modulated to stabilise the patient's temperature at constant values • Core temperature is kept stable (isothermic) • Risk of shivering appears reduced
Arterial blood pressure biofeedback	• A feedback control linking arterial pressure to ultrafiltration • Alters ultrafiltration rate according to periodic measurements of arterial pressure and its trend during treatment to maintain an adequate blood volume • Further studies are required to evaluate the clinical utility of this tool

Table 33.6: Pharmacological Agents to Prevent Intradialytic Hypotension

Pharmacological Agents	Doses
Midodrine	• Oral prodrug alpha 1 adrenergic receptor agonist — improves venous return and reduces intradialytic hypotension • 2.5–10 mg given 15–30 minutes before haemodialysis (half-life 3 hours) • Observational data suggest that midodrine use is associated with higher mortality and all-cause/cardiovascular hospitalisation, but the interpretation of the data is limited by confounding factors
L-carnitine	• Required for mitochondrial energy metabolism in skeletal and cardiac muscle • Data on its efficacy is limited and its use may result in increased formation of uraemic toxin trimethylamine N-oxide
Setraline	• Augmentation of central serotonergic pathways • Small studies showing efficacy
Fluid administration	• Albumin or hyperosmolar solutions to enhance plasma refill by increasing intravascular osmotic pressure
Antihypertensive medications	• Timing of antihypertensive medication administration should be individualised, taking into account interdialytic BP and the frequency of intradialytic hypotension • Avoid nondialysable antihypertensive medications if episodes of intradialytic hypotension are frequent

References

Chan CT, Chertow GM, Daugirdas JT, *et al.* (2014). Effects of daily hemodialysis on heart rate variability: Results from the Frequent Hemodialysis Network (FHN) Daily Trial. *Nephrol Dial Transplant* **29**(1): 168–178.

Daugirdas JT (2001). Pathophysiology of dialysis hypotension: An update. *Am J Kidney Dis* **38**(4 Suppl 4): S11–S17.

Flythe JE, Chang TI, Gallagher MP, *et al.* (2020). Blood pressure and volume management in dialysis: Conclusions from a Kidney Disease: Improving Global Outcomes (KDIGO) Controversies Conference. *Kidney Int* **97**(5): 861–876.

Kanbay M, Ertuglu LA, Afsar B, *et al.* (2020). An update review of intradialytic hypotension: Concept, risk factors, clinical implications and management. *Clin Kidney J* **13**(6): 981–993.

Kooman JP, Katzarski K, van der Sande FM, *et al.* (2018). Hemodialysis: A model for extreme physiology in a vulnerable patient population. *Semin Dial* **31**(5): 500–506.

Monardo P, Lacquaniti A, Campo S, *et al.* (2021). Updates on hemodialysis techniques with a common denominator: The personalization of the dialytic therapy. *Semin Dial* **34**(3): 183–195.

Reeves PB and Mc Causland FR (2018). Mechanisms, clinical implications, and treatment of intradialytic hypotension. *Clin J Am Soc Nephrol* **13**(8): 1297–1303.

Sars B, van der Sande FM and Kooman JP (2020). Intradialytic hypotension: Mechanisms and outcome. *Blood Purif* **49**(1–2): 158–167.

Interventional Nephrology

Tan Chee Wooi, Tan Ru Yu

Introduction

- Haemodialysis (HD) vascular access can be categorised into temporary and permanent vascular access and are distinguished by their type, ease of creation, and performance (Table 34.1).

Table 34.1: Characteristics of Vascular Accesses to Perform Haemodialysis

Characteristics	Arteriovenous Fistula	Arteriovenous Graft	Catheter
Type of vascular access	Permanent	Permanent	Temporary
Maturation time	4 to 12 weeks	May be immediately or 2 weeks, depending on the material it is made of	Can be used immediately
Ease of creation	Technically demanding	Technically demanding	Easy
Initial success rate	Low	High	High
Long-term patency rate	High	Moderate	Lowest
Blood flow rate (Qb)	High	High	Low
Infection rate	Lowest	Moderate	High
Overall maintenance cost	Low	High	High

- Arteriovenous fistula (AVF) and arteriovenous graft (AVG) are preferred over HD catheters for their lower complication and superior long-term patency rates.

Arteriovenous Fistula

- An AVF can be surgically created by anastomosing a vein to an artery such as anastomosing the radial artery to the cephalic vein (radiocephalic), the brachial artery to the cephalic vein (brachiocephalic), and the brachial artery to the basilic vein (brachiobasilic) (Figure 34.1). Brachiobasilic AVF often needs transposition before it is useable for dialysis.

- Compared to AVG and tunnelled dialysis catheter, AVF provides the best outcome in terms of patency rate, infection rate, as well as overall maintenance cost.

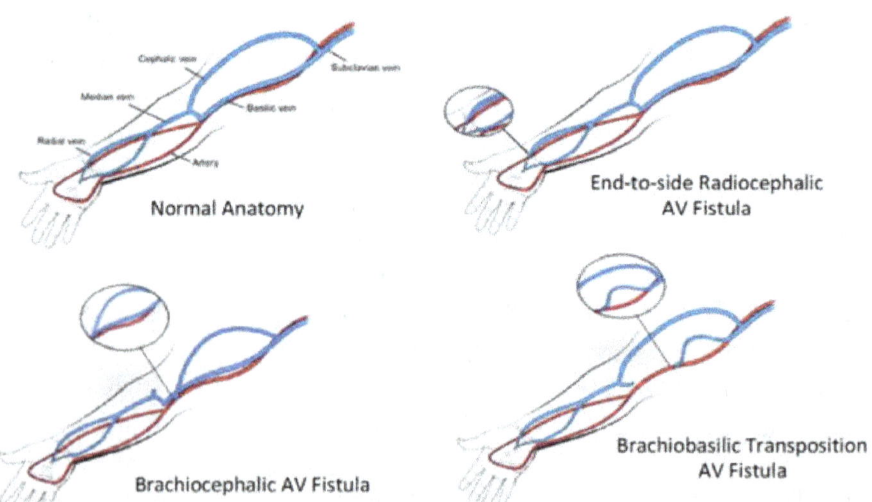

Figure 34.1:   Types of Arteriovenous Fistulas

Adapted from Baylor Medicine (https://www.bcm.edu/healthcare/specialties/cardiovascular-medicine/vascular-health/hemodialysis). Credit: Scott Holmes.

- However, creating an AVF can be technically challenging due to the lack of optimal vessels, especially with HD increasingly offered to older patients with more co-morbidities such as diabetes mellitus and peripheral vascular disease. In particular, pre-operative vessels with a diameter of less than 2 mm have been associated with high failure rates.

- There are multiple factors that could contribute to successful AVF creation and maturation, such as:

  - Timely referral to vascular surgeon for access planning

  - Preservation of veins by avoiding peripherally inserted central catheters and transvenous cardiac implantable devices, whenever possible

  - Pre-operative vein mapping

- Recently, an endovascular approach to AVF creation has increasingly gained acceptance as an alternative to the surgical creation of AVF. Several devices have been approved for use in Singapore where endovascular AVF (EndoAVF) (Figure 34.2)

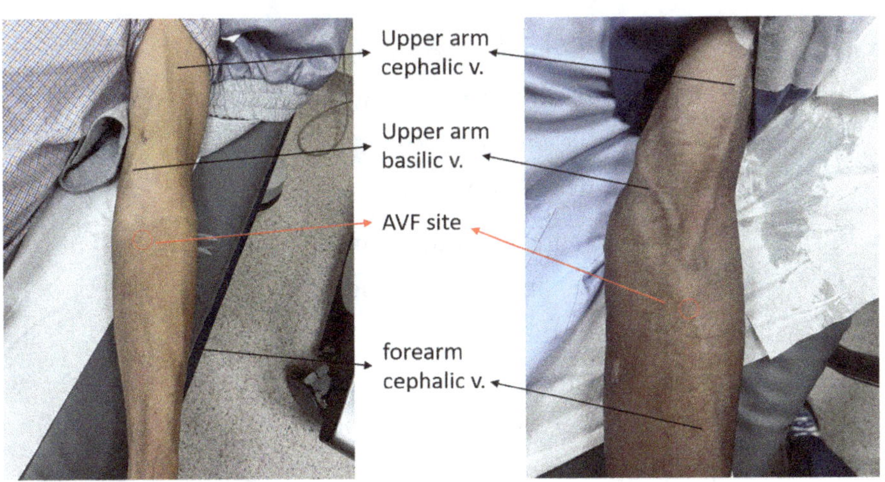

Figure 34.2:   Endo-arteriovenous Fistulas

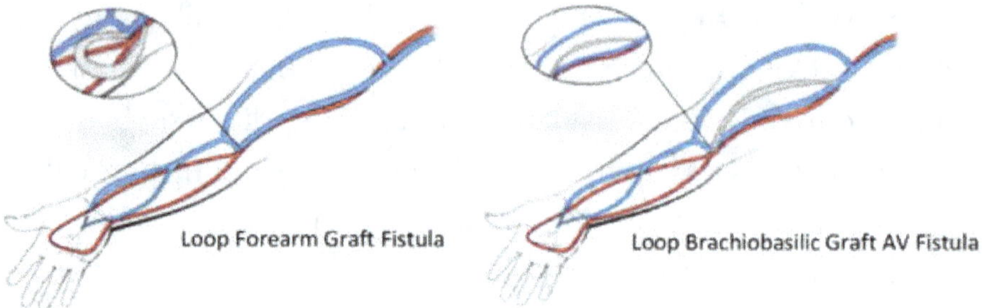

Figure 34.3: Types of Arteriovenous Grafts

Adapted from Baylor Medicine (https://www.bcm.edu/healthcare/specialties/cardiovascular-medicine/vascular-health/hemodialysis). Credit: Scott Holmes.

is created in the upper forearm by anastomosing the radial or ulnar artery to a deep vein via radiofrequency (WavelinQ device) or the radial artery to a perforating vein using thermal anastomosis (Ellipsys device). The blood flows via perforating veins into superficial veins after anastomosis, resulting in multiple superficial vessel dilatations for cannulation.

Arteriovenous Graft

- When veins are too small to support an AVF, an AVG is the next best option. Instead of connecting an artery to a vein, AVG is surgically constructed by interposing a graft (prosthetic or biologic) between an artery and vein.

- Graft configuration can be straight or looped and located at the forearm, upper arm, and thigh. The main benefit of AVG is that there is no maturation time, so it can be used for dialysis as soon as 24 hours after its creation, depending on the type of graft used. However, AVGs are associated with higher infection rates and patency maintenance costs than AVFs.

Haemodialysis Catheter

- Haemodialysis catheters (HDC) usually have two main lumens attached to two ports (blue and red coloured) and can be categorised into tunnelled or non-tunnelled HDCs (Table 34.2). Non-tunnelled HDCs may have a third lumen present for blood draws and drug-delivery (Figure 34.4).

- By convention, the red port is used as the "arterial" lumen to draw blood from the body and the blue port is used as the "venous" lumen for the return of blood from dialysis machines to the patients. The flow direction may occasionally be reversed on dialysis if blood flow is limited in the conventional direction, but this increases the risk for recirculation, reduced solute clearance, and possibly inadequate dialysis.

Table 34.2: Characteristics of Non-Tunnelled and Tunnelled Dialysis Catheters

Non-tunnelled Dialysis Catheters	Tunnelled Dialysis Catheters

<ul><li>Shorter extra-vascular segment, emerged from the skin at the site of entry into the vein</li><li>Short term usage depending on the insertion site (<7 days for the femoral vein and up to 14 days for the internal jugular vein)</li><li>General guide for the length
  – Right internal jugular vein: 16 cm
  – Left internal jugular vein: 19–20 cm
  – Femoral vein: 20–24 cm</li><li>Not for chronic, long-term, or outpatient haemodialysis</li></ul>
	<ul><li>Presence of a Dacron cuff ensures subcutaneous anchoring and reduces risk of infection</li><li>Tunnelled under the skin from the point of insertion in the vein to an exit site some distance away</li><li>Right internal jugular is the preferred site of insertion unless contraindicated followed by the left internal jugular vein and femoral veins</li><li>Longer term usage (>14 days)</li></ul>

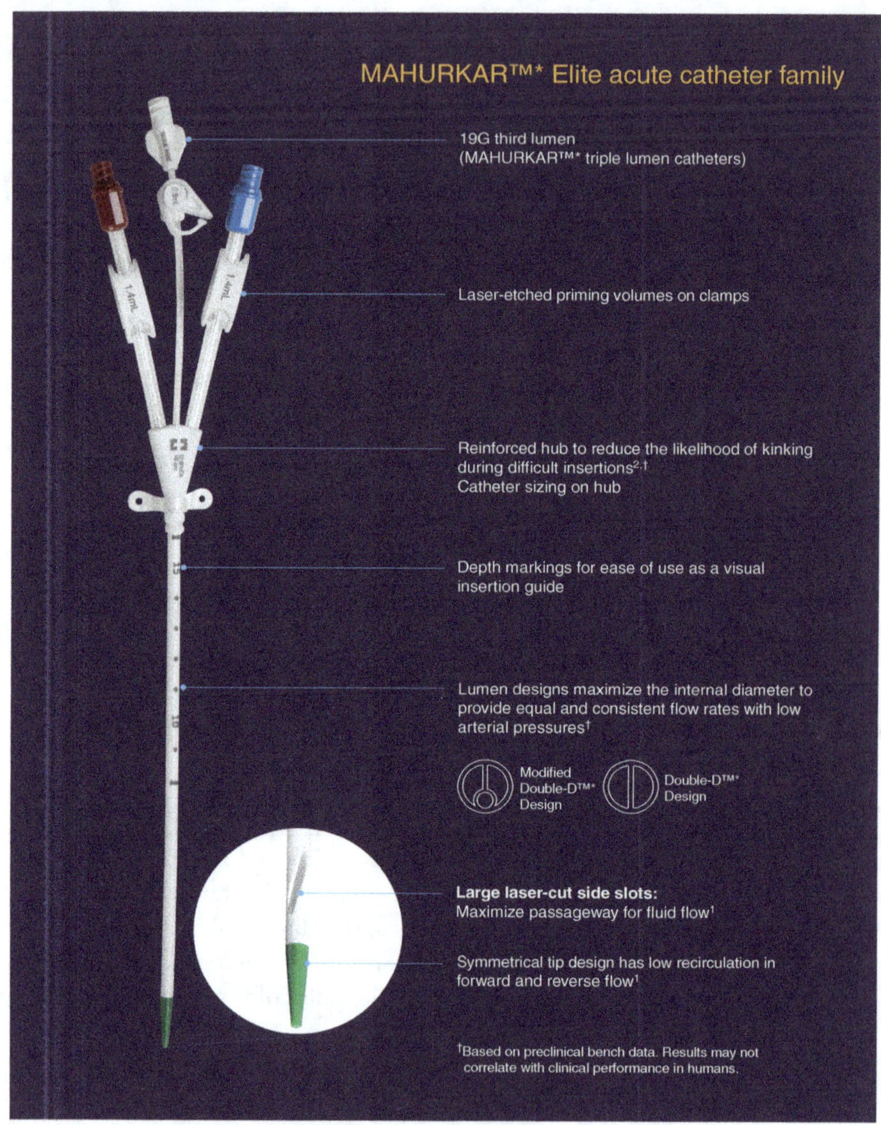

Figure 34.4: Non-tunnelled Dialysis Catheters

Photocredit: Medtronic (with permission)

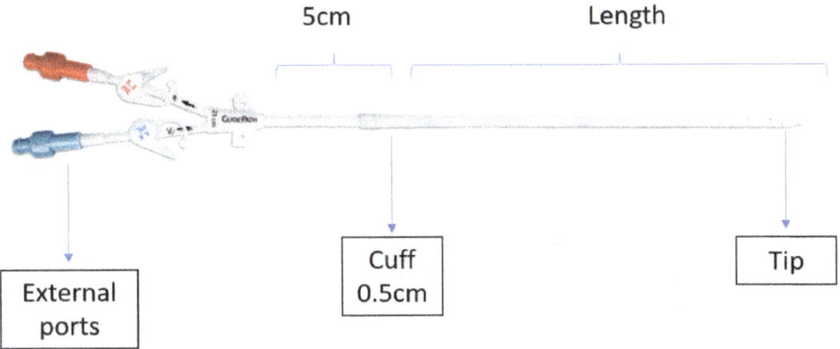

Figure 34.5:   Tunnelled Dialysis Catheters

The risk of recirculation during the reversal of flow direction is minimised in a HDC with a symmetrical tip.

- The selection of the appropriate catheter type is at the discretion of the practitioner. The operator should consider the need, requirements, and duration for the catheter, as well as access site location.

References

Canaud, B. *et al.*, 2019, 'Vascular Access Management for Haemodialysis: A Value-Based Approach from NephroCare Experience', in A. E. Berezin (ed.), Vascular Access Surgery — Tips and Tricks, IntechOpen, London. 10.5772/intechopen.84987.

Wu S, Kalva S, Park H, *et al.* (2021). *Dialysis Access Management 2nd ed.* Springer, Switzerland.

35 Haemodialysis Catheter Complications

Gan Chye Chung

- Haemodialysis catheter (HDC) complications can be classified according to the time it occurred (immediate or at the time of insertion and delayed or >1 week) (Table 35.1) or the type of complication — catheter-related infection, catheter dysfunction, and central vein stenosis.

Table 35.1: Short- and Long-Term Complications of Haemodialysis Catheters

Immediate Complications	Delayed Complications
• Bleeding	• Infection
• Arterial puncture	– localised catheter infection
• Venous laceration	– catheter-related blood stream infection

• Haematoma (haemothorax, haemopericardium, haemomediastinum)	• Mechanical dysfunction
	  – kinking
	  – bending

• Pneumothorax	– breakage
• Pneumopericardium	• Thrombosis
• Cardiac arrhythmia	– intraluminal
• Air embolism	– mural
	– atrial
	• Fibrin sheath formation
	• Central vein stenosis
	• Inadequate dialysis

Post-insertion Bleeding

- Persistent bleeding from the exit site following insertion of a HDC is common and exacerbated by uraemia-induced platelet dysfunction and possible use of antiplatelet agents for cardiovascular diseases. Methods to secure haemostasis include:
  - Manual compression or pressure dressing of both the subcutaneous tract and venotomy site
  - Desmopressin if the patient is uraemic
  - Placement of a purse string suture around the exit site of the HDC

Vascular Injuries

- Insertion of HDC under ultrasound (US) guidance has significantly reduced the incidence of vascular injury during HDC insertion but may still occur in <1% of patients.
- Accidental carotid artery puncture may occur, potentially causing haemorrhage, airway obstruction by a haematoma, arteriovenous malformation, and stroke.
- Pulsatile flow from the cannulating needle or catheter is a sign that an arterial puncture has occurred.
- In the event of an inadvertent carotid artery puncture, the management will depend on whether dilation of the venotomy site has been performed or not:
  - Pre-dilatation — If the dilatation of the venotomy site is not employed yet, the needle can be removed and the arterial puncture site should be compressed for at least 10–15 minutes.

- Post-dilatation — If the dilatation has been performed or the HDC has been inserted, the dilator or HDC should not be removed as it serves as a tamponade for the injured vessel. An urgent surgical consult needs to be obtained so that the artery can be repaired with open surgical repair or an endovascular arterial closure device.

- Venous injuries may not be immediately apparent and present themselves later as haemorrhagic shock, haemothorax, haemomediastinum, haemopericardium, or cardiac arrest. The patient should be resuscitated and urgent surgical consult should be sought.

Air Embolism

- Air embolism is a potentially fatal complication that can occur when the catheter ports are open to air during insertion or removal.

- The patient may present with tachypnoea, tachycardia, chest pain, cough, and hypoxia. If air has entered into the heart, a churning sound ("mill wheel murmur") may be auscultated.

- When air embolism is suspected clinically, the following manoeuvres should be performed:

  - Place the patient in the left lateral and Trendelenburg position to allow air bubbles to move out of the right ventricular outflow tract and into the right atrium.

  - Provide high-flow 100% oxygen therapy.

  - Attempt to remove air from the systemic circulation by aspirating from the central venous catheter.

- In the event of cardiopulmonary collapse, basic cardiac life support (BCLS) and advanced cardiac life support (ACLS) protocol should be employed accordingly.

- The patient should be transferred to the ICU for close monitoring and management.

- Hyperbaric oxygen therapy or extracorporeal membrane oxygenation (ECMO) can be considered.

Cardiac Arrhythmia

- Cardiac arrhythmias seen during insertion of HDCs are usually due to irritation by the tip of the guidewire at the atrial and ventricular endocardium.

- Most arrhythmias are benign premature ventricular contractions, but non-sustained or sustained supraventricular or ventricular tachycardias may occur.

- It is often self-limiting when the guidewire is pulled out by a few centimetres. When repassing the guidewire again, the tip of the guidewire should pass into the inferior vena cava.

- If arrhythmia is sustained despite adjusting the guidewire, the guidewire should be removed completely and basic or advanced cardiac life support protocols should be applied.

- In the event of difficulty passing the guidewire into the desired place, it is advised that the catheter placement should be done under fluoroscopic guidance.

Catheter Malposition

- Catheter malposition occurs if the catheter tip is in an unintended anatomical location such as in the mediastinum, arterial system, or venous system (not at the intended venous location such as the superior vena cava or mid-atrium) (Figures 35.1 and 35.2).

- In the event of a catheter malposition:

  - Do not use or remove the catheter as it serves as a tamponade for the injured vessel.

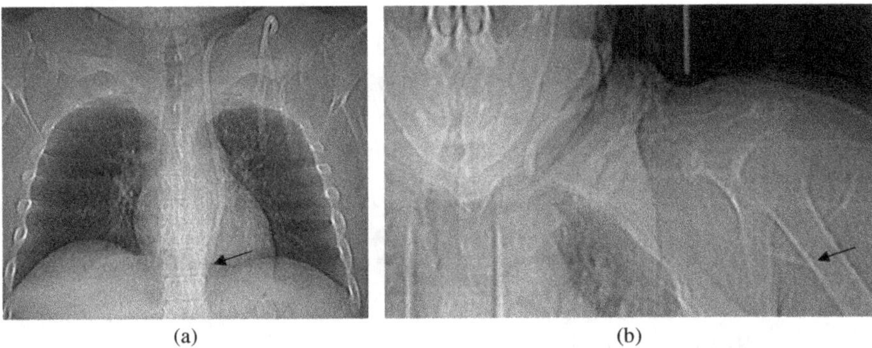

(a) (b)

Figure 35.1: Catheter misadventure: (a) The tip of the left IJV haemodialysis catheter did not cross the midline and is in the mediastinum, (b) The left IJV haemodialysis catheter did not cross the midline and is in the subclavian artery.

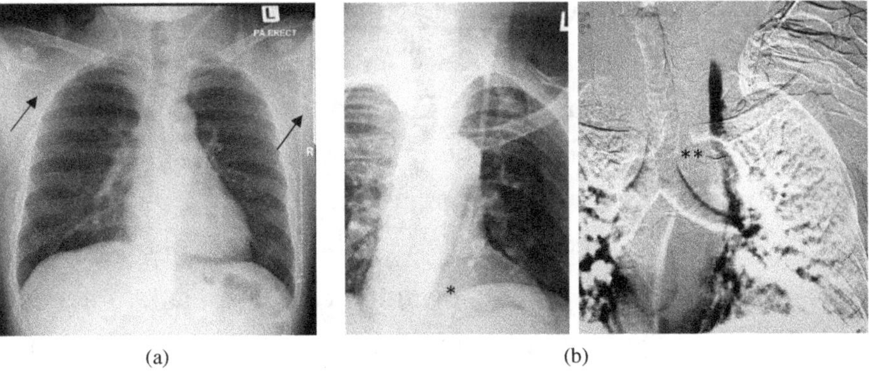

(a) (b)

Figure 35.2: (a) Both the tip of the right and left IJV haemodialysis catheter in the right subclavian vein and left axillary vein respectively, (b) The left IJV haemodialysis catheter did not cross the midline and travels from persistent left SVC into the coronary sinus* with the absence of left brachiocephalic vein**.

- Do not infuse fluids or medications if the catheter has no backflow of blood upon drawing from the catheter ports. Both ports should be clamped and recapped to prevent air embolism, pneumothorax, or pneumomediastinum.

- The patient should be monitored closely and resuscitation be given if necessary.

- An urgent surgical consult needs to be obtained.

Haemodialysis Catheter-related Infections

- Catheter-related infections are the most common complication of HDCs with their frequency depending on the site of insertion and type of catheter used:

  - Infections are more common with femoral vein insertions than jugular vein insertions.

  - Non-tunnelled HDCs have a higher incidence of catheter-related blood stream infection (CRBSI) at 3.8 to 6.5 episodes/1,000 catheter-days compared to 1.3 to 5.5 episodes/1,000 catheter-days for tunnelled dialysis catheter.

- Risk factors for catheter-related infections include older age, diabetes mellitus, malnutrition, iron overload, long duration of catheter use, peripheral atherosclerosis, previous episodes of bacteraemia, frequent manipulation of catheters, colonisation with bacteria, and contamination of the dialysis solutions.

- The most common pathogen causing catheter-related infection is *Staphylococcus aureus*, which can cause significant morbidity and mortality via its tendency for secondary metastatic infections.

- Catheter-related infections should be suspected in a patient with HDC whenever there is:

- Fever or chills

- Exit site or tunnel infection

- Potential metastatic infection (e.g., endocarditis, osteomyelitis, epidural abscess, septic arthritis)

- Septic shock

- Raised inflammatory markers

Among elderly patients, the symptoms and signs may be subtle such as altered mental state, hypothermia, hypotension, or abnormal glucose levels.

Catheter-related Bloodstream Infection

- When a patient is suspected to have a CRBSI, the following will need to be addressed:
  - Septic work-up
  - Antibiotic therapy
  - Removal of HDC
  - Response to culture and sensitivity (C/S) results

Septic Work-up for CRBSI

- When a patient is suspected to have a CRBSI, cultures and other tests should be performed prior to administration of antibiotic therapy:
  - Blood culture ideally from a peripheral vein and the HDC (discard the line lock; i.e., first 3 mL of blood using a separate syringe) — blood culture can be obtained from the HD circuit blood line (instead of the peripheral vein) if the patient develop symptoms and signs of CRBSI just before or during HD

- Swab any purulent discharge from the exit site of HDC for C/S

- FBC

- Inflammatory markers — procalcitonin, CRP

- Exclude other sources of infection (e.g., CXR, urine C/S, echocardiogram)

Empirical Antibiotic Therapy

- Empirical antibiotic covering gram-positive cocci and gram-negative bacilli should be given as soon as possible after the blood culture is taken, for example:

Gram positive cover:	Loading dose of IV vancomycin at 20 mg/kg followed by 500 mg given at the last minutes of each subsequent dialysis session. Pre-dialysis trough levels may be obtained to guide further dosing. If patient is allergic to vancomycin, daptomycin is an alternative.
Gram negative cover:	IV piperacillin/tazobactam 4.5 g q 12 h (over 4 h) or IV ceftazidime 1 g after each dialysis session. IV gentamicin 1 mg/kg is an alternative but associated with ototoxicity, especially when given together with IV vancomycin.

Removal of Haemodialysis Catheter

- If the patient has an urgent indication for dialysis at the time of presentation (e.g., acute pulmonary oedema), the HDC can be used once to stabilise the patient before any removal.

- For patients with non-tunnelled HDC, the HDC should be removed and its tip sent for culture. Whenever possible, the patient should be left "line-free" for as long as possible before reinserting a new HDC.

- Tunnelled HDC may or may not be left *in situ* depending on the clinical presentation. Tunnelled HDC should be removed if there is:

  - Severe sepsis (e.g., septic shock)

  - Exit site infection (e.g., purulent discharge, erythema/pain at the exit site)

  - Suspected metastatic infection (e.g., murmur, bone pain, arthritis)

  If possible, the patient should be left line-free for a defined period before insertion of a non-tunnelled HDC to continue HD while awaiting the C/S results.

Response to Blood Culture Results

- Antibiotic therapy should be adjusted to blood and other culture results when they are made available. For example, for patients with methicillin-sensitive staphylococcus (MSSA) infection, IV vancomycin can be switched to IV cefazolin 2 g after each HD session.

- If the tunnelled HDC has not been removed yet and the blood C/S shows *Staphylococcus aureus*, *Pseudomonas* spp, fungi, or multi-drug resistant bacteria, the HDC should be removed and a non-tunnelled HDC can be inserted after a line-free period to provide interim vascular access for HD.

- If the tunnelled HDC is left *in situ* and the patient clinically improves with antibiotics, a new catheter can be exchanged over the guidewire to replace the pre-existing catheter. Alternatively, the pre-existing catheter can be left *in situ* by the concurrent use of an antibiotic lock after each dialysis session for at least 2 weeks after completing 2 weeks of IV antibiotics.

- If the tunnelled HDC is left *in situ* and the patient does not clinically improve after 48–72 hours with antibiotics to which the identified pathogen is susceptible to, the tunnelled HDC should also be removed.

- A new tunnelled HDC should only be inserted after the patient clinically responds and there is clearance of bacteraemia.

- Blood cultures should be obtained to document clearance of bacteraemia during antibiotic therapy.

- The total duration of antibiotics is dependent on the type of pathogen, clinical response, and severity of infection, such as 4–6 weeks for uncomplicated *Staphylococcus aureus*, 1–2 weeks for gram-negative bacilli or *Enterococcus*, and at least 2 weeks for *Candida* species. Infective endocarditis should be treated for 4–6 weeks while osteomyelitis should be treated for at least 6–8 weeks.

Exit Site Infection

- Exit site infection is a localised infection at the site of insertion of a HDC or distal to the cuff of a tunnelled HDC. If left untreated, it may cause ascending infection into the tunnel tract and blood stream.

- In an exit site infection, there may be erythema, crusting and discharge, which should be swabbed for C/S.

- Most infections can be treated with either PO or IV antibiotics and catheter removal may not be needed.
- However, if the infection does not improve despite antibiotics, catheter removal is indicated.

Tunnel Tract Infection

- Tunnel tract infection is defined as an infection along the tunnel tract from the venotomy site to the outer border of the cuff.
- It presents with erythema and tenderness along the tunnel tract and there may be discharge from the exit site which should be swabbed for C/S.
- Tunnel tract infection is an indication for removal of HDC. Antibiotics should be given for at least 2 weeks.

Haemodialysis Catheter Dysfunction

- HDC dysfunction is defined as the inability to maintain the prescribed extracorporeal blood flow required to ensure adequacy of haemodialysis without increasing the duration of the haemodialysis session. It can occur early (within 1–2 weeks of insertion) or later after insertion.

Early Haemodialysis Catheter Dysfunction

- Early HDC dysfunction is usually due to technical problems such as suboptimal tip positioning, migration, kinking of the catheter, or a tight exit site suture that constricts the catheter. The HDC may also be inserted into a wrong blood vessel or into a pre-existing fibrin sheath if exchange over a guidewire is performed.

- A chest X-ray should be performed to determine the position of the tip of the HDC and identify any kinking of the catheter at the venotomy site due to acute angulation of the catheter upon entry into the internal jugular vein or at the exit site. Management is dependent on what is found on the chest X-ray (Table 35.2)

- For femoral HDC, an AXR should be performed to check that the tip is at least above the pelvic brim for the common iliac vein or at the L2–L3 lumbar vertebrae level for IVC placement.

Table 35.2:   Approach to Early Haemodialysis Catheter Malfunction

Early Haemodialysis Catheter Malfunction	Intervention
Tip of HDC below the middle of the atrium level	For non-tunnelled HDC, withdraw HDC to obtain appropriate tip position. Tunnelled HDC can also be withdrawn, provided the cuff is still within 1–2 cm proximal to the exit site after adjustment. Otherwise, a shorter tunnelled HDC needs to be exchanged over the guidewire.
Tip of HDC above the middle of the atrium level	This requires an exchange of the HDC over a guidewire, using a longer HDC.
Kinking of HDC at the venotomy site	Exchange of HDC over the guidewire is indicated and a new, less angulated subcutaneous tract should be created for tunnelled HDC insertions.
Tip in the correct position	For non-tunnelled HDC, this may be due to intraluminal clot and a new catheter should be inserted. For tunnelled HDC, thrombolysis could be attempted to lyse the potential intraluminal clot.

Late Haemodialysis Catheter Dysfunction

- Late HDC dysfunction is usually due to extra luminal obstruction from fibrin sheath formation around the catheter tip or a thrombus at the catheter tip or within the lumen of the catheter. Thrombus can also involve the entire vein (mural thrombus) or form in the right atrium.

- To prevent thrombosis between dialysis sessions, catheter locks with heparin or citrate have been used.

- In the event of intraluminal thrombosis of a HDC, a trial of thrombolytic dwell can be attempted for a tunnelled HDC (Table 35.3), but if this is unsuccessful, then exchanging the HDC over the guidewire with or without balloon fibrin sheath disruption should be arranged.

- For extraluminal thrombosis associated with a HDC where central veins are thrombosed, the patient may complain of pain, localised tenderness, and upper extremity swelling. CT and venography can confirm the diagnosis, which should then

Table 35.3: Thrombolytic Treatment of Thrombosed Tunnelled Haemodialysis Catheter

1. The catheter and surrounding area should be cleaned and draped under sterile conditions.
2. The caps of the catheter ports are removed and 5 mL of blood from each lumen is aspirated to remove the catheter lock.
3. 2 mL of tissue plasminogen activator (1 mg/mL) is instilled into each lumen and allowed to dwell for 30 minutes. Alternatively, urokinase can be used (60,000 IU diluted in 10 mL of normal saline to make a 6,000 IU/mL concentration).
4. At the end of the thrombolytic dwell time, 5 mL of blood is aspirated and discarded from each catheter port.
5. Catheter flow is then tested with a 20 mL syringe — if flow remains poor, catheter exchange over a guidewire should be performed.

trigger removal of the HDC and commencement of anticoagulation for at least 3 months.

- HDC-related atrial thrombosis is often asymptomatic but can present as cardiogenic shock, heart failure, tricuspid regurgitation, pulmonary embolism, and infection. The HDC should be removed and options for treatment of HDC-related atrial thrombus include thrombolysis, thrombectomy, or anticoagulation. The choice will depend on the individual patient's condition and availability of expertise.

References

Beathard G (1999). Management of bacteremia associated with tunneled-cuffed hemodialysis catheters. *J Am Soc Nephrol* **10**(5): 1045–1049.

Kairaitis L (1999). Outcome and complications of temporary hemodialysis catheters. *Nephrol Dial Transplant* **14**(7): 1710–1714.

Little M, O'Riordan A, Lucey B, *et al.* (2001). A prospective study of complications associated with cuffed, tunneled haemodialysis catheters. *Nephrol Dial Transplant* **16**(11): 2194–2200.

Oliver M, Callery S, Thorpe K, *et al.* (2000). Risk of bacteremia from temporary hemodialysis catheters by site of insertion and duration of use: A prospective study. *Kidney Int* **58**(6): 2543–2545.

Saad T (1999). Bacteremia associated with tunnelled cuffed hemodialysis catheters. *Am J Kidney Dis* **34**(6): 1114–1124.

Salgado OJ, Urdaneta B, Colmenares B, *et al.* (2004). Right versus left internal jugular vein catheterization for hemodialysis: Complications and impact on ipsilateral access creation. *Artif Organs* **28**: 728–733.

Schillinger F, Schillinger D, Montagnac R and Milcent T (1991). Post catheterisation vein stenosis in haemodialysis: Comparative angiographic study of 50 subclavian and 50 internal jugular accesses. *Nephrol Dial Transplant* **6**: 722–724.

Wu S, Kalva S, Park H, *et al.* (2021). *Dialysis Access Management 2nd ed.* (pp. 314–318). Springer International Publishing.

Chapter

36 Insertion and Removal of Haemodialysis Catheter

Alvin Tng

Indications for Non-tunnelled Haemodialysis Catheter Insertion

- Insertion of a haemodialysis catheter (HDC) is indicated for patients requiring:
  - HD or continuous kidney replacement therapy, but do not have any existing dialysis access such as arteriovenous fistula (AVF), arteriovenous graft (AVG), or a tunnelled HDC *in situ*
  - HD but placement of a tunnelled HDC is contraindicated due to presence of bacteraemia or sepsis
  - HD but placement of a TDC is contraindicated due to deranged coagulation parameters
  - Rest from an existing HD vascular access that failed cannulation or require further intervention

Sites of Insertion

- In the absence of previous history of central vein stenosis or the use of pacemakers, the right internal jugular vein (IJV) is the preferred side due to its direct anatomy, lower rates of infection, and convenience to the patient.

■ 389

Table 36.1: Equipment for Insertion of Non-Tunnelled Haemodialysis Catheter

1. A 12.5F non-tunnelled dialysis catheter set (16 cm for right IJV, 20 cm for left IJV or femoral; 24 cm for femoral insertion in patients with large body habitus) which will contain an 18G introducer needle, a 0.035' guidewire, and a set of 10 and 12F dilators
2. Line insertion kit which should contain (1) a sterile tray, (2) gauze, (3) cotton balls, (4) needle holder, (5) tissue forceps, (6) scissors, (7) and syringes (2 × 10 cc syringe and 1 × 20 cc syringe)
3. 1% lignocaine or lidocaine
4. Normal saline
5. 1 mL heparin 5000 IU/mL vial
6. Chlorhexodane cleaning solution
7. 2/0 non-absorbable suture × 1
8. Ultrasound (US) probe with sterile cover and gel

- The 2nd choice would be the left IJV followed by the femoral veins due to their higher risk of infection. It is important to note that the femoral catheter should not be placed on the same side of the transplanted kidney as it can injure the vasculature of the transplanted kidney and result in venous obstruction or thrombosis of the transplanted kidney.

Insertion of Right IJV Non-tunnelled Haemodialysis Catheter

- The insertion of a HDC under US guidance increases the likelihood of successful insertion and is associated with lower risks of arterial puncture. US imaging helps in the localisation of the target vein and detection of any abnormal anatomy or intraluminal thrombosis. Hence, it is important to combine both knowledge from anatomic landmark techniques and US guidance to achieve successful and safe dialysis catheter placement.

Table 36.2: Steps in Insertion of Right Internal Jugular Venous Non-Tunnelled Haemodialysis Catheter

1. Informed consent should be obtained from the patient before proceeding to insert the catheter.
2. Equipment and cardiac monitoring should be made ready for dialysis catheter insertion in the IJV.
3. The proceduralist should review the indications for non-tunnelled dialysis catheter insertion and plan the site of placement.
4. Standing at the head of the bed, the proceduralist should scan both IJVs to assess their patency and decide on the site of placement of the catheter.
   - If the vein appears small or collapsed, the patient should be placed in the Trendelenburg position to distend the vein and reassess its size. If the vein appears large with multiple collateral veins in the neck, central vein stenosis may be present and the proceduralist may wish to choose a femoral insertion site instead.
   - If the vein is non-compressible, colour-doppler mode on the US should be used to ensure that the vessel is patent and not thrombosed.
5. The insertion site should be cleaned and draped.
6. The US probe should be placed within the sterile sleeve and positioned at the apex of the anatomical triangle (formed by the two heads of the sternocleidomastoid muscle and the clavicle) (Figure 36.1). A transverse view of the IJV should also be obtained by placing the US probe perpendicular to the IJV (Figure 36.2).

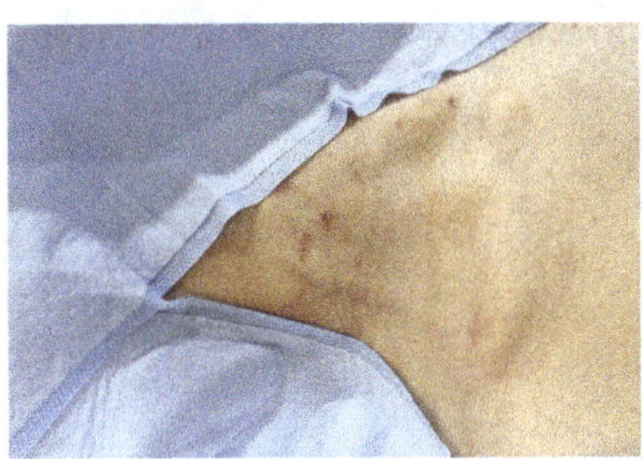

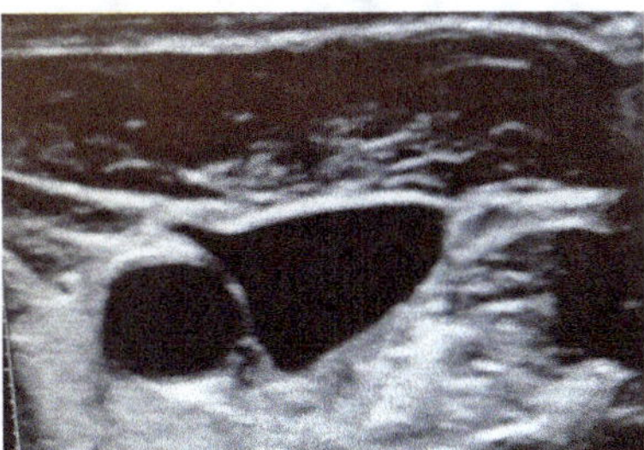

Figure 36.1   **Figure 36.2**

7. The skin is then anaesthetised over the insertion site with 1% lidocaine (Figure 36.3).
8. The 18G introducer needle is inserted into the vein under real-time US guidance. Avoid puncturing through the muscle as this would result in discomfort when the patient turns their head.
9. After successful cannulation, the guidewire is inserted through the introducer needle into the IJV (Figure 36.4).

(Continued)

Table 36.2:　(*Continued*)

- If there is any resistance, the guidewire should not be forced in. Instead, the guidewire should be removed and blood should be aspirated via the needle with a syringe. This is to check for smooth blood flow to ensure that the needle had not dislodged during the insertion of the guidewire. If needed, the needle should be repositioned under US guidance.
- If there is persistent resistance and the guidewire is unable to advance adequately into the vein despite ensuring that the introducer needle is indeed in the vein, there may be underlying central vein stenosis. In such a situation, the guidewire should not be forced through. The needle and guidewire should be removed, and pressure applied for haemostasis. Another site for catheter insertion should be selected.

10. Cardiac monitoring should be observed for ectopic rhythms. The presence of atrial ectopics signify that the guidewire has entered the right atrium and will need to be pulled back slightly until the ectopic beats have resolved.

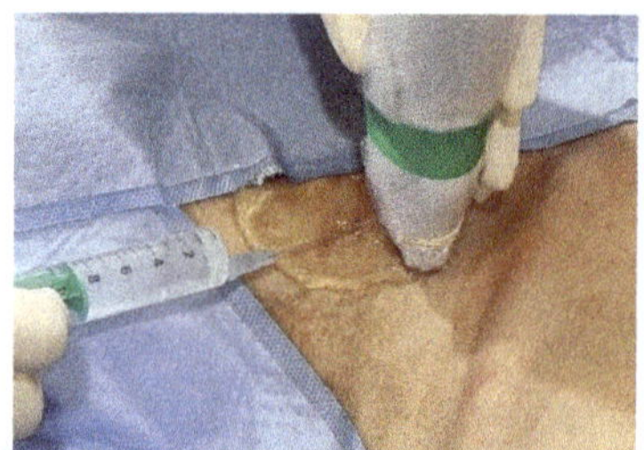

Figure 36.3

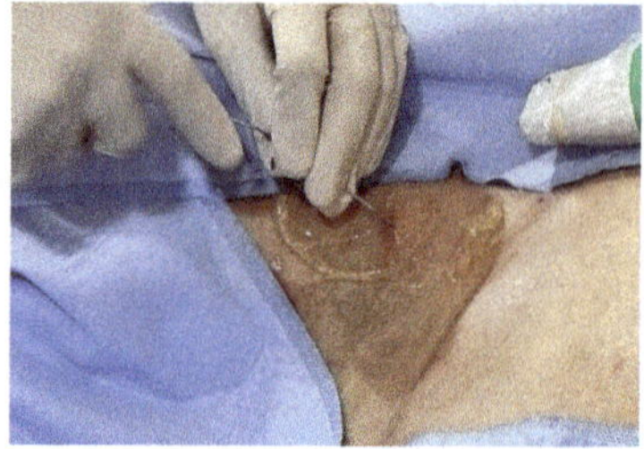

Figure 36.4

11. The introducer needle should now be removed over the guidewire. A small incision is made along the guidewire to enlarge the venotomy site (Figure 36.5). The venotomy tract is serially dilated by inserting a 10F dilator over the guidewire, followed by the 12F dilator (Figure 36.6).

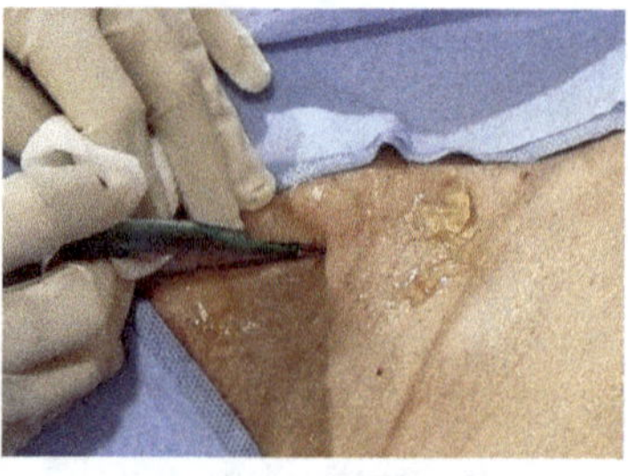

Figure 36.5

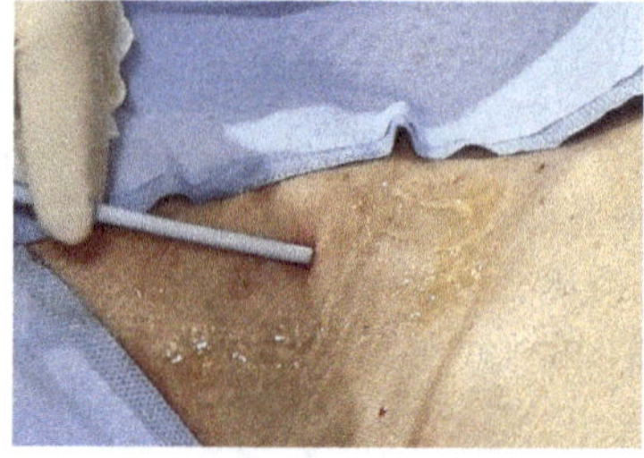

Figure 36.6

Table 36.2:   (*Continued*)

12. The 12F dilator is then exchanged for the 12.5F dialysis catheter (Figure 36.7).

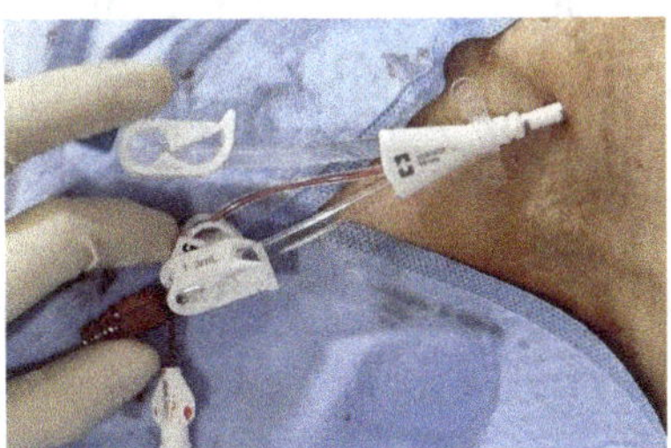

Figure 36.7

13. The guidewire is removed and the flow of the catheter is tested using a 20 mL syringe. On aspiration, the syringe should fill up rapidly within 3 seconds without much resistance and there should not be any resistance encountered during flushing. If the flow is not smooth, the dialysis catheter should be rotated to test the flow again.
14. The catheter is flushed with normal saline.
15. 1 mL of heparin 5000 IU/mL solution is diluted with normal saline to a total of 5 mL. The catheter is locked with the diluted heparin solution to prevent thrombus formation within the catheter.
16. The wings of the catheter are sutured to the skin with non-absorbable sutures. The wound and catheter are covered with sterile breathable dressings.
17. The dressing should be changed whenever it is moist or wet. Water impermeable dressings should be used when showering to keep the wound dry.

Table 36.3:   Equipment for Removal of Tunnelled Haemodialysis Catheter

1. Toilet and suture set should contain:
    - sterile tray
    - gauze
    - cotton balls
    - artery forceps
    - haemostat
2. 1% lignocaine or lidocaine
3. Chlorhexodane cleaning solution
4. Blade

Removal of Tunnelled Haemodialysis Catheter

- Tunnelled HDC should be removed once the patient's vascular access is ready for cannulation, as prolonged catheter usage is associated with risks of central vein stenosis and increased line sepsis.

Table 36.4:   Steps in the Removal of Tunnelled Haemodialysis Catheter

1. Medication records should be reviewed to ensure the patient is not on any anticoagulation.
2. The cuff of the catheter should be located — this should be palpable approximately 2 cm from the exit site (Figure 36.8). The purse string stitch may be present if the catheter was recently placed.
3. The patient should be cleaned and draped (Figure 36.9).

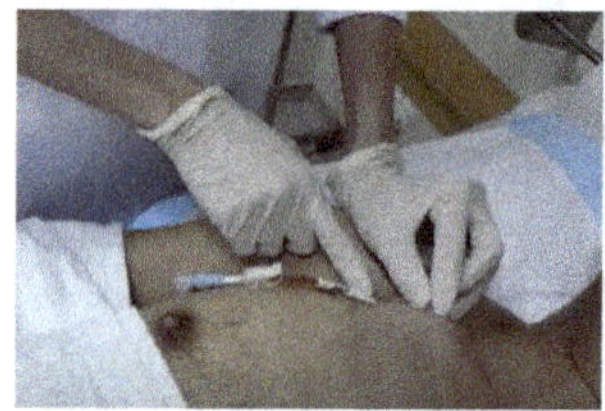

Figure 36.8

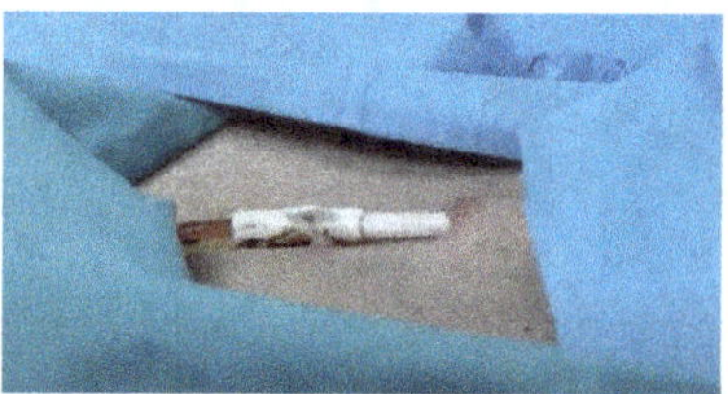

Figure 36.9

4. Lidocaine is injected at the exit site and around the cuff using a 23G needle (Figure 36.10).

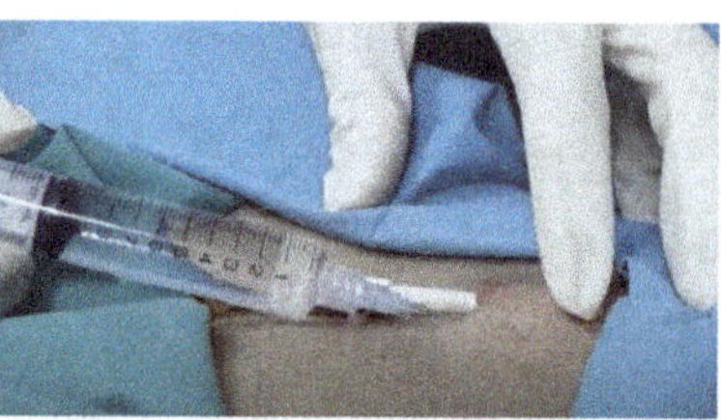

Figure 36.10

5. Stitches are removed (Figure 36.11).
6. Using a combination of gentle traction and blunt dissection with a haemostat or artery forceps (facing upwards), the cuff is separated from the surrounding tissue (Figure 36.12).

Table 36.4:   (Continued)

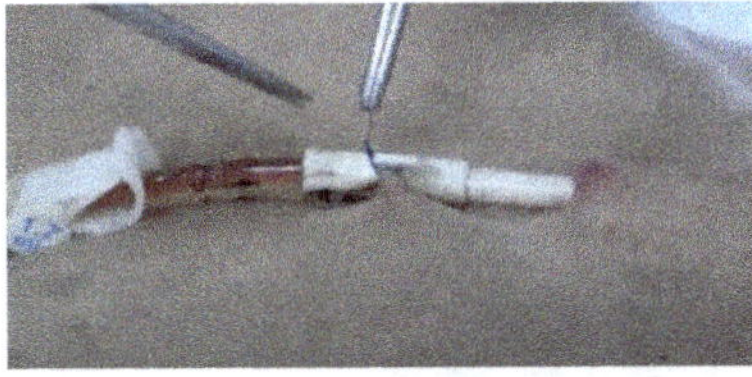

Figure 36.11

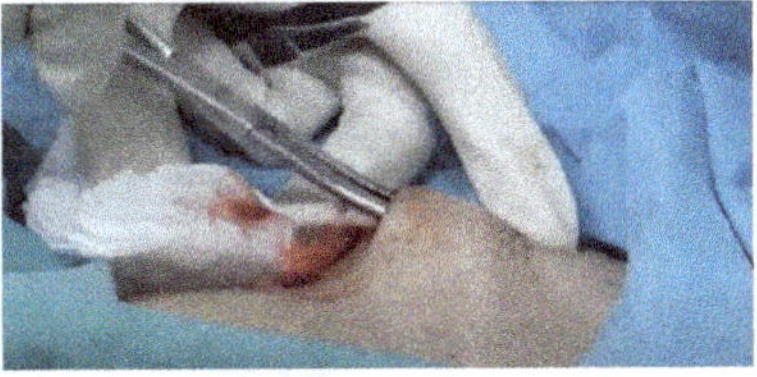

Figure 36.12

7. If the cuff is placed too far from the exit site and the cuff cannot be reached with the haemostat, a small incision is made over the cuff and blunt dissection is performed through the incision to free the cuff. (Figures 36.13 and 36.14).

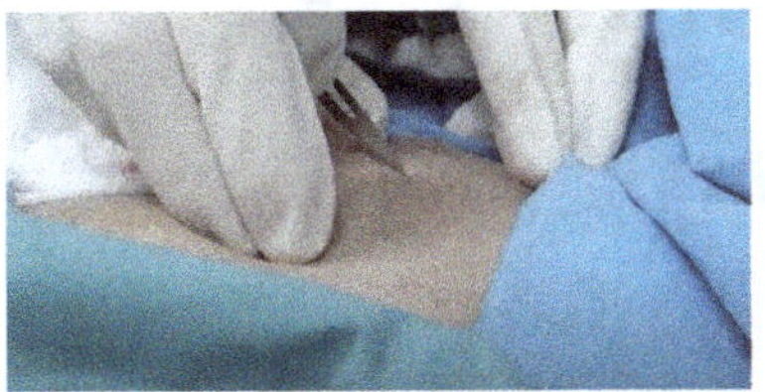

Figure 36.13

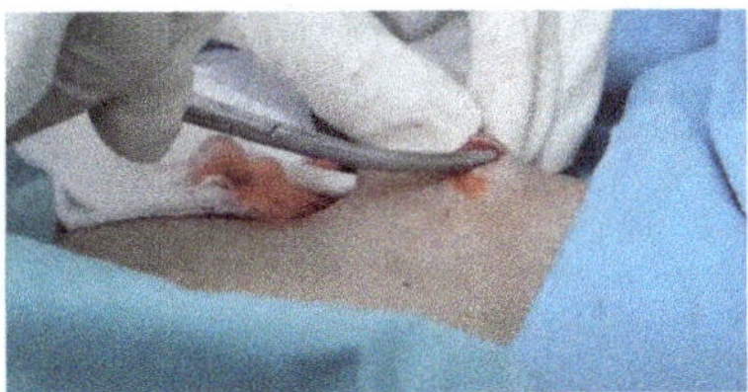

Figure 36.14

8. The cuff is the only part of the catheter that is tethered to the body. Once it is free, the catheter can be easily removed (Figure 36.15). Compress the IJV at the base of the neck while removing the catheter.

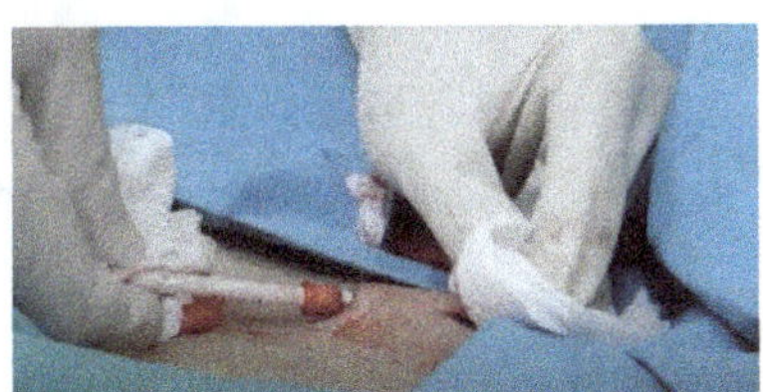

Figure 36.15

9. If the cuff becomes separated from the catheter and was left behind in the subcutaneous tunnel after the removal of the catheter, the cuff should be palpated and a small incision is made over the cuff. The cuff can then be removed using a haemostat and forceps using the blunt dissection technique.

(Continued)

Table 36.4:   (*Continued*)

10. The IJV at the root of the neck should be compressed after removal for
    3–5 minutes (Figure 36.16).

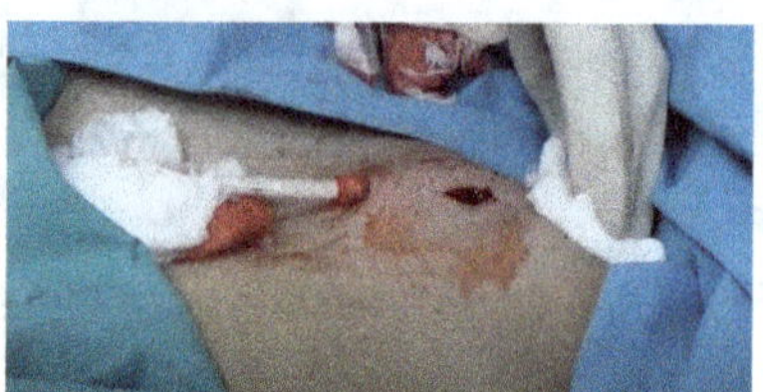

Figure 36.16

11. Observe for any bleeding complications after removal.
12. Stitches are usually not required unless an incision was made at the cuff
    which would then need to be sutured. The wound should be covered with
    dressing.

References

Maecken T, Marcon C, Bomas S, *et al.* (2011). Relationship of the internal jugular vein to the common carotid artery: Implications for ultrasound-guided
vascular access. *Eur J Anaesthesiol* **28**(5): 351–355.

Prabhu MV, Juneja D, Gopal PB, *et al.* (2010). Ultrasound-guided femoral
dialysis access placement: A single-center randomized trial. *Clin J Am Soc
Nephrol* **5**(2): 235–239.

Yevzlin AS, Song GU, Sanchez RJ and Becker YT (2007). Fluoroscopically
guided vs modified traditional placement of tunneled hemodialysis catheters: Clinical outcomes and cost analysis. *J Vasc Access* **8**(4): 245–251.

37 Arteriovenous Dialysis Access Complications

Pang Suh Chien

Introduction

- Vascular access is the "Achilles Heel" of haemodialysis (HD), with its most common complications being (1) stenosis, (2) thrombosis, (3) infection, and (4) aneurysm.

- The frequency of complications is related to the type (e.g., arteriovenous graft (AVG) > arteriovenous fistula (AVF)) and anatomical location of the arteriovenous (AV) access (e.g., elbow > upper arm > forearm).

Arteriovenous Access Flow Dysfunction

- AV access flow dysfunction is a common complication of patients on HD and includes (1) failure to mature, (2) stenosis, and (3) thrombosis.

- The success rate of an AV access can be defined by patency rates (Table 37.1).

Failure to Mature

- AVF usually requires a maturation time of 1–4 months before it can be used for HD.

- However, AVF may fail to mature where it remains unsuitable to use for HD or thrombose before it can ever be used.

Table 37.1: Definitions of Patency of Arteriovenous Access

Patency Term	Definition
Primary patency (unassisted patency)	• The period from time of access creation to first access thrombosis or any intervention to maintain or restore access blood flow • Time calculated is either from the time of creation (thus includes primary failures) or from first use
Secondary patency (assisted or cumulative patency)	• The period from time of access creation to abandonment of the access • Time calculated is either from the time of creation (thus includes primary failures) or from first use

- AVF has a primary non-functional rate of about 20% (range 10–50%).

- Compared to AVF, AVG has lower primary failure rates with a reported rate of about 10% (6–20%).

Stenosis of AV Access

- Stenosis is the most common complication after AV access creation, where a clinically significant stenosis is defined as more than 50% reduction in the lumen of the blood vessel.

- Stenosis is usually associated with clinical abnormalities on physical examination or functional abnormalities during dialysis (Table 37.2). Ultrasound (US) can also help diagnose a stenosis.

- Venous stenosis is most common, often develops because of neointimal hyperplasia, and may occur at any time after the creation of the AV access and at different sites of the AV access (Figure 37.1), such as the:

  - Juxta-anastomotic (JA) segment — the first 2 cm of the vein after artery-vein anastomosis

Table 37.2: Signs and Symptoms Suggesting Clinically Significant Stenosis in Arteriovenous Access

Domain	Clinical Indicators
Physical examination	• Ipsilateral extremity swelling • Pulsatile, difficult to compress fistula • Weak thrill • Bruit is high pitched and systolic only on auscultation • Lack of pulse augmentation (inflow stenosis) • Failure of the fistula to collapse on arm elevation (outflow stenosis) • Excessive collapse of the fistula upon arm elevation
Dialysis related	• Cannulation difficulty • Aspiration of clots • Inability to achieve prescribed dialysis blood flow (Qb) • Abnormal negative arterial and venous pressures • Prolonged bleeding after dialysis needle removal × 3 sessions • Unexplained drop in delivered dialysis clearance

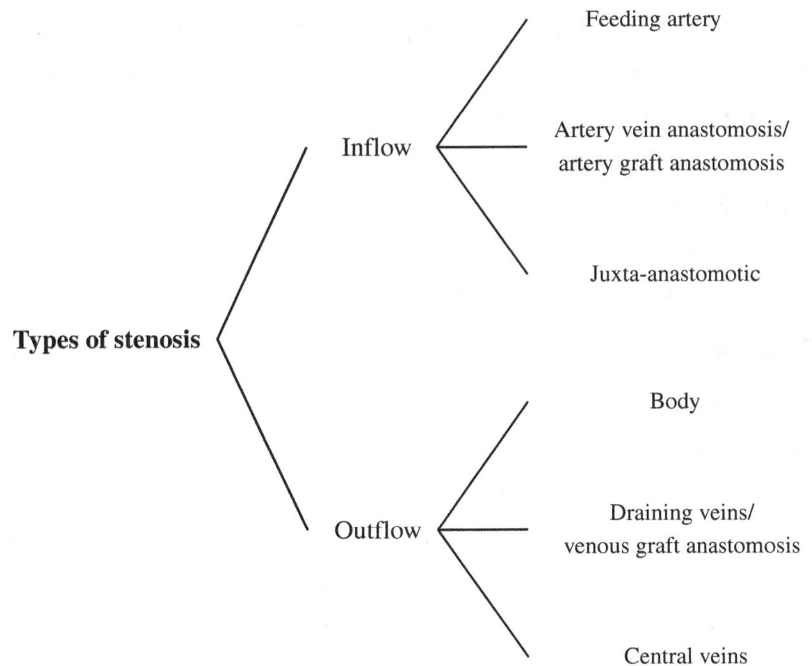

Figure 37.1:   Type of stenosis in arteriovenous fistula.

- Body of the AVF — the segment of the venous limb where cannulation for dialysis is made

- Draining veins — the segments that drain the AV access towards the heart (inclusive of the cephalic arch)

- Central veins — includes the axillary, subclavian, brachiocephalic veins, and superior vena cava

- Stenosis can cause primary failure of AVF to mature and may be due to an inflow stenosis, caused by neointimal hyperplasia at the juxta-anastomotic segment. Late fistula failure is caused primarily by neointimal hyperplasia that results in venous stenosis.

- In comparison to AVF, AVG has lower primary failure rates but inferior long-term patency with 1-year primary and cumulative patency reported locally of 34.1% and 54.3% respectively. The site of stenosis is usually at the graft-vein anastomosis or within 6–10 cm of the anastomosis.

- Angioplasty of AV access can potentially accelerate neointimal hyperplasia and lead to vessel injury. As a result, the decision for angioplasty should be guided by the presence of signs and symptoms suggestive of clinically significant stenosis. These clinical features can be identified through routine AV access monitoring and surveillance by the patient and/or dialysis care provider (Tables 37.2 and 37.3).

- Two endovascular techniques are valuable in the management of AV access:

  - **Angiogram** — This is a diagnostic procedure to visualise blood vessels using contrast material. Angiograms of AVF and AVG are called the fistulogram and graftogram respectively and can confirm the presence and severity of stenosis.

Table 37.3: Clinical Features Suggestive of Possible Sites of Stenosis in an AVF Access

Clinical Presentation	Possible Site of Stenosis and Associated Causes	Physical Examination
Failure to mature	Inflow stenosis Presence of accessory veins or collateral	Flat AVF Multiple dilated veins
Difficult cannulation	Inflow and body stenosis No stenosis, AVF too deep or tortuous for cannulation	Flat AVF with weak thrill Good thrill
Decreased thrill	Inflow and body stenosis	Flat AVF
High dynamic or static venous pressure	Outflow stenosis	Pulsatile AVF
Prolonged bleeding after removal of dialysis needle	Outflow stenosis	Pulsatile AVF
Upper limb swelling (same side as AVF)	Central vein stenosis	Swollen arm with or without visible chest vein

Abbreviation: AVF, arteriovenous fistula

- **Angioplasty** — This is a procedure to dilate stenosed or occluded blood vessels. It is synonymous with percutaneous transluminal angioplasty (PTA), which involves entry through the skin (percutaneous) and going through the vessels (transluminal) to the site of the lesion and dilation of the narrowed or occluded blood vessel (angioplasty).

Central Vein Stenosis

- The development of central vein stenosis or occlusion can compromise AV access function and preclude the creation of an ipsilateral AV access.

- The development of central vein lesions is likely caused by an initial injury to the vascular endothelium which precipitates a local inflammatory response, leading to fibrosis.

- Factors associated with the development of central vein stenosis include deep vein thrombosis, previous or existing central venous catheters (CVC), peripherally inserted central catheters (PICC), and pacemakers.

- The true incidence of CVC-induced stenosis or occlusion is unknown. They can be asymptomatic or symptomatic.

- Signs and symptoms of central vein stenosis in patients on HD include:

  - Arm swelling on the same side as the access

  - Breast swelling with or without arm swelling on the same side as the access

  - Prominent or visible veins on the chest wall

  - Prolonged bleeding following the removal of the dialysis needle

  - Elevated venous pressure during dialysis

  - High AV access recirculation

- Asymptomatic central vein stenosis should be left untreated as angioplasty of asymptomatic stenosis has been shown to be associated with a more rapid progression to a symptomatic lesion. Current vascular access guidelines recommend no intervention for asymptomatic lesions or those associated with minimal symptoms as collateral veins will develop over time.

- Angioplasty is the first line of treatment for symptomatic central vein stenosis. It is associated with a high early technical success rate but poor long-term patency rate. Stenting of central veins and open surgical options (e.g., axillary-axillary bypass) are usually reserved for severe and recurrent cases.

Thrombosis of AV Access

- Thrombosis of AV access is considered a renal "emergency" that requires urgent intervention as a thrombosed AV access is not useable for HD. It accounts for 65–85% of all AV access abandonments.

- Thrombosis most commonly occurs due to stasis of blood secondary to flow-restricting stenoses within the AV circuit. Therefore, treatment of a thrombosed AV access requires thrombolysis and angioplasty of the underlying stenosis.

- Other causes of AV access thrombosis include infection, large haematoma, and prothrombotic states. At the end of a HD session, low blood pressure, haemoconcentration due to excessive ultrafiltration, and prolonged, firm compression of the access are contributing factors.

- Percutaneous declotting of AV access is minimally invasive and well tolerated by most patients. It can be easily arranged and performed in an outpatient setting. As a result, it is the preferred technique for salvaging thrombosed AV accesses compared to traditional open surgical thrombectomy.

- There are generally two percutaneous methods of declotting (Table 37.4). The method chosen depends on operator experience, available resources, and patient factors.

- Open surgical repair is generally reserved for lesions:
    - that are recurrent

Table 37.4: Percutaneous Methods of Declotting the Arteriovenous Access

Pharmacological	Mechanical
• Lysis and wait	• Mechanical device
• Pulse spray technique	• Thrombo-aspiration

- that are not amenable to endovascular treatment

- where the outcomes associated with the endovascular approach are poor

AV Access Infection

- Infection of AV access is a frequent cause of hospitalisation among HD patients, occurring at a rate of 0.56–5% per year for AVFs and 4–20% per year for AVGs. It is also the 2nd most common cause of AV access failure and is potentially fatal.

- AV access infections can occur any time from the initial surgical creation to the frequent needle punctures required for HD. It is mostly caused by *Staphylococcus* spp followed by coagulase-negative staphylococci and polymicrobial infections with gram-negative bacteria.

- The spectrum of potential sequelae of AV access infections are broad and can manifest as:

  - Fever, chills

  - Localised infection — cellulitis, abscess, purulent discharge, exposed access, sinus tract

  - Other complications of AV access — pseudoaneurysm, haematoma, thrombus

  - Bacteraemia, septicaemia with possible septic emboli

  - Septic shock

- Sometimes AV access may be difficult to diagnose, so US imaging to detect fluid collection or tagged white blood cell scans may be helpful.

- AV access infections can be prevented by:

  - Avoiding the creation of lower extremity AV access

  - Using appropriate prophylactic peri-operative antibiotics

- Practicing strict sterile and appropriate techniques of handling the AV access
- Regular monitoring of AV access for any evidence of infection
- Avoiding routine use of buttonhole cannulation technique
- Having a low threshold for treatment
- Management of AV access infection can be medical and/or surgical

Medical Treatment

- Blood cultures should always be obtained whenever an AV access infection is suspected.
- Also obtain cultures from any infected skin, soft tissue, AV access site, tunnel track (e.g., obvious abscess or purulent drainage), or tissue sample obtained during surgery.
- Immediate initiation of broad-spectrum antibiotics for both gram-positive and gram-negative organism coverage after obtaining relevant cultures.
- Avoid the use of infected AV access for dialysis.
- Antibiotics alone may be adequate treatment for limited localised AV access infections (e.g., buttonhole track infection in AVF).
- Consult infectious diseases experts for guidance in complex cases (e.g., disseminated infection, infective endocarditis).

Surgical Treatment

- Surgical treatment options can be broadly categorised as strategies to either salvage the AV access or excise the AV access. The choice depends on several factors:

- Extent of infection (e.g., localised vs. extensive)
- Type of AV access (e.g., AVF vs. AVG)
- Bacterial aetiology (e.g., aggressive bacteria like *Pseudomonas* spp)
- Functional status of the AV access (e.g., occluded vs. patent)
- Type of presentation (e.g., bleeding, discharge, cellulitis, fever of unknown origin)

- Salvage option — This may be possible if the infection is localised, such as graft replacement with excision of the involved segment for an AVG infection as long as the adjacent segments are uninvolved. Close follow-up and surveillance are mandatory because of the risk of recurrent infection and the potential for anastomotic disruption with significant bleeding.

- Excision option — This includes subtotal or total AV access excision and are considered for infections involving the full length of the AVG.

- Other options — Depending on the extent of infection and circumstances, vein patch angioplasty, vein bypass and ligation are other options.

AV Access Aneurysm

- After creation of an AV access, the haemodynamic changes lead to vessel dilatation and localised enlargement of the AV. These haemodynamic changes are likely exacerbated by (1) repeated cannulations and injury to the vein or graft material and (2) increased intraluminal pressures from any outflow stenosis. As a result, aneurysms or pseudoaneurysms may develop with an incidence rate of 5–60% or 0.04 per 1,000 patient days.

- True aneurysm is a circumscribed dilation of all 3 layers of the vessel wall. They commonly occur in the outflow vein but can develop anywhere along the course of the AV access circuit, including the inflow artery.

- Pseudoaneurysm is an extraluminal "blood flow through" defect in the vessel or prosthetic AV access that is walled off or contained by the surrounding soft tissue. They more commonly occur in AVGs than AVFs. It usually occurs due to vessel wall defects from repeated cannulations in the same location but can also develop at the site of vascular anastomosis (which should raise the suspicion of an infectious aetiology).

- Aneurysms or pseudoaneurysms present as a localised mass and can lead to skin erosion with haemorrhage, AV access dysfunction, pain, and difficulties with cannulation. Those with skin erosion, ulceration, or haemorrhage are associated with an increased risk of life-threatening emergency which warrants immediate surgical assessment and treatment.

- US examination may be useful and perianeurysmal inflammation or fluid collections suggest co-existent infection.

- The absolute size of an AVF aneurysm alone is not an indication for surgical treatment but there should be routine monitoring for symptoms, such as rapidly enlarging and development of complications (e.g., ulceration).

- Worrisome signs and symptoms should be checked to determine if aneurysm/pseudoaneurysm is symptomatic (e.g., rapidly expanding and/or at risk for ulceration or bleeding or infection), which then require intervention (Tables 37.5 and 37.6).

Table 37.5:   Signs and Symptoms of Aneurysms and Pseudoaneurysms That May Need Intervention

Physical Examination Findings	Close Monitoring	Urgent Intervention
Size	Not enlarging	Enlarging
Overlying skin	Can be pinched easily	Thin, shiny, depigmented
Skin erosion	None	Ulcers, scabs
Arm elevation sign	Collapse	May not collapse
Bleeding from puncture sites	Uncommon	Often prolonged

Table 37.6: Decision Making for Urgent Intervention of Aneurysm/Pseudoaneurysm

<u>Expectant management</u>
- Involved segment should not be used for cannulation
- Use optimal cannulation technique to prevent aneurysm formation (e.g., rope ladder)
- If there is no alternative annulation site available, cannulate the side of the aneurysm/pseudoaneurysm by creating a longer tract using a lateral approach (Figure 37.2)

<u>What to do with a bleeding aneurysmal AVF</u>
- Apply direct pressure on the site of bleeding
- Occlude the AVF access inflow by applying direct pressure at the anastomosis
- Apply purse string suture by incorporating the surrounding soft tissue (to be done by a trained surgeon only)
- Avoid compression of AV access outflow (as it increases the intraluminal access pressure and increases bleeding)
- Call the vascular surgeon for definite repair

<u>Interventions</u>
- Endovascular — intraluminal covered stent (Figure 37.3)
- Open surgical repair — aneurysmorrphaphy, interpositional graft, ligation ± excision

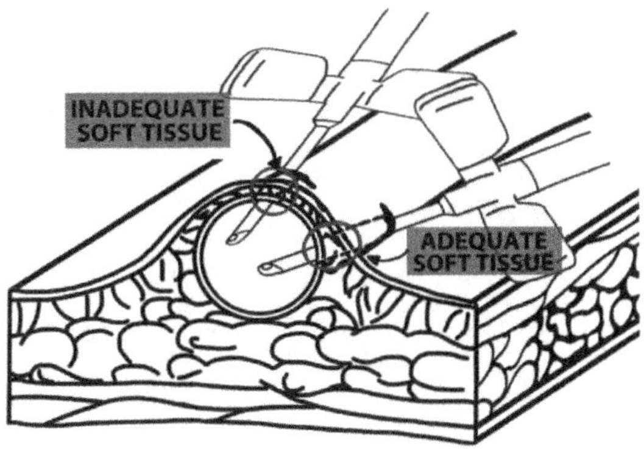

Figure 37.2: Cannulate area with adequate soft tissue (lateral side) of aneurysm/pseudoaneurysm.

Source: Lok CE, Huber TS, Lee T, *et al.* (2020). KDOQI Clinical practice guideline for vascular access: 2019 update. *Am J Kidney Dis* **75**(4 Suppl 2): S1–S164.

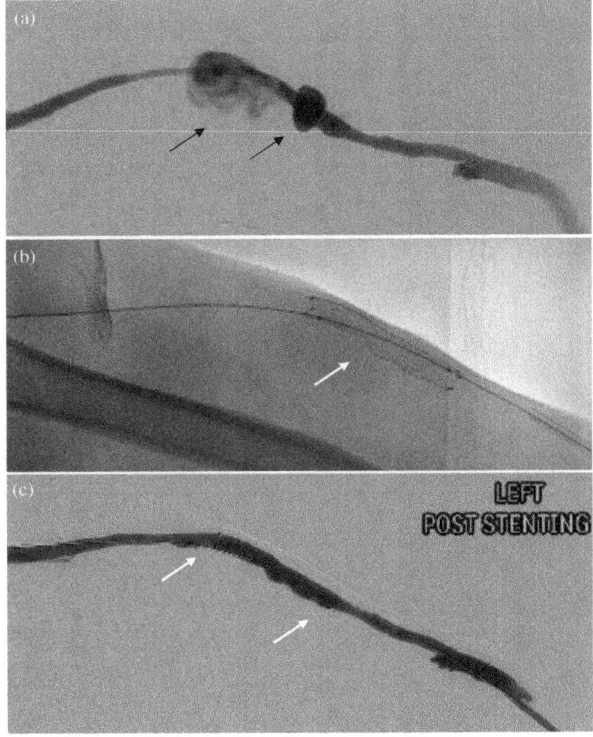

Figure 37.3: Stenting of pseudoaneurysms in a patient with a left brachio-cephalic AVF. (a) the pseudoaneurysms (arrows), (b) deployment of covered stent (arrow) across the lesion, and (c) lesion after stent placement (the stent lies between the two arrows).

AV Access Steal

- When a dialysis vascular access is created, blood flow is immediately diverted into the low pressure, low resistance venous connection and results in a decrease of perfusion pressure distal to the anastomosis. This pressure gradient results in a reversal of blood flow in the artery distal to the access which is called an AV access steal.

- AV access steals affect most patients who remain asymptomatic (i.e., the AV access steal phenomenon). However, among patients where the AV access steal is symptomatic, this is called AV access steal syndrome. Symptoms may be neurological, ischaemic, or musculoskeletal.

- The natural history of steal syndrome is poorly defined, but moderate to severe symptoms rarely resolve without definitive treatment. Timely recognition and treatment are crucial to avoid long-term complications. It is important to be familiar with clinical signs and symptoms because the diagnosis is largely a clinical one (Table 37.7). While hand pain is a common complaint in steal syndrome, other possible differential diagnoses should be considered and looked out for (Table 37.8).

Table 37.7: Clinical Signs and Symptoms of Arteriovenous Access Steal Syndrome

Grade	Severity	Clinical Presentation	Treatment
1	Mild	Cool extremity with few symptoms	None
2	Moderate	Intermittent symptoms during dialysis Claudication	Intervention sometimes
3	Severe	Ischaemic rest pain Digital cyanosis or gangrene Finger contracture Amputation	Intervention mandatory

Table 37.8: Differential Diagnoses of Arteriovenous Access Steal Syndrome

Differential Diagnosis	Clue
Carpal tunnel syndrome	Usually bilateral
Diabetic neuropathy	Usually bilateral
Iatrogenic nerve damage e.g., haematoma compressing a nerve	Symptom begins immediately after creation, resolves within first 2–4 weeks
Arthropathy	Symptom present before access creation
Ischaemic monomeric neuropathy	Excruciating pain immediately after creation Neurological signs and symptoms predominate Hand is warm with no ischaemic changes

- The risk factors of an AV access steal include:
  - Peripheral artery disease
  - Brachial artery anastomosis
  - Diabetes mellitus
  - High access blood flow
  - Female gender
  - Age >60 years
  - Multiple previous access procedures
- The investigation for AV access steal syndrome includes a doppler US, finger pressure (Figure 37.4), and nerve conduction study.
- The treatment goal is to correct haemodynamic changes and potentially reverse the symptoms:
  - Ligation (if symptoms are severe, limb at risk of loss, or no other option available) — will require alternative AV access
  - Banding to narrow venous outflow but often complicated by thrombosis

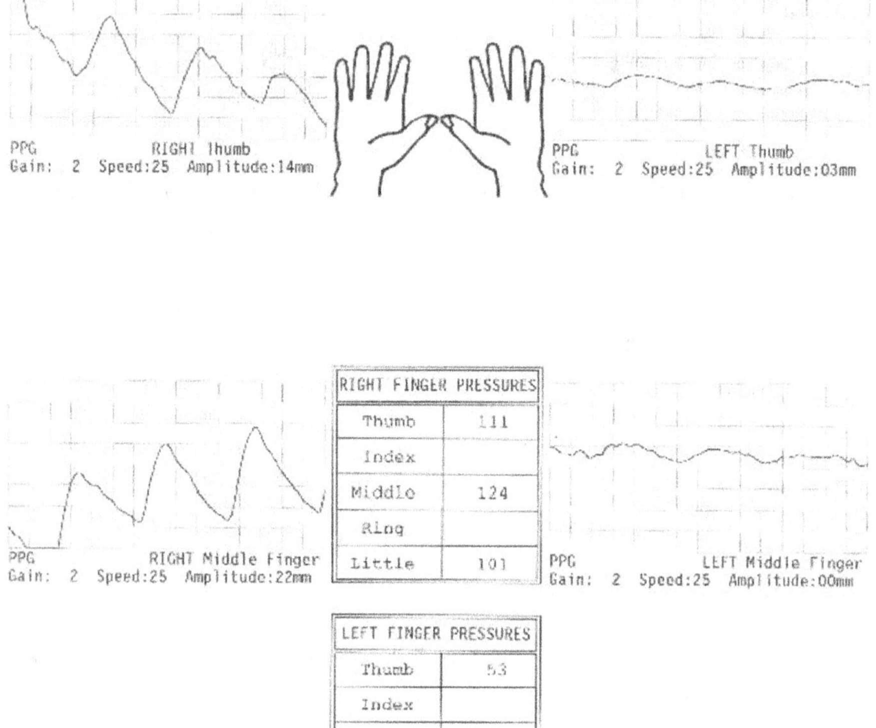

RIGHT FINGER PRESSURES	
Thumb	111
Index	
Middle	124
Ring	
Little	101

LEFT FINGER PRESSURES	
Thumb	53
Index	
Middle	67
Ring	
Little	73

Figure 37.4: Bilateral plethysmographic waveforms and finger pressures during a diagnostic steal study (photoplethysmography). The left arm waveforms are blunted and diminished in amplitude compared to the right. The digital pressures are lower in the left arm which is suggestive of steal.

- Correction of arterial inflow stenosis

- Rerouting of arterial inflow

- Distal revascularisation and interval ligation (DRIL), which include a bypass (between the artery proximal and distal to

AV access anastomosis) and interval ligation of the artery distal to the AV access

High-flow AV Access

- The creation of an AV access is a non-physiological process that joins the high-flow arterial circuit to the low-flow, low-resistance venous pathway. The systemic vascular resistance decreases immediately after anastomosis and the cardiac output increases to accommodate the shunting effect of the AV access.

- High-flow AV access primarily occurs with AVFs where increased flow rates through an AV access can potentially lead to high output cardiac failure and other complications (Table 37.9).

- The exact threshold to define high-flow access is not unified. For instance, an arterial flow rate (Qa) of 1–1.5 L/min or Qa of >20% of the cardiac output (Qa/CO) has been suggested. Patients may develop symptoms of congestive heart failure at lower thresholds if they have an underlying heart disease.

- Monitoring and management for high-flow AV access include:

  - 6–12 monthly echocardiograms to look for cardiac decompensation and changes in Qa/CO

Table 37.9: Potential Problems Associated With High-Flow AVF Access

• High-output congestive heart failure
• Pulmonary hypertension
• Central vein stenosis
• Venous hypertension
• Aneurysmal formation in AVF
• AV access-related hand ischaemia

Abbreviation: AVF, arteriovenous fistula; AV, arteriovenous

- Flow-reducing therapies (e.g., bandings)
- Angioplasty to arterial inflow stenosis
- Ligation
- Revision

- Very often, patients have co-existing cardiac disease which may present similarly, and confirmation that a high-flow AV access is the cause of symptoms is when they resolve with treatment of the AV access.

References

Al-Jaishi AA, Liu AR, Lok CE, *et al.* (2017). Complications of the arteriovenous fistula: A systematic review. *J Am Soc Nephrol* **28**(6): 1839–1850.

Balaz P and Björck M (2015). True aneurysm in autologous hemodialysis fistulae: Definitions, classification and indications for treatment. *J Vasc Access* **16**(6): 446–453.

Inston N, Mistry H, Gilbert J, *et al.* (2017). Aneurysms in vascular access: State of the art and future developments. *J Vasc Access* **18**(6): 464–472.

Levit RD, Cohen RM, Kwak A, *et al.* (2006). Asymptomatic central venous stenosis in hemodialysis patients. *Radiology* **238**(3): 1051–1056.

Lok CE, Huber TS, Lee T, *et al.* (2020). KDOQI Clinical practice guideline for vascular access: 2019 update. *Am J Kidney Dis* **75**(4 Suppl 2): S1–S164.

Lok CE, Sontrop JM, Tomlinson G, *et al.* (2013). Cumulative patency of contemporary fistulas versus grafts (2000–2010). *Clin J Am Soc Nephrol* **8**: 810–818.

MacRae JM, Dipchand C, Oliver M, *et al.* (2016). Arteriovenous access failure, stenosis, and thrombosis. *Can J Kidney Health Dis* **3**: 2054358116669126.

MacRae JM, Dipchand C, Oliver M, *et al.* (2016). Arteriovenous access: Infection, neuropathy, and other complications. *Can J Kidney Health Disease* **3**: 2054358116669127.

Padberg FT Jr, Calligaro KD and Sidawy AN (2008). Complications of arteriovenous hemodialysis access: Recognition and management. *J Vasc Surg* **48**(5 Suppl): 55S–80S.

Quencer KB and Friedman T (2017). Declotting the thrombosed access. *Tech Vasc Interv Radiol* **20**(1): 38–47.

Renaud CJ., Francois M, Nony A, *et al.* (2012). Comparative outcomes of treated symptomatic versus non-treated asymptomatic high-grade central vein stenoses in the outflow of predominantly dialysis fistulas. *Nephrol Dial Transplant* **27**(4): 1631–1638.

Roy-Chaudhury P, Kelly BS, Melhem M, *et al.* (2005). Vascular access in hemodialysis: Issues, management, and emerging concepts. *Cardiol Clin* **23**(3): 249–273.

Sidawy AN, Gray R, Besarab A, *et al.* (2002). Recommended standards for reports dealing with arteriovenous hemodialysis accesses. *J Vasc Surg* **35**(3): 603–610.

Voorzaat BM, van der Bogt KEA, Janmaat CJ, *et al.* (2018). Dutch Vascular Access Study Group: Arteriovenous fistula maturation failure in a large cohort of hemodialysis patients in The Netherlands. *World J Surg* **42**: 1895–1903.

Peritoneal Dialysis

38 Basic Concepts in Peritoneal Dialysis

Elizabeth Oei

Introduction

- Peritoneal dialysis (PD) is a remarkably effective mode of renal replacement therapy. Solutes such as urea and excess fluid in the blood circulation move across the peritoneal membrane and into PD fluid in the peritoneal cavity during a dwell.

Anatomy of PD

- The first requirement for PD is for blood containing solutes and excess fluid to be within diffusable distance of the PD fluid.

- For diffusion to occur across the membrane, solutes and excess fluid must first be transported to the peritoneal membrane via peritoneal capillaries. Areas of peritoneum that are too far away from a capillary do not contribute significantly to the dialysis process, giving rise to the concept of effective peritoneal surface area.

- The second requirement for PD is for dialysis fluid to be in contact with the peritoneal membrane. Once the solutes and excess fluid are transported to the peritoneum, these cross the areas of the peritoneal membrane that are in contact with PD fluid and diffuse (or osmose) into the dialysate.

- By increasing fill volume, more effective peritoneal surface area is recruited, thus maximising area available for diffusion and hence solute clearance.

Physiology of PD

- The three-pore model summarises the movement of solutes and water across the peritoneal membrane:
  - Large pores are fewest in number and transport macro molecules. These are clefts between endothelial cells.
  - Small pores are the most numerous and allow transport of solutes and water. These have been postulated to be clefts in the endothelium.
  - Ultrasmall pores (aquaporins) are numerous and exclusively transport water.
- People with more pores will have a faster diffusion rate and are known as high transporters. They tend to have excellent solute clearance, but they also absorb glucose faster from the dialysis fluid. Thus, high transporters may lose their osmotic gradient quickly and tend to have less ultrafiltration (UF) when compared to low transporters.

Processes in Peritoneal Dialysis

Solute clearance

- Solutes such as potassium and urea diffuse out of the patient's body along a diffusion gradient. This gradient decreases over time, and solute clearance becomes less efficient with prolonged dwell times.

- Whenever the patient or the automated PD machine drains out the dialysate and instills fresh PD solution for the next exchange, the original (maximal) diffusion gradient is restored.

- While superior clearance of small molecules such as potassium and urea can be achieved, multiple exchanges or cycles with a short dwell time are not performed because clearance of substances that diffuse more slowly (e.g., larger middle molecules and phosphate) will be compromised. Additionally, short, and frequent exchanges (or cycles) may give rise to sodium sieving, resulting in salt and water overload.

Sodium sieving

- Early in a dwell when the osmotic gradient is greatest, water moves into the peritoneal cavity via aquaporins before any significant solute transport has taken place via the small or large pores. Exclusive movement of water into the peritoneal cavity is demonstrated as a decrease in the dialysate sodium concentration.

- As the dwell progresses past 90 minutes, sodium diffuses into the peritoneal cavity and the dialysate sodium concentration increases back to its original value. If the peritoneum is drained early (i.e., if the dwell is shorter than 90 minutes) while the dialysate sodium is low, this results in loss of free water, sodium retention, and ultimately hypernatraemia.

Fluid removal

- Water movement into the PD fluid, or UF, mainly occurs by osmosis and occasionally by convection.

- Glucose is the most commonly used osmotic agent in PD. The higher the tonicity of the PD fluid (e.g., 4.25% vs. 1.5%), the higher the osmotic gradient, and the larger the UF expected. Alternative osmotic agents include amino acids (e.g., in Nutrineal PD fluid).

- Notably, even as solutes diffuse into the dialysis fluid, osmotic agents such as glucose diffuse from the dialysis fluid and into the blood. The reduction in the absolute number of osmotically active particles in dialysis fluid, compounded by dilution due to UF, results in a decrease in osmotic gradient over time.

- The larger the number of osmotically active particles (e.g., higher tonicity and a larger dwell volume), the longer an osmotic gradient can be maintained. Once the osmotic gradient is lost, UF stops and fluid may even begin to move from the dialysate back into the patient's circulation. Hence, larger dwell volumes of higher tonicity over shorter dwell times will yield more UF.

- Another important factor to consider is when excessively large dwell volumes are used in PD. This increases intraperitoneal pressure to the extent that the osmotic pressure exerted by the dialysis fluid is overcome by the opposing hydrostatic pressure, resulting in minimal movement of fluid from the blood into the peritoneal space and poor UF. This is of particular significance in those who may have polycystic kidneys already occupying a large intra-abdominal volume, and careful attention to PD prescription usually can circumvent most difficulties.

- Finally, icodextrin is a starch that generates colloidal oncotic pressure rather than an osmotic gradient. UF is achieved through convection rather than osmosis. This takes place more slowly than osmosis, and icodextrin (7.5%) is conventionally used as the last fill. The peritoneal membrane is relatively impermeable to such a large molecule and the oncotic gradient does not diminish significantly over time, unlike the osmotic gradient generated by glucose described earlier.

Reference

Khanna R (2017). Solute and water transport in peritoneal dialysis: A case-based primer. *Am J Kidney Dis* **69**(3): 461–472.

39 Initiation and Prescription of Peritoneal Dialysis

April Toh, Htay Htay

Introduction

- In stable chronic kidney disease (CKD) patients who have opted for peritoneal dialysis (PD), placement of the PD catheter should be scheduled in a timely manner so that PD can be electively initiated when the estimated glomerular filtration rate (eGFR) falls below 10 mL/min/1.73 m² (planned-start PD).

- However, patients who are unstable, such as those who are experiencing frequent fluid overload or with cirrhotic ascites that require frequent paracentesis, should initiate PD earlier.

- PD is usually started after 2 weeks of PD catheter placement to allow healing of the abdominal wound and thus mitigate the risk of dialysate leak. However, if there are indications for urgent or early initiation of dialysis, PD can be started earlier (urgent-start PD).

Types of Peritoneal Dialysis

- PD therapy can be delivered through manual exchanges (continuous ambulatory PD or CAPD) or via a machine (automated PD or APD).

- There are conflicting results on whether APD is superior to CAPD in terms of technique and patient survival. As a result, the modality of PD is usually decided based on the patient's preference, lifestyle, and in some cases, clinical conditions (Table 39.1).

Components of PD Prescription

- PD prescription (Table 39.2) is dependent on:
  - **Unadjustable parameters** — body size, residual kidney function (RKF), peritoneal membrane transporter status
  - **Adjustable parameters** — fill volume, therapy time, type of dialysate, number of exchanges

General Considerations for PD Prescription

- Diuretics are usually prescribed for incident end-stage kidney disease patients to preserve residual urine volume and achieve fluid balance.

Table 39.1:   Comparison of Continuous Ambulatory Peritoneal Dialysis Versus Automated Peritoneal Dialysis

	CAPD	APD
Technique	• Performed manually throughout the day by the patient or a care giver. • Uses gravity to instil and drain dialysate, called an exchange. • 3 to 4 exchanges per day are performed.	• Performed overnight while the patient sleeps using an automated cycler machine. • More frequent exchanges can be performed.

Table 39.1: *(Continued)*

	CAPD	APD
Factors influencing choice of PD modality	• CAPD may be preferred for patients who do not want to be connected to a machine for several hours. • CAPD offers flexibility in the timing of exchanges. • CAPD is performed in an upright position which may increase the risk of discomfort, hernias, and leaks due to increased IPP. • Risk of non-adherence to exchanges may be higher in CAPD.	• APD may offer patients more time for work, family, and social activities during the day. • APD may be preferred for the elderly who are dependent on a caregiver as it reduces the daily workload of the caregiver. • Patients with high peritoneal membrane permeability (fast transporters) may be better suited for APD due to shorter dwell times. • High doses of PD can be achieved with frequent APD exchanges over 8–10 hours during the night with an additional daytime dwell — this is called continuous cycling peritoneal dialysis (CCPD). • APD is performed in a supine position which may be better tolerated by patients who cannot tolerate high IPP. For urgent-start PD in hospital, APD reduces the risks of leak due to lower IPP and requires less nursing time. • Adherence to exchanges may be better in APD.

Abbreviations: APD, automated peritoneal dialysis; CAPD, continuous ambulatory peritoneal dialysis; IPP, intraperitoneal pressure

Table 39.2:   Adjustable Parameters of Peritoneal Dialysis Prescription

Adjustable Parameters of PD Prescription	Factors Affecting Parameter Adjustment
Fill volume Volume of dialysate instilled in the peritoneal cavity per exchange or cycle — usually prescribed between 1500–2000 mL.	The fill volume can be modified based on: • Body size • IPP not exceeding 18 cmH20 • Tolerance to different volumes
Number of exchanges or cycles Frequency of filling and draining of PD fluid in and out of the abdomen.	The number of exchanges is adjusted to achieve adequate clearance.
Therapy time Total duration of time that the patient is connected to the cycler for APD. This is usually ordered between 8 and 10 hours.	Therapy time is adjusted to target solute clearance and lifestyle factors.
Type of PD solutions Type of PD solutions available commercially are: • Dianeal — dextrose based with 1.5%, 2.5% and 4.25% dextrose concentrations • Balance — biocompatible PD solutions with low levels of glucose degradation products (GDP) • Extraneal — glucose-based PD solutions suitable for long dwells	• Low dextrose concentration PD solution is prescribed initially during incremental PD therapy but when RKF declines, a higher dextrose concentration PD solution is used to ensure fluid balance. • Neutral pH and low GDP solutions are preferred over conventional PD dialysate for better preservation of RKF. • Icodextrin (extraneal) is particularly useful for patients who are (1) high transporters or (2) fluid overloaded where better ultrafiltration can be achieved with icodextrin.

Abbreviations: GDP, glucose degradation products; IPP, intraperitoneal pressure; KT/V, "K" is dialyser urea clearance, "T" is total dialysis session time, and "V" is volume of distribution of urea; PD, peritoneal dialysis; RKF, residual kidney function

- Low tonicity (containing low concentration of dextrose) PD solution should be prescribed to preserve peritoneal membrane function when there is still RKF.

- Avoid prescribing an inappropriately long dwell time especially when using low dextrose concentration PD solution to prevent fluid retention and subsequent fluid overload.

- Some patients experience drain pain when spent dialysate is drained from the abdomen. The drain pain is usually due to the sucking of the catheter tip on abdominal viscera such as the bowels, bladder, or peritoneum. The pain can be mitigated by clearing the bowel and using tidal PD therapy for patients on APD. In tidal PD therapy, usually 20–30% or (200–300 mLs) of PD fluid is left in the peritoneal cavity instead of draining out completely at the end of each cycle. Estimated UF should be as close to final UF to avoid overfill during therapy.

- Patients who have high or fast solute transport characteristics of the peritoneal membrane are more suitable for shorter dwell times with APD therapy to mitigate the risk of fluid retention, especially when there is loss of RKF.

Types of PD Solutions

- There are generally 2 different types of dialysates — biocompatible and non-biocompatible (Table 39.3).

- Biocompatible PD solutions are pH neutral, have less glucose degradative products (GDP), and exert less oxidative stress on the membrane. The product comes in 2 compartments — acidic (containing glucose and electrolytes) and alkaline (containing buffer and electrolytes). The 2 compartments are "mixed upon use" allowing for dialysate generation on the spot.

Table 39.3:   Types of Peritoneal Dialysis Solutions

Components of PD Solutions	Conventional Solution	Biocompatible PD Solutions			
		Balance	Physioneal	Extraneal	Nutrineal
pH	5.5	7.0	7.0–7.4	5.5-6.0	6.7
Osmotic agent	Glucose	Glucose	Glucose	Icodextrin	Amino acids
Dextrose or Icodextrin (%)	1.5/2.5/4.25	1.5/2.5/4.25	1.5/2.5/4.25	7.5	1.1
Osmolarity (mOsmol/L)	345–483	356–511	344–483	284	365
Lactate (mmol/L)	35–40	35	10-15	40	40
Bicarbonate (mmol/L)	0	0	25	0	0
Sodium (mmol/L)	132–134	134	132–134	132	132
Chloride (mmol/L)	95–102	100–101.5	95- 101	96	105
Calcium (mmol/L)	1.25/1.75	1.25/1.75	1.25/1.75	1.75	1.25
Magnesium (mmol/L)	0.25/ 0.5	0.5	0.25	0.25	0.25
3-DG (mmol/L)	167 ± 0.3	17.6 ± 0.3	93.3 ± 5.0	7.5 ± 0.4	< 0.1
3,4 DGE (mmol/L)	11.3 ± 0.5	< 2.4	14.3 ± 2.5	< 2.4	Not tested

DG = Deoxyglucosone; 3,4-DGE = di-deoxyglucosone-3-ene; GDP = glucose degradation products, PD = peritoneal dialysis
Table adapted from Htay H, Johnson DW, Strippoli GFM, *et al.* Evidence. In *Evidence-based Nephrology.* (https://doi-org.libproxy1.nus.edu.sg/10.1002/9781119105954.ch47)

- The non-biocompatible solutions are acidic (pH 5.2) and have higher levels of GDPs. The osmotic agent generally used for these solutions is glucose. The higher the concentration of glucose, the more UF can be generated. However, more glucose will also be absorbed into the patient and can worsen diabetic control in those with diabetes mellitus.

Urgent-start PD

- Urgent-start PD is the initiation of PD within 2 weeks of catheter placement. The scenarios in which urgent-start PD take place include:
  - Starting PD as the initial and long-term kidney replacement therapy for selected patients who present to the hospital emergently with uraemia and fluid overload requiring urgent dialysis ("crash landers").
  - Switching to PD in crash landers who are treated initially with emergent haemodialysis (HD) — the PD catheter is inserted once the patient is stabilised with HD, and PD can start 48–78 hours after PD catheter insertion. Although PD can be prescribed as early as 24 hours post-catheter placement, there is a risk of dialysate leak and clinicians should balance the risk and benefit of immediate PD initiation.
- CAPD or APD can be used to start PD urgently, but APD is preferred because it allows nephrologists to order higher dialysis doses by increasing the number of cycles without needing to increase the fill volume.
- For urgent-start PD, prescribe a low fill volume (600–800 mL) for the first 2–3 days and gradually increase the fill volume (~30% every 2–3 days) if there is no sign of dialysate leak.

Table 39.4: Advantages and Disadvantages of Incremental PD

Advantages	Disadvantages
• Fewer connections need to be performed, reducing risk of peritonitis, reducing care delivery, and improving quality of life. • Less solution is used which reduces not only healthcare cost but exposure of the peritoneal to glucose, hence prolonging the longevity of peritoneal membrane function. • Reduces PD carbon footprint (e.g., packaging materials).	• Risk of inadequate dialysis (presenting with uraemia and fluid overload) when RKF declines and is unaccompanied by an increase in PD dose. • Patients may be unwilling to increase PD dose when clinically required to.

- Instruct the patient to be in a supine position during dialysis to mitigate the risk of dialysate leak.

Incremental PD

- Incremental PD is a strategy of prescribing less than the standard "full-dose" of PD when initiating PD. The rationale is that RKF is still sufficient to provide adequate solute clearance when combined with a lower dose of PD. However, when RKF declines, the dose of PD needs to be increased. It has some proposed advantages (Table 39.4).

- An incremental PD prescription may be:

  - CAPD with fewer than 4 dwells per day, <2 L dwell volume or <7 d/week (e.g., 3 exchanges per day with or without night dwell), dextrose 1.5% exclusively or in combination with one bag of dextrose 2.5%, fill volume 1200–1800 mL/ exchange.

  - APD with no day dwell, <10 L total daily dose or <7d/ week, e.g., 3 to 5 cycles over 6 to 9 hours at night with no day dwell or dialyse 6 days per week with one day break, usually dextrose 1.5% alone, fill volume 1200 to 1800 mL/cycle.

- Incremental PD is usually prescribed for kidney failure patients who still have significant RKF. For patients who have no RKF or those who are transferred from HD due to running out of vascular access, full-dose PD rather than incremental PD should be prescribed.

Implementing Incremental PD

- Educate patients about the need to increase dialysis dose when kidney function declines
- Preserve RKF:
  - Use angiotension-converting enzyme inhibitor or angiotensin receptor blocker to treat hypertension
  - Avoiding nephrotoxic drugs
  - Avoid hypotension
  - Use a biocompatible PD solution
- Prescribe loop diuretics to preserve residual urine volume
- Monitor RKF regularly (every 3–6 months) and increase the dialysis dose as appropriate when RKF declines
- Monitor the patient's clinical conditions and laboratory investigations regularly for any signs of inadequate dialysis
- Increase dialysis dose when RKF declines or clinical features and/or laboratory parameters indicate inadequate dialysis
- Address inadequate solute clearance by:
  - Increasing fill volume
  - Increasing the number of exchanges
  - Adding a long day-dwell or overnight dwell with icodextrin

- Address inadequate fluid clearance by:
  - Increasing the dose of diuretics
  - Adding icodextrin in the long dwell
  - Adjusting dwell times to avoid fluid retention
  - Educating on salt and fluid restriction
  - Increasing dextrose concentration of PD fluid

References

Blake PG, Dong J and Davies SJ (2020). Incremental peritoneal dialysis. *Perit Dial Int* **40**(3): 320–326.

Htay H, Johnson DW, Craig JC, *et al.* (2020). Urgent-start peritoneal dialysis versus conventional-start peritoneal dialysis for people with chronic kidney disease. *Cochrane Database Syst Rev* **12**(12): CD012913.

Htay H, Johnson DW, Wiggins KJ, *et al.* (2018). Biocompatible dialysis fluids for peritoneal dialysis. *Cochrane Database Syst Rev* **10**(10): CD007554.

Liu Y, Ma X, Zheng J, *et al.* (2017). Effects of angiotensin-converting enzyme inhibitors and angiotensin receptor blockers on cardiovascular events and residual renal function in dialysis patients: A meta-analysis of randomised controlled trials. *BMC Nephrol* **18**(1): 206.

Medcalf JF, Harris KP and Walls J (2001). Role of diuretics in the preservation of residual renal function in patients on continuous ambulatory peritoneal dialysis. *Kidney Int* **59**(3): 1128–1133.

Morelle J, Stachowska-Pietka J, Öberg C, *et al.* (2021). ISPD recommendations for the evaluation of peritoneal membrane dysfunction in adults: Classification, measurement, interpretation and rationale for intervention. *Perit Dial Int* **41**(4): 352–372.

Ng AKH, Tan SN, Tay ME, *et al.* (2022). Comparison of planned-start, early-start and deferred-start strategies for peritoneal dialysis initiation in end-stage kidney disease. *Ann Acad Med Singap* **51**(4): 213–220.

Roumeliotis A, Roumeliotis S, Leivaditis K, *et al.* (2021). APD or CAPD: One glove does not fit all. *Int Urol Nephrol* **53**(6): 1149–1160.

40 Assessment and Management of Peritoneal Dialysis Adequacy

Marjorie Foo

Introduction

- The definition of adequacy in peritoneal dialysis (PD) has recently been revised by the International Society of Peritoneal Dialysis (ISPD) in 2020 with the overarching aim of not only targeting the fundamentals of dialysis, such as Kt/V, bone disease, anaemia, and managing complex diseases (e.g., diabetes mellitus), but also increasing the emphasis on high quality and goal-directed treatment.

- Assessment of adequacy should be person-centric, focusing on well-being and life participation in addition to assessment of solute clearance, volume, and nutritional status, anaemia and mineral bone disease management, and optimisation of glycaemic control.

- The sense of wellbeing can be monitored subjectively (e.g., eating and sleeping well, gaining weight, absence of itch) and more objectively using quality of life (QOL) questionnaires (e.g., Kidney Disease Quality of Life (KDQOL) instrument).

- The fundamentals of dialysis adequacy can be categorised as follows:

Mineral Bone Disease

- The aim of treatment of mineral bone disease is to prevent or reduce the risk of osteoporosis and fracture by maintaining normal serum calcium (Ca) and targeting lower serum phosphate (PO4) levels (Table 40.1).

- Evaluation should also include serum isonised parathyroid hormone (iPTH) and alkaline phosphatase (ALP).

- PD dialysate use of lower Ca content of 1.25–1.5 mmol/L will allow for higher doses of Ca-based phosphate binders to be used and ameliorate the risk of hypercalcaemia and metastatic calcification in the long term.

Table 40.1: Targets to Control in Mineral Bone Disease

	Target	**Treatment Suggestion**
iPTH	2–9 times the normal range	If iPTH is above the recommended range, the following can be used to reduce iPTH: – calcitriol – vitamin D analogs – calcimimetics or – a combination of calcimimetics and calcitriol or vitamin D analogs If iPTH falls below 2 × the normal upper limit, calcitriol, vitamin D analogs, and/or calcimimetic should be reduced or stopped.
Ca	Normal range — avoid hypercalcaemia	Use PD solution with dialysate Ca concentration of 1.25–1.5 mmol/L.
PO4	Normal range — avoid hyperphosphataemia	Ensure adherence to PO4 binders and dietary restrictions of PO4.

Abbreviations: Ca, calcium; iPTH, ionized parathyroid hormone; PD, peritoneal dialysis; PO4, phosphate

Anaemia

- The aim of treatment of anaemia is to ensure a sufficient level of haemogloblin (Hb) to reduce the risk of cardiovascular disease and improve quality of life (Table 40.2).

- Anaemia should be assessed with a full blood count (with red cell indices, white blood cell differentials, and platelet count), absolute reticulocyte count, serum ferritin, transferrin saturation (TSAT), vitamin B_{12}, and folate.

- One of the most serious complications of the use of erythropoietin-stimulating agents (ESA) is the development of pure red cell aplasia (PRCA), presenting as a rapid drop in Hb of 0.5 to 1 g/dL per week or needing transfusion every 1–2 weeks with normal platelet and white cell count and absolute retic count of $<10^3$/uL.

Volume Status Assessment and Management

- Optimal volume management in PD will result in better survival from cardiovascular disease.

- The assessment of fluid status is based on a combination of clinical and biochemical parameters. Clinical assessment includes the monitoring of blood pressure, varying degrees of anasarca, respiratory rate, and presence of lung crepitations on auscultation. Biochemically, there may be a dilutional effect on albumin and haematocrit, thus lowering these parameters. The use of a bioimpedance monitor can provide information on hydration status as well as body composition (e.g., lean and fat mass). Serial monitoring using a combination of the above methods will enhance the quality of dialysis.

Table 40.2:   Targets to Control in Anaemia

	Target	Treatment Suggestion	Remarks
Haemoglobin	10–12 g/dL	Individualised to the patient's needs (e.g., activities and lifestyle)	
Ferritin	>500 ng/mL	In patients with or without ESA, IV iron 1–3 monthly if TSAT <30% or Ferritin <500 ng/mL	Avoid iron infusion in active infection
TSAT	>30%		
ESA	Aim for a Hb increase of 1 to 2 g/dL per month (response is dependent on initial dose, dose frequency, and route of administration) Starting dose: Epoetin α or β: SC 20–50 IU/kg body weight, 3× /week Darbepoetin: SC/IV 0.45 ug/kg body weight weekly or SC 0.75 ug/kg body weight every 2 weeks CERA (Mircera) SC/IV 0.6 ug/kg fortnightly or 1.2 ug/kg monthly	Start when Hb 9–10 g/dL Dose adjustment according to Hb, present ESA dose, and clinical circumstance	Watch out for hypertension in the first 3 months of initiation If Hb increased by >1 g/dL in a 2-week period, consider reducing the dose by 25% Change in dose should not be more than once a month Exercise caution when treating patients with malignancy aiming for lower range

Abbreviations: CERA, continuous erythropoietin receptor activator; ESA, erythrocyte stimulating agents; Hb, haemoglobin; IV, intravenous; SC, subcutaneous; TSAT, transferrin saturation

- On a practical note, it is essential to set a "dry weight" for the patient so that they can monitor any rapid increase or decrease in weight and adjust their treatment accordingly.

- Volume management should consider the net balance between intake and output in the form of UF, urine output and insensible losses, e.g., sweat, respiration. Maintenance of neutral balance is essential to preserve residual kidney function (RKF) and minimise the use of hypertonic solution which can increase the longevity of the membrane. Treatment with renin-angiotensin-aldosterone blockers can help to slow the rate of decline in RKF.

- Increasing UF in PD can be done by increasing the tonicity of dialysate, increasing the number of exchanges, or increasing the fill volume per exchange. In the latter, it is important not to "overfill" the abdomen as this will lead to back filtration, resulting in fluid retention or the development of hernia or leaks. To optimise fluid removal, apart from UF, increasing the dose of diuretics is another option to reduce the metabolic burden of treatment.

- The use of icodextrin for UF is suitable for chronic overload requiring slow removal and should not be used in conditions of acute overload. In situations where fluid removal is urgent, a high tonicity dialysate should be used.

Small Solute Clearance

- Small solute clearance (SCC) should be routinely measured 3–4 times monthly in anticipation of loss of RKF during the early phase of PD and where incremental dialysis is being prescribed. The loss of RKF will result in a reduction of SCC and this will need to be compensated by increasing the dose of dialysis.

- SSC can be measured using weekly urea clearance (Kt/V urea) or weekly creatinine clearance (CrCl). This will need to consider clearances from both dialysate and kidney components.

Total Kt/V urea = Peritoneal Kt/V urea + Renal Kt/V urea

The recommended range is between 1.7 and 2.0 with a minimal target of 1.7 as recommended by the ISPD. The results of Kt/V urea can be affected by variation in volume (approximately equal to total body water). It does not consider differences in fat content between gender or in patients who are overweight where fat contains less water than muscle. As such, patients with high BMI (hence large V) will result in lower Kt/V urea, giving the impression of inadequate clearance. In cases where the BMI is high, it is preferable to use ideal body weight in the Watson formula for volume calculation.

Total CrCl = Peritoneal CrCl + Renal CrCl

The minimum target is 45 L normalised to 1.73 m^2 of body surface area according to European guidelines. For accurate calculation of V, fat-free body weight should be used. Serum creatinine can be used as a surrogate for kidney creatinine clearance if there is no recent change in body mass or PD prescription.

- The adjustment of solute clearance will be determined mainly by the dialysis dose (i.e., volume of therapy). The dose can be increased by increasing the volume per exchange or the number of exchanges (Table 40.3).

Table 40.3: Ways to Increase Dose of Peritoneal Dialysis According to Clinical Scenarios

Clinical Scenarios	Increase Tonicity	Reduce Tonicity	Increase Dialysis Dose	Reduce Dialysis Dose	Increase Exchanges or Volume	Reduce Exchanges or Volume	Diuretics
Low SSC			+		+		
High SSC				+		+	
Dehydrated		+		+		+	
Overloaded	+		+		+		+

Metabolic and Glycaemic Control

- Good lifestyle changes, such as smoking cessation, regular exercise (at least 30 minutes, 5 times per week), and salt restriction (<2 g sodium or 5 g sodium chloride daily), are recommended.

- There is no good evidence of cardiovascular risk reduction on lipid control in dialysis patients. The magnitude of relative risk reduction among patients on dialysis appears to be substantially smaller than in the earlier stages of CKD and hence initiation of statin treatment is not recommended for most prevalent dialysis patients.

- For glycaemic control, KDIGO recommends a HbA1c target of 7–8% (53–69 mmol/mol), with older diabetic patients on PD aiming for the higher target. Similarly, good nutritional status is essential and should be monitored at least twice a year.

Dialysis related symptom complication

Symptoms control, e.g., itch, insomnia, appetite should be assessed at each clinic session and QOL enquiry at least once a year for holistic person-centric care.

Conclusion

Dialysis adequacy assessment is more than just managing the fundamentals of disease as it should also encompass the assessment of overall wellbeing, life participation, and treatment goals.

References

Auguste BL and Bargman JM (2023). Peritoneal dialysis prescription and adequacy in clinical practice: Core curriculum 2023. *Am J Kidney Dis* **81**(1): 100–109.

Boudville N and de Moraes TP (2020). 2005 guidelines on targets for solute and fluid removal in adults being treated with chronic peritoneal dialysis: 2019 update of the literature and revision of recommendations. *Perit Dial Int* **40**(3): 254–260.

Brown EA, Blake PG, Boudville N, *et al.* (2020). International Society for Peritoneal Dialysis practice recommendations: Prescribing high-quality goal-directed peritoneal dialysis. *Perit Dial Int* **40**(3): 244–253.

Kidney Disease: Improving Global Outcomes (KDIGO) CKD-MBD Work Group (2009). KDIGO clinical practice guideline for the diagnosis, evaluation, prevention, and treatment of chronic kidney disease-mineral and bone disorder (CKD-MBD). *Kidney Int Suppl* (113): S1–S130.

Locatelli F, Nissenson AR, Barrett BJ, *et al.* (2008). Clinical practice guidelines for anemia in chronic kidney disease: problems and solutions. A position statement from Kidney Disease: Improving Global Outcomes (KDIGO). *Kidney Int* **74**(10): 1237–1240.

Rivara MB and Patel A (2022). Living life on PD to its fullest: Towards a PD-focused life participation measure. *Perit Dial International* **42**(6): 549–551.

Wang AY, Brimble KS, Brunier G, *et al.* (2015). ISPD cardiovascular and metabolic guidelines in adult peritoneal dialysis patients part I: Assessment and management of various cardiovascular risk factors. *Perit Dial Int* **35**(4): 379–387.

Wang AY, Dong J, Xu X and Davies S (2020). Volume management as a key dimension of a high-quality PD prescription. *Perit Dial Int* **40**(3): 282–292.

Wanner C, Tonelli M and Kidney Disease: Improving Global Outcomes Lipid Guideline Development Work Group Members (2014). KDIGO clinical practice guideline for lipid management in CKD: Summary of recommendation statements and clinical approach to the patient. *Kidney Int* **85**(6): 1303–1309.

41 Peritoneal Dialysis Catheter Malfunction and Flow Pain

Elizabeth Oei

- Complications that may occur after the insertion of a peritoneal dialysis (PD) catheter include (1) catheter malfunction, (2) peri-catheter leakage, and (3) flow pain.

- PD catheter malfunction is a common cause of technique failure and occurs when there is a problem with PD fluid inflow, outflow, or both.

- Inflow and outflow problems are characterised by:

  - Prolonged flow times — Typically, inflow of 2 L of dialysis solution requires 10–15 minutes to complete while draining out effluent usually takes 20–30 minutes. Longer inflow and outflow times are considered poor flow.

  - PD catheter malfunction may lead to poor small solute clearance and ultrafiltration — in automated PD (APD), PD catheter malfunction may lead to the machine spending a longer filling and/or draining time, resulting in lesser dwell time. Hence, the dialysis dose delivered is less than expected.

Diagnosis of Peritoneal Dialysis Catheter Malfunction

- PD catheter malfunction may be patient- or catheter-related, with extra- or intra-luminal occlusion of the drainage holes of the catheter (Table 41.1).

- PD catheter malfunctions are most commonly due to outflow problems, often due to constipation.

- Differential diagnosis is greatly aided by good history taking — is it poor inflow, poor outflow, or both? Patients on continuous ambulatory PD (CAPD) may have prolonged fill or drain times whereas those on APD might report frequent machine alarms, which may disturb sleep.

- Physical examination and watching a patient perform an exchange may also be helpful (Figure 41.1).

- A bladder scan should be performed to assess post-void residual urine volume to exclude a distended bladder.

- An X-ray of the kidney/ureter/bladder (KUB) is often ordered to check catheter tip position. Faecal loading may also been seen on a KUB X-ray.

- Catheter kinks are not well visualised on a KUB X-ray and a lateral X-ray or computed tomorgraphy (CT) abdomen may be indicated.

Table 41.1:   Causes of Peritoneal Dialysis Catheter Malfunction

Patient-related	Catheter-related
• Constipation	• Migration of catheter tip
• Bladder distension	• Kinking of catheter
• Other intra-abdominal space-occupying lesions	• Intraluminal occlusion by clots or fibrin
• Omental wrapping	
• Adhesions	

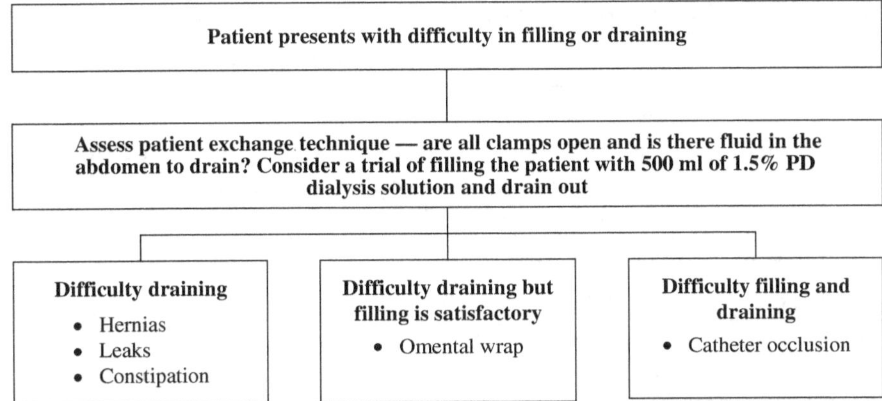

Figure 41.1:   Approach to Peritoneal Dialysis Catheter Flow-related Problems

Source: Modified from http://www.bcrenal.ca/resource-gallery/Documents/RR_PD-Flow-related_ Complications.pdf

Prevention and Management of Peritoneal Dialysis Catheter Malfunction

- Good surgical technique is important in preventing PD catheter malfunction.

- Following the insertion of a PD catheter, the catheter should be irrigated with saline on a weekly basis to prevent clots.

- Constipation should be avoided or managed with diet and laxatives (e.g., polyethylene glycol laxative).

- Management of PD catheter malfunction is dependent on the underlying cause of malfunction (Table 41.2).

Table 41.2:   Management of Peritoneal Dialysis Catheter Malfunction

Cause	Intervention
Constipation	Laxatives
Fibrin or clot	Irrigation using saline or thrombolytic agents with use of wires under fluoroscopic guidance to dislodge intraluminal material or surgical PD catheter exchange
Omental wrap	Omentectomy
Adhesions	Adhesiolysis
Catheter kink or migration	Fluoroscopic/surgical repositioning or PD catheter exchange

Abbreviation: PD, peritoneal dialysis

Pain During Inflow and Outflow of Peritoneal Dialysis Fluid

- Patients may also experience pain during inflow, outflow, or both. Management is dependent on the specific cause (Table 41.3).

Table 41.3:   Management of Inflow and Outflow Pain

Type of Flow Pain	Causes	Intervention
Occurs at the beginning of filling	• Brisk filling rate • Acidity of dialysis solution • Temperature of dialysis solution	• Reduce filling rate by semi-occluding line with finger pressure • Use a biocompatible PD solution • Warm the PD solution before filling in
Occurs throughout the filling process	• Catheter impingement on intra-abdominal organs	• Reposition the catheter
Occurs at the end of filling	• Over-distension of the abdomen	• Incremental PD • Reduce the fill volume • Convert to APD
Occurs at the end of drainage	• Contact of PD catheter with the peritoneal membrane	• Incremental PD • Convert to APD • Tidal APD

Abbreviations: APD, automated peritoneal dialysis; PD; peritoneal dialysis

Reference

Diaz-Bux JA (1998). Management of peritoneal catheter malfunction. *Perit Dial Int* **18**(3): 256–259.

42 Fluid Management in Peritoneal Dialysis Patients

Carolyn Tien, Marjorie Foo

Introduction

- Ultrafiltration (UF) or removal of fluid during peritoneal dialysis (PD) is dependent on several factors such as:
  - Peritoneal membrane characteristics — hydraulic permeability, effective surface area
  - Pressure gradients between the peritoneal blood and intraperitoneal dialysate compartments — transmembrane osmotic, hydrostatic pressure
  - Lymphatic absorption of fluid from the abdominal cavity

  Fluid overload occurs when one or more of these factors reduce transcapillary movement of water into the peritoneal cavity.

- Fluid overload is frequent in PD patients and is an important predictor of increased all-cause as well as cardiovascular mortality and morbidity.

- As a result, it is important to ensure that patients remain euvolaemic and adhere to an appropriate prescribed diet and fluid restriction during maintenance PD.

■ 451

- Optimal fluid management in PD includes a regular review of fluid removal from dialysate and urine with adjustment made over time to increase UF to compensate for eventual declines in kidney function.

- Prescription of PD should focus on optimising UF, exposing the peritoneal membrane to the lowest metabolic burden (glucose exposure), and optimising the use of diuretics. Furthermore, renin-angiotensin-aldosterone system (RAAS) blockers can be used to retard the loss of residual kidney function (RKF).

Causes of Fluid Overload in Peritoneal Dialysis Patients

- Fluid overload in PD patients can be related as well as unrelated to PD (Table 42.1)

Table 42.1:   Causes of Fluid Overload in Peritoneal Dialysis Patients

Related to Peritoneal Dialysis	Unrelated to Peritoneal Dialysis
• Non-adherence to PD regimen — skipping exchanges, shortening or lengthening dwell times, using incorrect PD solution, shortening drain time which allows reabsorption of undrained fluid • Mismatch between PD prescription and peritoneal membrane transport characteristics — high transporters need short dwell times while low transporters need longer dwell times • PD catheter malfunction • Leak of peritoneal dialysis fluid • Peritonitis • Peritoneal membrane failure	• Non-adherence to dietary salt and fluid intake • Loss of residual kidney function • Hypoalbuminaemia • Uncontrolled hyperglycaemia • Cardiac failure • Inadequate doses of diuretics

Abbreviation: PD, peritoneal dialysis

Assessment of Fluid Status

- Patients on PD should have their fluid status reviewed regularly and weight documented. The assessment of fluid status (over-, normo-, and dehydration) in PD relies on clinical and other examinations as follows:
  - Blood pressure (BP) — systolic and diastolic hypertension
  - Raised jugular venous pressure
  - Oedema of the extremities and sacrum
  - Increased weight
  - Respiratory distress
  - Auscultations of the lung fields — pulmonary crepitations, reduced air entry from pleural effusions
  - Chest X-Ray — cardiothoracic ratio, pulmonary oedema, pleural effusion
  - Non-invasive studies — bioimpedance analysis device and lung ultrasound (Table 42.2)

Table 42.2:   Non-Invasive Studies to Assess for Volume Overload in Peritoneal Dialysis Patients

	Bioimpedance Analysis Device	**Lung Ultrasound**
Description	Estimate body fluid volumes by measuring the resistance to electrical current (inversely proportional to TBW)	Detect B lines (pulmonary oedema) and pleural effusion
Advantages	Non-invasive	Non-invasive
Disadvantages	Less accurate in malnourished patients or with hypoalbuminaemia due to distribution between ICW and ECW being altered Measurements must be adjusted for patients with limb amputations	Requires a trained operator and findings are operator-dependent

Abbreviations: TBW, total body water; ICW, intracellular water; ECW, extracellular water

Approach to Fluid Overload

- Exclude medical complications (e.g., acute coronary syndrome, cardiac failure, poorly controlled diabetes mellitus, hypertensive urgency/emergency)

- Review patient factors
  - Dietary and fluid intake
  - Adherence to performing PD treatments
  - Medications that may contribute to oedema or fluid overload (e.g., calcium channel blockers, nephrotoxic agents, inappropriate doses of diuretics)
  - Loss of RKF

- Exclude PD-related issues — dialysate leaks (e.g., pleural, peritoneal, or subcutaneous leaks, inguinal hernias), catheter dysfunction, prescription mismatch, peritoneal membrane dysfunction, PD-related peritonitis.

Investigations for Fluid Overload in Peritoneal Dialysis Patients

- Laboratory tests — Renal panel, glucose, haemoglobin, calcium, phosphate, albumin, HbA1C, cardiac enzymes

- Electrocardiogram

- Echocardiogram

- 24-hour urine volume

- PD effluent appearance, cell count (to exclude PD peritonitis)

- Chest X-Ray — to detect pleural-peritoneal leak, pulmonary oedema

- X-ray kidney, ureter, bladder (KUB) — to detect catheter migration and faecal loading

Management of Fluid Overload in Peritoneal Dialysis Patients

Acute management

- Stabilisation of patient — there may be a need to transfer to the high dependency or intensive care unit according to the clinical condition.

- Assess clinically and decide if there is a need for rapid removal of fluid (using 4.25% to dwell for 2 hours, fill volume 1–1.5 L).

- Treat any PD peritonitis according to the hospital's peritoneal dialysis programme protocol.

Chronic management

- Measure BP daily as a surrogate measure of fluid balance.

- Assess the patient's daily need for fluid intake and counterbalance with output from UF and urine — if fluid balance is achieved, the net daily weight will not change significantly (+/– 0.5 kg).

- Restrict fluid and salt intake (<2 g/day) — reducing salt will lower the sensation of thirst.

- Optimise glycaemic control in patients with diabetes.

- Use diuretics to enhance urine output (if spontaneous pre-existing urine output is > 100 mL/day).

- Preserve peritoneal membrane function — using a biocompatible PD solution, reducing risk of PD peritonitis.

- Start or titrate RAAS blockers to preserve RKF.

- Avoid nephrotoxins.

- Adjust current PD prescription by altering tonicity, dwell time, and fill volume to achieve the daily target UF — Consider APD rather than CAPD for patients who have high solute transfer rates.

- Empower patients to do minor alterations of their prescription tonicity to allow for more or less UF — in patients who are anuric, UF from PD should be at least 750 mL/day to reduce the risks of fluid overload.

- Consider the addition of icodextrin rather than hypertonic solution to help with increasing UF, as meta-analysis shows that icodextrin increases UF and reduces episodes of fluid overload, especially in those who have a high peritoneal solute transfer rate (PSTR).

- In cases of dehydration, it is preferable for the patient to increase their fluid intake rather than to alter their PD prescription or stop PD. Stopping dialysis runs the risk of hyperkalaemia and other electrolyte imbalances.

- Consider kidney replacement treatment modality conversion as per the membrane characteristics assessed by a peritoneal equilibration test (PET) test, e.g., CAPD, APD or explore haemodialysis or transplantation if adequacy cannot be achieved.

Peritoneal Equilibration Test

- Prior to starting PD, the solute and fluid transport characteristics of the peritoneal membrane in an individual patient is unknown and changes over time once when PD begins. As such, the PET is a method of assessing solute and fluid transport characteristics at the time of initiating PD and during PD.

- PET is usually performed 4–6 weeks after starting PD to allow time for equilibration and stabilisation of the patient's condition and PD regimen.

- PET measures the PSTR for urea, creatinine, and glucose based on their concentrations in the dialysate and plasma at specific times (t) during the dialysate dwell. Calculation of PET uses the 4-hour dialysate/peritoneal (D/P) creatinine ratio and glucose concentration (Table 42.3). There are new and shorter versions of PET that can also provide fluid and solute assessment e.g., Mini-PET test.

- The PSTR is a continuum and generally is classified into 4 categories based on the rate of solute equilibration between the blood and dialysate compartments (Table 42.4). In general,

Table 42.3:   Standard Peritoneal Equilibration Test

1. Perform an overnight 8–12-hour exchange with 2.5% dialysate to stabilise the membrane
2. Drain the overnight exchange to completion (facilitated by an upright position) and send sample for creatinine and glucose.
3. Infuse up to 2 L of 2.5% dialysate in supine position, allow for adequate membrane exposure by turning to the sides at regular intervals, dwell time 4 hrs
4. Blood is sampled for creatinine at 2 hrs and dialysate sample for creatinine and glucose at 0, 2, 4 hours

Table 42.4:   Categories of Peritoneal Equilibration Test Results

4H D/P Cr	PET Status	Implication
0.81–1.03	High	• Fast transport for solutes but loses glucose gradient rapidly, so UF can be limited especially with long dwells.
0.65–0.8	High average	• Will do best with more frequent exchanges with shorter dwells to avoid reabsorption. • Consider the use of APD with addition of icodextrin for long dwells if UF is needed.
0.5–0.65	Low average	• Slow transport for solutes and equilibrates slowly so UF is good even with longer dwells.
0.34–0.5	Low	• Will do best with longer dwells and higher volume exchanges to get adequate solute clearance • CAPD

Abbreviations: APD, automated peritoneal dialysis; CAPD, continuous ambulatory peritoneal dialysis; UF, ultrafiltration

a high PSTR will provide patients with good solute transfers but poor UF, while the reverse is true for a low PSTR. This knowledge is helpful for the prescriber to decide the modality of PD treatment (CAPD/APD), dwell time, and tonicity of PD solution for the patient.

References

Brown EA, Davies SJ, Rutherford P, *et al.* (2003). Survival of functionally anuric patients on automated peritoneal dialysis: The European APD Outcome Study. *J Am Soc Nephrol* **14**(11): 2948–2957.

Cho Y, Johnson DW, Badve S, *et al.* (2013). Impact of icodextrin on clinical outcomes in peritoneal dialysis: A systematic review of randomized controlled trials. *Nephrol Dial Transplant* **28**(7): 1899–1907.

Mistry CD, Gokal R and Peers E (1994). A randomized multicenter clinical trial comparing isosmolar icodextrin with hyperosmolar glucose solutions in CAPD. MIDAS Study Group. Multicenter Investigation of Icodextrin in Ambulatory Peritoneal Dialysis. *Kidney Int* **46**(2): 496–503.

Wang AY, Brimble KS, Brunier G, *et al.* (2015). ISPD Cardiovascular and metabolic guidelines in adult peritoneal dialysis patients part I: Assessment and management of various cardiovascular risk factors. *Perit Dial Int* **35**(4): 379–387.

Twardowski ZJ, Nolph KD, Khanna R, *et al.* (1987). Peritoneal equilibration test. *Perit Dial Bull* **7**: 138–147.

La Milla V, Di Filippo S, *et al.* (2005). Mini-peritoneal equilibration test: A simple and fast method to assess free water and small solute transport across the peritoneal membrane. *Kidney Int* **68**(2): 840–846.

43 Peritoneal Dialysis-Related Peritonitis

Cai Jiashen, Htay Htay

Introduction

- Peritoneal dialysis (PD)-related peritonitis is a common and serious complication and can potentially lead to:
    - Removal of PD catheter and switch to haemodialysis
    - Fluid overload due to disruption in membrane permeability
    - Injury and fibrosis to the peritoneal membrane
    - Significant morbidity and occasionally mortality
- PD-related peritonitis can develop through the inoculation of intraperitoneal fluid by pathogens via several routes:
    - Intraluminal — touch contamination
    - Periluminal — exit site infections or tunnel infections
    - Transmural — gut translocation

<u>Calculation of peritonitis episodes per patient year</u>
- Determine years at risk — number of patient days (days on peritoneal dialysis × number of patients)/365 (e.g., 120 days × 150 patients/365 = 43,800/365 = 120)
- Divide the number of reported episodes by years at risk = 65/120 = 0.54 episodes per year

---

- Haematogenous — blood stream
- Transvaginal — through the vagina

- PD programmes should monitor the peritonitis rate at least on a yearly basis, preferably as number of episodes per patient-year.

Diagnosis

- Peritonitis is defined as per the International Society of Peritoneal Dialysis (ISPD) recommendation including at least two of the following:
  - Clinical features consistent with peritonitis — abdominal pain and/or cloudy effluent
  - Dialysis effluent white cell count >100 cells/μL (after dwell time of $\geq$ 2 hours) with > 50% neutrophils
  - Positive dialysis effluent culture
- The most common pathogen is bacteria while fungal and mycobacteria rarely cause PD-related peritonitis. Sometimes, multiple bacteria can be isolated from dialysis effluent culture.
- PD-related peritonitis can be classified according to its pathogenesis (Table 43.1).
- There are other causes of cloudy dialysis effluent which need to be considered if infective peritonitis is unlikely:
  - Chemical peritonitis
  - Eosinophilia of the effluent
  - Haemoperitoneum
  - Malignancy
  - Chylous effluent

Table 43.1: Peritoneal Dialysis Peritonitis According to Pathogenesis

Types of PD Peritonitis	Definition
Pre-PD peritonitis	An episode that occurs after insertion of PD catheter and prior to commencement of PD
PD catheter insertion-related peritonitis	An episode that occurs within 30 days of PD catheter insertion
Catheter-related peritonitis	An episode that occurs in temporal conjunction with a catheter infection (either exit site or tunnel) with the same organism at the exit site and in the effluent
Enteric peritonitis	Peritonitis arising from an intestinal source involving inflammation, perforation or ischaemia of intra-abdominal organs

Abbreviation: PD, peritoneal dialysis

Assessment

- All PD patients presented with abdominal pain or cloudy effluent should be managed as peritonitis until proven otherwise (Figure 43.1).

- Assessment of a PD patient suspected to have peritonitis should include assessing the severity of infection (Table 43.2), possible risk factors or causes of peritonitis (Table 43.3), and complications of PD-related peritonitis.

Management of PD-Related Peritonitis

- PD-related peritonitis episodes can be managed in the outpatient setting. However, patients should be admitted for close monitoring and treatment if they have the following conditions:
  - Unstable haemodynamics
  - Signs of systemic inflammation (e.g., fever)

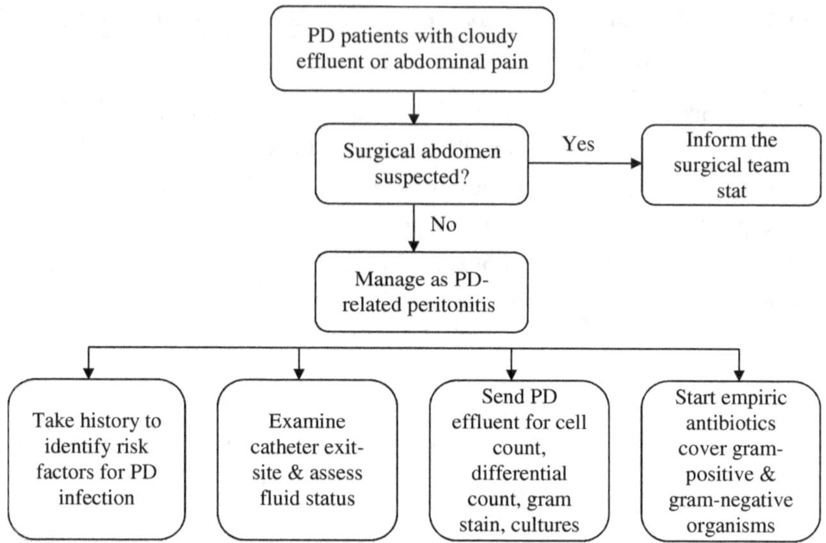

Figure 43.1: Approach to Patients with PD Peritonitis

Table 43.2:   Assessment of PD-Related Peritonitis

Assessment	Clinical Parameters
Severity of infection	• Vital signs for haemodynamic stability
Risk factor/causes	• History of touch contamination, adherence to sterile technique • Recent invasive procedures (e.g., colonoscopy) • Changes in bowel habits (e.g., diarrhoea or constipation) • Exit site or tunnel tract infection
Complications	• Fluid overload
Laboratory tests	• PD effluent tests (before antibiotics are started) — gram stain, cell count and differential, aerobic and anaerobic culture (using blood culture bottles) • Blood cultures if patient appears septic or an acute surgical abdomen is suspected

Abbreviations: CRP, C-reactive protein; FBC, full blood count; PD, peritoneal dialysis

Table 43.3:   Risk Factors for Peritoneal Dialysis Peritonitis

	Non-modifiable	**Modifiable**
Patient-related	• Older age • Female • Black ethnicity • Lower socioeconomic status • Diabetes mellitus • Coronary artery disease • Chronic lung disease • Hypertension • Poor residual kidney function	• Obesity • Smoking • Depression • Hypoalbuminaemia • Hypokalaemia • Constipation • Medical procedures (e.g., colonoscopy) • No vitamin D supplement • Bioincompatible fluids • Nasal *Staphylococcus aureus* carrier • Previous exit site infection • Touch or wet contamination
Technique-related	• Centre effect	• Method of patient training • Connecting system • Prophylactic antibiotics for nasal carriage • Prophylactic antibiotics for exit site care
Environment-related	• Hot and humid climate	• Living distantly from PD unit • Household pets

Adapted from Cheuk-Chun S (2017). Peritonitis in peritoneal dialysis patients. In Nissenson AR and Fine RN (eds.) *Handbook of Dialysis Therapy* (Elsevier, Philadelphia), pp. 435–447.

- Severe abdominal pain

- Concomitant exit site infection

- Elderly or immunocompromised patients

- Unable to continue self-care or perform self-administration of antibiotic therapy or there is no caregiver to help otherwise

- Suspected relapse or recurrent peritonitis
- Polymicrobial peritonitis with multiple gram-negative organisms or anaerobic organisms
- Pre-existing conditions increasing the risk for secondary peritonitis (e.g., diverticular disease)

- Antibiotics should be administered as soon as possible without waiting for a confirmation of diagnosis.
- The intraperitoneal (IP) route is preferred over the IV route to treat PD-related peritonitis.
- The empiric antibiotics should be decided based on:
  - Types of common micro-organisms and sensitivity results of the PD centre
  - Ability to cover both gram-positive and gram-negative organisms
- The subsequent choice and duration of antibiotics are based on causative organisms (Table 43.4).
- Majority of PD-related peritonitis episodes respond to antibiotics therapy, but removal of the PD catheter should be considered in the following conditions:
  - Fungal peritonitis (urgent removal is required within 24 hours)
  - Refractory peritonitis (Table 43.5)
  - Relapsed peritonitis (Table 43.5)
  - Peritonitis with concomitant exit site or tunnel infection
  - Exit site or tunnel tract infection that led to subsequent peritonitis
  - Refractory exit site and tunnel tract infection (Table 43.5)

Table 43.4: Choice of Antibiotics and Duration of Therapy for PD-Related Peritonitis

Organisms	Antibiotics and Duration
Gram-positive Organisms	
Streptococcus species	IP cefazolin for 2 weeks if susceptible
Staph aureus	IP cefazolin for 3 weeks if susceptible If MRSA — IP vancomycin for 3 weeks
Coagulase negative Staph	IP cefazolin for 2 weeks if susceptible Methicillin resistant — IP vancomycin for 2 weeks
Corynebacterium species	IP vancomycin for 2 weeks
Enterococcus species	IP vancomycin for 3 weeks or PO amoxicillin 3 weeks VRE — refer to the infectious disease physician for linezolid or daptomycin
Other Gram-positive	IP cefazolin for 2 weeks if susceptible
Gram-negative Organisms	
Pseudomonas species	IP amikacin for 2 weeks and PO ciprofloxacin 3 weeks; if resistant to one of these antibiotics, change to IP ceftazidime for 3 weeks if resistant but give 2 antibiotics
Stenotrophomonas species	PO bactrim — 3 weeks and levofloxacin — 3 weeks (give 2 drugs, monitor neutropenia)
Other gram-negative	IP amikacin or gentamicin if susceptible, or third generation cephalosporin-based regimen 2–3 weeks
ESCAPM	As per culture — 3 weeks
Polymicrobial	
Multiple gram-positive	As per culture sensitivity — 3 weeks
Multiple gram-negative	Consider surgical abdomen, treat as per culture sensitivity — 3 weeks, add metronidazole if anaerobic organisms are identified
Culture negative	Improvement — IP cefazolin or vancomycin for 2 weeks No improvement — re-culture, AFB, fungal smear, and culture

(Continued)

Table 43.4: (*Continued*)

Organisms	Antibiotics and Duration
Fungal species	Immediate PD catheter removal Commence anti-fungal therapy — for 2 weeks as per sensitivity
Mycobacterial species	
Non-tuberculous species	Refer to ID physician, macrolides, and aminoglycoside, arrange for catheter removal
Tuberculous peritonitis	Refer to ID physician, anti-TB therapy, may not need to remove catheter

Notes:

- All patients must receive Nystatin 500,000 units qds for the length of antibiotics treatment plus additional 2 days after the last dose of aminoglycoside, 7 days after the last dose of vancomycin
- Add PO acetylcysteine 600 mg bd if order aminoglycoside to prevent ototoxicity
- If no improvement at 72 hours, reevaluate, review antibiotics and culture, repeat culture including fungal and AFB, consider catheter removal if no clinical improvement by day 5

Abbreviations: AFB, acid-fast bacilli; ESCAPM, Enterobacter, Serratia, Citrobacter, Aeromonas, Acinetobacter, Providencia, Proteus, Morganella; ID, infectious disease; IP, intraperitoneal; PO, per oral; PD, peritoneal dialysis; TB, tuberculosis

Table 43.5: International Society of Peritoneal Dialysis Recommendation for Management of Different Types of PD-Related Peritonitis

Types of Peritonitis	Definition as per International Society for Peritoneal Dialysis (ISPD) Guidelines	ISPD Recommendation
Relapsing peritonitis	Peritonitis episode occurs within 4 weeks of completion of antibiotics therapy for a prior episode with the same organism or one sterile episode	Recommend timely PD catheter removal Simultaneous catheter removal and reinsertion can be considered if culture is negative, effluent cell count <100/uL, and there are no concomitant exit site or tunnel infections
Recurrent peritonitis	Peritonitis episode occurs within 4 weeks of completion of antibiotics for a prior episode with different organisms	
Repeat peritonitis	Peritonitis episode occurs > 4 weeks after completion of antibiotics therapy for a prior episode with the same organism	

Table 43.5:   (*Continued*)

Types of Peritonitis	Definition as per International Society for Peritoneal Dialysis (ISPD) Guidelines	ISPD Recommendation
Refractory peritonitis	Failure of the effluent to clear after 5 days of appropriate antibiotics	Recommend catheter removal, however, observation for >5 days is appropriate if cell count trends downwards towards normal

Prevention of PD-Related Peritonitis

- Prophylactic antibiotics should be prescribed to prevent peritonitis in PD patients before certain procedures such as dental procedures and scopes (Table 43.6).

- Patients should be advised to seek medical attention from the PD team immediately if contamination occurs during dialysis exchange so that appropriate measures can be taken to prevent peritonitis (Table 43.7).

- Conditions including constipation, persistent hypokalaemia, and use of histamine 2 blockers (H2 blockers) are reported to increase the risks of peritonitis and should be avoided as much as possible.

- Adoption of proper exit site care including application of topical antimicrobial cream is crucial to prevent peritonitis.

- Education and re-training should be considered for all PD patients who developed PD peritonitis.

Table 43.6: Prophylactic Antibiotics Prior to Procedures to Prevent PD-Related Peritonitis

Type of Procedures	Prophylactic Antibiotics
PD catheter placement	IV cefazolin 2 g (IV vancomycin 15–20 mg/kg if allergic to vancomycin or MRSA carrier) just before procedure
Dental procedures	PO amoxicillin 2 g to be given 2 hours before procedure or PO clindamycin 600 mg if allergic to penicillin
Cholecystectomy, colonoscopy, cystoscopy, ureteroscope, hysteroscopy, IUCD insertion	IV ampicillin 1 g (IV vancomycin 15–20 mg/kg if allergic to penicillin) and IV gentamicin 240 mg just before procedure. The abdomen should be empty prior to abdominal or pelvic procedures

Table 43.7: Types of Contamination and Management

Types of Contamination	Conditions	Antibiotics Therapy
Dry contamination (contamination outside a closed PD system)	Disconnection distal to closed clamp	Not need antibiotics
Wet contamination (contamination with an open PD system)	Catheter set left open for extended period, dialysis fluid is not infused	IP vancomycin one dose only
	Dialysis fluid is infused after contamination (physical defect in tubing or leak from dialysis bag during dialysis)	Send effluent for tests. IP vancomycin one dose and IP gentamicin for 3 days or till effluent results are out

Change transfer set immediately before dialysis for all contaminations.

References

Li PK, Chow KM, Cho Y, *et al.* (2022). ISPD peritonitis guideline recommendations: 2022 update on prevention and treatment. *Perit Dial Int* **42**(2): 110–153.

Li PK, Szeto CC, Piraino B, *et al.* (2016). ISPD peritonitis recommendations: 2016 update on prevention and treatment. *Perit Dial Int* **36**(5): 481–508.

44 Peritoneal Dialysis Catheter-Related Infections

Mathini Jayaballa

Introduction

- Peritoneal dialysis (PD) involves the insertion and maintenance of a catheter that extends from the external abdominal surface into the peritoneal cavity through the layers of subcutaneous fat and muscle in the abdominal wall (Figures 44.1 and 44.2).

- PD catheter-related infections refers to both exit site infection (ESI) and/or tunnel infection. These two conditions can occur on their own or simultaneously.

- Catheter-related infection is one of the most common PD-related complications and can lead to peritonitis, permanent loss of the PD catheter, and transfer to haemodialysis.

- Therefore, the primary goal of exit site care is to prevent infections in PD.

Pathogenesis

- Soon after insertion of a PD catheter, the catheter and exit site often get colonised with microorganisms. These microorganisms often produce a biofilm which further encourages bacterial growth as well as protects themselves from the immune

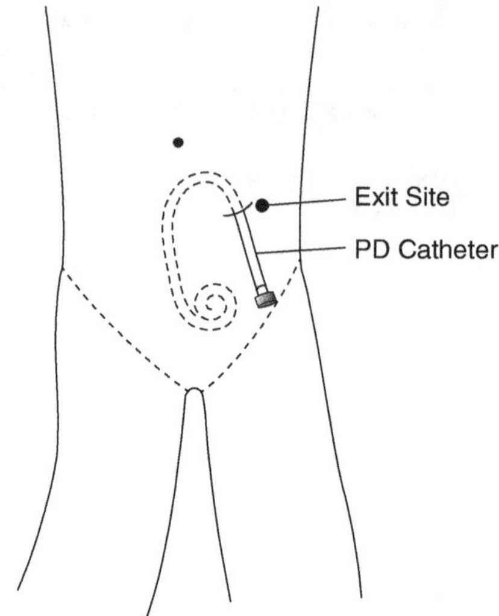

Figure 44.1

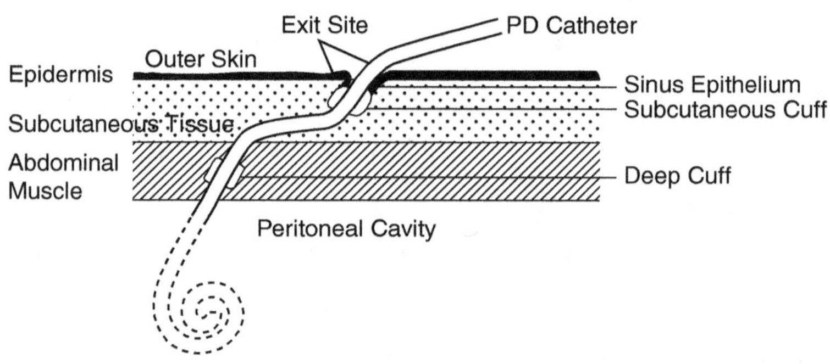

Figure 44.2

system and antimicrobial agents. Although microbial colonisation does not always mean a clinical infection, it does pre-dispose PD patients to ESI, especially following any mild exit site trauma. The infection may involve just the exit site and/or the tunnel tract of the catheter.

- Some of the common pathogens to cause PD catheter-related infections are gram-positive organisms (commonly

Staphylococcus aureus and *coagulase negative Staphylococcus*) and gram-negative organisms (commonly *Pseudomonas aeruginosa and Escherichia coli*).

- The pathogens that cause PD catheter-related infections have shifted over time with the routine use of antibiotic prophylaxis for exit site care in PD patients. Most infections are still caused by gram-positive organisms, but the relative percentage caused by *Staphylococcus aureus* seems to have reduced with relative increase in other gram-positive organisms and gram-negative organisms. There is also an occurrence of unusual organisms such atypical mycobacteria, corynebacteria, burkholderia species, as well as fungal pathogens.

Risk Factors

- Risk factors for PD catheter-related infections can be related to catheter placement and exit site self-care (Table 44.1).

- Factors such as age, sex, race, and clinical factors such as diabetes or insulin dependence do not predict infection rates.

Table 44.1: Risk Factors for Peritoneal Dialysis Catheter-Related Infection

Peritoneal Dialysis Catheter Placement	Peritoneal Dialysis Catheter Self-Care
• Poor catheter immobilisation • Catheter-pulling injury	• Poor competency of exit site care • Swimming • Presence of pets during exchanges • Mechanical stress on the exit site by the waist belt or peritoneal dialysis catheter bag

Diagnosis

Exit site infection

- PD catheter exit site infection is characterised by purulent discharge from the exit site which may be associated with:
    - Erythema of the skin at the catheter-epidermal surface
    - Tenderness
    - Exuberant granuloma
    - Oedema
- Peri-catheter erythema without purulent discharge is sometimes an early indication of infection but can also be a normal skin reaction to a recently implanted PD catheter or an exit site trauma. Crusting alone or positive cultures from exit site without signs of inflammation is not indicative of infection.

Tunnel infection

- Most, but not all, PD catheter tunnel infections occur in conjunction with exit site infections. Of note, exit site infections caused by *Staphylococcus aureus* or *Pseudomonas aeruginosa* are often associated with concomitant tunnel infections. The presence of a tunnel infection increases the risk for peritonitis.
- PD catheter tunnel infection is characterised by:
    - Clinical inflammation — erythema, oedema, induration, tenderness
    - Intermittent or chronic purulent, bloody, or gooey discharge which discharges spontaneously or after pressure on the cuff
    - Ultrasonographic evidence of a fluid collection along the catheter tunnel

- However, PD catheter tunnel infection is often occult and often only unveiled with ultrasound.

Severity Classification of Peritoneal Dialysis Catheter Exit Site Infection

- Proper assessment of the exit site requires gross inspection of the exit site including the:

  - External skin and sinus epithelium

  - Palpation of the tunnel tract and expression of discharge from the exit site

- There are different grading systems that have been proposed to document the clinical severity of ESI. The severity of infection is often graded based on the presence of swelling, crust, redness, pain, and drainage (Table 44.2).

Table 44.2: Classification of Exit Site Infection According to Appearance

Perfect exit site	A perfect exit site is usually achieved 6 months after catheter placement but can occur as early as 3 months after. With a perfect exit site, there is normal skin with natural skin colour. There is mature and dry epithelium in the sinus where crust formation occurs no more than once every 7 days. There should be no pain, swelling, pink or red skin, granulation tissue, external exudation, or any internal secretion.
Good exit site	A good exit site usually takes more than 6 weeks of healing time to occur. The skin is natural in colour and redness should not extend more than 13 mm from the catheter, including the width of the catheter. There should be no pain, swelling, bright pink or red colour, exuberant granulation tissue, external exudation, or abundant internal secretion.

(Continued)

Table 44.2:   (*Continued*)

Equivocal exit site	An equivocal exit site is neither a good exit site nor an obvious infection. Purulent or bloody drainage is only present in the sinus, cannot be expressed outside, and is accompanied by regression of the epithelium and slight exuberant granulation tissue in the sinus. There might be some mild redness but there is no pain, swelling, or external drainage. Crust usually develops every one to two days. This crust may occur in the form of a cuff that is large or difficult to detach. Equivocal sites often suggest low-grade infections that may improve spontaneously or progress if left untreated.
Acute infection	Characterised by redness, swelling, and tenderness. The area of redness is greater than 13 mm in diameter. The erythema is more than twice the diameter of the catheter, and there is regression of the epithelium in the sinus. The exit site may be painful and a scab and/or daily crust might be present. Crusting alone does not mean infection. External drainage is purulent or bloody. This drainage may be spontaneous or expressed after pressing on the sinus and is often in the form of a white, yellow, or green liquid. Of note, a large amount of serous drainage may indicate a sign of infection.
Chronic infection	Characteristics of exit site are similar to that of an acute infection but the duration of infection is more than 4 weeks. Granulation tissue is typically present both externally and in the sinus of the exit site in chronic infections. The exit is sometimes covered by a large, persistent crust or scab. There is usually no pain, redness, or swelling, and the skin is often hyper-pigmented.
Traumatised exit site	This is not an infection but may involve pain, bleeding, scab development, and deterioration of the exit site. It may be a pre-disposition to developing an exit site infection.

Management (Figure 44.3)

Prevention of ESI

- Proper care of the exit site is paramount in the prevention of ESI and hence peritonitis, and overall outcomes of PD patients.

Exit site infection

1. Clinical examination
2. Swab and send for culture
3. ± Ultrasound to assess for tunnel tract infection

1. Initiate empirical antibiotics
2. Ensure appropiate daily exit site care
3. ± Shaving of extruded/protruded external cuff
4. Modify antimicrobials once culture and
sensitivity results return

Consider catheter removal if

- ESI refractory to medical treatment
- Recurrent ESI with the same organism
- Concurrent tunnel tract infection
- Peritonitis occurring simultaneously or as
  a consequence

Figure 44.3:   Summary of Management of Exit Site Infections in Peritoneal Dialysis Patients

Proper exit site care involves the use of cleansing agents, topical antiseptic/antibiotics, and local dressing.

- During the early post-operative (first 2 weeks), keep exit site dry until it is well healed. It should be covered with sterile dressing. This dressing change should only be performed by an experienced PD nurse before the patient is trained to do so.

- Once the patient or caregiver is properly trained, they should wash the exit site with anti-septic cleansing agents (e.g., povidone iodine or chlorhexidine). This should be done at least twice weekly or after every shower; if not, daily in the presence of an ESI.

- Prophylactic topical antibiotic cream/ointment (e.g., gentamycin cream, mupirocin ointment) should be applied to exit site daily.

- Exit sites should be examined daily by the patient/caregiver at home or by a PD nurse in the hospital and be constantly covered in sterile dressing.

- Two topical antibiotics that have been shown to be effective in reducing ESI and hence are commonly used for exit site care in PD patients are gentamicin and mupirocin. Some PD centres choose either one whilst others alternate between the two, though the latter is shown to have a higher rate of fungal peritonitis. Gentamicin is as effective as mupirocin against *Staphylococcus aureus* and other gram-positive organisms and may be more effective against gram-negative organisms such as pseudomonas. Usually, gentamicin is less costly than mupirocin. Other alternative topical antimicrobial agents, including medihoney, have been studied but have yet to be proven to be as effective in the prevention of ESI.

- Hand hygiene plays an integral part in reducing the risk of ESI. All who are handling the PD catheter including the patient/caregiver and healthcare professionals need to have proper hand hygiene practices before and after handling the PD catheter and its exit site using a hand sanitising agent. The most effective is 70% alcohol-based hand rub or anti-microbial soap.

Treatment of ESI

- The exit site discharge should be sent for microscopy, gram stain, culture, and sensitivity pattern. This should be taken first before the initiation of empirical antibiotics.

- Do an abdominal wall ultrasonography of the exit site region if there is any suspicion of local collections or tunnel tract collections.

- Exit site infection should be treated right away with empirical anti-microbial therapy.

- Start oral cefuroxime 250 mg BD. The initial choice of treatment with empirical antibiotics is usually from a centre-based protocol (which should be based on local antibiograms) and initial gram-stain; it should have appropriate *Staphylococcus aureus* cover. It is also important to account for any previous infections and the profile of those organisms. In general, first-generation cephalosporin or penicillinase-resistant penicillin (e.g., dicloxacillin or flucloxacillin) can be used as initial treatment for ESI in PD patients.

- Once the microbiological swab culture results which identify the culprit organisms and their antibiotic susceptibility profile are available, the choice of appropriate antibiotics and duration of therapy should be modified accordingly.

- If the patient has a prior infection or colonisation with methicillin-resistant *S. aureus* (MRSA) and gram stain showing gram-positive organisms, they should also receive empiric treatment for MRSA; we use intraperitoneal vancomycin (15–20 mg/kg as first dose) and vancomycin levels should be checked prior to redosing with a goal to achieve a therapeutic serum level of 15–20 mcg/mL.

- If the patient has prior infection or colonistion with pseudomonas and gram stain showing gram-negative organisms, they should also receive empiric treatment for pseudomonas; we use oral ciprofloxacin 250 mg BD. Pseudomonas aeruginosa ESI can be difficult to treat and may require two antibiotics to be given concurrently with longer duration.

- Note that when giving intermittent dosing of intraperitoneal antibiotics, it is important to ensure that the dwell time is at least 6 hours in order to allow adequate absorption.

- Effective antibiotic treatment duration for ESI should be at least 2 weeks. However, for tunnel infection or ESI caused by pseudomonas species, the duration of treatment should be 3 weeks. Antibiotic therapy should be continued until the exit site appears entirely normal. Patients with ESI and/or tunnel infection should be closely followed up to ascertain if they do respond to therapy.

- If the external cuff is partially or fully protruding outside the exit site, trimming or shaving of the external cuff can be considered.

- Whenever systemic antibiotics are prescribed in PD patients, concurrent use of antifungal prophylaxis (e.g., oral nystatin) might be beneficial to lower the risk of fungal peritonitis. However, there is no data that directly supports the use of anti-fungal prophylaxis during the treatment of catheter-related infection.

Refractory exit site infection

- Refractory ESI is defined as failure to respond after 3 weeks of effective antibiotic therapy.

- Those with refractory ESI/tunnel infection without concurrent peritonitis should have the catheter removed and have a new catheter inserted simultaneously with a new exit site under antibiotic coverage.

- However, those with ESI/tunnel infection and concurrent peritonitis need to have their catheter removed and most would go on to require temporary haemodialysis whilst awaiting another catheter reinsertion. In such circumstances, it is recommended that any reinsertion of a PD catheter be performed at least 2 weeks after catheter removal and complete resolution of peritoneal symptoms.

- Some indications for PD catheter removal:
  - Refractory catheter related infection — ESI and/or tunnel infection
  - Catheter-related infection that occurs simultaneously with a peritonitis episode
  - Catheter-related infection that leads to a subsequent peritonitis episode

- ESI that is caused by atypical mycobacteria can be challenging to treat, requiring at least two or more systemic antimicrobial agents (e.g., parenteral aminoglycosides, fluoroquinolones, tetracyclines, and macrolides) and a prolonged therapy duration of at least 6 weeks. Despite that, less than half the patients will respond to medical therapy and will require catheter removal for refractory ESI.

- ESI caused by fungi is rare and there is limited evidence to recommend its optimal treatment. When fungi are isolated from an exit site swab, it may be wise to exclude contamination of the swab as a cause for this. However, if a true fungal ESI is confirmed, then removal of the PD catheter should be considered to avoid progression to fungal peritonitis, of which the latter entails high risk of morbidity and mortality.

References

Bernardini J, Bender F, Florio T, *et al.* (2005). Randomized, double-blind trial of antibiotic exit site cream for prevention of exit site infection in peritoneal dialysis patients. *J Am Soc Nephrol* **16**(2): 539–545.

Kwan TH, Tong MK, Siu YP, *et al.* (2004). Ultrasonography in the management of exit site infections in peritoneal dialysis patients. *Nephrology* **9**(6): 348–352.

Lee A (2019). Swimming on peritoneal dialysis: Recommendations from Australian PD units. *Perit Dial Int* **39**(6): 527–531.

Li PK, Szeto CC, Piraino B, *et al.* (2010). Peritoneal dialysis-related infections recommendations: 2010 update. *Perit Dial Int* **30**(4): 393–423.

Lin J, Ye H, Li J, *et al.* (2020). Prevalence and risk factors of exit-site infection in incident peritoneal dialysis patients. *Perit Dial Int* **40**(2): 164–170.

Lo MW, Mak SK, Wong YY, *et al.* (2013). Atypical mycobacterial exit-site infection and peritonitis in peritoneal dialysis patients on prophylactic exit-site gentamicin cream. *Perit Dial Int* **33**(3): 267–272.

Lo WK, Chan CY, Cheng SW, *et al.* (1996). A prospective randomized control study of oral nystatin prophylaxis for Candida peritonitis complicating continuous ambulatory peritoneal dialysis. *Am J Kidney Dis* **28**(4): 549–552.

Nadeau-Fredette AC and Bargman JM (2015). Characteristics and outcomes of fungal peritonitis in a modern North American cohort. *Perit Dial Int* **35**(1): 78–84.

Piraino B, Bailie GR, Bernardini J, *et al.* (2005). Peritoneal dialysis-related infections recommendations: 2005 update. *Perit Dial Int* **25**(2): 107–131.

Piraino B, Bernardini J, Brown E, *et al.* (2011). ISPD position statement on reducing the risks of peritoneal dialysis-related infections. *Perit Dial Int* **31**(6): 614–630.

Renaud CJ, Subramanian S, Tambyah PA and Lee EJ (2011). The clinical course of rapidly growing nontuberculous mycobacterial peritoneal dialysis infections in Asians: A case series and literature review. *Nephrology* **16**(2): 174–179.

Scalamogna A, De Vecchi A, Maccario M, *et al.* (1995). Cuff-shaving procedure. a rescue treatment for exit-site infection unresponsive to medical therapy. *Nephrol Dial Transplant* **10**(12): 2325–2327.

Szeto CC, Li PK, Johnson DW, *et al.* (2017). ISPD catheter-related infection recommendations: 2017 update. *Perit Dial Int* **37**(2): 141–154.

Tsai CC, Yang PS, Liu CL, *et al.* (2018). Comparison of topical mupirocin and gentamicin in the prevention of peritoneal dialysis-related infections: A systematic review and meta-analysis. *Am J Surg* **215**(1): 179–185.

Twardowski ZJ and Prowant BF (1996). Classification of normal and diseased exit sites. *Perit Dial Int* **16**(Suppl 3): S32–S50.

Wong PN, Tong GM, Wong YY, *et al.* (2016). Alternating mupirocin/gentamicin is associated with increased risk of fungal peritonitis as compared with gentamicin alone: Results of a randomized open-label controlled trial. *Perit Dial Int* **36**(3): 340–346.

Critical Care Nephrology

45 Acute Kidney Injury

Teo Su Hooi

Introduction

- Acute kidney Injury (AKI) is a heterogeneous syndrome characterised by a sudden and often reversible reduction in kidney function as measured by the glomerular filtrate rate (GFR). This results in the retention of nitrogenous waste products, fluid overload, and the dysregulation of electrolytes.

- AKI is a common condition and can be seen in up to 7% of hospital admissions. It can be serious and accounts for 30% of admissions to the intensive care unit (ICU).

- AKI is defined as a range of acute kidney diseases which can also lead to chronic kidney disease (CKD).

- AKI is defined as any one of the following:

  - Increase in serum creatinine (sCr) by $\geq 26.5\,\mu$mol/L within 48 hours

  - Increase in sCr to ≥ 1.5 times the baseline, which is known or presumed to have occurred within the last 7 days

  - Urine volume < 0.5 mL/kg/hr for 6 hours

"

Diagnosis

- The Kidney Disease: Improving Global Outcomes (KDIGO) stages the severity of AKI from stage 1 (mild) to stage 3 (severe) (Table 45.1).

Types of Acute Kidney Injury

- AKI can be classified into three types based on the location and mechanism of injury (Figure 45.1):
    1. Pre-renal
    2. Intrinsic
    3. Post-renal
- Many patients have more than one overlapping aetiology.

Pre-renal AKI

Pre-renal AKI conditions that can cause kidney injury include:

- Hypovolaemia

Table 45.1:   KDIGO Staging of Acute Kidney Injury

Stage	Serum Creatinine	Urine Output	Other
1	1.5–1.9 times baseline or $\geq 26.5\,\mu$mol/L increase	<0.5 mL/kg/hr for 6–12 hours	
2	2.0–2.9 times baseline	<0.5 mL/kg/hr for ≥ 12 hours	
3	3.0 times baseline or Increase in serum creatinine to $\geq 354\,\mu$mol/L	<0.3 mL/kg/hr for ≥ 24 hours or Anuria for ≥ 12 hours	Initiation of renal replacement therapy

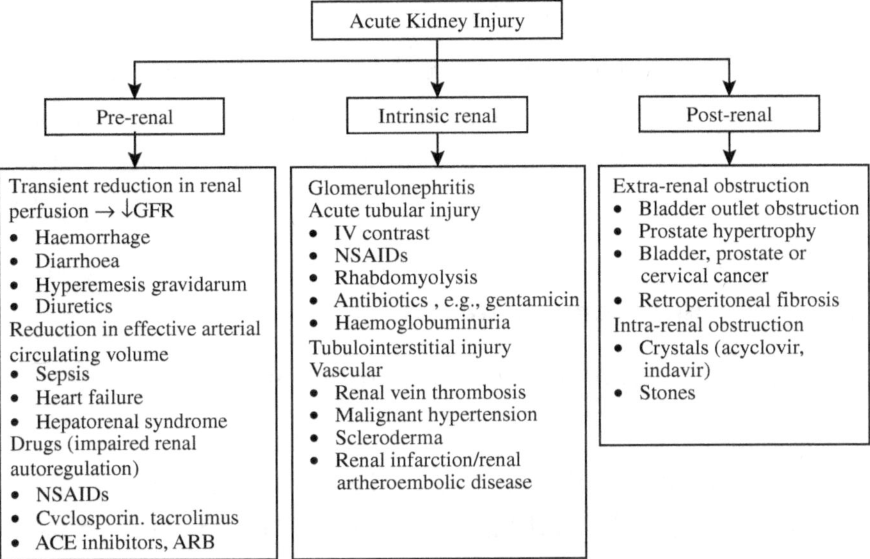

Figure 45.1:   Aetiologies of Acute Kidney Failure

- Gastrointestinal (e.g., reduced oral intake, vomiting, diarrhoea)

- Haemorrhage

- Unreplenished insensible losses (e.g., burns)

- Over-diuresis

- Hypervolaemic states with reduced effective arterial volume causing low renal perfusion pressure:

  - Heart failure with reduced ejection fraction

  - Decompensated liver disease with portal hypertension

- Abdominal compartment syndrome

- Hypercalcaemia

- Systemic vasodilation (e.g., sepsis)

- Intrarenal vasoconstriction
  - Medications: nonsteroidal anti-inflammatory drugs (NSAIDs), renin-angiotensin-aldosterone (RAAS) blockers, cyclosporine, tacrolimus, iodinated radiocontrast media

Intrinsic renal vascular disease

- Glomerular: nephrotic or nephritic pattern
- Vascular:
  - Small vessel vasculitis and disease that cause micro-angiopathy and haemolytic anaemia (MAHA), thrombotic thrombocytopenic purpura/haemolytic uraemic syndrome (TTP/HUS), scleroderma, atheroembolic kidney disease, malignant hypertension
  - Larger vessels: kidney infarction from aortic dissection, kidney artery aneurysm, acute kidney vein thrombosis, systemic thromboembolism
- Interstitial and tubular disease
  - Acute tubular necrosis (ATN) from ischaemia or a nephrotoxic exposure (e.g., RAAS blockers with NSAIDs)
  - Medications (e.g., immune checkpoint inhibitors for cancer immunotherapy, crystalline nephropathy associated acyclovir, acute phosphate nephropathy following a phosphate-containing bowel preparation)
  - Cast nephropathy in multiple myeloma or other monoclonal gammopathies
  - Infections (e.g., dengue virus, leptospirosis, candidiasis)

- Systemic disease (e.g., sarcoidosis, lupus)
- Tubular injury in the setting of COVID-19

Post-renal disease

Post-renal disease is caused by obstructive uropathy. A substantial reduction in GFR suggests bilateral obstruction (or unilateral obstruction of a single functioning kidney).

- Bladder outlet obstruction, prostatic pathology (prostate hypertrophy or cancer), bladder, cervical, or metastatic cancer, retroperitoneal fibrosis, etc.

Approach to Evaluating a Patient with Acute Kidney Injury

- The initial assessment of a patient with AKI should include a detailed history and physical examination. The timing of onset of AKI is important because the timing of onset often suggests the contributing cause(s) of the AKI.

- In hospitalised patients, the date of onset can be precisely timed if the sCr had been measured frequently. For example, if sCr only begins to rise on day 5 of hospital admission in a patient with a prior stable sCr, one should review the course of hospitalisation in the medical notes to ascertain any precipitating event(s) on day 3 or 4 (e.g., hypotension and/or radiocontrast exposure may have occurred).

- Review of historical progress of the patient should include:
  - Exposure to nephrotoxic medications or other nephrotoxins (e.g., NSAIDs)

- Inciting events (e.g., diarrhoea, nausea, vomiting causing volume depletion)
- Pre-existing chronic medications (particularly RAAS blockers) that render patients vulnerable to AKI from ATN or pre-renal causes of AKI

- Physical examination should emphasise assessing the patient's volume status, for example:
  - Assessing intravascular volume status for signs of volume contraction (pre-renal aetiologies)
  - "Drug rash" suggests acute tubulointerstitial nephritis
  - Significant volume overload and signs of volume overload suggests cardio-renal syndrome
  - "Blue toes" suggests cholesterol emboli
  - Livedo reticularis, digital ischaemia, and purpura suggest vasculitis

- The initial laboratory evaluation should include:
  - Renal panel
  - Full blood count
  - Urine microscopy
  - Quantification of urine protein or albumin
  - Urine electrolytes such as measurement of fractional excretion of sodium (FE_{Na}) which is helpful in distinguishing pre-renal from intrinsic renal causes of AKI
  - Imaging studies to exclude obstruction

- Further testing includes:
  - Serologic testing — anti-neutrophil cytoplasmic antibodies (ANCA), anti-nuclear antibodies (ANA), anti-double-

stranded deoxyribonucleic acid antibodies (anti-dsDNA), anti-streptolysin titer (ASOT), complement levels (C3, C4)

- Virology testing — hepatitis B, hepatitis C, HIV serology
- Myeloma panel — to look for monoclonal spikes
- Kidney biopsy

Overview of the Management of Acute Kidney Injury in Adults

- The current strategies of managing AKI are focused on alleviating poor outcomes by emphasising clinical risk identification, early detection of injury, modifying clinician behaviour to avoid harm, and providing surveillance among survivors for the longer-term sequelae of CKD.

Initial management

- If fluid overload is not a concern, patients with AKI should receive a fluid challenge with close monitoring of urine output and renal panel.
- If the renal function improves with fluids, this points towards a pre-renal cause of AKI. AKI due to ATN does not improve or improves only slowly.
- Complications of AKI should also be addressed such as fluid overload and hyperkalaemia:
  - High doses of IV furosemide may be needed to correct volume overload in patients with AKI. However, not all patients will respond to diuretics. A frusemide stress test can be performed by administering 1–1.5 mg/kg of frusemide. If the urine output is less than 200 mL within 2 hours of

the furosemide dose, the patient should be prepared for kidney replacement therapy without further delay.

- Hyperkalaemia should also be treated. Initial medical therapy for hyperkalaemia includes:
  - IV calcium gluconate 10 mL in 100 mL normal saline over 1 hour
  - IV insulin soluble (actrapid) 10 u with IV dextrose 50% 40 mL over 20 minutes (if eGFR >15 mL/min and not on dialysis)
  - PO resonium (sodium polystyrene sulfonate) 15 g stat or PO lokelma (sodium zirconium cyclosilicate) 10 g stat

- Kidney replacement therapy is indicated for:
  - Fluid overload/acute pulmonary oedema not responding to diuretics
  - Severe hyperkalaemia (serum K > 6.0 mmol/L or associated with ECG changes of hyperkalaemia) — haemodialysis is preferred
  - Persistent hyperkalaemia refractory to medical therapy
  - Signs of uraemia (e.g., pericarditis, asterixis, decline in mental status)
  - Severe metabolic acidosis (pH <7.1)
  - Acute poisoning

Subsequent management

- Subsequent management of AKI includes:
  - Treating reversible causes (e.g., hypotension, volume depletion, urinary obstruction)

- Avoiding nephrotoxin medications

- Removing any active insult to avoid perpetuating the progression of AKI

- Adjusting dosages of drugs excreted by the kidneys according to prevailing kidney function

Specific Causes of AKI

Sepsis-associated AKI

- Sepsis is the most common precipitant of severe AKI and portends a high burden of morbidity and mortality in critically ill patients. Sepsis-associated AKI represents a distinct subset of AKI attributed by haemodynamic, inflammatory, and immune mechanisms.

Rhabdomyolysis

- AKI develops in 10–40% of patients with severe rhabdomyolysis. The mechanism of kidney damage in patients with rhabdomyolysis is the massive release of myoglobin into the circulation alongside myoglobinuria. Myoglobinuria is visible when urine myoglobin excretion exceeds 100–300 mg/dL, causing cast formation and accumulation of iron in the proximal tubules. This results in intratubular obstruction and proximal tubular cell injury.

- Laboratory markers of rhabdomyolysis include:

  - Elevated plasma creatinine kinase (CK) levels (values from 5–10 times the upper limit of normal)

  - Elevated lactate dehydrogenase

  - Elevated serum transaminase level

  - Presence of myoglobinuria

- The electrolyte abnormalities below can occur due to release of cellular constituents from damaged muscles:
  - High anion gap metabolic acidosis
  - Hyperkalaemia
  - Hyperphosphataemia
  - Hyperuricaemia
  - Hypocalcaemia (a result of calcium deposition in damaged muscles)
- The mainstay of treatment strategies focuses on the prevention of AKI:
  - Maintaining fluid hydration — saline solutions to expand intravascular volume aimed at increasing urine flow (about 200–300 mL/hour)
  - Treatment of underlying causes of rhabdomyolysis
  - Dialysis in severe AKI — haemofiltration on continuous kidney replacement therapies is more effective than conventional haemodialysis filters because they provide much greater clearance of myoglobin

Tumour lysis syndrome

- Tumour lysis syndrome (TLS) is an oncologic emergency caused by massive tumour cell lysis which releases large amounts of potassium, phosphate, and nucleic acids into the systemic circulation (Table 45.2).
- AKI occurs as a result of catabolism of the nucleic acid to uric acid leading to hyperuricaemia. The marked increase in uric

Table 45.2:   Clinical and Electrolyte Abnormalities Associated with Tumour Lysis Syndrome

Clinical	Electrolyte
Acute kidney injury	Hyperkalaemia
Arrythmias	Hyperphosphataemia
Muscle cramps and weakness	Hyperuricaemia
Seizures	Secondary hypocalcaemia

acid excretion can result in the precipitation of uric acid in the renal tubules leading to renal vasoconstriction, impaired auto-regulation, decreased renal blood flow, and inflammation.

- Other electrolyte abnormalities include that of hyperphosphataemia with calcium phosphate deposition in the renal tubules.

- TLS can occur spontaneously or after treatment of non-haematology solid tumours such as highly aggressive lymphomas (Burkitt subtype) and T-cell acute lymphoblastic leukaemia.

- Management of TLS includes:

  - Aggressive intravenous hydration

  - Hypouricaemic agents — allopurinol, rasburicase (recommended for those with impaired renal or cardiac function)

  - Kidney replacement therapy for:
    - Hyperkalaemia refractory to medical therapy
    - Symptomatic uraemia
    - Metabolic acidosis
    - Fluid overload refractory to medical therapy

References

Chatzizisis YS, Misirli G, Hatzitolios AI and Giannoglou GD (2008). The syndrome of rhabdomyolysis: Complications and treatment. *Eur J Intern Med* **19**(8): 568–574.

Chawla LS, Davison DL, Brasha-Mitchell E, *et al.* (2013). Development and standardization of a furosemide stress test to predict the severity of acute kidney injury. *Crit Care* **17**(5): R207.

Esposito P, Estienne L, Serpieri N, *et al.* (2018). Rhabdomyolysis-associated acute kidney injury. *Am J Kidney Dis* **71**(6): A12–A14.

Kellum JA, Lameire N, Aspelin P, *et al.* (2012). Kidney disease: Improving global outcomes (KDIGO) acute kidney injury work group. KDIGO clinical practice guideline for acute kidney injury. *Kidney Int Suppl* **2**(1): 1–138.

Zimmerman JL and Shen MC (2013). Rhabdomyolysis. *Chest* **144**(3): 1058–1065.

46 Kidney Replacement Therapy for Patients with Critical Illness and Acute Kidney Injury

Manish Kaushik, Liew Zhong Hong, Tan Han Khim

Introduction

- The AKI-EPI study, a multi-national, cross-sectional study, identified acute kidney injury (AKI) in more than 50% of patients admitted to the intensive care unit (ICU), with one-third of them in AKI KDIGO Stage 3.

- Kidney replacement therapy (KRT) was required in 13.5% of ICU patients or 23.5% of patients with AKI.

- Continuous kidney replacement therapy (CKRT) was used in 75.2% while intermittent haemodialysis (HD) and peritoneal dialysis (PD) was used in 24.1% and 0.7% respectively (Figure 46.1).

Timing for Initiation of Kidney Replacement Therapy

- In recent years, well-designed randomised studies have addressed the question of timing of initiation of KRT in patients with critical illness (Table 46.1).

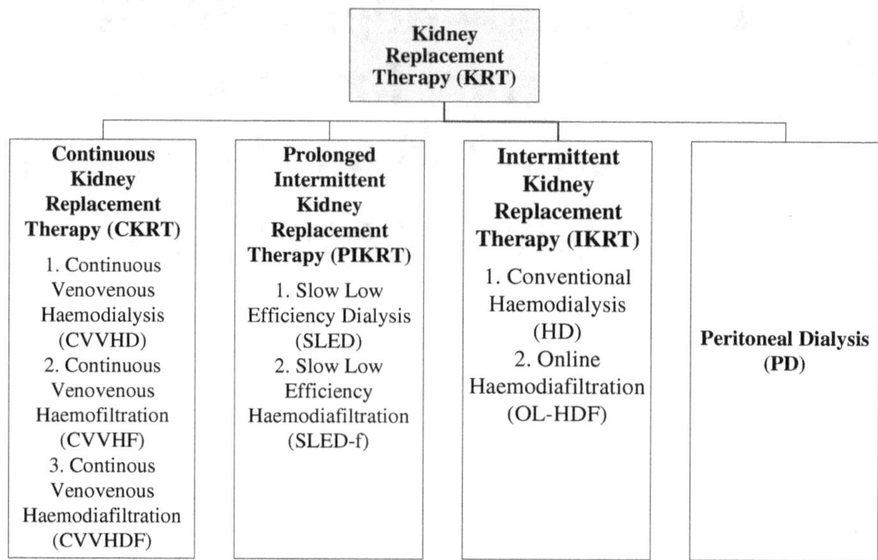

Figure 46.1: Options for Kidney Replacement Therapy (KRT) in Patients with Critical Illness

- KRT should be initiated immediately in the presence of emergent indications of hyperkalaemia, metabolic acidosis, or fluid overload.

- In patients with advanced AKI, and in the absence of emergent indications for KRT, medical management of complications of AKI can be continued, such as:

  - Hyperkalaemia — dextrose-insulin, potassium binders, limiting potassium intake

  - Metabolic acidosis — isotonic bicarbonate drip

  - Fluid overload — diuretics

  with close monitoring of clinical and laboratory parameters.

- In patients without hypovolaemia, a dose of intravenous furosemide (1 mg/kg if diuretic naïve or 1.5 mg/kg if the patient has received a dose of diuretic in the preceding 7 days) may

Table 46.1: **Summary of Studies in Timing of Kidney Replacement Therapy Initiation in Patients with Critical Illness**

Characteristic	ELAIN Study	AKIKI Study	IDEAL-ICU Study	STARRT-AKI Study	AKIKI 2 Study
Year	2016	2016	2018	2020	2021
Region	Germany	France	France	Global	France
Study population size	231	620	488 (terminated after second interim analysis)	2927	278
Patient profile (medical surgical)	– / 95%	80%/20%	Not specified	67%/33%	Not specified
Patient with burn/ trauma	12%	Not specified	Not specified	Not specified	Not specified
Septic shock	32%	67%	100%	43.8%	63% (average)
SOFA score	16	11	12.4	11.8	11
Early start group	Within 8 hours of AKI KDIGO Stage 2	Within 12 hours of AKI KDIGO Stage 3	Immediately upon diagnosis of AKI (maximally within 12 hours of AKI diagnosis)	Within 12 hours of AKI KDIGO Stage 2	AKI KDIGO Stage 3 or oliguria for 72 hours or serum urea > 40 mmol/L
Delayed start group	Within 12 hours of AKI KDIGO Stage 3 or development of emergent indication for KRT	Development of emergent indication to commence KRT or oliguria for >72 hours after randomisation	Initiation of KRT at least 48 hours after diagnosis of AKI or development of an emergent indication for KRT	Standard initiation of KRT or persistence of AKI for >72 hours	Development of emergent indication to commence KRT

(Continued)

Table 46.1: *(Continued)*

Characteristic	ELAIN Study	AKIKI Study	IDEAL-ICU Study	STARRT-AKI Study	AKIKI 2 Study
Emergent indications for KRT (also indications for KRT initiation in delayed group)	• Serum urea: >36 mmol/L • Serum K > 6 mmol/L with ECG changes • Serum Mg: >4 mmol/L • Urine output: <200 mL/12 hours • Anuria • Organ oedema in the presence of AKI resistant to diuretic	• Serum urea: >40 mmol/L • Hyperkalaemia: Serum K > 6 mmol/L or persistent 5.5 mmol/L despite medical Rx • Metabolic acidosis with pH: <7.15 (pCO_2 < 35) or mixed (pCO_2 > 50 and cannot be ↓ by MV) • APO due to FO requiring O_2 > 5 L/min to keep SpO_2 > 95% or FiO_2 > 0.5 on NIV/MV, and despite diuretics • Oliguria > 72 hours after randomisation	• Serum K ≥ 6.5 mmol/L with ECG changes • Metabolic acidosis defined as pH < 7.15 and base deficit > 5 mEq/L or HCO_3 ≤ 18 mmol/L • APO	• Serum K > 6 mmol/L • Metabolic acidosis with ≤10 mmol/L • PaO_2/FiO_2 < 200 with infiltrates on CXR compatible with APO • Persistent AKI for ≥72 hours	• Serum urea: >50 mmol/L • Metabolic acidosis with HCO_3 = or < 10 • Serum K > 6 mmol/L • Persistent K = 5.5 mmol/L despite medical Rx • Metabolic acidosis with pH: <7.15 (pCO_2 < 35) or mixed (pCO_2 > 50 and cannot be ↓ by MV) • APO due to FO requiring O_2 > 5 L/min to keep SpO_2, >95% or FiO_2 > 0.5 on NIV/MV, and despite diuretics
Time to start (early vs. delayed)	6 hours vs. 25.5 hours	2 hours vs. 57 hours	7.6 hours vs. 51.5 hours	6.1 hours vs. 31.1 hours	3 hours vs. 33 hours
First KRT modality (IKRT/CKRT)	0/100%	55%/45%	44%/56%	31.5%/68.5%	59%/40%
Percentage of patients who received KRT in the delayed group	91%	51%	62%	61.8%	79%

Mortality (early vs. delayed)	39.3% vs. 54.7% at 90d	48.5% vs. 49.7% at 60d	58% vs. 54% at 90d	43.9% vs. 43.7% at 90d	44% vs. 55% at 60d
Percentage patients requiring emergent KRT at randomisation	Not specified	19.3%	19.6%	18.5%	Not specified
Comments	• Predominantly surgical patients, with approximately 50% cardiac surgery patients • Separation between early and delayed group was <24 hours • Low fragility index • Single centre study	• Cautioned "wait and see" approach may not be safe for all patients and careful surveillance is mandatory when choosing to delay initiation of KRT • Follow up: AKIKI-2 Study (2021)	In the delayed strategy group, 27.5% patients needed to commence KRT due to an emergency indication and the mortality was the highest in this group at 68.3%	• Allowed clinicians to use judgement in confirming full eligibility and this may have introduced patient heterogeneity between groups • Among eligible patients, 66.5% were not randomized as clinicians felt KRT initiation or KRT deferral was mandated based on clinical judgement	In severe AKI patients with oliguria > 72 hrs or blood urea > 40 mmol/L and no severe complication that would mandate KRT, longer postponing of KRT did not confer any additional benefit and was associated with potential harm (HR 1.65 CI 1.09–2.50 for 60-day mortality)

Abbreviations: AKI KDIGO, Acute Kidney Injury Kidney Disease Improving Global Outcomes stage; APO, acute pulmonary oedema; CI; confidence intervals; CXR, chest X-ray; d, days; ECG, electrocardiogram; FO, fluid overload; HCO3; bicarbonate; hrs, hours; SOFA, Sequential Organ Failure Assessment score; KRT, kidney replacement therapy; K, potassium; Mg, magnesium; MV, mechanical ventilation; NIV, non-invasive ventilation; PaO_2/FiO_2, ratio of arterial oxygen partial pressure to fractional inspired oxygen; Rx, treatment; SpO_2, oxygen saturation

be considered to pre-empt the need for KRT. In a randomised study, 13.5% of responders to IV furosemide (urine output >200 mL over 2 hours) required KRT as opposed to 75% of non-responders, for an emergent indication.

Modality Selection for Kidney Replacement Therapy in Patients with Critical Illness

- There is no high-quality randomised study that has shown a survival benefit of continuous over prolonged intermittent or intermittent KRT.

- In general, the choice of continuous vs. intermittent KRT is influenced by several factors including haemodynamic instability, fluid balance goals, underlying medical issues, availability of resources, and institutional experience.

- In certain clinical scenarios, for example in patients with cerebral oedema, acute liver failure, hyperammonaemia, or severe hypo- or hyper-natraemia, CKRT may be preferred over intermittent forms of therapy.

- The various prescriptions and technical characteristics of different acute KRT options are summarised in Table 46.2.

Vascular Access for Continuous Kidney Replacement Therapy (Table 46.3)

- In patients who have a tunnelled cuffed haemodialysis catheter (HDC) *in situ*, CKRT can be performed using the existing HDC.

Table 46.2:   Prescription and Technical Characteristics of Kidney Replacement Therapy

Variable	Intermittent Haemodialysis (IHD)	Prolonged Intermittent Kidney Replacement Therapy (PIKRT)	Continuous Venovenous Haemodialysis (CVVHD)	Continuous Venovenous Haemofiltration (CVVH)	Continuous Venovenous Haemodiafiltration (CVVHDF)
Session time (hours)	3–6	6–16	24/day	24/day	24/day
Solute transport mechanism	Predominantly diffusion	Predominantly diffusion (and convection if slow low efficiency diafiltration — SLED-F)	Predominantly diffusion	Predominantly diffusion	Convection and diffusion
Blood flow rate (mL/min)	200–500	200–400	100–300	100–300	100–300
Dialysate flow rate (mL/min)	300–800	100–300	17–100	0	17–50
Replacement flow rate (mL/min)	0	40–100 (in SLED-f)	0	17–100	17–50

(*Continued*)

Table 46.2: (*Continued*)

Variable	Intermittent Haemodialysis (IHD)	Prolonged Intermittent Kidney Replacement Therapy (PIKRT)	Continuous Venovenous Haemodialysis (CVVHD)	Continuous Venovenous Haemofiltration (CVVH)	Continuous Venovenous Haemodiafiltration (CVVHDF)
Urea clearance (mL/min)	>150	50–200	<100	<100	<100
Target dose delivered/ session	Single-pool KT/V >1.2	Single pool KT/V 0.7–0.9	Effluent dose: 10–80 mL/min	Effluent dose: 10–80 mL/min	Effluent dose: 10–80 mL/min
Anti-coagulation	Nil Unfractionated heparin Low molecular weight heparin	Nil Unfractionated heparin Low molecular weight heparin Citrate	Nil Citrate Unfractionated heparin Low molecular weight heparin	Nil Citrate Unfractionated heparin Low molecular weight heparin	Nil Citrate Unfractionated heparin Low molecular weight heparin
Vascular access	AVF AVG Non-tunnelled or tunnelled dialysis catheter	AVF AVG Non-tunnelled or tunnelled dialysis catheter	Non-tunnelled or tunnelled dialysis catheter	Non-tunnelled or tunnelled dialysis catheter	Non-tunnelled or tunnelled dialysis catheter

Abbreviations: AVF, arteriovenous fistula; AVG, arteriovenous graft

Table 46.3: Non-Tunneled Non-Cuffed Vascular Access Options for Continuous Kidney Replacement Therapy

Choice	Catheter Site	Catheter Size	Tip Position	Scenarios Favouring Choice
1	Right IJV	16 cm	Cavo-atrial junction	BMI > 28.4 Ambulation/ rehabilitation
2	Femoral vein (right or left)	24 cm	Inferior vena cava	BMI < 24.2 Tracheostomy/neck surgery Emergency KRT or inadequate operator
3	Left IJV	20 cm or 16 cm in small-sized patients	Cavo-atrial junction	Contraindications for right IJV or femoral veins
4	Subclavian vein	16–20 cm	Cavo-atrial junction	Contraindications to IJV or femoral sites

Abbreviations: BMI, body mass index; IJV, internal jugular vein; KRT, kidney replacement therapy

- In patients on extracorporeal membrane oxygenation (ECMO), consider integrating CKRT with ECMO (only in institutions with adequate support and experience).

- In patients who do not have a pre-exiting vascular access, establish a new vascular access with a non-tunnelled non-cuffed HDC, with insertion performed under ultrasound (US) guidance.

- Every attempt to secure an appropriately sized and appropriately sited vascular access must be made.

Effluent Dose of Continuous Kidney Replacement Therapy

- Effluent is all waste that exits the CKRT filter, and the total effluent flow rate (QE) is the sum of the following flow rates:

$$QE = QD + QRF + QNetUF + QCitrate + QCalcium$$

QD   = Dialysate flow rate in mL/hr

QRF   = Replacement or substitution fluid flow rate in mL/hr

QNet UF = Net ultrafiltration rate in mL/hr

QCitrate = Citrate anticoagulation flow rate in mL/hr

QCalcium = Calcium replacement flow rate during citrate anticoagulation (when calcium pump is integrated in circuit) in mL/hr

- The AKI KDIGO 2012 guidelines recommend a delivered effluent dose of 20–25 mL/kg/hour over a 24-hour period (based on ATN and RENAL studies).

- However, to account for CKRT downtime due to interruptions for procedures, bag changes, filter clotting, and loss of filter efficiency secondary to membrane fouling, the prescribed dose is usually higher at 30 mL/kg/hour.

- The RENAL study excluded patients weighing less than 60 kg or more than 100 kg. In the ATN study, patients weighing more than 128.5 kg were excluded, and for patients whose actual body weight was >30% of their ideal body weight, the CKRT effluent dose was calculated based on adjusted body weight as follows:

$$\text{Adjusted body weight} = [\text{IBW} + 0.25 \times (\text{Actual body weight} - \text{Ideal body weight})]$$

$$\text{Ideal body weight} = 50 \text{ (in men) or } 45.5 \text{ (in women)} + (0.91 \times [\text{height in cm} - 152.4])$$

- Effluent dosing must be dynamic and may be temporarily adapted to account for clinical situations of severe hyperkalaemia (e.g., rhabdomyolysis, tumour lysis syndrome), metabolic acidosis (e.g., mesenteric ischaemia awaiting surgery), high obligate fluid or nutrition requirements, hyper catabolic states (e.g., severe burn injuries), etc.

Modality of CKRT

- Modalities of CKRT are based on the primary mechanism of solute clearance: diffusion and/or convection (Table 46.4). Adsorption is inherent to all CKRT modality. It is influenced by membrane structure/composition and surface area while limited by saturation of the adsorptive surface.

- Diffusion removes small solutes, while convection removes small and middle molecular weight solutes. Though most inflammatory mediators are middle molecules, studies have not demonstrated any survival advantage of purely convective modalities over diffusive modalities.

- On the other hand, convective modalities are associated with shorter filter life spans as compared to diffusive modalities.

Table 46.4: Modalities of Continuous Kidney Replacement Therapy

Modality	Diffusive Dose	Convective Dose		
	Dialysate	Replacement Fluid/ Substitution Fluid	Anticoagulant (Citrate or Other)	Net Ultrafiltration
CVVHD	++++	0	+/–	+
CVVH	0	++++	+/–	+
CVVHDF	++	++	+/–	+

Abbreviations: CVVHD; continuous veno-venous haemodialysis; CVVH; continuous veno-venous haemofiltration; CVVHDF; continuous veno-venous haemodiafiltration; + to ++++; quantitative contribution from minimal to maximal

- In convective modalities, replacement fluid may be administered either pre-filter or post-filter.

- Pre-filter administration of replacement fluid dilutes the solute concentrations presented to the filter and hence compromises the effluent dose delivered. The extent of dilution may be estimated by the dilution fraction (DF), calculated as:

$$\text{Dilution fraction} = [\text{QPlasma}/(\text{QPlasma} + \text{QRF})]$$

QPlasma is the plasma flow rate in mL/min, obtained as [QBlood in mL/min × (1 − haematocrit)]

QRF is the replacement fluid flow rate in mL/min

- Pre-filter replacement fluid, by virtue of dilution, may prolong filter life.

- Post-filter administration of replacement fluid is constrained by blood flow rate. To minimise the risk of filter clotting, it is suggested to keep the filtration fraction < 0.20–0.25.

- Filtration fraction (FF) is the ratio of total ultrafiltration to the plasma flow rate and is estimated by the equation:

$$\text{Filtration Fraction (FF)} = [\text{QTotalUF}/\text{QPlasma}]$$

QTotalUF in mL/min is the todal ultrafiltration across the membrane and is equal to QRF + QNetUF

QPlasma is the plasma flow rate in mL/min, obtained as [QBlood in mL/min × (1 − haematocrit)]

- In clinical practice, continuous venovenous haemodiafiltration (CVVHDF), which combines diffusion and convection, offers a good compromise to maximise effluent dose delivery in CKRT.

- In CKRT, with regards to small solutes like urea, given the relatively slow effluent flow rate as compared to blood flow rate, the effluent is saturated as it exits the filter (i.e., the concentration of solute in effluent is equal to the concentration of solute in plasma; CEffluent/CPlasma = 1)

- The clearance of any solute in CKRT may be estimated by the following equation:

$$\text{Clearance of solute X} = [\text{CXEffluent/CXPlasma}] \times \text{QEffluent (mL/min)}$$

CXEffluent is the concentration of solute X in the effluent

CXPlasma is the concentration of solute X in the plasma

Anticoagulation Choice in CKRT

- Despite a good vascular access and non-anticoagulant options to minimise filter clotting, CKRT circuits are interrupted due to clotting.

- Regional citrate anticoagulation (RCA) has been shown to improve filter life and decrease risk of bleeding when compared to heparin. A multi-centre, randomised RICH study compared 300 patients receiving CKRT with RCA (titrating post-filter ionised calcium between 0.25–0.35 mmol/L) to 296 patients receiving CKRT with heparin anticoagulation (titrated to activated partial thromboplastin time of 45–60 seconds). Patients receiving RCA had a filter life of 47 hours and bleeding complications in 5.1% as compared to a filter life of 26 hours and bleeding complications in 16.9% in patients receiving heparin.

- RCA works by chelating calcium in the blood and decreasing the level of ionised calcium to 0.25–0.35 mmol/L, which inhibits coagulation.

- Citrate dose (defined as the concentration of citrate achieved in blood required to achieve target post-filter ionized calcium of 0.25–0.35 mmol/L) is between 2.5 to 4 mmol/L.

- For any given citrate fluid, the citrate dose is a ratio between citrate flow rate, QCitrate (mL/hour), and blood flow rate, QB (mL/min). With current modern generations of CKRT machines where the blood and citrate pumps are coupled, any change in QB will automatically induce a proportional change in QCitrate to maintain the prescribed citrate dose and hence anticoagulation efficiency constant.

- As the citrate calcium complex (CCC) traverses the filter, between 30–60% is lost in the effluent, depending on the CKRT effluent dose.

- The remainder of the CCC and citrate entering the circuit minus the citrate lost in the effluent enters the patient's body and constitutes the citrate load that the patient has to metabolise to generate bicarbonate (1 mmol citrate generates 3 mmol bicarbonate upon metabolism). Therefore, citrate load influences the acid base status of the patient.

- The metabolism of citrate also releases the complexed calcium and partially replenishes the patient's calcium pool. Additional intravenous calcium has to be administered to replace the calcium lost in the effluent and thus replete completely the calcium body pool.

- Citrate load, if not metabolised completely, leads to citrate toxicity.

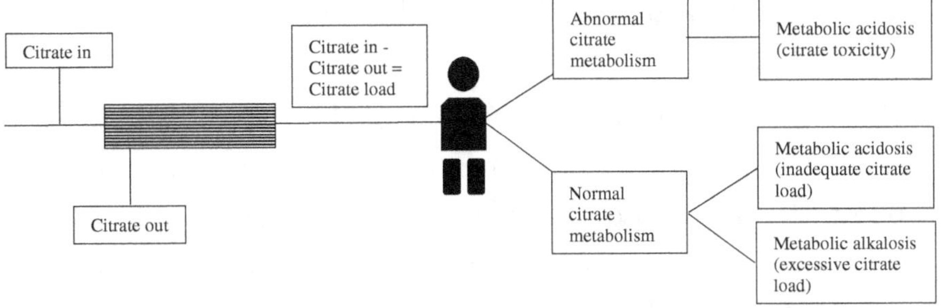

Figure 46.2:   Metabolic Complications of Regional Citrate Anticoagulation

- During global deterioration of a patient's condition with worsening haemodynamics and/or liver dysfunction, citrate toxicity is diagnosed by presence of the following triad (Figure 46.2):

  - Worsening high anion gap metabolic acidosis

  - Decreasing systemic ionised calcium with increasing intravenous calcium requirement

  - Total calcium to systemic ionised calcium ratio increased to >2.5 (do not correct calcium for albumin)

- In situations of citrate toxicity or metabolic alkalosis due to excessive citrate load, the strategy is to decrease citrate load. This is achieved by decreasing the QB or increasing the QD, with reassessment of metabolic parameters in 1–2 hours. In extreme situations, RCA may have to be discontinued.

- In metabolic acidosis due to inadequate citrate load, the strategy is to increase citrate load by increasing the QB.

Fluid Management During CKRT

- Both hypovolaemia and fluid overload are associated with worse outcomes in patients with AKI requiring KRT. Hence, assessing and achieving the fluid balance target is important during CKRT.

- Frequent multi-modal assessment of fluid status, if possible, with clinical examination, dynamic haemodynamic parameters, point of care ultrasound, bioimpedance analysis and possibly biomarkers have been suggested to help guide fluid management during CKRT.

- Retrospective studies have identified ultrafiltration rates < 1.0 mL/kg/hr or >1.75 mL/kg/hr to be associated with adverse outcomes.

Drug Dosing and Nutrition Management During CKRT

- CKRT drug or toxin clearance is considered significant when CKRT contributes to >25% of the total body clearance of the drug or toxin.

- Water soluble drugs or toxins with low molecular weight (<500 Da), low protein binding (<80%), and low volume of distribution (<0.8–1 L/kg) are likely to be cleared significantly by CKRT.

- Drug dosing, especially maintenance doses, must be adjusted based on the CKRT effluent dose.

- Like with drugs, CKRT also augments the clearance of many vitamins, essential minerals, and amino acids.

- Nutrition planning during CKRT should take into account losses via CKRT. For example, amino acid supplementation should be increased by about 10%, ascorbic acid should be replaced if the patient develops scurvy-like symptoms, etc.

- Caloric intake is 25–30 kCal/kg/day and protein intake 1.2–1.5 g/kg/day.

Monitoring During CKRT

- During CKRT, perform regular monitoring of laboratory parameters for solute, electrolyte, and acid-base control every 6–12 hourly (e.g., urea, creatinine, sodium, potassium, chloride, bicarbonate, glucose, calcium, phosphate, albumin, arterial blood gas, full blood counts, and coagulation parameters).
- When possible, monitoring therapeutic drug monitoring should be performed to ensure adequate drug levels.

References

Barbar SD, Clere-Jehl R, Bourredjem A, *et al.* (2018). Timing of renal-replacement therapy in patients with acute kidney injury and sepsis. *N Engl J Med* **379**(15): 1431–1442.

Gaudry S, Hajage D, Martin-Lefevre L, *et al.* (2021). Comparison of two delayed strategies for renal replacement therapy initiation for severe acute kidney injury (AKIKI 2): A multicentre, open-label, randomised, controlled trial. *Lancet* **397**(10281): 1293–1300.

Gaudry S, Hajage D, Schortgen F, *et al.* (2016). Initiation strategies for renal-replacement therapy in the intensive care unit. *N Engl J Med* **375**(2): 122–133.

Gaudry S, Palevsky PM and Dreyfuss D (2022). Extracorporeal kidney-replacement therapy for acute kidney injury. *N Engl J Med* **386**(10): 964–975.

Kellum JA, Lameire N, Aspelin P, *et al.* (2012). Kidney disease: Improving global outcomes (KDIGO) acute kidney injury work group. KDIGO clinical practice guideline for acute kidney injury. *Kidney Int Suppl* **2**(1): 1–138.

Neyra JA, Yessayan L, Thompson Bastin ML, *et al.* (2020). How to prescribe and troubleshoot continuous renal replacement therapy: A case-based review. *Kidney 360* **2**(2): 371–384.

STARRT-AKI Investigators, Canadian Critical Care Trials Group, Australian and New Zealand Intensive Care Society Clinical Trials Group, *et al.* (2020). Timing of initiation of renal-replacement therapy in acute kidney injury. *N Engl J Med* **383**(3): 240–251.

Zarbock A, Kellum JA, Schmidt C, *et al.* (2016). Effect of early vs delayed initiation of renal replacement therapy on mortality in critically ill patients with acute kidney injury: The ELAIN randomized clinical trial. *J Am Med Assoc* **315**(20): 2190–2199.

47 Extracorporeal Therapies in Acute Kidney Injury and Critically Ill Patients

Riece Koniman

Introduction

- Extracorporeal therapies, such as therapeutic plasma exchange (TPE), double filtration plasmapheresis (DFPP), and immunoadsorption (IA), can be used as either a principal or adjunct therapy in a variety of diseases. The principles, mechanisms and indications of these therapies are summarised in Table 47.1.

- During these therapies, the blood of the patient is passed through an extracorporeal device, which separates the components of blood (e.g., immunoglobulins, proteins, immune complexes) to treat a disease.

- The properties of the target substances, such as molecular weight, electric charge, hydrophilic or hydrophobic properties, rate of transfer between compartments, half-life, and production rate, determine the selection of extracorporeal modality, dose and frequency of therapies, and efficacy of their removal.

- As therapies aimed at suppression of their production may take weeks or months to be effective and some of these pathogenic substances have long half-lives, extracorporeal therapy allows

Table 47.1:   Principles, Mechanisms, and Indications of Extracorporeal Therapies

Modalities	Principles	Mechanisms	Examples of Diseases
Therapeutic plasma exchange (TPE) using membrane separation technique	• Plasma is separated and removed from the whole blood and during this process, pathogenic molecules (e.g., antibodies, antibody complexes, immune complexes, or antigens) are also removed from the body. • An equal volume of replacement fluids such as fresh frozen plasma and/or albumin are returned back into the patient to prevent haemodynamic compromise. The ideal target molecules should ▪ be identified ▪ be of high MW (>=15,000 Da) ▪ have a slow rate of production and low turnover ▪ have a low volume of distribution ▪ have a high rate of transfer into the intravascular compartment	• Blood drawn from a dialysis catheter is passed through a highly permeable filter with large pore sizes (0.3–0.5 μm), and plasma is separated from the cellular components of blood and filtered out. • As plasma is filtered out, an equal volume of replacement fluids is replaced simultaneously.	• Anti-glomerular basement membrane disease • ANCA-associated vasculitis • Desensitisation for kidney transplantation • Treatment of antibody-mediated rejection • TTP

	• Can also be used for the supplementation of certain substances, such as coagulation factor replacement in liver failure, ADAMTS-13 in TTP.	

Double filtration plasmapheresis (DFPP)	• Plasma is separated from the whole blood and pathogenic molecules are selectively removed and discarded before the rest of the plasma is returned to the patient.
	• As the majority of the processed plasma is returned to the patient, the need for replacement fluid is minimal.
	• Ideal target molecules for DFPP:
	  ▪ Identified target molecule
	  ▪ High molecular weight [≥15,000 Da, and greater than the cut-off level of the second filter (plasma fractionator)]
	  ▪ Slow rate of production
	  ▪ Low turnover
	  ▪ Low volume of distribution
		• The first filter (plasma separator) separates plasma from the whole blood.
		• The filtered plasma then passes through the second filter (plasma fractionator) where larger molecules are selectively removed and discarded. Smaller molecules are returned to the patient.
			• Desensitisation for kidney transplantation
			• Treatment of antibody-mediated rejection

(*Continued*)

Table 47.1:   (*Continued*)

Modalities	Principles	Mechanisms	Examples of Diseases
Immunoadsorption – Plasma adsorption	• Plasma components are separated by adsorber systems. • Selective plasma components (e.g., immunoglobulins, immune complexes, auto-antibodies, endotoxins, cytokines and/or a host of other inflammatory mediators) bind to the adsorption column, while other plasma proteins are preserved.	• The first filter (plasma separator) separates plasma from the whole blood and the filtered plasma passes through an adsorption column, which allows the adsorption of selective pathogenic molecules from the plasma. The treated plasma is then returned to the patient. • There are many commercially available adsorption columns, each with a different active ligand to which the molecule of interest attaches, thus allowing for selectivity in the molecules removed.	• Desensitisation for kidney transplantation • Treatment of antibody-mediated rejection
Immunoadsorption – Haemoperfusion	• Direct adsorption of circulating endotoxin by perfusion of the blood through the adsorption column.	• Direct perfusion of the whole blood through the adsorption column, which allows the adsorption of circulating endotoxin and inflammatory cells and mediators.	• Endotoxic or gram-negative septic shock

Abbreviations: ADAMTS13, ADAM metallopeptidase with Thrombospondin Type 1 Motif 13; ANCA, anti-neutrophil cytoplasmic antibody; MW, molecular weight; Da, daltons; TTP, thrombotic thrombocytopenic purpura

for the rapid removal of these pathogenic substances to prevent ongoing organ damage, thus reducing morbidity and mortality.

References

Agishi T, Kaneko I, Hasuo Y, *et al.* (2000). Double filtration plasmapheresis. 1980. *Ther Apher* **4**(1): 29–33.

Ahmed S and Kaplan A (2020). Therapeutic plasma exchange using membrane plasma separation. *Clin J Am Soc Nephrol* **15**(9): 1364–1370.

Noiri E and Hanafusa N (2014). *The Concise Manual of Apheresis Therapy.* Springer, Japan.

Padmanabhan A, Connelly-Smith L, Aqui N, *et al.* (2019). Guidelines on the use of therapeutic apheresis in clinical practice: Evidence-based approach from the Writing Committee of the American Society for Apheresis: The eighth special issue. *J Clin Apher* **34**(3): 171–354.

Williams ME and Balogun RA (2014). Principles of separation: Indications and therapeutic targets for plasma exchange. *Clin J Am Soc Nephrol* **9**(1): 181–190.

48 Extracorporeal Treatment for Poisoning and Drug Overdoses

Riece Koniman, Manish Kaushik

Introduction

- Poisoning and drug overdoses are associated with significant morbidity and mortality. Although their treatment mainly involves supportive care, extracorporeal removal treatment (ERT) may aid in the elimination of the drug or poison (referred here as xenobiotics or chemical substances not naturally produced by the human body), especially in life-threatening situations or when endogenous elimination mechanisms are impaired.

- The choice of which ERT to use (Table 48.1) depends on:

  - the characteristics of the xenobiotic to be removed

  - the availability of suitable ERT technologies

  - risks-benefits analysis — ERTs are expensive, invasive, and associated with their own set of treatment-related complications. For example, ERTs require vascular access (with risk of infection, bleeding, and injury to surrounding structures), anticoagulation, and haemodynamic stability (hypotension may occur during treatment).

Table 48.1:　Use of Extracorporeal Therapies for Drug Overdose and Toxicities

ERCT	Xenobiotic Characteristics			Example	Remarks
	MW (Da)	Vd (L/kg)	Protein Binding		
HD	Up to 10,000 to 15,000	$\leq$1.5–2	$\leq$80%	Salicylates Lithium Theophylline Metformin Toxic alcohols (e.g., ethylene glycol, methanol, ethanol, isopropanol)	• More readily available • Can treat electrolyte/acid base disturbances and fluid overload • Anticoagulation usually required • Haemodynamic instability may occur • Rebound may occur as HD is intermittent and removes only free drug in the plasma • May remove therapeutic drugs that need top up doses after HD
CKRT	Up to 15,000 to 25,000	$\leq$1.5–2	$\leq$80%	Lithium Theophylline Vancomycin Ethylene glycol	• Can treat electrolyte/acid-based disturbances and fluid overload • Slow clearance but useful for xenobiotics with slow redistribution that can lead to rebound

ECRT	MW	Vd		Indicative xenobiotics	Comments
HP (usually activated charcoal)	Unclear but high — xenobiotics need to be adsorbed by charcoal	≤ 1.0	Any	Valproic acid Carbamazepine Phenobarbitone Theophylline Phenytoin Salicylate	• Limited availability • Saturation of adsorbent by xenobiotics, cellular debris and proteins develop over time, and change of the HP column would be required to maintain clearing effectiveness • Anticoagulation required • Potential complications include clotting, hypocalcaemia, thrombocytopenia and charcoal embolisation
PLEX	No limit	≤ 1.0	Any	Monoclonal antibodies Arsine poison	• Limited availability • Evidence based mainly on case reports • Rapid clearance • Anticoagulation required • Like HD, rebound can occur when PLEX is discontinued

Abbreviations: CKRT, continuous kidney replacement therapy; ECRT, extracorporeal removal treatment; HD, haemodialysis; HP, haemoperfusion; MW, molecular weight; PLEX, plasma exchange; Vd, volume of distribution

Modified from King JD, Kern MH and Jaar BG (2019). Extracorporeal removal of poisons and toxins. *Clin J Am Soc Nephrol* **14**(9): 1408–1415.

- Peritoneal dialysis can be used to remove xenobiotics but it is technically not considered an ERT as removal of xenobiotics does not occur in a blood circuit outside the body. Besides, clearance of xenobiotics by PD is poor and too slow to be clinically useful.

Indications for Extracorporeal Removal Treatments

- First aid and supportive treatments (e.g., oral administration of activated charcoal) should always be initiated first while awaiting extracorporeal removal treatment (ECRT).

- ECRT should be considered when:
  - the drug implicated can be removed by ECRT
  - life-threatening toxicity does not improve with supportive measures
  - normal routes of elimination are impaired
  - the total body clearance of the xenobiotic can be increased by at least 30% above normal excretory routes through ECRT (e.g., drugs with low endogenous clearance [<4 mL/min/kg] like toxic alcohols, lithium, salicylate, and theophylline are suitable for ECRT)
  - Some of the common drug overdoses, toxicities, indications for ECRT and preferred modality are listed in Table 48.2

Table 48.2: Indications and Preferred Extracorporeal Treatment of Some Drug Overdoses and Toxicities

Drugs	Risk Factors for Toxicities	Clinical Presentations or Laboratories	Indications for Extracorporeal Treatment	Preferred Kidney Replacement Therapy Modality
Metformin	• Impaired kidney function • Acute or high dose ingestion	• Serum lactate > 5 mmol/L • Serum pH < 7.35 (metformin-associated lactic acidosis)	• Lactate concentration > 20 mmol/L • pH < or = 7.0 • Failure of standard supportive treatment • Threshold for initiating extracorporeal treatment is lower in patients with impaired kidney function, shock, liver failure, decreased level of consciousness	• HD (preferred) • CKRT
Vancomycin	• Advanced age • Impaired kidney function • Dehydration • Female • Hypoalbuminaemia • Sepsis	• AKI • Elevated serum vancomycin concentration	• AKI	• HD (high-flux) • HDF

(Continued)

Table 48.2: *(Continued)*

Drugs	Risk Factors for Toxicities	Clinical Presentations or Laboratories	Indications for Extracorporeal Treatment	Preferred Kidney Replacement Therapy Modality
	• Concomitant administration with other nephrotoxic agents • Long treatment duration • High dose treatment			
Cefepime	• Impaired kidney function • ESKD	• Confusion • EEG findings (generalised periodic discharge with triphasic morphology)	• Confusion	• HD (preferred) • CKRT
Acyclovir	• Impaired renal function • ESKD • Hypovolaemia • Concurrent use of other nephrotoxic agents	• Neurotoxicity • Nephrotoxicity	• Neurotoxicity • Nephrotoxicity	• HD
Lithium	• Impaired renal function • Drug-drug interaction that impairs elimination	• Neurotoxicity • Arrhythmias • Nausea, vomiting • Hypotension	• Impaired renal function and [Li+] > 4.0 mmol/L	• HD (preferred) • CKRT

			• Decreased level of consciousness, seizures, or life-threatening arrythmias irrespective of [Li+]	
Acetaminophen	• Massive ingestions	• Altered mental status	• APAP > 1000 mg/L (6620 μmol/L) and NAC is not administered	• HD (preferred) • CKRT
		• Metabolic acidosis with elevated lactate concentrations (typically within 12 hours post ingestion and often prior to biochemical or clinical evidence of hepatotoxicity) • Hepatotoxicity • AKI	• Altered mental status, lactic acidosis and APAP >700 mg/L (4630 μmol/L) and NAC is not administered • Altered mental status, lactic acidosis and APAP > 900 mg/L (5960 μmol/L) even if NAC is administered	
Carbamazepine	• Carbamazepine-naïve • Massive ingestions	• Neurotoxicity • Respiratory depression • Arrythmias • Hypotension	• Multiple seizures refractory to treatment • Life threatening arrhythmias	• HD (preferred) • CKRT

Abbreviations: AKI, acute kidney injury; APAP, acetaminophen; CKRT, continuous kidney replacement therapy; ESKD, end-stage kidney disease; HD, haemodialysis, HDF, haemodiafiltration; EEG, electroencephalography; Li+, Lithium; NAC, N-acetylcysteine

Characteristics of Xenobiotics Removed by Extracorporeal Removal Treatments

- The effectiveness of ECRT in clearing a xenobiotic depends on the physicochemical and pharmacokinetic characteristics of the xenobiotic:

  - **Molecular mass**

    - For haemodialysis (HD) and continuous kidney replacement therapies (CKRT), removal of xenobiotics is limited by the molecular weight (MW) of the molecule and the pore sizes in the semi-permeable membranes. This is less likely a problem with haemoperfusion (HP) and plasma exchange (PLEX).

  - **Volume of distribution**

    - Volume of distribution (Vd) is the total amount of xenobiotic in the body divided by its concentration in plasma.

    - As a result, Vd describes the extent to which a xenobiotic is present in the extravascular tissues rather than in the plasma. For example, a xenobiotic with a high Vd has a low plasma concentration because it tends to leave the plasma and enter the extravascular tissues. This is the case for lipophilic substances which distribute into body fat and hence less is available in the plasma for extracorporeal removal.

    - Xenobiotics with a large Vd > 1.0 L/kg are not suitable for ECRT (e.g., digoxin).

  - **Plasma protein binding**

    - Xenobiotics that bind to plasma proteins are less likely to diffuse or transverse membranes used for HD or

CKRT. However, protein-bound xenobiotics can be removed by HP or PLEX.

- **Rate of endogenous clearance**

  – ECRT is unlikely to provide further therapeutic benefit if the endogenous clearance is high (>4 mL/kg/min). However, it will benefit the removal of xenobiotics associated with low endogenous clearance or when endogenous clearance is impaired.

- **Rate of redistribution**

  – If the rate of redistribution from extravascular to plasma compartment is slow, then rebound increase in the plasma level of the xenobiotic can occur following discontinuation of ERCT.

Haemodialysis

- HD removes xenobiotics through diffusion across a semi-permeable membrane from the plasma (where xenobiotic concentration is higher) to the dialysate (where xenobiotic concentration is lower).

- Xenobiotic clearance is dependent on (1) dialysate flow rate, (2) blood flow rate, (3) membrane characteristics — pore size, surface area — and (4) molecular weight of the xenobiotic.

- The flow rates, duration, and frequency of HD prescription depends on the type of xenobiotic to be cleared and the hae-modynamic condition of the patient. The availability of high-flux dialysers with larger pores and surface areas are useful for xenobiotics that are not easily removed by standard dialyser membranes.

- HD is preferred whenever there is a need for rapid removal of the xenobiotic, but HD also requires a haemodynamically stable patient.

Continuous Kidney Replacement Therapies

- Continuous venovenous haemofiltration (CVVH) removes xenobiotics in plasma by the movement of plasma across a semipermeable membrane under a hydrostatic pressure gradient (convection).

- Xenobiotic removal can be augmented by adding dialysate (continuous venovenous haemodiafiltration; CVVHDF). Therefore, xenobiotics are removed by both convection and dialysis.

- CVVH or CVVHDF is used when patients are not haemodynamically stable enough to tolerate HD. It is not preferred over HD because of its slower removal of xenobiotics.

- A potential advantage of CVVH or CVVHDF is that the membranes used in these ECRTs have larger pores and hence can clear xenobiotics of larger molecular weight than those cleared by HD.

- CVVH or CVVHDF is also used as a continuous treatment to remove xenobiotics that are associated with rebound or xenobiotics which continue to be absorbed from the gastrointestinal tract.

Charcoal Haemoperfusion

- Charcoal HP involves pumping blood through a perfusion column containing a large surface area of adsorbent (usually activated charcoal) that can adsorb xenobiotics which are otherwise bound to plasma proteins. Protein binding, water solubility, and molecular size are not limiting factors.

Plasma Exchange

- In nephrology units, PLEX is performed using a standard haemodialysis or continuous kidney replacement therapy machine fitted with a semipermeable membrane filter that separates plasma from its cellular components. The filtered plasma is discarded and replaced by replacement fluid or plasma products which are returned back to the patient with the cellular components.

- As a result of plasma removal, PLEX can rapidly remove xenobiotics regardless of its size and protein-binding characteristics. It may be advantageous in certain situations where the xenobiotics generate toxic by-products in the plasma, which either can be removed by PLEX or the replacement with new plasma products restore normal physiology that was disrupted by abnormal exposure to xenobiotic.

References

Calello DP, Liu KD, Wiegand TJ, *et al.* (2015). Extracorporeal treatment for metformin poisoning: Systematic review and recommendations from the Extracorporeal Treatments in Poisoning workgroup. *Criti Care Med* **43**(8): 1716–1730.

Decker BS, Goldfarb DS, Dargan PI, *et al.* (2015). Extracorporeal treatment for lithium poisoning: Systematic review and recommendations from the EXTRIP workgroup. *Clin J Am Soc Nephrol* **10**(5): 875–887.

Fertel BS, Nelson LS and Goldfarb DS (2010). Extracorporeal removal techniques for the poisoned patient: A review for the intensivist. *J Intensive Care Med* **25**(3): 139–148.

Fleischer R and Johnson M (2010). Acyclovir nephrotoxicity: A case report highlighting the importance of prevention, detection, and treatment of acyclovir-induced nephropathy. *Case Rep Med* **2010**: 602783.

Ghannoum M, Yates C, Galvao TF, *et al.* (2014). Extracorporeal treatment for carbamazepine poisoning: Systematic review and recommendations from the EXTRIP workgroup. *Clin Toxicol* **52**(10): 993–1004.

Gosselin S, Juurlink DN, Kielstein JT, *et al.* (2014). Extracorporeal treatment for acetaminophen poisoning: Recommendations from the EXTRIP workgroup. *Clin Toxicol* **52**(8): 856–867.

King JD, Kern MH and Jaar BG (2019). Extracorporeal removal of poisons and toxins. *Clin J Am Soc Nephrol* **14**(9): 1408–1415.

Lee SJ (2019). Cefepime-induced neurotoxicity. *J Neurocrit Care* **12**(2): 74–84.

Schutt RC, Ronco C and Rosner MH (2012). The role of therapeutic plasma exchange in poisonings and intoxications. *Semin Dial* **25**(2): 201–206.

Zamoner W, Prado IRS, Balbi AL and Ponce D (2019). Vancomycin dosing, monitoring and toxicity: Critical review of the clinical practice. *Clin Exp Pharmacol Physiol* **46**(4): 292–301.

Transplantation

Liew Ian Tatt

Introduction

- Kidney transplantation (KT) is the kidney replacement therapy (KRT) of choice for end-stage kidney disease (ESKD) as it offers the best patient survival outcomes and quality of life. Living kidney donor transplant (LDKT) is preferred over deceased kidney donor transplant (DDKT) because of its superior likelihood of graft and patient survival.

- Whenever possible, pre-emptive LDKT should be performed before maintenance dialysis (defined arbitrarily as dialysis ≥ 3 months) as it offers the best graft and patient survival.

- Patients should be referred for transplant evaluation as follows:

  - Within 6–12 months of expected start of dialysis

  - When glomerular filtrate rate (GFR) is <20 mL/min

  - Within 6 months after stabilising on maintenance dialysis

- Patients with Type I or II diabetes mellitus (DM) should also be reviewed for suitability to receive simultaneous kidney and pancreas transplantation from a deceased donor.

- The goal of evaluation (Table 49.1) is to ensure that harm is minimised and benefit is maximised with a KT so that the optimal use of the donated kidney can be assured (i.e., graft survival is not limited by premature death or avoidable graft loss).

Table 49.1:   Goals of Evaluation

- Will the patient benefit from transplantation with an improved quality and quantity of life?
- Are the surgical risks reasonable and acceptable?
- Is the surgery technically possible?
- Are there any conditions that may worsen with immunosuppression or surgery?
- What measures need to be taken to minimise peri- and post-operative complications?
- Is the patient psychosocially and financially ready?

Evaluation of the Potential Kidney Transplant Candidate

- There are few contraindications to KT (Table 49.2).

Table 49.2:   Contraindications to Kidney Transplantation

1. Active cancer
2. Active and uncontrolled infection
3. Systemic disease with anticipated poor graft outcomes, e.g., Primary hyperoxalosis, uncontrolled amyloidosis
4. Other end-organ failure where transplant is not an option
5. Other conditions with a poor prognosis, regardless of transplantation (e.g., progressive neurodegenerative disease)
6. Other active conditions that render the patient unable to tolerate surgery or immunosuppression (e.g., symptomatic cardiovascular disease)
7. Active substance misuse
8. Uncontrolled psychiatric disease
9. Inability for self-care and/or adherence to medical follow-up and treatment

Note: Age is not by itself a contraindication to KT and depends on the fitness of the individual as well as the availability of a suitably aged kidney donor.

- Evaluation of a potential KT candidate requires a multidisciplinary team, which at the minimum in Singapore would be a physician, surgeon, transplant coordinator, medical social worker, and psychiatrist.

Evaluation of Primary Kidney Disease

- Recurrence of primary kidney disease accounts for 15% of all graft loss. As far as possible, the primary kidney disease should be determined to allow accurate prognostication of the recurrence risk (Table 49.3). This is to assist in determining prevention and monitoring measures for recurrence after KT.

- The primary disease should be quiescent before transplantation for two purposes:

  - Allow time for possible recovery of kidney function to declare itself, hence avoiding KT.

  - Allow any circulating pathogenic antibodies to fall to lower levels or disappear to reduce the risk of recurrence after KT (e.g., anti-glomerular basement membrane (GBM) disease).

Table 49.3: Risks of Recurrence of Specific Glomerulonephritis and 10-Year Risk for Allograft Loss

Disease	Risk of Recurrence (%)	10-year Risk of Allograft Loss (%)
IgA nephropathy	40–50	5–15
Membranous nephropathy	10–50	10–25
FSGS	20–30	8–15
ANCA-associated vasculitis	10–15	5
Anti-GBM (in presence of circulating antibodies)	100	80
C3 glomerulopathy	70	50 (5-year graft loss)
Dense deposit disease	50–100	45 (5-year graft loss)
Lupus nephritis	5	1

Note: Alport's syndrome, ADPKD and Fabry's disease do not recur after KT while primary hyperoxalosis and anti-GBM disease with detectable circulating anti-GBM antibodies are absolute contraindications to KT.

Abbreviations: FSGS, focal segmental glomerulosclerosis; ANCA, anti-neutrophil cytoplasmic antibodies; GBM, glomerular basement membrane

- Determining the natural history and treatment of primary kidney disease is also important, for example:

  - Focal segmental glomerulosclerosis (FSGS) with acute nephrotic syndrome and rapid progression to ESKD requires close surveillance post-transplant to detect early recurrence of FSGS that can lead to graft loss.

  - The type, dose, duration, and adverse effects to any immunosuppressive agents used to treat the primary kidney disease is important (e.g., evaluation should include cystoscopy to exclude bladder cancer for those treated with cyclophosphamide).

Malignancy Evaluation

- KT recipients have at least a 2-fold higher risk of cancer and cancer-related death than age- and sex-matched individuals in the general population. Therefore, KT candidates must be evaluated for unsuspecting cancers prior to KT according to age and sex (Table 49.4).

Table 49.4:   Screening Routine Investigations to Exclude Cancer Prior to Transplantation

1. Chest X-ray
2. CT abdomen and pelvis (will also examine for patency and calcifications of iliac arteries)
3. Stool occult blood
4. Cervical smear
5. Mammogram
6. Prostate-specific antigen
7. Other investigations as required (e.g., oesophago-gastro-duodenoscopy, colonoscopy)

Abbreviation: CT, computerised tomography

- KT candidates with a history of malignancies also have a higher hazard ratio of all-cause mortality after KT and need to be evaluated for:

  - Clearance of cancer prior to transplantation

  - Risks of recurrence of cancer after transplantation

  - Risks of secondary cancers from previous cancer treatment (e.g., radiation-induced tumours, tamoxifen-related uterine malignancies)

- Guidelines advocate a wait time of 2–5 years from cancer remission to transplantation depending on the type of cancer (Table 49.5). This wait time allows for surveillance of disease recurrence and occult metastasis to manifest prior to transplantation.

Table 49.5: Recommended Wait Times Required Prior to Kidney Transplantation for Individuals with a History of Specific Cancers According to Different Transplant Guidelines

Cancer Site	AST	CST	CARI
Lung	>2 years	>2 years	Not stated
Colorectal			
Duke A or B1	>2 years	>2 years	>2 years
Duke C	>5 years	>5 years	>5 years
Duke D	Not for transplant	Not for transplant	Not for transplant
Kidney			
Incidental/small	0 years	0 years	0 years
Large/invasive	5 years	5 years	>5 years
Bladder			
In situ	0 years	0 years	0 years
Invasive	>2 years	>2 years	>2 years
Breast			
In situ	>2 years	>2 years	>2 years
Advanced	>5 years	Not for transplant	Not for transplant

(Continued)

Table 49.5:   (Continued)

Cancer Site	AST	CST	CARI
Prostate			
Low grade/ localised	0 years	0	0
Invasive	>2 years	>2 years	>2 years
Advanced	Not for transplant	Not for transplant	Not stated
Uterine	>2 years	Not stated	Not stated
Cervix			
In situ	Not stated	≤2 years	0 years
Localised	>2 years	>2 years	>5 years
Invasive	Not stated	>5 years	Not stated
Thyroid	>2 years	>2 years	>2 years
Skin cancer			
Basal	0 years	0 years	0 years
Squamous	Not stated	>2 years	0 years
In situ melanoma	>2 years	>2 years	>2 years
>*In situ* melanoma	>5 years	>5 years	>5 years
Lymphoma	>2 years	>2 years	>years
Leukaemia	>2 years	>2 years	Not stated
Myeloma	Not stated	Not for transplant	Not for transplant
Testicular cancer	>2 years	>2 years	>2 years

Note: The table is just a guide as it is important to discuss the state of cancer remission and exact risk of cancer after KT always with a medical oncologist.

Abbreviations: AST; American Society of Transplantation, CST; Canadian Society of Transplantation. CARI; Caring for Australians and New Zealanders with Kidney Impairment.

Infective Evaluation

- Screening is performed to detect specific infections that need to be cleared before KT or prevented after KT (Table 49.6).

- Immunisation history should be obtained to identify vaccines that need to be given or updated (Table 49.7).

Table 49.6: Common Screening Tests for Infection at the Singapore General Hospital

1. Hepatitis B — HbsAg, anti-HBs Ab, anti-HBc Ab, HBV DNA
2. Hepatitis C — Anti-HCV Ab, HCV RNA
3. HIV — anti-HIV Ab, HIV PCR
4. Anti-HAV IgG
5. Hepatitis E — anti-HEV IgG, HEV RNA
6. CMV IgG
7. VZV IgG
8. EBV IgG
9. Measles IgG
10. TB-SPOT
11. Treponema pallidum particle agglutination assay (TPPA)
12. Multi-drug resistant organism screening — MRSA, CRE, VRE
13. Urine culture and sensitivity

Abbreviations: HIV, human immunodeficiency virus; HAV, hepatitis A virus; CMV, cytomegalovirus; VZV, varicella zoster virus; EBV, Epstein–Barr virus; TB, tuberculosis; MRSA, methicillin-resistant staphylococcus aureus; CRE, carbapenem-resistant enterobacterales; VRE, vancomycin-resistant enterococci

Table 49.7: Common Vaccinations Required Before Kidney Transplantation

Vaccination	Immunisation Regimen
Tdap (tetanus, reduced diphtheria, acellular pertussis)	1 dose before transplantation, if Tdap was not given in the last 10 years
Influenza	At least 1 dose annually or per season
Pneumococcal	Pneumococcal conjugate vaccine (PCV13) is given first followed by pneumococcal polysaccharide vaccine (PPSV23) 2 months later, if not given before
Hepatitis B	3 doses at 0, 1 and 6 months later if not immune to HBV — an accelerated course can be given at 0, 7, and 21–30 days later
Varicella	2 doses at 0 and 4–8 weeks later for those not immune
Measles, mumps, rubella (MMR)	2 doses at 0 and 4 weeks later for those not previously vaccinated or not immune

Note: Patients should also be vaccinated against COVID-19 according to prevailing national guidelines.

Table 49.8: Cardiovascular Screening Prior to Kidney Transplantation at the Singapore General Hospital

1. Electrocardiogram
2. Chest X-ray
3. 2D echocardiogram
4. Stress test (treadmill or pharmacologic) (e.g., Myocardial perfusion imaging scan, dobutamine stress echo)
5. Coronary angiogram (for all diabetics, those with positive stress test)

Cardiac Evaluation

- Potential KT candidates may have pre-existing cardiovascular disease (CVD) and remain at risk of CVD post-KT. CVD is a common cause of patient death after KT.

- CVD history and risk factors (e.g., family history, diabetes mellitus, hypertension, hyperlipidaemia, smoking, obesity) should be determined.

- Cardiovascular evaluation varies between transplant centres (Table 49.8).

Surgical Evaluation

- Potential KT candidates should be assessed by the transplant surgeon. Areas to be addressed include:
    - Space considerations for implantation — native kidney nephrectomy may be considered for patients with large polycystic kidneys. Nephrectomy can be performed prior to KT or simultaneously with KT, though the latter is less frequently practiced.
    - Nephrectomy for other indications — nephrectomy may be performed for native kidneys with (1) infections, (2)

suspicious masses, (3) haemorrhage, and (4) symptomatic stones. Patients who need nephrectomy and are not yet on dialysis will need to be prepared to initiate dialysis after nephrectomy.

- Bladder dysfunction — further assessment by the transplant surgeon may be required for patients with bladder dysfunction or previous complex bladder anatomy (e.g., bladder reconstruction or augmentation).

- Vascular anastomosis — the iliac vessels should be evaluated with a CT while patients should be clinically examined for peripheral vascular disease.

- Obesity — patients may need to lose weight (aiming for a BMI < 30–35 kg/m^2) prior to KT as obesity increases the risk of delayed graft function and problems with wound healing. Obesity also increases the risk of obstructive sleep apnoea, CVD, and hyperfiltration injury to the allograft.

Psychosocial Evaluation

- All potential KT candidates should be reviewed by medical social workers. Both potential living kidney donors and recipients should also be reviewed by a psychiatrist. This is to identify potential problems such as:
  - Non-adherence to follow-up and treatment
  - Poor psychosocial support
  - Insufficient financial resources for KT
  - Substance misuse (e.g., alcohol, recreational drugs)
  - Psychiatric illness

References

AlBugami M and Kiberd B (2014). Malignancies: Pre and post transplantation strategies. *Transplant Rev* **28**(2): 76–83.

Chadban SJ, Ahn C, Axelrod DA, *et al.* (2020). Summary of the Kidney Disease: Improving Global Outcomes (KDIGO) clinical practice guideline on the evaluation and management of candidates for kidney transplantation. *Transplantation* **104**(4): 708–714.

50 Histocompatibility Assessment in Kidney Transplantation

Ho Quan Yao

Introduction

- In kidney transplantation (KT), histocompatibility antigens expressed in the kidney tissue from the donor are recognised as "non-self" (Table 50.1) and will generate an allo-immune cell-mediated or antibody-mediated response in the recipient that can lead to rejection and possibly allograft dysfunction or failure.

- The objective of histocompatibility tests (Table 50.2) is to detect the presence of pre-formed antibodies against non-self antigens (i.e., ABO blood group antigens and human leukocyte antigens (HLAs) that can cause antibody-mediated rejection (ABMR)). Antibodies to non-HLA antigens (e.g., anti-endothelial antibodies) can also cause ABMR but are not routinely screened prior to KT.

- There is no test to assess the T-cell memory and hence predict the risk of routinely T-cell-mediated rejection. Fortunately, modern immunosuppression is strong enough to suppress or treat T-cell responses in most cases.

547

Table 50.1:   Major Histocompatibility Antigens

Major Histocompatibility Antigen	Description
ABO blood group antigens A, B, or AB — ABO blood group O do not express A or B antigens	ABO antigens are expressed not only in red blood cells but also the endothelial and epithelial cells of organs like the kidney. Humans start developing antibodies against non-self A or B antigens in the first year of life due to cross-reactivity between the A/B antigens and gut bacteria.
Human leukocyte antigens **Class I** HLA-A, -B, and -C **Class II** HLA-DRB1, -DQB1, and -DPB1	Class I HLAs are expressed in all nucleated cells (including T and B lymphocytes) and platelets while class II HLAs are expressed only in antigen-presenting cells such as B-lymphocytes. The HLA system is highly polymorphic with >30,000 HLA allelic variants, and potential KT candidates develop anti-HLA antibodies after pregnancy, during blood transfusions, or after a tissue/organ transplant.

Abbreviations: HLA, human leukocyte antigen; KT, kidney transplant

Table 50.2:   Goals of Histocompatibility Assessment

Goals	Clinical Relevance
Identify events of sensitisation	Sensitisation events where anti-HLA antibodies may be generated such as exposure to blood product transfusion, pregnancy, and transplantation.
Determine ABO compatibility	Kidney donors and their recipients should preferably be ABO compatible. ABO-incompatible kidney transplantation can be performed with desensitisation but with potentially higher risks of rejection, infections and, other complications.
Assess degree of HLA matching	The higher the degree of HLA matching, the lower the risk of rejection and graft loss. However, trying to find a fully matched kidney donor is rare and the focus has shifted to finding a kidney donor where the potential KT recipient does not have antibodies against the HLA of the donor.

Table 50.2:   (*Continued*)

Goals	Clinical Relevance
Identify the presence of pre-formed antibodies against the HLA of the donor	Graft survival is poorer in KT recipients who have preformed DSAs compared to those without, even with a negative crossmatch result. Augmented immunosuppression for KT is required to avoid ABMR.
Determine the immunological risk and treatment options required to perform KT	Patients with an ABO- or HLA-incompatible kidney donor should try to find a more compatible donor, failing which they can opt for a paired kidney donor exchange (provided there is a compatible kidney donor). In many cases, there are no other suitable donors and the patient either gets listed for a DDKT or undergoes desensitisation to enable ABO- or HLA-incompatible KT.
Counsel the patient on the risks of rejection, graft loss, complications, and high costs of desensitisation treatments	If the patient decides to proceed with an ABO- or HLA-incompatible KT, he/she would need to be carefully counselled and given informed consent.

Abbreviations: ABMR, antibody-mediated rejection; DDKT, deceased donor kidney transplant; DSA, donor-specific antibodies; HLA, human leukocyte antigen; KT, kidney transplant

Determination of ABO Compatibility

- ABO compatibility for KT follows the ABO blood group rules for blood transfusion (i.e., O individuals are universal donors, AB individuals are universal recipients) (Table 50.3).

- For blood group A donors, check for the presence of ABO blood group subtype A2 because it is less immunogenic and therefore associated with a lower risk of ABMR. Unfortunately, A2 subtypes are uncommon in the Asian population.

- The titre of the relevant anti-A or anti-B antibodies should be measured to determine the risk of ABMR after KT — a titre of ≥1:256 confers a higher risk of ABMR (Table 50.4).

Table 50.3:   ABO Blood Group Compatibility Table

Donor Blood Group	Recipient Blood Group	Interpretation	Antibody to Screen in the Recipient
O	O, A, B, AB	ABO-compatible	Not necessary
A	O, B	ABO-incompatible	Anti-A
A	A, AB	ABO-compatible	Not necessary
B	O, A	ABO-incompatible	Anti-B
B	B, AB	ABO-compatible	Not necessary
AB	O	ABO-incompatible	Anti-A and anti-B
AB	A	ABO-incompatible	Anti-B
AB	B	ABO-incompatible	Anti-A
AB	AB	ABO-compatible	Not necessary

Table 50.4:   Methods to Measure Anti-ABO Antibodies

Test	Samples/ Reagents	Result	Interpretation
Conventional tube titration	• Recipient serum • Reagent RBCs	Titre of recipient serum which causes agglutination and/or haemolysis (1:1, 1:2, 1:4, 1:8 etc)	Higher titre indicates higher levels of anti-A/B IgM antibodies in the recipient's blood
Indirect antiglobulin (Coombs) test	• Recipient serum • Reagent RBCs • Anti-human IgG	Titre of recipient serum which causes agglutination and/or haemolysis	Higher titre indicates higher levels of anti-A/B IgG +/− IgM antibodies in the recipient's blood

Abbreviations: RBC, red blood cells; Ig, immunoglobulin

Matching of Donor and Recipient HLA

- In general, 1 set of HLA genes is inherited from each parent. Therefore, there will be 2 copies of each HLA gene (2 × HLA-A, 2 × HLA-B etc).

- If only 1 HLA allele is detected in a particular locus, it generally means that the patient is homozygous for a particular HLA gene.

- HLAs found on the donor tissue that are not found in the recipient (i.e., non-self) will likely generate an allo-immune response in the recipient.

- The degree of HLA mismatch is typically presented as the number of donor HLA-A, B, and DR alleles not found (i.e., mismatched) in the recipient (i.e., X of 6 mismatch, see example below).

Locus	Donor	Recipient	Mismatch
A	A*02, A*11	A*02	1 of 2
B	B*13, B*41	B*13, B*41	0 of 2
DR	DRB1*01	DRB1*01, DRB1*08	0 of 2
Total HLA mismatches			1 of 6

Panel-reactive Antibodies

- The purpose of this test is to detect antibodies against a panel of HLAs and therefore estimate the general degree of sensitisation and the risk that the recipient may have donor-specific antibodies (DSAs) against any potential donor.

- The result is usually expressed as a percentage of antigens in the panel that reacted with the recipient's serum. A higher percentage will mean that the recipient is more likely to have DSAs against any potential donor.

Detection of donor-specific antibodies

- Patients who are HLA-mismatched may or may not have DSAs — the presence of pre-formed DSAs increase the risk of rejection and graft loss. There are several methods to detect DSAs (Table 50.5). Solid bead assays are the most sensitive and specific of all but they have their limitations too (Table 50.6).

Table 50.5:   Methods to Detect Donor-Specific Antibodies

Method	Test Category	Description	Advantages	Disadvantages
Complement-dependent cytotoxic cross-match Requirements: • Recipient's serum • Donor's lymphocytes • Complement	Cell-based assay	Recipient's serum is mixed with donor's lymphocytes. The complement is then added.If there are significant levels of complement-fixing DSAs, activation of complement will occur and lead to lysis of the donor's lymphocytes.	• Strong predictor of hyperacute rejection • Cheaper than flow cytometry and solid bead assays • Semi-quantitative measurement of antibody concentration (reported as titre of the recipient's serum that causes cell lysis; e.g., 1:2 with a higher titre representing a higher concentration of antibodies) • DTT can be added to inactivate IgM so that the CDCXM only detects IgG • AHG can be added to increase the sensitivity of the test by enhancing complement fixation	• Only detects complement-fixing antibodies • Detects both HLA- and non-HLA antibodies • Autoantibodies can cause a positive CDCXM which can be detected by performing an auto-crossmatch (the recipient's lymphocyte is mixed with the recipient's serum) • May not detect antibodies at low levels • False positive reactions may occur if the patient was treated with prior antibodies (e.g., thymoglobulin, rituximab, IVIG)

| Flow cytometry cross-match

Requirements:
• Recipient's serum
• Donor's lymphocyte
• Anti-human immunoglobulin (IgG) with fluorescence label | Cell-based | The recipient's serum is mixed with the donor's lymphocytes. Then anti-human IgG is added and if there are significant levels of lymphocyte-binding DSAs, the antibodies will be detected by a flow cytometer through the shift in fluorescence caused by the anti-human IgG binding to the DSAs. | • More sensitive than CDCXM in detecting low level of antibodies
• Detects both complement-fixing and non-complement-fixing antibodies
• More expensive than CDCXM
• Results are reported as channel shift which is the change in fluorescence compared to a control sample | • Depending on the lab, will only detect IgG antibodies and not IgM antibodies that may be generated during a recent sensitisation event
• Detects both HLA- and non-HLA antibodies
• Like CDCXM, autoantibodies may be detected which requires an auto FCXM to determine
• False positive reactions may occur if the patient was treated with prior antibodies (e.g., thymoglobulin, rituximab, IVIG — however pronase can be added to remove or reduce the effect of rituximab) |

(Continued)

Table 50.5:   *(Continued)*

Method	Test Category	Description	Advantages	Disadvantages
Single antigen bead assay Requirements: • Recipient's serum • Single antigen polystyrene beads impregnated with different ratios of two fluorescent marker dyes to provide a unique identity to each bead • Anti-human immunoglobulin (IgG) with fluorescent label	Solid phase (non-cell-based)	Recipient serum is mixed with a panel of single antigen microbeads and anti-human IgG. Both bead and bound antibody are detected by a fluoroanalyser, which can identify the bead and binding antibody	• Most specific method to detect DSA — does not detect non-HLA antibodies • Semi-quantitative measurement of antibody concentration (reported as mean fluorescence index (MFI)) • Addition of C1q may identify complement-fixing antibodies but this is not routinely practised	• Most expensive method to detect DSAs • Defects in the beads can lead to false positive or false negative reactions (see Table 50.6) • There is no agreed MFI cut-off representing a clinically significant concentration of DSA — in Singapore, a cut off <1,500 is accepted as not having significant DSAs • MFI measurements can vary from one time point to another — a variation of <25% is considered not clinically significant • Comprehensive donor typing is required to correctly match the antibodies detected as

| Virtual crossmatch Requirements:
• Donor HLA typing
• Recipient anti-HLA antibody profile | Non-cell-based | The patient's anti-HLA antibody profile can be first characterised. It can then be later cross-referenced to any donor HLA-typing result to determine if DSAs are present (i.e., a virtual crossmatch), such as when a deceased donor becomes available. | • Can quickly short-list potential recipients or donors for KT by determining the presence of DSAs — short-listed donors and recipients can then undergo a crossmatch to confirm their immunological eligibility for KT
• Can reduce cold ischaemia time during DDKT activation by avoiding "wet" crossmatches | DSA — some HLAs expressed by the donor may not be represented by the panel
• Accuracy of the VCXM depends on the accuracy of the SAB
• Not all patients have an anti-HLA antibody profile
• Past HLA antibody profile may not reflect current antibody profile
• Would still need a physical crossmatch to determine the immunological significance of DSAs |

Abbreviations: AHG, anti-human globulin; CDCXM, complement-dependent cytotoxic crossmatch; DDKT, deceased donor kidney transplant; DSAs, donor-specific antibodies; DTT, dithiothreitol; FCXM, flow cytometric crossmatch; HLA, human leukocyte antigen; IVIG, intravenous immunoglobulin; MFI, mean fluorescence index; SAB, single antigen bead; solid VCXM, virtual crossmatch

Table 50.6:   Limitations of Solid Bead Assays

False Positive or Falsely High Measurements	False Negative or Falsely Low Measurements
Denaturing of HLA protein bound on the microbead can expose non-native HLA epitopes which lead to spurious binding of antibodies Higher antigen density on beads may lead to over-estimation of antibodies	Prozone effect due to: 1. High concentration of antibodies that agglutinate in suspension — can be addressed with serial dilution 2. Binding of complement C1 to the Fc portion of the antibody — can add EDTA to prevent binding of C1 3. Competitive binding to the bead antigen by IgM — can add DTT Lower antigen density on the beads or saturation of binding sites may lead to under-estimation of antibodies

Abbreviations: EDTA, ethylenediaminetetraacetic acid; DTT, dithiothreitol

- A flow cytometric crossmatch (FCXM) result will report a negative/positive IgG B- and T-cell crossmatch. The interpretation of a complement-dependent cytotoxic crossmatch (CDCXM) is more complicated (Table 50.7).

Cross-reactive Groups

- Anti-HLA antibodies bind to an area of the HLA known as an epitope, rather than the entire HLA molecule. Each HLA molecule may have more than 20 epitopes.

- Different HLAs may have shared epitopes that react with the same antibody. HLAs which are known to have antibodies that cross-react are classified into groups called cross-reactive groups (CREGs).

- CREGS are not associated with ABMR but DSAs may bind on CREG beads instead of the actual DSA bead, leading to a falsely low MFI on the actual DSA bead.

Table 50.7:   Interpretation of the Complement-Dependent Cytotoxic Crossmatch Result

CDCXM Test	Result 1	Result 1	Result 2	Result 3	Result 4
Normal T-cell	Negative	Positive	Negative	Negative	Positive
Normal B-cell	Negative	Positive	Negative	Positive	Positive
DTT-treated T-cell	Negative	Negative	Negative	Negative	Positive
DTT-treated B-cell	Negative	Negative	Negative	Positive	Positive
AHG DTT-treated T-cell	Negative	Negative	Negative	Negative	Positive
AHG DTT-treated B-cell	Negative	Negative	Positive	Positive	Positive
Possible interpretations	No antibodies or antibodies too low a concentration to activate complement	IgM antibodies (autoantibodies, weak antibodies, or recent sensitisation)	Low level DSAs Non-HLA antibodies	Low level Class I or Class II DSAs Non-HLA antibodies Drugs (e.g., rituximab)	Class I DSAs or Class I and II DSAs Non-HLA antibodies Drugs (e.g., thymoglobulin)

Note: An isolated positive T-cell CDCXM without a concurrent B-cell CDCXM may be a laboratory issue such as poor T-cell lymphocyte viability, causing a false positive T-cell CDCXM. The histocompatibility laboratory should be consulted for advice.

Abbreviations: AHG, anti-human immunoglobulin; CDCXM, complement dependent cytotoxic crossmatch; DSA, donor-specific antibodies; DTT, dithiothreitol; HLA, human leukocyte antigen

Assessing Overall Immunological Risk

- Components of the histocompatibility assessment should be interpreted together with an understanding of the use and limitations of each test.

- Patients are usually classified into risk categories based on the results of the histocompatibility assessment, though the ideal risk classification system and their corresponding treatment regimens are unclear.

- Immunological risk due to histocompatibility is more likely a continuum rather than discrete categories (Tables 50.8 and 50.9).

Table 50.8: Risks Associated with HLA-Incompatible Kidney Transplantation

Factor	Higher Risk	Lower Risk
Antibody level	CDCXM positive	CDCXM negative
Antibody level	Microbead MFI >10,000	Microbead MFI <500
Antibody level	FCXM positive	FCXM negative
DSA specificities	Class I plus Class II	Single DSA
DSA specificities	Class I and DR	DP, DQ, and DRB3,4,5
Sensitisation history	Pregnancy-induced sensitisation, donor is patient's child or father of a child	Transplant-induced sensitisation with low DSA levels
Antibody characteristics	Complement-binding microbead positive	Complement-binding microbead negative
ABO donor-recipient status	ABO incompatible	ABO compatible
Donor source	Deceased donor	Living donor

Source: British Transplantation Society Guidelines on Antibody Incompatible Transplantation

Abbreviations: CDCXM, complement-dependent cytotoxic crossmatch; MFI, mean fluorescence index; FCXM, flow cytotoxic crossmatch; DSA, donor specific antibody

Table 50.9: Risks Associated with ABO-Incompatible Kidney Transplantation

Factor	Higher Risk	Lower Risk
Haemagglutination titre	>1/256	<1/256
If donor is group A	Group A1	Group A2
Donor type	Deceased donor	Living donor
HLA antibody incompatibility	Yes	No

Source: British Transplantation Society Guidelines on Antibody Incompatible Transplantation

Table 50.10: Immunosuppression Protocol According to HLA- and ABO-Incompatible Status

Risk Category	Test Results	Possible Treatment Regime
Standard/ low	ABO compatible, XM and DSAs negative	Basiliximab induction Cyclosporine-based maintenance
Moderate	ABO compatible, XM negative with low-level DSAs	Thymoglobulin induction Tacrolimus-based maintenance
High risk	ABO incompatible OR	Plasmapheresis and rituximab desensitisation Basiliximab induction Tacrolimus-based maintenance
	CDC or FCXM positive with DSAs on SAB assay OR XM negative but high level DSAs	Plasmapheresis, IVIG, rituximab desensitisation Thymoglobulin induction Tacrolimus-based induction

Abbreviations: CDC, complement-dependent cytotoxic crossmatch; DSA, donor specific antibody; FCXM, flow cytotoxic crossmatch; SAB, single antigen bead; IVIG, intravenous immunoglobulin; XM, crossmatch

- Other factors such as age, co-morbidities, risk of infection or malignancy, and potential tolerance to immunosuppression need to be considered before estimating the outcomes of the transplant and individualising the treatment regime (Table 50.10).

- If there are inconsistencies amongst the various tests, experts familiar with histocompatibility testing and/or the HLA lab should be consulted.

References

British Transplantation Society Guidelines on Antibody Incompatible Kidney Transplantation. Retrieved on 26th March 2023, from https://bts.org.uk/guidelines-standards/.

Tait BD, Süsal C, Gebel HM, *et al.* (2013). Consensus guidelines on the testing and clinical management issues associated with HLA and non-HLA antibodies in transplantation. *Transplantation* **95**(1): 19–47.

51 Assessment of Deceased Donor

Carolyn Tien, Terence Kee

Introduction

- There are 2 types of deceased donors (Table 51.1).

- There are also 2 types of donors under donation after brain death (Table 51.2).

- Expanded criteria donors (ECDs) have a higher risk of graft failure than standard criteria donors (SCDs) and are reserved for older recipients (≥50 years) who are at lower immunological risk for rejection. In Singapore, explant biopsies are performed to assess the histological quality of the kidneys and to determine if single or dual kidney transplantation should be performed (Table 51.3). It has improved graft survival of ECD KT, which are now comparable to SCD KT.

- Another type of deceased donor, which could be a SCD or ECD, is an increased risk donor (IRD), which is defined as a donor with increased risk for specific infections based on donor demographic and behavioural characteristics (Table 51.4).

Assessment of a deceased donor

- The eligibility of a potential deceased donor to donate kidneys for transplant is determined by

  - Medical suitability of the donor to donate any organ or tissue — exclude infection and cancer

Table 51.1:   Types of Deceased Donors

	Donation after Circulatory Death (DCD)	Donation after Brain Death (DBD)
Criteria for death certification	• By circulatory criteria — donor does not meet all criteria for brain death	• By neurologic criteria for brain death
When is death certified	• After 5 minutes of continuous asystole following withdrawal of life support	• On completion of brain death testing protocol
When is organ donation discussed with the family	• Organ donation is discussed before the diagnosis of death — the physician first decides on futility of care, determines inability of donor to survive without ventilatory support and establishes an agreement with the family to extubate • Consent is taken from the next of kin if the organ donor was not a prior organ pledger	• Organ donation is discussed after donor meets all criteria for brain death and is certified brain dead • Consent is taken from the next of kin if the organ donor was not a prior organ pledger
Organ recovery	• After extubating, there is observation of asystole and no touch time of 5 minutes • Donor is certified dead and then transferred to operating theatre (OT) for organ recovery • Usually only the kidney and liver can be recovered	• Organ donor is transferred to OT where organ recovery take place while the donor remains on ventilator • Kidney, liver, heart, lungs, pancreas, and intestines can be recovered
Warm ischaemia time	• Occurs — increase risk for delayed graft function but graft survival has been shown to be similar to donation after brain death donors	• Does not occur

Table 51.2:   Types of Donors under Donation after Brain Death

Expanded Criteria Donor (ECD)	• Any donor aged ≥60 years
	• Donor aged 50–59 years with at least 2 of the following
	  – serum creatinine >133 μmol/L
	  – history of HTN
	  – death by CVA
	• Singapore's specific criteria
	  – Any donor with DM
	  – Any donor with other specific conditions that may be associated with a poorer outcome after transplantation

Standard Criteria Donor (SCD)	Any other donor not meeting ECD criteria

Table 51.3:   Remuzzi Scoring System

Kidney Compartment	Remuzzi Score Allocation
Glomerular global sclerosis	0 — no glomeruli globally sclerosed 1 — <20% global glomerulosclerosis 2 — 20 to 50% global glomerulosclerosis 3 — >50% global glomerulosclerosis
Tubular atrophy	0 — absent 1 — <20% of tubuli affected 2 — 20 to 50% of tubuli affected 3 — >50% of tubuli affected
Interstitial fibrosis	0 — absent 1 — <20% of renal tissue replaced by fibrous connective tissue 2 — 20 to 50% of renal tissue replaced by fibrous connective tissue 3 — >50% of renal tissue replaced by fibrous connective tissue
Arterial and arteriolar narrowing	0 — absent 1 — increased wall thickness but to a degree that is less than the diameter of the lumen 2 — wall thickness that is equal or slightly greater to the diameter 3 — wall thickness that far exceeds the diameter of the lumen with extreme luminal narrowing or occlusion

(Continued)

Table 51.3:   (*Continued*)

Kidney Compartment	Remuzzi Score Allocation
Total score	Each kidney will have its score from individual compartment summated over a total possible score of 12 or less (if one compartment is not present on biopsy for scoring).

<u>Final score (range from 0 to 12) and allocation according to Singapore's criteria</u>

0 to 3	mild	Ok for single kidney transplant
4 to 7	moderate	Ok for dual kidney transplant
≥8	severe	Should not be transplanted

Table 51.4:   Criteria for Increased Risks Donors

1. Men who have sex with men (MSM) in the preceding 12 months.
2. Nonmedical injecting drug users (IDU) in the preceding 12 months.
3. People who have had sex in exchange for money or drugs in the preceding 12 months.
4. People who have had sex with a person known or suspected to have HIV, HBV or HCV infection in the preceding 12 months.
5. Women who have had sex with a man with a history of MSM behaviour in the preceding 12 months.
6. People who have had sex with a person who had sex in exchange for money or drugs in the preceding 12 months.
7. People who have had sex with a person who injected drugs by IV, IM or SC route for nonmedical reasons in the preceding 12 months.
8. A child ≤18 months old who was born to a mother known to be infected with, or at an increased risk for HIV, HBV or HCV.
9. A child breastfed within the preceding 12 months, and the mother is known to be infected with, or at an increased risk for HIV infection.
10. People incarcerated in prison or juvenile correctional facility for 72 consecutive hours in the preceding 12 months.
11. People on HD in the preceding 12 months.
12. Any patient who's medical/behavioural history cannot be obtained or who's blood specimen is haemodiluted.

Abbreviation: HBV, hepatitis B virus; HCV, hepatitis C virus; HD, haemodialysis; HIV, human immunodeficiency virus; IV, intravenous; IM, intramuscular; SC, subcutaneous.

- ■ Suitability of the kidney for transplantation — assess kidney structure and function

- Assessment of a deceased donor is based on "2nd hand" information, and hence there is always a risk that such information would be incomplete (Table 51.5).

Table 51.5: Areas to Assess a Potential Deceased Kidney Donor

General evaluation	• Age
	• Gender
	• Occupation
	• Country of birth
	• Recent travels and residences including places of outbreaks
Lifestyle risks	• Smoking
	• Alcohol
	• Sexual promiscuity
	• Non-medical drug use
	• Exposure to animals including pets
Past medical history	• Surgeries and diseases, noting those which may affect kidney structure and function
	• Recent vaccinations
	• Diabetes — complications, treatment, extend of control and HbA1c
	• Hypertension — check for LVH on ECG or echo
	• Coronary or cerebral or peripheral arterial disease
	• Cancer — histology, stage, treatment, current status
	• History of cancer screening tests and their results
	• Bloodborne infections — HBV, HCV, HIV
	• Sexually transmitted diseases
	• Risk factors for Transmissible Spongiform Encephalopathies (TSE) — family history of early dementia, use of pituitary hormone extract
	• Multi-drug resistant organism (MDRO) status — MRSA, VRE, CRB
Symptoms prior to admission	• Screen for symptoms especially for those relating to infection or cancer, e.g., fever, weight loss
	• Exposure to COVID-19 or other contagious infections

(Continued)

Table 51.5:   (*Continued*)

Current presentation	• Presentation of current illness • Any trauma and cardiovascular collapse • Vital signs at presentation and during admission • I/O balance • Trend of daily urine output • Ventilatory support • Volume of fluids and blood products — to identify haemodilution • Inotropes — dose, escalating or de-escalating • Other medications especially antibiotics given • Exposure to contrast • Invasive procedures, e.g., surgery • Imaging procedures and their results • Clinical progress in hospital • Need for renal replacement therapy • Eventual cause of death — to exclude infective and cancer causes, vaccine-induced thrombosis and thrombocytopenia may be associated with post-transplant thrombosis • Complications of brain death, e.g., diabetes insipidus

Physical examination	• Height and weight
	• BMI
	• Signs of cachexia or recent weight loss, e.g., skin folds
	• Full physical examination including
	  – Skin for cancer and infections
	  – Needle track marks
	  – Tattoos
	  – Injuries
	  – Rashes
	  – Surgical scars
	  – Wounds
	  – Masses including palpation of breasts, scrotum
	  – Lymphadenopathy — neck, axilla, groin
	  – Genitalia
	  – Vaginal and rectal examination
	• Catheters/drains

Table 51.5:   (*Continued*)

Laboratory tests	• Renal function — sCr, eGFR prior to admission, on admission, peak and terminal • Urine FEME or dipstick • Urine PCR or dipstick • Urine albumin: creatinine ratio • Liver panel • Full blood count • Procalcitonin • C-reactive protein • HbA1c • Beta human chronic gonadotrophin hormone (for women of reproductive age to detect metastatic choriocarcinoma)
Radiological examination	• Chest X-ray • Ultrasound abdomen or abdomen/pelvis computerised tomography

Microbiological work-up	• Culture and sensitivity (should be done prior to organ recovery)
	  – urine
	  – blood
	  – endotracheal/bronchoscopic
	  – other relevant sites
	• HBV — HbsAg, anti-HBs Ab, anti-HBc IgM/total Ab, HBV DNA
	• HCV — anti-HCV Ab, HCV RNA
	• HIV — HIV Ag-Ab screen, HCV PCR
	• VDRL
	• Anti-CMV IgG
	• Anti-EBV IgG
	• Dengue, Zika and Chikungunya NAT (in Singapore)
	• ART or NAT for SARS-CoV-2 as indicated

Immunological work-up	• ABO and human leukocyte antigen typing • Class 1 and 2 flow panel reactive antibodies • Crossmatches • Donor-specific antibodies

(Continued)

Table 51.5:   (*Continued*)

Surgical assessment (performed at time of organ recovery)	• Examine kidneys and other organs for clinically occult malignancies • Explant biopsy — histopathological assessment according to the Remuzzi scoring system

Abbreviations: ART, antigen rapid test; BMI, body mass index; CMV, cytomegalovirus; CRB, carbapenem-resistant bacteria; EBV, Epstein–Barr virus; eGFR, estimated glomerular filtration rate; ECG, electrocardiogram; HbA1C, Haemoglobulin A1C; HBV, hepatitis B virus; HCV, hepatitis virus; HIV, human immunodeficiency virus; I/O, input and output; LVH, left ventricular hypertrophy; MRSA, methicillin resistant staphylococcus aureus; NAT, nucleic acid test; PCR, protein creatinine ratio; sCr, serum creatinine; UFEME, urine full examination and microscopy; VDRL, venereal disease research laboratory; VRE, vancomycin resistant enterococcus

- As a result, there is always a risk (though low) that a potential donor may harbour an infection or cancer that may be transmitted to the recipient.

- Unlike heart, lung and liver transplantation, kidney transplantation is not immediately life-saving as patients can continue on dialysis. The threshold to accept kidneys for transplantation is, therefore, higher to allow a greater margin of safety.

References

Aubert O, Kamar N, Vernerey D, *et al.* (2015). Long term outcomes of transplantation using kidneys from expanded criteria donors: Prospective, population based cohort study. *BMJ* **351**: h3557.

Gagandeep S, Matsuoka L, Mateo R, *et al.* (2006). Expanding the donor kidney pool: Utility of renal allografts procured in a setting of uncontrolled cardiac death. *Am J Transplant* **6**(7): 1682–1688.

Lau, KO, Vathsala A, Kong S, *et al.* (1999). Preliminary results of heart-beating and non-heart-beating donor kidney transplants — the Singapore experience. *Ann Acad Med Singap* **28**(2): 222–226.

Merion RM, Ashby VB, Wolfe RA, *et al.* (2005). Deceased-donor characteristics and the survival benefit of kidney transplantation. *JAMA* **294**(21): 2726–2733.

Ojo AO, Hanson JA, Meier-Kriesche HU, *et al.* (2001). Survival in recipients of marginal cadaveric donor kidneys compared with other recipients and wait-listed transplant candidates. *J Am Soc Nephrol* **12**(3): 589–597.

Remuzzi G, Cravedi P, Perna A, *et al.* (2006). Long-term outcome of renal transplantation from older donors. *N Engl J Med* **354**(4): 343–352.

Summers DM, Watson CJ, Pettigrew GJ, *et al.* (2015). Kidney donation after circulatory death (DCD): State of the art. *Kidney Int* **88**(2): 241–249.

Yap YT, Ho QY, Kee T, *et al.* (2021). Impact of pre-transplant biopsy on 5-year outcomes of expanded criteria donor kidney transplantation. *Nephrology (Carlton)* **26**(1): 70–77.

52 Evaluation for Living Kidney Donation

Sobhana Thangaraju

Introduction

- The first successful living kidney donor transplant (LDKT) was performed between identical twin brothers in 1954.

- LDKT is preferred over a deceased kidney donor transplant (DDKT) because of its superior patient and graft survival.

- Other benefits of LDKT include:

  - Shorter waiting time to transplantation, with potential for pre-emptive transplantation and avoidance of dialysis

  - Allows for selection of the most suitable donor if there are multiple potential donors

  - Planned surgery with adequate time for optimisation of potential donor and recipient

- Outcomes such as life expectancy and quality of life for living kidney donors (LKDs) are generally good.

- Nonetheless, immediate and longer term surgical, medical, financial, and psycho-emotional risks need careful consideration.

- The goal of evaluation (Table 52.1) is to ensure that ethical principles (e.g., autonomy, non-maleficence) are adhered to while endeavouring to minimise risks to the potential donor.

- Stringent donor assessment and individualised counselling are essential in ensuring donor safety.

Table 52.1:   Goals of Evaluation

- Is the potential donor's willingness to donate voluntary and without coercion?
- Are the individualised benefits and risks of donation acceptable?
- Has the potential donor received adequate education and counselling for informed consent for donation?
- Does the transplant program have clear policies to guide the acceptance or refusal of potential donors?
- Does the accepted potential donor have care plans for donation and subsequent follow up?
- Does the ineligible potential donor have appropriate care plans and support in place after a failed assessment?

Evaluation of the potential kidney donor

- Eligibility criteria vary between various existing clinical practice guidelines (CPG) and/or national guidelines, such as those by the Organ Procurement and Transplantation Network (OPTN) in the United States of America (USA). Individual transplant programs may also have different thresholds for acceptable post-donation risks, where the acceptance criteria may not be clearly prescribed by guidelines.

- For example, the legal age for donation in Singapore is 21 years. However, some CPGs (e.g., USA, England) allow for donors 18 years or older if they can make an informed decision (*'Gillick* competent') and do not have any mental incapacity.

- The following are absolute contraindications practised at the Singapore General Hospital (Table 52.2).

- Evaluation of a potential donor requires a multidisciplinary team, which at the minimum in Singapore, be a physician who is not involved in the care of the recipient, surgeon, transplant coordinator, medical social worker, and psychiatrist.

Table 52.2: Absolute Contraindications to Kidney Donation

- Age <21
- Metabolic conditions:
  - Diabetes Mellitus Type I and II
  - Hypertension that is uncontrolled or with evidence of end organ damage
  - Obesity (BMI $\geq$35 kg/m^2)
- Renal abnormalities
  - Impaired or suboptimal kidney function
  - Presence of persistent proteinuria or haematuria
  - Bilateral kidney stones, recurrent stone disease or nephrocalcinosis
  - Vascular or urological abnormalities that preclude donation
- Infections
  - Active and uncontrolled infection, unless treated
  - HIV infection
  - Hepatitis C infection
- Active or past history of malignancies such as melanoma, solid organ cancers or haematological cancers
- Chronic illnesses such as cardiac, liver, pulmonary, neurologic, or autoimmune diseases
- Genetic predisposition
  - Two apolipoprotein L1 (APOL1) risk alleles
  - Other genetic mutations associated with increased risk of kidney disease
- When pregnant
- Psychosocial conditions
  - Uncontrolled psychiatric disease
  - Mental incompetence
  - Active substance and/or alcohol abuse
  - Concerns for donor coercion or commercial transaction between potential donor and recipient
- Any other condition that the transplant program policies deem unsuitable for donation based on individual risk assessment

Note: There is no upper age limit as long as there are no absolute contraindications

Evaluation of kidney function

- Assessment of renal function includes estimated glomerular filtration rate (eGFR) in mL/min per 1.73 m^2, followed by measured GFR (e.g., ^{51}Cr-EDTA, Tc99m DTPA). Where measured

Table 52.3:   Local Guidelines on Pre-donation GFR Thresholds

Age (Years)	GFR (mL/min/1.73 m^2)
<30	≥90
30–59	≥80
60–64	≥76
65–69	71
70–74	67
≥75	63

GFR is not available, confirmation with 24-hour creatinine clearance can be used if performed accurately.

- If kidney sizes are discrepant by >10% or there are vascular or urological abnormalities, differential kidney function should be obtained with radionuclide scans.

- GFR ≥90 mLs/min/1.73 m^2 is an acceptable level of kidney function for donation.

- GFR ≤60 mLs/min/1.73 m^2 is an absolute contraindication to donation.

- For donors with GFR between 61 and 89 mLs/min/1.73 m^2, recommendations vary between CPG. Local guidelines are shown in Table 52.3.

- However, in conjunction with GFR thresholds, additional risk factors should be considered for an individualised approach to determine post-donation risks of kidney failure.

Evaluation of pre-donation albuminuria

- Urine albumin-creatinine ratio (UACR) or albumin excretion rate (UAER) should be performed using early morning samples.

- Persistent UACR ≥30 mg/g or UAER ≥30 mg/day are contraindications to transplantation due to their association with CKD and increased cardiovascular mortality.

Evaluation of pre-donation microscopic haemturia

- Urine analysis for microscopic haematuria should be performed on at least 2 separate occasions.

- Persistent microscopic haemturia (more than 3 red blood cells per high-powered field) warrants further investigation to identify possible causes such as urinary tract infections, malignancies, nephrolithiasis, or glomerular disease (e.g., thin basement membrane disease, IgA nephropathy, Alport syndrome).

- Further investigations may include phase contrast microscopy, 24-hour urine stone studies, urine culture, cystoscopy, and imaging.

- Presence of dysmorphic urinary red blood cells may indicate glomerular causes of microscopic haematuria. Kidney biopsy should be considered only if less invasive tests do not preclude donation. Genetic testing should be considered if there is a family history for haematuria and/or presence of thin basement membrane on biopsy.

- Donors with IgA nephropathy and X-linked Alport syndrome are prohibited from donation.

Evaluation of pre-donation hypertension

- Blood pressure should be measured at clinic visits.
- Ambulatory blood pressure monitoring can be performed if the presence of or control of pre-existing blood pressure is uncertain.

- In the absence of end-organ damage, potential donors with pre-existing hypertension can be considered if:
  - Age ≥50 years, and
  - Well controlled blood pressure with one or two antihypertensive agents, and
  - Individualised risk is not deemed unacceptably high

Evaluation of pre-donation history for nephrolithiasis

- Prior history of renal stone disease should be ascertained. Medical records pertaining to the episode(s) should be reviewed.

- Presence of uncorrectable metabolic abnormalities identified through repeated 24-hour urine studies and/or persistence of nephrolithiasis (e.g., bilateral or large stones) on renal imaging are absolute contraindications to donation

- Donation of a kidney with a small renal stone may be permitted in the absence of metabolic abnormalities with informed consent from both donor and recipient. Where feasible, stone removal ex-vivo is recommended prior to implantation.

Malignancy Evaluation

- Cancer screening is required to prevent donor-derived malignancy in the recipient as well as to protect the health of the donor candidate.

- Donor-derived malignancy is associated with poor prognosis in the kidney transplant recipient (KTR).

- Potential donors should undergo cancer screening prior to donation according to age, gender, family history and personal risk factors such as smoking and occupational exposure (Table 52.4).

Table 52.4: Screening Routine Investigations to Exclude Cancer Prior to Donation

1. Chest X-ray
2. CT Angiogram (which is performed to also ascertain renal vasculature)
3. Stool occult blood
4. Cervical smear
5. Mammogram
6. Prostate specific antigen
7. Other investigations as required, e.g., Oesophago-Gastro-Duodenoscopy (OGD), colonoscopy, CT thorax

- Guidelines allow for potential donors with a history of treated malignancy to be considered on a case-by-case basis if there is a low risk of transmission or recurrence. Incidental renal tumours (<4 cm) may also be permissible. However, informed consent from recipient is required.

- Singapore General Hospital does not accept donors with any prior history for malignancy.

Infective Evaluation

- Screening is performed to detect specific infections that may preclude donation or require treatment before donation can proceed. Serostatus for prior infections (e.g., CMV) are important in ascertaining risk and prophylaxis strategy in the KTR (Table 52.5).

- Vaccination recommendations follow that of age-appropriate recommendations in the general population. Additional vaccination in donors who are household contacts (e.g., Varicella or MMR vaccination) can be recommended.

Table 52.5:   Common Screening Tests for Infection at the Singapore General Hospital

1. Hepatitis B — HbsAg, anti-HBs Ab, anti-HBc Ab, HBV DNA
2. Hepatitis C — Anti-HCV Ab, HCV RNA
3. HIV — Anti-HIV Ab, HIV PCR
4. HEV — Anti-HEV IgG, HEV RNA
5. CMV IgG
6. VZV IgG
7. EBV IgG
8. Measles IgG
9. Treponema pallidum particle agglutination assay (TPPA)
10. Multi-drug resistant organism screening — MRSA, CRE, VRE
11. Urine culture and sensitivity
12. Chest X-ray

Table 52.6:   Cardiovascular Screening Prior to Kidney Donation at the Singapore General Hospital

1. ECG
2. CXR
3. 2D Echocardiogram
4. Stress test (treadmill or dobutamine stress echo)

Cardiac Evaluation

- Potential donors should be screened for occult cardiovascular disease (CVD)

- CVD history and risk factors (e.g., family history, DM, HTN, HLD, smoking, obesity) should be determined.

- Cardiovascular evaluation varies between transplant centres (Table 52.6).

Surgical Evaluation

- Potential living kidney donors must be assessed by the transplant surgeon.
- The following investigations are required for selection of the most appropriate kidney:
    - Detailed imaging of donor kidneys, collecting systems and vascular anatomy using CT renal angiography or magnetic resonance angiography (MRA)
    - Split kidney function using radionuclide renography or CT renal volumes
- The kidney with poorer function should be selected for nephrectomy. Where split kidney function and anatomy are similar, the left kidney should be preferentially procured as the longer venous pedicle allows for technical ease.
- Laparoscopic donor nephrectomy is preferred to open nephrectomy as it allows for reduced hospitalisation days, faster recovery, and reduced pain. However, open nephrectomy can be considered for technical reasons such as adhesions, complex renal anatomy, or a lack of expertise for laparoscopic technique.
- Risks of major perioperative complications are less than 1%. The potential living kidney donor should be counselled regarding these risks (Table 52.7).

Table 52.7: Perioperative Risks of Living Donor Nephrectomy (Non-Exhaustive).

1. Death (0.03%)
2. Complications related to anaesthesia (<2%)
3. Complications requiring re-operation or blood transfusion (0.5% to 0.1%)
4. Injury to internal organs, ileus, or intestinal obstruction (0.05% to 0.1%)
5. Chylous ascites (<1%)
6. Deep vein thrombosis or pulmonary embolism (0.1%)
7. Prolonged wound pain or wound infections (<5%)

Psychosocial Evaluation

- All potential living kidney donors should be reviewed by an independent MSW and psychiatrist, who are not involved in the care of the recipient, for the following:

  - To ascertain willingness, and absence of coercion in reasons for donating

  - To assess the donor's mental capacity to make an informed decision

  - To ascertain if the donor has the appropriate understanding of the potential outcomes for the donor, recipient, and transplant procedure

  - To identify mental health conditions, high-risk behaviour, substance abuse, or other psychosocial issues which may influence motivation to donate and post-donation recovery

  - To facilitate consideration of donation decision on employment, insurance, and other life goals

  - To ascertain if appropriate social support is available or recovery

- To review needs and facilitate access to financial assistance when needed

Risks Post-donation

- All potential donors should be counselled on long-term risks of kidney donation as part of informed consent.
- Long-term risks include the following:
  - Permanent loss of GFR (up to 35%)
  - Potential increase in blood pressure (increases of 6 mmHg observed within 10 years of donation)
  - Increased risk of proteinuria after donation (incidence 10%)
  - Slightly increased risk of end-stage kidney disease (ESKD) post-donation (0.3% in living kidney donors as compared to 0.03% in healthy non-donors)
- Risk factors for increased risk of ESKD after donation include:
  - Non-adherence to a healthy lifestyle
  - Non-adherence to regular follow up
  - Genetic relationship with the recipient

Post-donation follow up

- Guidelines recommend a follow up at 6 weeks, followed by 6 and 12 months after donation.
- Longer-term follow up is strongly recommended thereafter. In Singapore General Hospital, donors are reviewed annually (Table 52.8).

Table 52.8:   Post-donation follow up at Singapore General Hospital

	Parameters
Lifestyle	Healthy diet, exercise, smoking cessation, avoidance of nephrotoxic medications and supplements
Renal function	eGFR, UACR, urine analysis and renal imaging every 2–5 years.
Obesity	Weight, BMI
Hypertension	Blood pressure measurements
Diabetes	Fasting glucose, HbA1c, OGTT
Other metabolic complications:	
Dyslipidaemia	Lipid panel
Non-alcoholic	Liver panel
Gout	Uric acid
Psychological and emotional assessment	Anxiety, depression, high risk behaviour

Abbreviations: BMI, body mass index; eGFR, estimated glomerular filtration rate; HbA1c, haemoglobulin A1c; UACR, urine albumin:creatinine ratio; OGTT, oral glucose tolerance test

References

Andrews PA and Burnapp L (2018). British Transplantation Society / Renal Association UK guidelines for living donor kidney transplantation 2018: Summary of updated guidance. *Transplantation* **102**(7): e307.

Lentine KL, Kasiske BL, Levey AS, *et al.* (2017). KDIGO clinical practice guideline on the evaluation and care of living kidney donors. *Transplantation* **101**(8S Suppl 1): S1–S109.

53 Immunosuppression for Kidney Transplant

Sobhana Thangaraju, Lim Rou Wei

Introduction

- Immunosuppression is required to prevent acute rejection and graft loss in all kidney transplant (KT) recipients, except when the donor kidney is from an identical twin sibling (Table 53.1).

- Induction immunosuppression refers to immunosuppression that is administered intravenously during the pre and peri-transplant period when the risk of rejection is at the highest. It is also given to provide adequate immunosuppression while awaiting maintenance immunosuppression given orally to reach steady state and effective concentrations.

- Maintenance immunosuppression refers to chronic immuno-suppression that is required for the duration of the functioning KT. As the risk of rejection decreases over time, maintenance immunosuppression required for sufficient suppression of

Table 53.1:   Goals of Immunosuppression

- Prevention of acute rejection,
- Achievement of maximal graft longevity,
- Prevention of mortality and morbidity from complications of immunosuppression such as diabetes mellitus, infections, cardiac disease, and cancers, and
- Prevention of other medical conditions that can affect quality of life, such as osteoporosis, obesity, and other changes in physical appearances

allo-recognition also decreases. However, it is not possible to eliminate the need for continued immunosuppression.

- Immunosuppressive drugs used for maintenance and induction may also be used in the treatment of rejection.

- Risks of infections and malignancy are increased because of the cumulative exposure to immunosuppression. Hence, it is prudent to achieve the lowest net state of immunosuppression.

- Immunosuppression protocol varies between countries, transplant centres and patient characteristics.

Induction immunosuppression

- Induction immunosuppression refers to immunosuppression that is administered at the time of transplant surgery (Table 53.2). It is recommended for most KT recipients except recipients of allografts from HLA-identical monozygotic twins

Table 53.2:   Type of Induction Agents

Types of Induction Agents	Medication (Brand Name)
Corticosteroids	Methylprednisolone
IL-2 receptor antagonists	Basiliximab (Simulect©)
Antilymphocyte antibodies	**Polyclonal** Rabbit antithymocyte globulin (rATG-Thymoglobulin©) Equine anti-thymoyte globulin (ATGAM©) **Monoclonal** Anti-CD52 monoclonal antibody — Alemtuzumab (Lemtrada©)
Anti-CD20 antibodies	**Monoclonal** Rituximab (Mabthera©, Truxima©)

who may not require induction immunosuppression, as the risk of rejection is low.

- Combination of interleukin-2 receptor antagonist (IL2-RA) and IV methylprednisolone (MP) are preferred for transplants that have a low immunological risk.

- Combination of antilymphocyte antibodies (ALA) and IV MP are preferred as induction agents for transplants that have a higher immunological risk of rejection. Risk factors for increased risk of rejection include:

  - Younger recipient and older donors

  - Strong sensitisation history, including re-transplant

  - Panel reactive antibody (PRA) > 3%

  - Mismatches in human leukocyte antigens (HLA)

  - Blood group incompatibility

  - Presence of pre-formed donor specific antibodies

  - Delayed graft function

  - Prolonged cold ischaemia time (>24 hours)

IL-2 receptor antagonists

- T-cell activation by donor antigens results in IL-2 production, which leads to T-cell proliferation. Hence, binding of IL2-RA to IL-2 receptors can mitigate this immune response and reduce the risk of cell-mediated rejection.

- Basiliximab is the only available IL2-RA and is a chimeric (murine/human) monoclonal antibody.

- Rejection rates, graft and patient survival are similar between basiliximab and antilymphocyte induction in low-risk KT. However, patients who received ALA induction had a higher incidence of cytomegalovirus (CMV) infection and cytopenia. Considering the benefits and risks of aggressive immunosuppression, basiliximab is the induction agent of choice for low-risk KT.

- Dose and administration:
  - First dose: IV 20 mg within 2 hours prior to transplant surgery
  - Second dose: IV 20 mg on postoperative day 4
- Basiliximab is generally well tolerated and has few adverse effects.

Antilymphocyte antibodies

- ALA include polyclonal and monoclonal antibodies, which induce lymphocyte depletion.
- Polyclonal ALA target a wide range of human T cell surface antigens, such as the major histocompatibility complex antigens.
- Thymoglobulin© (r-ATG) is produced by immunising rabbits with human thymocytes, whereas ATGAM© is produced by immunising horses with human thymocytes. The latter is rarely used due to its lower efficacy in preventing rejection compared to r-ATG.
- High immunological risk patients receiving r-ATG as compared to basiliximab induction experienced lower incidence of acute rejections, graft loss and death at 1- and 5-years post-transplant. Although infection rates were increased, risk of CMV disease and malignancy did not appear to be higher.
- As ALA are potent agents, the patient should be carefully reviewed for fitness to receive these drugs (Table 53.3).

Table 53.3:   Checklist for Administration of Antilymphocyte Antibodies

- Exclude prior sensitivity to r-ATG
- Active infections and malignancy have been ruled out
- Euvolaemic fluid status
- No significant electrolyte abnormalities
- No significant or unexplained cytopenias
- Baseline CD3 counts are available
- Baseline viral hepatitis status, CMV serostatus, and Epstein–Barr virus serostatus are known
- Central venous access has been established for infusion through a high-flow vein
- Patient has been counselled on the infusion side effects and longer-term increased risks for infection and malignancy
- Pre-medications comprising the following are administered at least 30 minutes prior to r-ATG infusion:
  a) PO Paracetamol 1 g once
  b) Antihistamine: IV Diphenhydramine 25–50 mg once
  c) IV Hydrocortisone 50–100 mg once
- Dose of r-ATG (1–1.5 mg/kg) is rounded to the nearest 25 mg and administered as an infusion over at least 6 hours (first dose) or at least 4 hours (subsequent doses if tolerated)
- Close monitoring of vital signs
- Emergency epinephrine and hydrocortisone should be readily available in the event of anaphylaxis
- Appropriate antiviral (including CMV prophylaxis), anti-fungal and antibacterial prophylaxis is prescribed

- Optimal cumulative dose of r-ATG is unknown. Hence, dose varies between centres. Doses between 3 and 6 mg/kg are felt to be optimal as there are no increased benefits for graft and patient survival seen above a cumulative dose of 6 mg/kg. However, doses lower than 3 mg/kg may not be adequate in prevention of rejection in high-risk patients.

- Doses of r-ATG should be adjusted according to white blood and platelet counts (Table 53.4).

Table 53.4: Dose Adjustment of Thymoglobulin© based on White Blood Cell and Platelet Counts

	WBC Count ($\times 10^9$/L)	Platelet Count ($\times 10^9$/L)
Reduce dose by 50%	2–3	50–75
Discontinue or hold off dose until recovery of counts	<2	<50

- Some centres monitor CD3⁺ lymphocyte count daily while on r-ATG. While it may not be used to determine dose of r-ATG for induction, suppressed counts (<25 cells/mm³) are reassuring if the dose is held off due to cytopenias or infection. Rising counts despite ongoing administration may also be suggestive of the formation of neutralising antibodies.

- Polyclonal ALA have significant short and long-term adverse effects that require close monitoring (Table 53.5).

- Cytokine release syndrome (CRS) is characterised by nausea, headache, tachycardia, hypotension, rash and/or shortness of breath. Severity grading of CRS is as follows:

  - Grade 1 — Fever with or without constitutional symptoms

  - Grade 2 — Fluid responsive hypotension, hypoxia responding to <40% fraction of inspired oxygen (FiO_2)

  - Grade 3 — Hypotension managed with one vasopressor, hypoxia requiring >40% FiO_2

  - Grade 4 — Life-threatening consequences; urgent intervention indicated

  - Grade 5 — Death

- Grades 1 and 2 are the commonly observed CRS. Management is largely supportive (Table 53.6). Symptoms of CRS usually abate with subsequent infusions.

Table 53.5:   Adverse Effects of Thymoglobulin©

Haematologic
Leukopenia (up to 63%) — lymphopenia may last up to 1 year
Thrombocytopenia (up to 37%)
Anaemia

Cardiovascular
Hypertension (up to 37%)
Tachycardia (up to 23%)

Gastrointestinal
Nausea, vomiting
Abdominal pain

Renal
Hyperkalaemia (up to 57%)

Neurologic
Chills (up to 57%)
Headache (up to 40%)

Musculoskeletal
Myalgia (up to 20%)

Increased risk of infection (up to 76%)
CMV infection (less than 15%)
Urinary tract infection

Malignancy (up to 4%)

Hypersensitivity
Serum sickness (up to 2%)

Rare but serious complications
Anaphylactic shock (<1%) and cytokine release syndrome,
    both of which can be fatal

Table 53.6:   Appropriate Action in the Event of an Infusion Reaction

1. Stop infusion
2. Ascertain if nature of reaction is anaphylaxis or cytokine release syndrome
   (CRS).
3. If anaphylaxis is confirmed, infusion should be permanently discontinued.
   Immediate rescue with epinephrine and hydrocortisone, alongside other
   resuscitative measures, should be instituted.
4. If CRS is suspected, supportive therapy should be instituted according
   to the severity grade. Infusion can be restarted at a slower rate after
   improvement of symptoms.

- C-reactive protein and procalcitonin are raised after r-ATG infusion, especially in CRS. Hence, they may not be useful in differentiating infection from CRS.

Anti-CD20 monoclonal antibodies

- Rituximab is an anti-CD20 monoclonal antibody that depletes B-cells.

- Rituximab is predominantly used as part of desensitisation protocols in HLA and ABO-incompatible transplants. Its use as antibody induction in ABO-compatible, non-sensitised recipients is not associated with significant improvement in rejection and graft/patient survival rates.

- The dose used for antibody induction varies with the centres, especially those from Asia, where lower fixed doses of 100–200 mg are used. However, the standard dose of 375 mg/m^2 is generally used for the treatment of rejection.

Maintenance immunosuppression

- Triple therapy with different classes of immunosuppressive drugs is recommended for initial maintenance therapy (Table 53.7). Through distinct mechanisms, the drugs work in synergy with benefits such as:
    - Lower doses of each immunosuppression, which then reduces the occurrence of side effects
    - Graft survival is maintained above 90%
    - Rejection rates are kept below 20%

- Immunosuppressive drugs can be used in different combination regimens according to the immunological risk for rejection, condition of the patient, and risks for certain complications

Table 53.7: Classes of Maintenance Immunosuppression

Drug Class	Medication (Brand Name)
Corticosteroids	Prednisone, Prednisolone
Calcineurin inhibitors	Cyclosporine (Neoral©) Immediate-release tacrolimus (Prograf©) Extended-release tacrolimus (Advagraf©)
Antimetabolite agents	Mycophenolate acid analogues (Cellcept©, Myfortic©) Azathioprine (Imuran©)
Mammalian target of rapamycin inhibitors	Sirolimus (Rapamune©) Everolimus (Certican©)

(Table 53.8). Most centres prescribe a combination of corticosteroids, calcineurin inhibitors (CNIs), and antimetabolite agents.

- Stable immunosuppression regimen and doses are usually reached between 3 and 6 months after transplantation. Further modifications should not be routinely performed if the graft function is stable, unless necessitated by other events such as complications (e.g., infection, cancer), pregnancy or the need for surgery. Complete withdrawal of all immunosuppression can only be considered in recipients of allografts from HLA-identical monozygotic twins.

- Adherence should be assessed at every follow up, as nonadherence is strongly associated with rejection risks and early graft loss. Reasons for nonadherence (if present) should be assessed. Modification of maintenance immunosuppression may be necessary to improve adherence (e.g., switch to once daily formulation of tacrolimus).

- Pharmacokinetic profile of generic formulations may differ, and hence switching between different preparations of the same drug should be avoided. Drug levels should be closely monitored if conversion is necessary.

Table 53.8:   Potential Combinations of Triple Immunosuppression

Triple Immunosuppression Combinations	Examples of Randomised Controlled Trials
Corticosteroids + CNI + MPA	Tricontinental Mycophenolate Mofetil Renal Transplantation study (1996) Elite-Symphony Trial (2009)
Corticosteroids + CNI + AZA	European Tacrolimus Multicentre Renal Study Group (1997) European Tacrolimus vs. Ciclosporine Microemulsion in Renal Transplantation Study Group (2002)
Corticosteroids + CNI + mTORi	Transform study (2015) Athena Study Group (2019)
Corticosteroids + mTORi + MPA	Spare the Nephron study (2011) Symphony study (2017)
Corticosteroids + Belatacept* + MPA	BENEFIT study (2010) BENEFIT-EXT study (2010)

*Belatacept is not available in Singapore and is not discussed in this chapter.

Abbreviations: AZA, azathioprine; CNI, calcineurin inhibitors; MPA, mycophenolate acid analogues (Cellcept© or Myfortic©); mTORi, mammalian target of rapamycin inhibitors

Choice of initial maintenance immunosuppression

- Choice of maintenance immunosuppression is primarily dependent on immunological risk for rejection. Risk factors for increased risk of rejection include:

  - Younger recipient and older donors

  - PRA > 3%

  - HLA mismatches

  - Blood group incompatibility

  - Presence of pre-formed donor specific antibodies

  - Delayed graft function

- Additional non-immunological factors that may be considered include:
    - Side effect profile (e.g., risk of post-transplant diabetes mellitus, cosmetic)
    - Prior intolerance
    - Primary disease or prior comorbidities
    - Cost of immunosuppression, which can otherwise lead to non-adherence
    - Patient preference
- Calcineurin inhibitors (CNIs) are the backbone of maintenance immunosuppression, as without them, the risk of rejection is very high. Complete CNI withdrawal (CAESAR study) or CNI-free regimens (Elite-Symphony study) have been associated with an increased risk of rejection.
- Between the CNIs, tacrolimus (TAC) is more effective than cyclosporine (CsA) in reducing acute rejection rates. Some studies have also suggested that long-term risk of allograft loss might be lower with TAC.
- Antimetabolite agents include azathioprine (AZA) and mycophenolate acid analogues (MPA). MPA is the preferred antimetabolite agent as it has significantly reduced risks of rejection and better adverse effect profile as compared to AZA.
- Mammalian target of rapamycin inhibitors (mTORi) may be an alternative to antimetabolite agents, but their use may be limited by the presence of delayed graft function and concerns for risk of poorer wound healing or lymphocele formation.
- Regardless of the choice of maintenance immunosuppression, all patients should receive the appropriate vaccination while on maintenance treatment.

- Long-term prophylaxis for *Pneumocystis jirovecii* is prescribed for all patients on mTORi and MPA-containing triple immuno-suppression.

Corticosteroids

- Corticosteroids (CS) inhibit a wide range of immune cells through multiple mechanisms, such as the redistribution of circulating lymphocytes (causing lymphopenia) and inhibition of cytokine production (reducing T-cell activation).

- Doses of prednisolone (PRED) vary with different centres and are tapered to a nadir of 5–10 mg daily unless a steroid avoidance or withdrawal protocol is employed where the PRED is not given or eventually weaned off. However, complete withdrawal or avoidance of CS from maintenance immunosuppression is associated with

  - Increased risk of acute rejections
  - Increased incidence of kidney fibrosis
  - Higher risks of recurrence of glomerulonephritis
  - Possible exacerbation of myelosuppressive effects of anti-proliferative drugs

- Alternate day dosing or doses of PRED below 5 mg/day are not recommended as they do not reduce the occurrence and severity of side effects (Table 53.9).

- Patients should be monitored for the development of adverse effects. Patients at higher risk should be identified. Prevention strategies should be instituted (e.g., bisphosphonates for osteoporosis, diet, and lifestyle management for metabolic complications, prophylaxis for infections).

Table 53.9: Adverse Effects of Corticosteroids

Metabolic and hormonal
Hyperglycaemia
Dyslipidaemia
Adrenal insufficiency

Cardiovascular
Hypertension
Atherosclerosis

Gastrointestinal
Gastritis, peptic ulcer disease
Fatty liver
Visceral perforation

Haematologic
Leukocytosis

Increased risk of infection

Neurologic
Mood disturbances
Insomnia
Akathasia

Bone and Muscle
Osteoporosis
Avascular necrosis

Ophthalmologic
Cataracts
Glaucoma
Central serous retinopathy

Dermatologic and cosmetic
Cushingoid appearance
Obesity
Acne, hirsutism
Thinning of skin, easy bruising and striae
Impaired wound healing

Calcineurin inhibitors

- CsA and TAC are the main CNIs available for clinical use (Table 53.10).

Adjustment of doses of calcineurin inhibitors

- Several factors should be considered in determining the initial doses of CNIs and their subsequent titration (Table 53.11).
- Accuracy of drug level results should be ascertained before any dose adjustments are made (Table 53.12).

Adverse effects of calcineurin inhibitors

- Adverse effects occurring at similar frequencies in both CNIs include risks of:
    - Nephrotoxicity — acute or chronic
    - Tubular dysfunction (e.g., hyperkalaemia. hypophosphataemia, hypomagnesaemia, metabolic acidosis)
    - Thrombotic microangiopathy
    - Infection
    - Malignancy
- Some adverse effects occur at a higher preponderance in CsA as compared to TAC (Table 53.13)
- Some of the adverse effects of TAC may be lower when taking extended-release formulations.
- Management of some adverse effects may include drug dose reduction or conversion to alternative classes of immunosuppression with the goal of maintaining adequate immunosuppression.

Table 53.10: Pharmacology of Calcineurin Inhibitors

Mechanism of action	CNI bind to immunophilins (CsA to cyclophilin and TAC to FKBP-12) and form a complex with calcium, calmodulin and calcineurin that leads to the inhibition of phosphatase activity of calcineurin. As a result, nuclear factor of activated T-cells (NF-AT) cannot be dephosphorylated and translocate to the nucleus to activate IL-2 gene transcription. The end-result is reduced IL-2 production, which leads to reduced T-cell proliferation.
Available formulations	Both CsA and TAC are available in oral and IV formulations. For oral formulation, CsA is available in Singapore as 10, 25 and 100 mg capsule or 100 mg/mL solution, while TAC is supplied as 0.5, 1 and 5 mg capsule. Non-PVC containers and tubings should be used to store and administer CNI to avoid leaching of DEHP and adsorption of CsA and TAC, respectively, which occurs with PVC. Both dextrose 5% and sodium chloride 0.9% solutions can be used as diluents.
Absorption	CNI are absorbed in the small intestines, but bioavailability is dependent on the presence of food, bile acids and gut motility. The microemulsion formulation of CsA (Neoral©) is preferred for its more consistent absorption and increased bioavailability as it is not dependent on bile salts for absorption. The bioavailability of TAC is also dependent on formulation — 7–32% (immediate release) vs. 12–19% (extended-release). TAC should preferably be administered on an empty stomach where absorption is better.
Time to tmax	CsA: 1.5–2 hours TAC: 0.5–6 hours
Elimination $t_{1/2}$	CsA: 8.4 hours TAC: 12 hours (immediate release), 38 hours (extended-release)
Time to steady state	CsA: ~2 days TAC: 2.5 days (immediate release), ~1 week (extended-release)

(Continued)

Table 53.10: *(Continued)*

Plasma protein binding	CsA: 90–98% TAC: 99% (primarily to albumin and alpha-1 acid glycoprotein)
Metabolism	CNI are metabolised by CYP3A4 and CYP3A5 systems with a half-life of 8.4 hours for CsA, 12 hours for immediate release TAC and 38 hours for extended-release TAC. Metabolism of CNIs vary between ethnic groups due to polymorphisms in the CYP3A genes. As a result, drug level monitoring is essential to ascertain the appropriate dose. Some centres will dose TAC according to CYP3A5 polymorphism, e.g., CYP3A5*1/*1 (extensive expressors) and CYP3A5*1/*3 (intermediate expressors) require higher doses of TAC than CYP3A5*3/*3 (low expressors).
Dosing	**<u>Oral dosing</u>** CsA — 2–2.5 mg/kg/dose BD TAC — 0.05–0.1 mg/kg/dose BD (immediate release) — 0.1–0.2 mg/kg/dose OM (extended-release) Immediate release and extended-release formulations of tacrolimus are comparable in safety and efficacy. If converting from immediate release to extended-release TAC, 1:1 dose conversion can be performed. It is important to ensure that drug level concentration with immediate release TAC is adequate before switching to extended-release TAC as TAC drug levels tend to be lower after conversion to extended-release TAC. **<u>IV dosing</u>** CsA — 1/3 of total daily oral dose given over 2–6 hours TAC — 1/3–1/4 of total daily oral dose given over 24 hours CNIs should be administered at a consistent time of the day and at 12-hour intervals unless using extended-release formulations, which are dosed once daily. Temporal relationship of CNI ingestion with meals should be consistent. Extended-release formulations of TAC should only be taken in the mornings, as area under the plasma drug concentration-time curve (AUC) is reduced when taken in the evening.

Elimination	CsA is mainly metabolised in the liver, and its metabolites are mostly excreted in bile, whereas TAC is metabolised in both the liver and intestine with faecal/urinary excretion of metabolites.
Sample for drug monitoring	Whole blood
Timing of drug sampling	CsA: 0 hour/trough (C0) or 2-hour/peak (C2) — C2 has better corelation with AUC as compared to C0 and is associated with reduced acute rejection rates in the 1st year. Hence, C2 monitoring is preferred over C0 in the 1st year. However, some patients may be slow absorbers, and the C2 may be low. In such cases, AUC may be needed to determine true CsA exposure. TAC: 0 hour/trough Steady state is achieved after at least 3 to 5 half-lives. Hence, drug levels should be monitored after at least 72 hours of initiation or following dose changes Drug level monitoring of CNI is essential as these drugs have a narrow therapeutic index. Monitoring of drug levels should be performed daily after a transplant while inpatient. Weekly drug level monitoring is recommended for the first 1–3 months of outpatient follow-up, followed by fortnightly until 6 months, and monthly thereafter for the first year. Subsequent drug levels should continue to be measured at routine clinic visits thereafter.
Target drug levels	Depends on antibody induction given and the other types of immunosuppression that CNI is combined with. Varies from centre to centre. CsA: Doses can be increased or decreased each time by 25–50 mg with subsequent close follow-up of serum creatinine and CsA level TAC: Doses can be increased or decreased each time by 0.5–1 mg with subsequent close follow-up of serum creatinine and TAC level.

Table 53.11:   Factors Affecting Dose Titration of Calcineurin Inhibitors

Factor	Decision on Determining Dose of Calcineurin Inhibitors (Examples)
Pharmacokinetics	CsA and TAC have significant intra and inter-individual variability. Hepatic dysfunction results in increased AUCs of CNIs, and close monitoring is required.
Time from transplantation	CNIs should be started just before transplantation or within the first 24 hours of transplantation, regardless of graft function. Doses are higher to achieve high drug concentration levels during the early period post-transplant, where the risk of rejection is high, and then subsequently reduced to achieve lower drug concentration levels to reduce long-term toxicity while maintaining efficacy in preventing rejection.
Presence of infection or rejection	Doses of CNI may be reduced during infection, e.g., BK virus or increased during rejection. When a rejection occurs at a certain level of CNI, the target drug level should be revised at a higher level.
Drug interactions	CNIs have a narrow therapeutic index, and drug-drug interactions require close monitoring to prevent subtherapeutic levels (causing rejection) or supratherapeutic levels (causing nephrotoxicity). Drugs such as diltiazem and ketoconazole increase CNI levels. Drug interactions can be used favourably to reduce CNI doses and hence, pill burden and cost for patient. Cessation of these drugs should prompt an empirical dose increase of CNI, followed by close drug level monitoring thereafter. If prescription of a strongly interacting drug is unavoidable due to a lack of alternatives, drug levels should be monitored closely, and drug doses adjusted accordingly.
Combinations with other immunosuppression	Higher doses of MPA or mTORi can help minimise doses of CNI to reduce risk of nephrotoxicity. This is especially useful in low immunological risk KT recipients with risks, e.g., expanded criteria donor or biopsy evidence of CNI nephrotoxicity.

Table 53.12: Questions to Ask When Determining Accuracy of Drug Levels

- Was CNI administered at the appropriate time in the preceding days?
- Was the CNI dose consumed accurate?
- Has there been a change in the relationship of meal timings to CNI administration?
- Were the meals in the preceding days typical of the patient's usual diet?
- Have any interacting medications or food been consumed concurrently?
- Was the blood draw for CNI drug level performed within 15 minutes before administration of the CNI dose?

Table 53.13: Common Adverse Effects of Calcineurin Inhibitors

	Cyclosporine	Tacrolimus
Hypertension	More common	Less common
Dyslipidaemia	More common	Less common
Post-transplant DM	Less common	More common
Hyperuricaemia/Gout	More common	Less common
Gastrointestinal	Less common	More common
Neurotoxicity	Less common	More common
<u>Cosmetic</u>		
Gingival hypertrophy	More common	Not observed
Alopecia	Not observed	More common
Hirsutism	More common	Not observed

- However, some adverse effects, such as malignancy and/or infections, may necessitate a reduction in overall immunosuppression, which, in turn, may compromise allograft function.

Mycophenolic acid analogues

- Mycophenolic acid analogues (MPA) are the preferred antiproliferative agents for immunosuppression. There are 2 formulations of MPA available — mycophenolate mofetil (MMF, Cell-cept©) and enteric-coated mycophenolate sodium (EC-MPS or MYF, Myfortic©). The rate and extent of absorption of these two products are not equivalent safety and efficacy profiles (Table 53.14).

Table 53.14:   Pharmacology of Mycophenolate Acid Analogues

Mechanism of action	MPA are selective reversible inhibitors of inosine-5`-monophosphate dehydrogenase, which inhibits *de novo* guanosine nucleotides preferentially in T and B lymphocytes, hence inhibiting their proliferation. This leads to the suppression of both cell-mediated immune responses and antibody formation.
Available formulations	MMF is available in oral (250, 500 mg capsules) and IV formulation, while MYF is only available in oral formulation (180, 360 mg capsules). MMF and MYF can be switched to each other formulation if there is intolerance to one formulation (500 mg MMF is equivalent to 360 mg MYF). When IV formulation is required, the dose is the same as the oral dose, e.g., PO MMF 500 mg BD or PO MYF 360 mg BD is equivalent to IV MMF 500 mg BD infused over at least 2 hours.
Absorption	MMF is absorbed in the stomach and small intestine and hydrolysed to mycophenolic acid (MPA). The bioavailability of MMF is 94%. MYF is absorbed in the small intestine with a lower bioavailability of 72%. MMF and MYF can be given with or without food as the effect on food on bioavailability is minor.
Time to tmax	MMF: 0.9–1.8 hours MYF: 1.5–2.5 hours
Elimination $t_{1/2}$	MMF: ~18 hours MYF: 8–16 hours
Time to steady state	~4 days
Plasma protein binding	MPA is highly protein bound (97% binding to albumin). When there is hypoalbuminaemia, there are higher levels of free MPA and, hence, greater clearance of MPA.

Table 53.14: (Continued)

Metabolism	MPA is metabolised to inactive mycophenolic acid glucuronide (MPAG) by uridine diphosphate-glucuronosyl transferases (UDP-glucuronosyltransferase) mainly in the gastrointestinal tract, liver and possibly kidney. The half-life of MMF and MYF is 18 and 12 hours, respectively. Enterohepatic recirculation of MPA occurs as excreted MPAG in the bile undergoes deglucuronidation by intestinal bacteria, which releases MPA that can be reabsorbed by the intestine. CsA inhibits this enterohepatic recirculation, and hence MPA levels may be lower in patients on CsA. MPA levels are higher in patients on TAC because enterohepatic recirculation is not inhibited. TAC also inhibits UDP-glucuronosyltransferase, which metabolises MPA.
Dosing	The standard dose is 1 g BD for MMF or 720 mg BD for MYF. Some centres, especially from Asia, will give lower doses at the time of transplantation or perform protocol dose reduction at a later time-point. When converting from CsA to TAC in patients who are concurrently on MPA, a dose reduction of MPA should be considered where appropriate to prevent adverse effects of MPA, such as diarrhoea and anaemia.
Elimination	MPAG is excreted in the urine and faeces. With kidney dysfunction, MPA levels may be higher as there is reduced protein binding. MPA exposure may be increased by 75% in the presence of significant renal impairment (eGFR < 25 mL/min/1.73 m^2)

Therapeutic drug monitoring and adjustment of doses of mycophenolate acid analogues

- Unlike CNIs, MPA trough readings do not corelate well to MPA AUC exposure, especially when taken in patients on MYF. Hence, it is not routine to monitor MPA trough readings.

However, if trough levels are obtained, the recommended target levels are ≥1.3 mg/L (with CsA) and ≥1.9 mg/L (with TAC).

- The gold standard to measure MPA exposure is to calculate MPA AUC using multiple blood samples, but this is not practical for outpatient settings. Therapeutic MPA AUC ranges from 30 to 60 mg h/L. However, MPA AUC increased 3 months after transplantation while on stable doses due to reduced drug clearance.

- Randomised controlled trials to examine the impact of therapeutic drug monitoring of MPA on clinical outcomes have yielded mixed results (Table 53.15), leading to consensus recommendations that therapeutic drug monitoring of MPA may be more beneficial in selected groups of patients:

  - Dual immunosuppression or CNI/steroid sparing regimens
  - High immunological risk for rejection
  - Delayed graft function
  - Altered gastrointestinal, hepatic or kidney function

Adverse effects of mycophenolate acid analogues

- MPA may be associated with several adverse effects (Table 53.16).

- EC-MPS may be associated with lower risk of gastrointestinal side effects in some patients. While conversion from MMF to EC-MPS can be performed safely, graft monitoring is recommended.

- If diarrhoea persists despite conversion, the following strategies can be considered:

  - MPA dose can be split to thrice daily administration
  - MPA dose can be further reduced
  - MPA can be replaced with Azathioprine

Table 53.15:   Summary of Landmark Randomised Studies on Therapeutic Drug Monitoring of Mycophenolic Acid

Study	N	Follow-up	Intervention	Primary End-point	Outcome
APOMYGRE study	137	12 months	Concentration controlled (using MPA AUC) vs. fixed dose of MMF.	Treatment failure (death, graft loss, acute rejection and MMF discontinuation).	Concentration controlled group had fewer treatment failure and rejections. No difference in adverse events.
FDCC study	901	12 months	Concentration controlled (using MPA AUC target 45 mg hr/L) vs. fixed dose of MMF.	Treatment failure (biopsy proven acute rejection graft loss, death of MMF discontinuation)	No difference in treatment failure but >35% of patients had AUC < 30 mg hr/L
Opticept trial	720	24 months	3 groups 1. Fixed dose of MMF with a standard dose of CNI 2. Concentration controlled (using trough level of 1.3 mg/L for CsA and 1.9 mg/L for TAC) with a standard dose of CNI 3. Concentration controlled (using trough level of 1.3 mg/L for CsA and 1.9 mg/L for TAC) with a reduced dose of CNI	Treatment failure (biopsy proven acute rejection, graft loss and death)	No difference in treatment failure

Table 53.16: Adverse Effects of Mycophenolate Acid Analogues

Gastrointestinal:
Diarrhoea, abdominal cramping (20–75%)
Mild elevation in liver enzymes

Bone marrow suppression:
Anaemia
Leukopenia
Thrombocytopenia

Increased risk of infection:
Viral infections (e.g., HSV, CMV)

Increased risk of malignancy:
Skin cancer in particular (>20%)

Rare but serious complications include:
Progressive multifocal leukoencephalopathy
Acute inflammatory syndrome

Azathioprine

- Azathioprine (AZA) was previously the main antiproliferative agent used for immunosuppression in KT but has been superseded by MPA due to the latter's superior efficacy in rejection prophylaxis (Table 53.17). However, it is an important alternative in the following scenarios:

  - Intolerance or hypersensitivity to MPA

  - To reduce the net state of immunosuppression in BK viraemia by switching from MPA to AZA

  - Pre-conception and during pregnancy

  - Low immunological risk

  - Financial constraints (however, immunological risk should be the predominant consideration)

Table 53.17:   Pharmacology of Azathioprine

Mechanism of action	AZA is a purine analogue and an imidazolyl derivative of 6-mercaptopurine (6-MP) — it inhibits purine synthesis through its conversion to 6-MP. 6-MP is converted to thioinosine monophosphate (TIMP) by hypoxanthine(guanine)phosphoribosyl transferase (HPRT). TIMP is then converted to 6-thioguanine deoxynucleoside triphosphate (dthioGTP), a thioguanine nucleotide (TGN), which incorporates into DNA (instead of DNA guanine) and interrupts DNA synthesis. This leads to decreased numbers of circulating B and T lymphocytes, reduced immunoglobulin, and IL-2 production. Another mechanism of immunosuppression includes induction of apoptosis of activated T lymphocytes by dthioGTP.
Available formulations	25 mg and 50 mg tablets are available in Singapore. Other countries may have IV formulation available.
Absorption	Readily absorbed in the gastrointestinal tract with a bioavailability of up to 90%.
Time to tmax	1–2 hours
Elimination $t_{1/2}$	~2 hours (biologic half-life of 24 hours)
Time to steady state	2–6 weeks (depending on metabolism)
Plasma protein binding	30% are bound to proteins, and notably, the drug is dialysable.
Metabolism	Thiopurine S-methyltransferase (TPMT) and nudix (nucleoside diphosphate linked moiety X)-type motif 15 (NUDT15) is responsible for the metabolism of thiopurines such as 6-MP into inactive metabolites. Genetic polymorphisms of the genes for TPMT and NUDT15 may result in the accumulation of active AZA metabolites, and hence lead to toxicity. Genotyping and/or functional assay screening for TPMT deficiency and a poor metaboliser phenotype of NUDT15 should be considered prior to AZA initiation. Another inactivation pathway is by xanthine oxidase, which converts 6-MP to 6-thiouric acid.

(Continued)

Table 53.17: (*Continued*)

Dosing	1.5 mg/kg when used with CNI and corticosteroids. Close monitoring of full blood count and liver function is recommended upon initiation and during dose escalation. Three monthly monitoring is recommended for stable patients on maintenance AZA.
Elimination	Metabolites are excreted in the urine. 6-thiouric acid (inactive metabolite) is excreted by the kidney and may contribute to the accumulation of 6-thioguanine and resultant toxicity in cases of kidney dysfunction.
Drug monitoring	Therapeutic drug monitoring is not performed for patients on AZA as its immunosuppressive effect is completely dependent on the activity of intracellular active metabolites.

Adverse effects of azathioprine

- AZA may cause macrocytosis, which is benign, but leukopenia is the most important adverse effect (Table 53.18). Temporary cessation of AZA is recommended if white cell counts fall below 3000 mm^3, and granulocyte colony stimulating factors may have to be administered. Recovery in white cell counts may take up to 2 weeks, after which low dose reintroduction can be performed, followed by dose increases as permitted by cell counts. Complete cessation of AZA is necessary when adverse effects are serious.

Table 53.18:   Adverse Effects of Azathioprine

Gastrointestinal:
Anorexia, nausea and vomiting soon after initiation (20%)
Diarrhoea (infrequent)
Mild elevation in liver enzymes

Bone marrow suppression:
Leukopenia (25%)
Thrombocytopenia (5%)

Increased risk of malignancy
Most commonly — skin cancer (>20%)

Rare but serious complications include:
Hypersensitivity syndrome characterised by rash, diarrhoea, vomiting, fever, myalgia, and deranged liver enzymes
Drug-induced pancreatitis

Mammalian target of rapamycin inhibitors

- There are 2 types of mammalian target of rapamycin inhibitors (mTORi) available — Sirolimus (SRL) is a macrolide antibiotic from a naturally occurring fungus found on Easter Island or Rapa Nui (hence its trade name Rapamune(c)), and Everolimus (ERL), which is a structural analogue to SRL (Table 53.19).

Table 53.19: Pharmacology of Mammalian Target of Rapamycin Inhibitors

Mechanism of action	Mammalian target of rapamycin (mTOR) is a serine-threonine kinase that is important for the regulation of cell proliferation, cell metabolism, and protein synthesis. It forms 2 complexes called mTORC1 and mTORC2. Both SRL and ERL bind to FK-binding protein (FKBP-12) and inhibit mTORC1. However, ERL is more potent than SRL in inhibiting mTORC2. mTORC2 is important in endothelial cell function and ERL may therefore be more beneficial in chronic antibody mediated rejection.
Available formulations	SRL — 0.5 and 1 mg (available in Singapore) ERL — 0.25 and 0.75 mg (available in Singapore) No IV formulation available
Absorption	Both SRL and ERL are rapidly absorbed in the intestinal tract, but the bioavailability differs — 14% for SRL and 30% for ERL. These differences are partly explained by the presence of an efflux system that specifically pumps SRL out from the intestinal epithelium. Drug absorption may be affected by food, so patients should be advised to take mTORi consistently with or without food to reduce unnecessary fluctuations in systemic exposure.
Time to tmax	1 to 2 hours for both SRL and ERL
Elimination $t_{1/2}$	SRL — 62 hours ERL — 28 hours The shorter $t_{1/2}$ makes ERL more practical to use and adjust — steady state and response to dose changes is faster; ERL is cleared faster than SRL if the drug is discontinued.
Time to steady state	SRL — 5 to 7 days (if a loading dose is not used) ERL — 4 days
Plasma protein binding	SRL — 92% ERL — 74%
Metabolism	SRL and ERL are metabolised by both the p-glycoprotein and CYP3A enzyme systems, but ERL is systemically cleared faster than SRL.

(Continued)

Table 53.19: **(*Continued*)**

Dosing	**<u>Loading dose with CsA</u>**
	SRL:
	6 mg (low immunological risk), 15 mg (high immunological risk)
	ERL:
	No loading dose required for ERL
	SRL needs to be given 4 hours post-CsA, but ERL can be given together with CsA
	<u>Initial maintenance dose with CsA</u>
	SRL — 2–5 mg/day
	ERL — 0.75 mg BD
	<u>Loading dose with TAC</u>
	No recommendations for SRL
	No loading dose required for ERL
	<u>Initial maintenance dose with TAC</u>
	No recommendations for SRL
	ERL — 1.5 mg BD
Elimination	SRL — 91% eliminated in faeces
	ERL — 80% eliminated in faeces
Sample for drug monitoring	Whole blood
Timing of drug sampling	Trough sampling is recommended:
	SRL — 5–7 days from initiation or dose adjustment
	ERL — 4 days from initiation or dose adjustment
Target drug levels with CNIs	SRL — 5–15 ng/mL
	ERL — 3–8 ng/mL

Both are categorised as proliferative signal inhibitors, but ERL was developed to improve the pharmacokinetic properties of SRL.

- There are many ways to use mTORi as maintenance immunosuppression, and many randomised controlled trials have concluded that mTORi are best used in combination with low dose CNI (Table 53.20):

Table 53.20: Some Landmark Trials on the Use of Mammalian Target of Rapamycin Inhibitors

Study	Intervention	FUP	Main Findings
***De novo* studies without CNI**			
SPEISSER (2007)	$n = 145$ randomised to #1 SRL (C0 10–15 ng/mL) + CS + MMF #2 CsA + CS + MMF All with ATG	12 m	Primary endpoint of GFR at 12 m — no difference on intent to treat analysis, but GFR was higher in those who remained on SRL. Adverse events and discontinuation rate with SRL higher than with CsA.
SYMPHONY (2007)	$n = 1645$ randomised to #1 sCsA + CS + MMF #2 rCsA + CS + MMF #3 rTAC + CS + MMF #4 rSRL (C0 4–8 ng/mL) + CS + MMF All with IL-2RA	12 m	Primary endpoint of GFR at 12 m — Highest in the low dose TAC group and lowest in the low dose SRL group. Higher rate of rejection and serious adverse events in the SRL group.
ORION (2011)	$n = 450$ randomised to #1 SRL (C0 8–20 ng/mL) + CS + TAC stop at 13 w #2 SRL (C0 5–15 ng/mL) + CS+ MMF #3 TAC + CS + MMF All with IL-2RA	12 m	Primary endpoint of GFR at 12 m was similar between groups. The SRL+CS+MMF group was sponsor-terminated due to a higher than expected rejection rate (which revised the target C0 of SRL to 8–15 ng/mL in the SRL+CS+MMF group). Rejection rate between group #1 and #3 was similar. Discontinuation rate with SRL was higher than with TAC.
***De novo* studies with CNI**			
Rapamune Maintenance Regimen (RMR) study (2001)	$n = 525$ on SRL (C0 $\geq$ 10 ng/mL) + CsA + CS then randomised at 3 m to continue SRL or stop CsA	12 m	Similar primary endpoint of graft survival between groups. The rejection rates were higher in the CsA withdrawal group.

Table 53.20:   *(Continued)*

Study	Intervention	FUP	Main Findings
A2309 (2010)	$n = 833$ randomised to #1 ERL (C0 3–8 ng/mL) + rCsA #2 ERL (C0 6–8 ng/mL) + rCsA #3 sCsA + MMF All with IL-2RA ± CS	12 m	No differences in composite efficacy failure (treated biopsy proven rejection, graft loss, death or loss to follow-up), kidney function, rejection and SAEs between groups.
TRANSFORM (2018)	$n = 2037$ randomised to #1 ERL (C0 3–8 ng/mL) + rCNI #2 MMF + sCNI All with IL-2RA + CS	12 m	Similar primary end-point (treated BPAR or eGFR < 50 mL/min/1.73 m^2 at M12). Study drug discontinuation was higher among ERL.
ATHENA (2019)	$n = 655$ randomised to #1 ERL (C0 3–8 ng/mL) + TAC #2 ERL (C0 3–8 ng/mL) + CsA #3 TAC + MMF	12 m	Primary end-point of GFR was lower (due to differences in CNI levels). Study drug discontinuation was highest among ERL.
Early conversion to mTORi (<3 months)			
CONCEPT (2009)	$n = 192$ randomised at 3 m to switch from CsA to SRL (C0 8–15 ng/mL). CS+MMF also given but CS discontinued at 8 m All received IL-2RA.	12 m	Primary end-point of CrCL at week 52 — Better in the SRL group but higher rejection rate among those on SRL, mainly occurring after withdrawal of CS. Serious adverse events also more frequent in the SRL group.
SMART (2010)	$n = 141$ randomised at 10–24 d to switching #1 CsA to SRL (C0 5–10 ng/mL) or #2 continuing CsA	12 m	Primary endpoint of GFR was better in the SRL group but significantly higher percentage of patients discontinuing SRL. Rejection rates were similar.

(Continued)

Table 53.20:   (*Continued*)

Study	Intervention	FUP	Main Findings
Spare the Nephron study (2011)	$n = 299$ at 30–180 d randomised to #1 switching CNI to SRL (C0 5–10 ng/mL) or #2 continuing CNI All received CS + MMF and IL-2RA or ALA	12 m	Primary endpoint of GFR at 2 years was better in the SRL/MMF group than the CNI/MMF group. Rejection rates were similar, but numerically more patients discontinuing SRL (but not statistically significant).
CENTRAL (2012)	$n = 202$ randomised at 7 w to #1 remain on sCsA #2 switch from CsA to ERL (C0 6–10 ng/mL) All on CS and MYF	12 m	Primary endpoint of GFR significantly better with ERL conversion, but rejection rate was higher. SAEs and discontinuation of ERL was more frequent.
ELEVATE (2017)	$n = 715$ randomised at 10–14 w #1 sCNI + MPA #2 switch from CsA to ERL (C0 6–10 ng/mL) at 10–14 w + MPA	24 m	Primary endpoint of change in GFR was similar. DSA and rejection rate was more frequent in the ERL group. SAE rate was similar, but discontinuation of ERL was more frequent.
Late conversion to mTORi (>3 months)			
CONVERT (2009)	$n = 830$ randomised at 6 to 120 m to switch from CNI to SRL (C0 8–20 ng/mL) and analysed according to GFR 20–40 vs. > 40 mL/min	24 m	Enrolment of GFR 20–40 mL/min subjects halted, as the primary safety endpoint of AR, graft loss or death reached by 16.7% of SRL patients vs. 0% of CNI patients. Among GFR > 40 mL/min, no difference in GFR at 12 and 24 m on intent to treat analysis but GFR was better on those who remained on SRL and rejection rates were similar although SRL discontinuation rates were higher. Post hoc analyses revealed that with baseline GFR > 40 mL/min and UPCR ≤ 0.11 benefit from conversion.

Table 53.20: (*Continued*)

Study	Intervention	FUP	Main Findings
ASCERTAIN (2011)	$n = 394$ randomised at >6 m (mean 5.6 years) #1 remain on sCNI ± CS ± AZA/MPA #2 switch from CNI to ERL (C0 8–12 ng/mL) — CNI withdrew when ERL C0 ≥ 8 ng/mL #3 switch from AZA/MPA to ERL (C0 3–8 ng/mL) + rCNI (dose reduced by 70–90%) when ERL C0 ≥ 3 ng/mL	24 m	Primary endpoint of GFR and rejection rate was similar between groups except among those with CrCL > 50 mL/min, where GFR was better. SAE and study discontinuation rate was higher in the ERL groups.
ZEUS (2011)	$n = 503$ randomised at 4.5 m to #1 remain on sCsA #2 switch from CsA to ERL (C0 6–10 ng/mL) All on CS, MYF and IL-2RA	12 m	Primary endpoint of GFR significantly better with ERL conversion, but rejection rate was higher. SAEs rate were similar.

Abbreviations: ALA, antilymphocyte antibodies; AR, acute rejection; ATG, antithymocyte globulin; AZA, azathioprine; BPAR, biopsy-proven acute rejection; C0, trough concentration level; CNI, calcineurin inhibitors; CrCL, creatinine clearance; CS, corticosteroids; CsA, cyclosporine; d, days; DSA, donor specific antibodies; eGFR, estimated glomerular filtration rate; ERL, everolimus; FUP, follow-up period; GFR, glomerular filtration rate; IL-2 RA, interleukin-2 receptor antagonist; m, months; M12, month 12; M24, month 24; MMF, Cellcept©; MPA, mycophenolate acid; MYF, Myfortic©; rCNI, reduced dose calcineurin inhibitors; rCsA, reduced dose cyclosporine; rSRL, reduced dose sirolimus; rTAC, reduced dose tacrolimus; sCNI, standard dose calcineurin inhibitors; sCSA, standard dose cyclosporine; SAEs, serious adverse events; SRL, sirolimus; TAC, tacrolimus; w, weeks; UPCR, urine protein:creatinine ratio

- *De-novo* immunosuppression in low immunological risk patients

- Facilitate CNI withdrawal or minimisation in patients with biopsy-proven CNI nephrotoxicity, and if concomitant rejection is excluded

- To permit CNI withdrawal in the presence of serious adverse effects (e.g., thrombotic microangiopathy, neurotoxicity, refractory BK or CMV infections)

- In tuberous sclerosis patients with angiomyolipoma as mTORi inhibit proliferation of smooth muscle cells

- In patients with malignancies such as Kaposi Sarcoma or a single episode of squamous cell carcinoma of the skin

Adverse effects with mammalian target of rapamycin inhibitors

- Adverse effects are common and may lead to discontinuation of mTORi. However, there are possible mitigation measures to ensure the continuation of mTORi for as long as possible (Table 53.21).

Surgery in patients treated with mammalian target of rapamycin inhibitors

- Due to the potential for impaired wound healing, it is important for patients to inform their physicians of any plans for surgery in case there is a need to stop mTORi (Table 53.22).

Table 53.21:   Adverse Effects of Mammalian Target of Rapamycin Inhibitors

Adverse Effect	Countermeasures
Impaired wound healing	*De novo* use of mTORi is not contraindicated in kidney transplant surgery though certain patients at risk of impaired wound healing may need to avoid it during the early postoperative period, e.g., obesity, elderly, concomitant steroids. mTORi impair wound healing in a dose-dependent manner by inhibiting angiogenesis and fibrosis. If mTORi is used, avoid loading doses (with SRL) and high-target trough levels (e.g., >10 ng/mL) Close surgical co-management is required with monitoring of wound healing and drainage. If impaired wound healing occurs, mTORi should be temporarily replaced with alternative immunosuppression until the wound is healed.
Lymphocele or productive surgical drainage	mTORi is associated with an increased risk of lymphoceles due to the impairment of lymphangiogenesis and postsurgical adhesion. During surgery, lymphatic vessels should be ligated, and extensive dissection should be avoided. Drains should be kept till drainage is <50 mL/day for 2 consecutive days. Loading doses and high-target trough levels should be avoided. If lymphocele develops, mTORi should be temporarily replaced with alternative immunosuppression until the lymphocele is resolved.
Thrombotic microangiopathy	In the presence of rejection, mTORi should be discontinued and replaced with alternative immunosuppression. Otherwise, dose can be adjusted to achieve lower trough levels. If mTORi is used in combination with CNI, the dose of CNI can be adjusted to achieve lower trough levels. Another alternative is to replace mTORi with alternative immunosuppression.
Pneumonitis	Pneumonitis due to mTORi is a diagnosis of exclusion but if this is diagnosed, usually indicate the need to replace mTORi with alternative immunosuppression.

(Continued)

Table 53.21:   (*Continued*)

Adverse Effect	Countermeasures
Proteinuria	This is a common complication and can be treated with a reduction of dose if the trough level is too high or adding angiotensin-converting enzyme inhibitor or angiotensin receptor blocker or other anti-proteinuria therapies. Biopsy should be considered to exclude other causes of proteinuria.
Haematological adverse effects, e.g., anaemia, leukopenia, thrombocytopenia	Reduce dose if trough levels permit; adjust other myelosuppressive drugs; use erythropoiesis-stimulating agents and granulocyte colony stimulating factor.
Post-transplant diabetes	Consider switching to alternative immunosuppression, or if on TAC, switch to CsA if this is appropriate.
Hyperlipidaemia	This is not a contraindication to continuing mTORi, but appropriate lipid lower therapy should commence, e.g., diet, weight loss, omega-3 fish oil, statins, etc.
Peripheral oedema	Compression stockings and diuretics may be helpful. If patients are on calcium channel blockers (that can cause oedema), consider switching to alternative anti-hypertensive drugs.
Gastrointestinal adverse effects, e.g., aphthous ulcers, diarrhoea	Adjust doses of mTORi and other drugs that can cause diarrhoea; triamcinolone for aphthous ulcers.
Dermatological adverse effects, e.g., acne	Reduce dose if trough levels permit. Topical dermatological treatments.

Table 53.22: **Guidelines on the Perioperative Management of Patients on Mammalian Target of Rapamycin Inhibitors**

Type of Surgery	Guidelines
Minor elective surgery or laparoscopic surgery	No need to discontinue mTORi unless there are other risk factors for impaired wound healing, e.g., concomitant corticosteroids, obesity, elderly.
Major elective surgery	Need to discontinue mTORi at least 1–2 weeks prior to the date of the surgery and replace with alternative immunosuppression. mTORi can be resumed once wound healing is completed (usually 1–3 months post-surgery), which is best advised by the surgeon.
Emergency surgery	mTORi should be discontinued immediately, and the surgeon should be informed of the risk of impaired wound healing (as there would not be time for wash-out).

Use of mammalian target of rapamycin inhibitors in malignancy

- Meta-analysis and large registry studies have demonstrated risk reduction of non-melanoma skin cancers in patients who are on immunosuppression combinations containing mTORi. There is no definitive influence on the risks of other cancer types.

- Antineoplastic properties of mTORi in the treatment of malignancy are typically at much higher doses than is prescribed for transplant immunosuppression and are often poorly tolerated.

- Routine conversion of CNI to mTORi after diagnosis or curative treatment of malignancy is not recommended due to increased discontinuation rates from adverse effects of mTORi and a potential increase in mortality risk.

Drug interactions with immunosuppression

Table 53.23:   Common Interacting Drugs with Calcineurin Inhibitors and Mammalian Target of Rapamycin Inhibitors

	Effect on CNI/mTORi Levels	Interacting Drugs
Cytochrome p450 3A4 inhibitors	Increased	Macrolide antibiotics (e.g., erythromycin, clarithyromycin) Azoles (e.g., itraconazole, ketoconazole) Amiodarone Diltiazem, verapamil Ritonavir-containing formulations HIV protease inhibitors Imatinib Grapefruit juice
Cytochrome p450 3A4 inducers	Decreased	Anti-seizure medications (e.g., carbamazepine, phenytoin) Rifampicin Dexamethasone St. John's wort
Inhibitors of P-glycoprotein	Increased	Macrolide antibiotics (e.g., erythromycin, clarithromycin) Azoles (e.g., itraconazole, ketoconazole) Amiodarone Diltiazem, verapamil Ritonavir-containing formulations Green tea (for tacrolimus)
Inducers of P-glycoprotein	Decreased	Anti-seizure medications (e.g., carbamazepine, phenytoin) Rifampicin St. John's wort
Competitive inhibition	Increased	Statins Colchicine mTORi with CNI

Table 53.24:   Drug Interactions with MPA Formulations

	Effect on MPA Levels	**Interacting Drugs**
Drugs that can decrease absorption but can still be administered at least 2 hours apart from MPA	Decreased	Antacids Magnesium supplements Phosphate binders (e.g., sevelamer) Proton pump inhibitors (not observed with EC-MPS)
Drugs that can decrease absorption and should be avoided	Decreased	Bile acid sequestrants (e.g., cholestyramine)

*Serum concentration of hormonal contraceptives may be decreased by MPA; hence additional or alternative contraception should be used to prevent pregnancy while on MPA formulations.

Drug interactions with azathioprine

- Most significant drug interaction relates to the use of allopurinol and febuxostat. Both are inhibitors of xanthine oxidase, which is required for the clearance of 6-MP. Hence concurrent administration with AZA results in its adverse effects (Table 53.18) and should be avoided.

- Drug interactions with other drugs should be checked prior to prescription in patients who are on AZA.

References

Cuadrado-Payán E, Diekmann F and Cucchiari D (2022). Medical Aspects of mTOR inhibition in kidney transplantation. *Int J Mol Sci* **23**(14): 7707.

Hardinger KL, Schnitzler MA, Miller B, *et al.* (2004). Five-year follow up of thymoglobulin versus ATGAM induction in adult renal transplantation. *Transplantation* **78**(1): 136–141.

Hwang SD, Lee JH, Lee SW, *et al.* (2018). Efficacy and safety of induction therapy in kidney transplantation: A network meta-analysis. *Transplant Proc* **50**(4): 987–992.

Le Meur Y, Borrows R, Pescovitz MD, *et al.* (2011). Therapeutic drug monitoring of mycophenolates in kidney transplantation: Report of the Transplantation Society consensus meeting. *Transplant Rev (Orlando)* **25**(2): 58–64.

Macklin PS, Morris PJ and Knight SR (2015). A systematic review of the use of rituximab as induction therapy in renal transplantation. *Transplant Rev (Orlando)* **29**(2): 103–108.

Steiner RW and Awdishu L (2011). Steroids in kidney transplant patients. *Semin Immunopathol* **33**(2): 157–167.

54 Early Post-operative Management of a Kidney Transplant Recipient

Terence Kee

Introduction

- After kidney transplantation (KT), the management of the KT recipient is divided into 2 periods, of which the goals are somewhat different:

  - Early post-operative period (arbitrary defined locally as 6 months), where prevention of rejection, achieving the best graft function, ensuring tolerance to immunosuppression and prevention of opportunistic infections are important goals.

  - Late post-operative period (>6 months) where maintaining graft function, ensuring adherence to immunosuppression, and prevention of toxicity of long-term immunosuppression, such as malignancy, cardiovascular complications and infections, are the main objectives.

Immediate post-operative care

- After completion of surgery and extubation, the patient is transferred to a recovery room for observation and to ensure

■ 623

recovery from general anaesthesia. A member of the KT team should review the patient there and check on the following:

- Operating theatre and anaesthesia records to check on medications given, haemodynamics, occurrence of any adverse intraoperative events (e.g., bleeding, technical complications) and any unusual surgical technique employed (as it may affect interpretation of KT images or post-operative management)

- Details of the donor kidney — nephrectomy information, any injury during organ recovery, benchwork required, etc.

- Stable airway, breathing and circulation — blood pressure, heart rate, respiratory rate, pulse oximetry, central venous pressure (CVP) reading, stridor, cardiopulmonary examination, patency of any arteriovenous dialysis access

- Cardiac telemetry for arrhythmias, tall T waves (of hyperkalaemia), myocardial ischaemia or any other ECG abnormalities

- Level of pain — severe post-operative pain is unusual after KT and warrants further attention

- IV lines for patency, bleeding or extravasation

- Urinary catheter for urine output and blockage — urine output in a previously anuric patient suggests a functioning KT, but if a patient has pre-operative residual urine output, then the urine output may be coming from either the native kidney, KT or both

- Drain and dressing for any active bleeding.

- If there is no or minimal urine output (<50 mL/hr) and the patient is clinically not in pulmonary oedema, IV fluid challenge can be ordered, e.g., normal saline 500 mL over 1 hour.

If there is still no diuresis, further fluid challenge may be given according to the fluid status, or IV furosemide 80–120 mg may be given to initiate a diuresis if there are no contraindications.

- Once the KT recipient is cleared to be transferred to the high dependency ward by the anaesthetist, the KT recipient would undergo a post-operative radionuclide perfusion scan or ultrasound doppler. This is to assess perfusion of the KT and ensure that there are no other structural abnormalities detected, e.g., haematoma. It is important that a physician accompany the patient for the imaging.

- Following imaging, the KT recipient is transferred to a high dependency isolation bed for monitoring during the next 24 to 48 hours. Upon arrival at the high dependency ward, the physician should check the following:

  - Airway, breathing and circulation — supplemental oxygen may be given

  - CVP measurement

  - Telemetry

  - Pain score

  - Status of IV lines — patency, bleeding and extravasation

  - Urinary catheter — urine output, leakage, blockage

  - Dressing and drain — bleeding

  - Arteriovenous dialysis access — thrill, bruit — a warning label should be placed on the arm where the arteriovenous dialysis access is located to avoid accidental venepuncture

  - Physical exam, including assessment for fluid overload, lung collapse, pneumothorax, ileus, possible perinephric haematoma, lower limbs for circulation, and deep venous thrombosis

- Post-operative chest X-ray — check position of CVP catheter, pneumothorax, collapse, pulmonary oedema, etc.

- Urgent blood tests — cardiac enzymes, renal panel, liver panel, CaPO4, Mg, FBC, urine, and blood culture (if KT is from a deceased donor or there is post-operative fever)

- ECG

- Immunosuppression regimen should be confirmed, ordered and informed to the nurse in charge.

- Following clinical and radiological assessment of fluid status, the IV fluid regimen should be ordered (see "Post-operative fluid management").

- Depending on the fluid balance and post-operative renal panel, post-operative dialysis may be required. Post-operative hyperkalaemia is common due to tissue trauma and resorption of intra-abdominal blood. It is often severe enough to require dialysis.

- In high immunological risk KT, post-operative plasma exchange may be ordered.

- Renal panel, Ca, PO4, Mg and FBC is repeated at 4–8 hourly interval to assess KT function, biochemical status, and the need for electrolyte replacement. If a patient requires post-operative dialysis, a renal panel is repeated 4 hours post-dialysis. As the patient's graft function and urine output stabilise, the frequency of laboratory testing can be reduced.

- Vital signs are monitored hourly for at least 24 hours after surgery, but the frequency can be stretched gradually to 2, 4 and finally 6 hours over the next few days, at the discretion of the KT physician.

- CVP reading may be performed daily if there is a CVP line *in-situ* but can be discontinued once the patient is stabilised.

CVP should be removed as soon as it is not required to avoid catheter related blood stream infections.

- The KT recipient would have a urinary catheter inserted for the next few days, which makes hourly monitoring of urine output easy. However, once the catheter is taken out, the patient should be advised to strictly chart his urine output for the nurses to record.

- Daily weight should be measured, with the general aim of returning the patient to the dialysis-prescribed dry weight if available.

- If there is a surgical drain, the type and volume of output should be monitored for bleeding, urinary leak, and lymphocele. Inspection of the wound and dressing should be performed on a daily basis. The surgeon will decide when to remove the surgical drain.

- Strict input and output charting is necessary to avoid fluid overload or dehydration. It is important to adjust IV and PO fluid intake accordingly. Patients should be tapered off IV fluids as soon as possible, especially once the kidney function stabilises and the patient is able to take orally.

- Diuretics and even ultrafiltration through dialysis may be required to achieve neutral fluid balance.

- Surgeon will decide when to remove the urinary catheter, but it is important not to leave a urinary catheter longer than surgically necessary to avoid catheter-related urinary tract infection.

- Some KT recipients, especially those who were anuric for many years, may suffer from bladder spasms once diuresis is established. Anti-spasmodic drugs may be prescribed after a discussion with the surgeon in charge.

- During post-operative recovery, the KT recipient should do the following:

  - Wean off IV fluids while avoiding fluid overload or dehydration (see below) — aim for a weight close to the pre-transplant dry weight

  - Undergo physical rehabilitation to ambulate and function independently upon discharge

  - Closely monitor laboratory and radiological parameters (Table 54.1)

  - Be monitored for surgical and medical complications (Table 54.2)

  - Achieve optimal immunosuppressive drug doses and levels to prevent rejection

Table 54.1:   Routine Post-operative Daily Monitoring of the Post-Kidney Transplant Recipient at the Singapore General Hospital

Laboratory Parameters

- Renal panel
- Blood glucose
- Liver panel
- CaPO4
- Mg
- Immunosuppressive drug level — cyclosporine, tacrolimus, sirolimus, everolimus
- FBC
- Urine FEME and C/S on alternate days

Radiological Parameters

- Post-operative chest X-ray as and when required
- US doppler at least once a week — more frequent if oliguric or anuric

Abbreviations: CaPO4, calcium phosphate; C/S, culture and sensitivity; FBC, full blood count; FEME, full examination and microscopy; Mg, magnesium; US, ultrasound

Table 54.2:   Common or Important Non-Infective Complications after Kidney Transplant Surgery

Complication	Diagnosis	Management
Delayed graft function (DGF)	Oligoanuria, KT dysfunction that require dialysis.	Exclude blocked urinary catheter, surgical complications, rejection and treat accordingly. A common cause of DGF is ATN due to prolonged cold ischaemia time and intraoperative hypotension.
Renal artery thrombosis	May occur during surgery or present post-operatively with oligoanuria and KT dysfunction. US doppler shows an absence of flow in renal artery and no perfusion in the KT.	Urgently consult surgeon for return to operating theatre and attempt surgical thrombectomy or, more often, nephrectomy if the graft is infarcted.
Renal artery stenosis	Oligoanuria, KT dysfunction, fluid overload, HTN, US doppler shows RAS (PSV >200 cm/s). CTA or MRA are alternatives to diagnose RAS.	Consult surgeon for advice on whether angioplasty or surgical revascularisation should be performed. However, suspected RAS on US doppler may be due to kinking or post-operative oedema, which may be left alone.
Renal vein thrombosis	Oligoanuria, macroscopic haematuria, pain and swelling over the graft, US doppler will show an absence of flow in renal vein and a reversal of diastolic flow in the renal artery. KT may look swollen or rupture on US doppler due to venous congestion.	Urgently consult surgeon for return to operating theatre and attempt surgical thrombectomy or nephrectomy if the graft is infarcted.

(Continued)

Table 54.2:   (*Continued*)

Complication	Diagnosis	Management
Haematoma	May be asymptomatic or severe with hypotension, tachycardia, abdominal/back pain, swelling over the graft, wound leaking blood, drain filling with blood, falling haemoglobin and US doppler or CT showing haematoma.	Small haematoma may not require intervention, but larger ones may require blood transfusion and surgical consultation for possible surgery to identify source of bleeding. Patients treated with antiplatelet agents are at a higher risk of bleeding.
Urinary leak	Oligoanuria, KT dysfunction, abdominal pain worse with voiding, urine seen in drain or leaking from wound, swelling over the graft, US doppler or CT or Tc-99m MAG3 scan showing urinoma, drain fluid Cr >sCr.	Keep or insert urinary catheter, consult surgeon for possible surgery to identify and repair urinary leak. Percutaneous nephrostomy and DJ stenting is an alternative. Urine leak can be from the renal pelvis, ureter or bladder.
Urinary tract obstruction	Oligoanuria, KT dysfunction, US doppler may show hydronephrosis and/or ureteral dilatation (suggesting distal obstruction). An empty bladder may suggest upper urinary tract obstruction, while a full bladder may suggest lower urinary tract obstruction due to bladder dysfunction.	Exclude blocked urinary catheter — blood clots in the urinary catheter can be flushed out with gentle irrigation. Otherwise consult surgeon to consider percutaneous nephrostomy with antegrade pyelogram and other interventions. Bladder dysfunction is common among diabetics and may be treated with alpha-blockers, e.g., tamsulosin.
Lymphocele	Lymphoceles are collections of lymphatic fluid leaking from transected lymphatic vessels in the recipient or from the KT. They are	Usually small, resolves on its own, and does not require any intervention. Large lymphoceles require a consult with the surgeon to

	usually asymptomatic and detected on US doppler as perinephric fluid collections.	determine need for percutaneous drainage or surgery, e.g., peritoneal window.
Rejection	Oliguria/anuria, KT dysfunction, elevated RI >0.8 on US doppler, biopsy of the KT is required for diagnosis.	Treat according to the type of rejection.
CNI toxicity	KT dysfunction, elevated concentration of CNI drug level, haemolytic anaemia and low platelet may occur with CNI induced thrombotic microangiopathy.	Reduce dose of CNI. If TMA occurs, dose of CNI may need to be reduced or replaced with alternative immunosuppression.
Electrolyte abnormalities	Hypokalaemia, hypomagesaemia and hypophosphataemia is common in KT with polyuria.	Replace electrolytes to keep K >4 mmol/L, Mg and PO4 >0.5 mmol/L. Oral supplementation may be required for prolonged periods even after discharge.
Hyperglycaemia	Detected by routine monitoring of blood glucose.	Post-operative stress, corticosteroid and CNI may trigger hyperglycaemia, which may require an oral hypoglycaemic agent or insulin to stabilise.
Liver dysfunction	Usually asymptomatic and detected by routine monitoring of a liver function test.	In the early post-operative setting, drugs are the most common causes of liver dysfunction, e.g., tacrolimus, antimicrobials, etc. Liver dysfunction due to tacrolimus may require a reduction of dose or switch to cyclosporine.

(*Continued*)

Table 54.2:   (*Continued*)

Complication	Diagnosis	Management
Anaemia	Usually asymptomatic and detected by routine monitoring of haemoglobin. Patients may look pale and have tachycardia.	Haemorrhage should be excluded first. Sometimes, bleeding is not from the KT but from a gastrointestinal source, e.g., stress gastric ulcer. Fluid overload may cause a dilutional anaemia, which improves with achieving negative fluid balance. Continuation of ESA is often required until the KT recovers sufficient function to produce erythropoietin on its own.

Abbreviations: ATN, acute tubular necrosis; CNI, calcineurin inhibitor; Cr, creatinine; CTA, computed tomography angiography; ESA, erythropoiesis stimulating agent; HTN, hypertension; K, potassium; KT, kidney transplant; Mg, magnesium; MRA, magnetic reasonance angiography; PO4, phosphate; PSV, peak systolic velocity; RAS, renal artery stenosis; RI, resistive indices; sCr, serum creatinine; TC-99 MAG3, technetium-99m mercaptoacetylglycylglycylglycine; TMA, thrombotic microangiopathy; US, ultrasound

- Undergo KT biopsy if the graft function does not recover or plateau at a higher-than-expected serum creatinine level or if it starts rising

- Be counselled and educated by allied health professionals on self-care and coping after a KT — osteoporosis nurse educator, transplant coordinator, dietician, physiotherapist, social worker

Post-operative fluid management

- Post-operative IV fluids are required to

  - Replace fluid losses, e.g., urine output, insensible fluid loss, fluid losses from drain and elsewhere

  - Maintain circulating volume — renal autoregulation is impaired in a transplanted denervated kidney and requires adequate intravascular volume to maintain renal perfusion

- The initial fluid of choice is dependent on the patient fluid status, hourly urine output, and biochemistry.

- Generally, the initial rate of fluid replacement is an hourly replacement of the previous hour of urine output with an additional 15–30 mL top-up. If the patient is hypovolaemic the top up can increase.

- Fluid boluses may be required to quickly improve haemodynamic parameters and urine output.

- Avoid over-replacement — reduce IV fluids accordingly, especially if the patient is more than 1 L positive fluid balance. Diuretics, e.g., frusemide 80–120 mg bolus or 10–30 mg/hr infusion may be started, and ultrafiltration may be required to quickly restore euvolaemia

- Sometimes, the patient may be oliguria or anuric and in a euvolaemic or hypervolaemic state. In such situations, post-operative IV fluids may be fixed at 500 mL/day and subsequently adjusted as urine output improves over the following days.

- IV fluids should be replaced and tapered off over the next few days. Fluid overload and hyperchloraemic metabolic acidosis may develop with inappropriate large volumes of saline administration. Patients who are fluid overloaded but asymptomatic should aim for negative fluid balance by at least 1 L/d till dry weight is restored.

- It is important to watch the electrolytes, especially when the patient is anuric or polyuric. Electrolyte abnormalities should be corrected. Maintenance potassium and other electrolyte supplementation may be required when urine output is >250 mL/hr.

- With improving renal function and high-volume urine output, IV fluids should be judiciously tapered, e.g., reduced by 1 L/d rather than maintained or increased, which will drive the diuresis rather than stabilise it. Patient should be encouraged to increase oral intake with close monitoring of fluid balance and electrolyte levels.

Post-operative Hypotension

- Appropriate blood pressure is a prerequisite for adequate graft perfusion as it ensures adequate oxygenation to an ischaemic allograft. Effective blood pressure must be maintained intra and post-operatively, ideally within 10–20 mmHg above the baseline blood pressure upon reperfusion and in the first 3 days post-operatively to ensure an effective graft perfusion.

- Hypotension must be quickly identified and corrected as it increases the risk of renal artery/vein thrombosis, acute tubular necrosis, and graft dysfunction.

- Common and/or important causes of hypotension that must be excluded include:

  - Haemorrhage, e.g., post-operative, gastrointestinal tract
  - Hypovolaemia
  - Opioid analgesia
  - Residual effects of anaesthesia
  - Anti-hypertensive medications
  - Ischaemia heart disease
  - Arrhythmia
  - Pulmonary embolism
  - Sepsis
  - Cytokine release syndrome from Thymoglobulin or Rituximab

- Always do a careful clinical examination and check ECG, cardiac enzymes, and FBC.

- Treat the identified cause(s) — IV fluid boluses and even IV dopamine may be required to increase blood pressure. However, be careful of over-zealous fluid administration and do note that high doses of IV dopamine and other inotropic agents can cause renal vasoconstriction.

Post-operative Hypertension

- Post-operative hypertension (HTN) may be due to pre-existing HTN or be related to include:

  - Excessive IV fluids (salt loading)
  - Corticosteroid related fluid retention
  - Pain
  - Transplant renal artery stenosis

- Previous reduction or discontinuation of anti-hypertensive drugs
- Calcineurin inhibitor therapy

- Immediately after the transplant surgery, a mild positive fluid balance and HTN (SBP <160 mmHg) is acceptable to ensure adequate perfusion of the KT

- Severe post-operative HTN may increase the risk for anastomotic leak.

- If post-operative HTN persists and >160/100 mmHg,
  - Correct fluid overload by fluid restriction, diuretics and ultrafiltration
  - Consider starting long-acting calcium channel blocker (CCB)
  - In severe and persistent hypertension, IV Glyceryl Trinitrate (GTN)/Labetalol may be started
  - Monitor carefully to avoid over-zealous reduction in blood pressure

Post-discharge care

- Upon discharge, the frequency of outpatient follow-up (Table 54.3) of uncomplicated KT recipients is as follows:
  - 1st month   – 1–2 times per week
  - 2nd month   – Once every 2 weeks
  - 3rd month   – Once every 3 weeks
  - 4th month to 12 months – Once every 4 weeks
  - After 12 months   – 2 to 6 months (interval between visits is stretched according to the stability of the patient's condition

Table 54.3: Areas of Ambulatory Care During the First 6 Months of Follow-Up after Surgery

Area of Care	Points of Consideration to Take Note
KT function	KT function may continue to improve and subsequently plateau to a baseline. Sometimes, KT function worsens after discharge due to dehydration or an elevated blood level of CNI. Otherwise, further investigation for urological causes, urinary tract infection, BK nephropathy and rejection may be required.
Immunosuppression	In steroid-based regimens, prednisolone is tapered over weeks till a nadir of 5 mg/d is reached. Doses of CNI are also adjusted down according to time-specific target drug levels, which are centre-specific. Some centres would also routinely reduce the dose of mycophenolate at specific time points.
Infection	Routine surveillance of urine culture is usually not required once the DJ stent is removed but monitoring for CMV, BK and sometimes EBV infection (for EBV D+/R- recipients) is required. Patients may be given prophylaxis against CMV according to centre protocol.
Metabolic	Post-transplant hyperglycaemia may persist and need to be managed as per diabetes mellitus. However, as corticosteroids improve, there may be a need for the adjustment of diabetes treatment to avoid hypoglycaemia.
Haematological	Post-operative anaemia usually improves over time and ESA may eventually be discontinued. Leukopenia and neutropenia are more common and be due to drugs like valganciclovir, which may need to be discontinued, or viral infections such as CMV which need to be excluded.

Abbreviations: CNI, calcineurin inhibitor; CMV, cytomegalovirus; EBV, Epstein–Barr virus; D+/R, seropositive donor seronegative recipient; DJ, double J; ESA, erythropoiesis-stimulating agent; KT, kidney transplant

- Upon discharge, patients would need to transit to a new lifestyle, e.g., taking medications strictly at specific timing, ensuring adequate fluids, modifying dietary intake, undergoing frequent blood taking, and visits to the clinic. This may be overwhelming, and they would need to be psychosocially supported and monitored during this transition period.

Reference

British Transplantation Society (2017). Post-operative care in the kidney transplant recipient. https://bts.org.uk/wp-content/uploads/2017/06/FINAL_PostOperative_Care_Guideline.pdf

55 Acute Kidney Injury in Kidney Transplantation

Terence Kee

Introduction

- After a successful kidney transplant (KT), most recipients achieve a baseline glomerular filtration rate (GFR) between 40 and 70 mL/min. This baseline GFR is achieved within the first 3 to 6 months after transplantation.

- Determinants of baseline GFR include both donor and recipient factors (Table 55.1).

- Acute kidney injury (AKI) in KT is a common problem, and appropriate management is critical for ensuring long-term graft survival and function. Thence, it is a medical emergency and needs to be attended to urgently.

Table 55.1: Determinants of Baseline Kidney Transplant Function

Donor	Recipient
• Age	• Pre-transplant sensitisation
• Gender	• Gender
• Comorbidities — DM, HTN	• Body habitus, e.g., obesity
• Pre-procurement kidney function	• Nephrotoxicity of immunosuppression
• Kidney size	• Early immunologic insults, e.g., rejection
• Baseline histology	• Early non-immunologic insults, e.g., infection

Abbreviations: DM, diabetes mellitus; HTN, hypertension

- There are no specific diagnostic criteria for kidney-transplant-related AKI. The definition of AKI follows those used for native kidneys, e.g., RIFLE and AKIN classifications for acute kidney injury.

Causes of acute kidney injury in kidney transplants

- The common causes of AKI in KT can be surgical or non-surgical in nature and varies with the time period after transplantation (Table 55.2).

Table 55.2: Common Causes of Acute Kidney Injury in Kidney Transplants

	Immediate (0 to 1 Week)	Early (1 to 12 Weeks)	Late (>12 Weeks)
Pre-renal causes			
Dehydration	XXX	XX	XX
Calcineurin inhibitor nephrotoxicity	XXX	XX	XX
Transplant kidney artery stenosis	X	X	X
Kidney artery or venous thrombosis	X	X	X
Renal causes			
Delayed graft function	XXX	0	0
Rejection	XXX	XX	XX
Urinary tract infection	XXX	XXX	XX
Polyomavirus BK virus nephropathy	0	XX	XX
Recurrent or de novo glomerulonephritis	XX	XX	XX
Thrombotic microangiopathy	XX	XX	XX

Table 55.2: *(Continued)*

	Immediate (0 to 1 Week)	Early (1 to 12 Weeks)	Late (>12 Weeks)
Interstitial nephritis	X	X	X
Exposure to nephrotoxic drugs/contrast	X	X	XX
Post-renal causes			
Obstruction	XX	XX	X
Urine leak	XX	XX	X

Note: XXX: common; XX: uncommon; rare: X; 0: does not occur

Diagnostic evaluation of acute kidney injury in kidney transplants

- AKI in KT is often asymptomatic and can only be diagnosed by laboratory monitoring (Table 55.3). Dysfunction of the KT can also manifest without a rise in serum creatinine (sCr) but a rise in proteinuria.

- KT function should be assessed when the patient starts reporting fever, new onset or worsening pre-existing hypertension, reduction in urinary frequency or urine output, changes in urinary flow, haematuria, weight gain, peripheral oedema and pain/swelling over the site of the kidney transplant.

Delayed graft function

- After KT surgery, functional status of the KT can be classified into 1 of 4 different categories (Table 55.4).

- Delayed graft function (DGF) is AKI usually due to ischaemia-reperfusion injury and increases the risk for poorer allograft function, rejection, longer hospital stay, higher health-care costs, and shorter graft/patient survival.

Table 55.3:   Practical Guide to Evaluation of Acute Kidney Injury in Kidney Transplants

History — screen symptoms for	• Infection — fever, dysuria • Bladder outflow obstruction • Fluid losses — vomiting, diarrhoea • Changes in urine output • Drug history — changes in doses of immunosuppressive drugs, addition of RAAS blockers/SGLT2I • Medication non-adherence
Physical examination	• Vital signs including postural hypotension or hypertension • Hydration status • Abdomen examination including palpation of kidney transplant and bladder • Rectal examination, especially men for prostate enlargement
Laboratory tests	• Renal panel including serum glucose • Liver panel • Calcium phosphate • Uric acid • Creatinine kinase • Full blood count • Coagulation profile • Group and crossmatch to standby for KT biopsy • Peripheral blood film • Reticulocyte count • Haptoglobin • Lactate dehydrogenase • C-reactive protein • Procalcitonin • Immunosuppressive drug level(s) • Urine FEME • Urine culture • Urine cytology (for eosinophils, decoy cells, cancer) • Urine protein or albumin:creatinine ratio • Blood BKV PCR • Blood CMV PCR • Donor specific antibodies • Optional — donor derived cell-free DNA (dd-cfDNA)

Table 55.3:   (*Continued*)

Radiological tests	• Bedside bladder scan to check post-void residual urine (>100 mL is abnormal) • Ultrasound doppler of kidney transplant • Optional investigations — CTKUB, Tc-MAG3 frusemide renogram
Biopsy	• Light microscopy • Electron microscopy • SV40 T-antigen immunohistochemical stain (for BKV) • C4d stain • Optional investigations — gene expression profiling

Abbreviations: BKV, BK virus; CMV, cytomegalovirus; CTKUB, computed tomography of the kidney, ureter and bladder; FEME, full examination and microscopy; PCR, polymerase chain reaction; RAAS, renal-angiotensin-aldosterone; SGLT2, sodium glucose co-transporter 2; SV40, Simian Virus 40; Tc-MAG3, Technetium-99m mercaptoacetyltriglycine

Table 55.4:   Categories of Post-operative Kidney Transplant Function

Type of Graft Function	Post-operative Presentation	Need for Post-operative Dialysis
Immediate graft function (IGF)	Daily improvement in serum creatinine with achievement of nadir creatinine within 1 week post-surgery	No
Slow graft function (SGF)	Daily improvement in serum creatinine but nadir creatinine is not achieved within 1 week post-surgery	No
Delayed graft function (DGF)	There is a delay in the onset of improvement in serum creatinine, and the patient needs dialysis to maintain biochemical stability	Yes
Primary non-function (PNF)	Failure of the kidney transplant to function at all — often defined as being dialysis dependent for 3 months post-operatively; this is a rare occurrence nowadays	Yes

- The most common definition of DGF is the requirement of haemodialysis (HD) during the first week of KT but may overestimate DGF when HD is performed to treat post-operative hyperkalaemia. Slow graft function (SGF) is a slow decline in KT function during the first week of KT surgery, but there is no requirement for HD.

- It is most common after a deceased donor kidney transplant (DDKT) (10–50%) and less common (5%) in a living donor kidney transplant (LDKT) where cold ischaemia times are shorter (Table 55.5).

- The combination of DGF or slow graft function (SGF) with acute rejection results in worst outcomes than either DGF/SGF or acute rejection alone. Therefore, prevention of rejection is of paramount importance in recipients with DGF or SGF.

Clinical presentation

- Post-operatively, there may be urine output seen, which then tapers off as ischaemic reperfusion injury sets in. As a result, there is anuria or oliguria, and the sCr does not fall. Complications like hyperkalaemia, acidosis and pulmonary oedema may occur and necessitate the need for dialysis.

- DGF may be masked by those with pre-transplant residual urine output — functional status of the KT will then be determined by trends in sCr change.

- The Organ Procurement and Transplantation Network database in the USA shows that 50% of patients with DGF start to recover kidney function by post-operative day (POD) 10, whereas 33% regain function by POD 10–20, while 10–15% do so subsequently.

Table 55.5: Risk Factors for Delayed Graft Function

Donor	Preservation	Recipient	Immunological
Graft quality • Older age • Female gender • Glomerulosclerosis • Vascular thickening • AKI • Size mismatch between recipient and donor **Donor comorbidities** • Obesity • DM, HTN • Deceased donation • DCD • High kidney donor profile index score **ICU events** • Hypoxic or CVA death • Brain death >24 hours • ICU stay >40 hours • Inotropic use	**Ischaemia times** • Cold ischaemia >15 hours • Warm ischaemia >45 minutes • Poor initial allograft reperfusion • Perioperative hypotension **Type of preservation** • Static cold perfusion vs. machine pulsatile perfusion • Preservation solution, e.g., UW or HTK vs. Euro-Collins	**Recipient comorbidities** • Older age • Frailty • Male • Obesity • DM, HTN • Cardiac function • Pre-transplant PO4, oliguria **Dialysis factors** • Pre-transplant dialysis/UF • Long dialysis time • Type of dialysis	• Higher peak PRA • Repeat transplant • Previous transfusion • Greater HLA mismatch • Higher CNI levels

Abbreviations: AKI, acute kidney injury; CNI, calcineurin inhibitor; CVA, cerebrovascular accident; DCD, donation after cardiac death; DM, diabetes mellitus; HLA, human leukocyte antigen; HTN, hypertension; UW, University of Wisconsin; HTK, histidine-tryptophan-ketoglutarate; PRA, panel reactive antibody; PO4, phosphate; UF, ultrafiltration

Prevention

- Careful assessment of allograft quality through a detailed review of medical records and histology of explant biopsies when they are performed.

- Cold static storage with preservation solution (HTK is used in Singapore), but machine perfusion may be better at reducing DGF.

- Minimise cold ischaemia time as much as possible by good wait-list management, expedited preparation of the candidate for surgery, and readily available surgical resources.

- Avoid excessive ultrafiltration during pre-op dialysis — keep the patient about 1 kg above dry weight.

- Ensure adequate intravascular volume and blood pressure during surgery.

- Keep warm ischaemia times short.

- Facilitate diuresis using intra-operative diuretics, e.g., mannitol given at the time of completion of vascular anastomoses, but this is no longer given at some centres (a recent randomised controlled trial of mannitol vs. normal saline showed that mannitol did not have an effect on post-operative graft function or biomarkers of ischaemia reperfusion injury in kidney transplantation).

- Pre- or intra-operative thymoglobulin, which may be logistically challenging due to the time constraints prior to surgery and is dependent on anaesthesia comfort levels to address the occurrence of possible cytokine release syndrome during surgery.

- Pre-operative methylprednisolone was shown in a randomised controlled trial as well as in a retrospective analysis to be associated with a lower incidence of DGF.

Management of delayed graft function

- Management of DGF is supportive and needs to investigate reversible causes, just like any AKI (Table 55.6).

Table 55.6:   Practical Guide to Managing Delayed Graft Function

1. Check for risk factors for delayed graft function (DGF)
2. Review operative notes for events that can cause DGF, e.g., hypotension
3. Examine patient for severe pain, bladder distension, excessive wound drainage, swelling over the wound, e.g., haematoma or swollen kidney transplant, fluid status
4. Check drains for excessive or unusual drainage, e.g., blood, urine
5. Check patency and position of the urinary catheter
6. Order chest X-ray, among other things exclude pulmonary oedema
7. Order ECG to check for perioperative coronary events and signs of electrolyte disturbances, e.g., tall T waves of hyperkalaemia
8. Order post-operative radionuclide perfusion scan or US doppler
9. Order post-operative bloods — renal panel, full blood count, CaPO4, Mg, liver panel, cardiac enzymes
10. Review CNI drug levels if recipient received CNI prior to kidney transplantation
11. Fluid challenge if the patient is not overloaded or assessed to be dehydrated — for patients with an acute fall in Hb, assess for bleeding and transfuse red blood cell
12. Trial of frusemide if patient is adequately filled with fluids, e.g., IV frusemide 80 mg bolus followed by 10–30 mg/hr infusion; if there is no diuretic response, frusemide can be discontinued
13. Adjust subsequent IV fluids to urine output and fluid status
14. Start inotropes if hypotensive and no other cause of hypotension found
15. Order HD as indicated, e.g., hyperkalaemia, acute pulmonary oedema — avoid heparin, excessive UF, hypotension
16. Immunosuppression should be optimised to prevent rejection — there is no strong evidence to support reducing or avoiding CNI during DGF
17. Consider a biopsy of kidney transplant by POD 5–7 to exclude acute rejection and other causes. Do the biopsy earlier if the patient is sensitised

---

Abbreviations: CaPO4, calcium phosphate; CNI, calcineurin inhibitor; ECG, electrocardiogram; Hb, haemoglobin; HD; haemodialysis; IV, intravenous; POD, post-operative day; UF, ultrafiltration; US, ultrasound; Mg, magnesium;

Rejection

- Rejection is inflammation and destruction of the KT, triggered by the recipient's immune system recognising nonself antigens on the KT. Risks of rejection can be related to donor, recipient and immunological characteristics (Table 55.7).

Table 55.7:   Risk Factors for Kidney Transplant Rejection

Donor	Recipient	Immunological
• Deceased donor • Older age • Long cold ischaemia time • Long warm ischaemia time	• Younger age • Black race • Delayed graft function • Prior rejection • Prior transplant • Non-adherence to immunosuppressive treatment • Intentional reduction of immunosuppression	• ABO incompatibility • HLA mismatch, especially DR/DQ • High panel reactive Abs • Positive crossmatch • Pre-formed DSAs • De novo DSAs

Abbreviations: Abs, antibodies; DSAs, donor-specific antibodies; HLA, human leukocyte antigen

- It presents clinically as an AKI. However, it can also be silent, presenting as asymptomatic proteinuria or without any abnormalities (called subclinical rejection or SCR).

- There are 4 general types of rejection as follows:

  - Hyperacute rejection: Occurs after surgical anastomosis is completed and due to preformed antibodies. It is now rare following the introduction of crossmatch tests.

  - Acute rejection: Usually occurs days to weeks after transplant but can also occur anytime later. It may be due to T-cell or antibody-mediated rejection.

  - Chronic rejection: Occurs several months after transplant and can be due to T-cell or antibody mediated rejection.

- Acute on chronic rejection: Occurs several months after transplant where there is a mix of acute rejection on a background of pre-existing chronic rejection.
- Rejection is associated with particular histopathological changes, and thence, the diagnosis of rejection is based on histopathological criteria set by The Banff Classification of Allograft Pathology (Table 55.8).
- In order to achieve a proper diagnosis, a minimum number of 10 glomeruli and 2 arteries should be seen on a microscopy of the biopsy tissue (considered as adequate sample). A sample is considered marginal if there are 7–10 glomeruli and 1 artery, while <7 glomeruli and no arteries is considered an inadequate sample.

T-cell mediated rejection

- T-cell mediated rejection (TCMR) is caused by activation and infiltration of T-cells to damage the KT through inflammatory processes.
- Acute TCMR (Table 55.9) is most frequently encountered during the first year of KT, approximately at a rate of 10%.
- It responds well to corticosteroids and lymphocyte depleting agents — it has little effect on graft survival unless it is associated with antibody mediated rejection (ABMR).
- However, chronic active TCMR (CA-TCMR) (Table 55.9) has a poorer prognosis — the 5-year graft survival rate of CA-TCMR is approximately 80%.
- Augmented baseline immunosuppression is important following a diagnosis of TCMR because TCMR may increase the risk of *de novo* DSA and subsequent AMR.

Table 55.8:   Definitions of Banff Lesion Scores

Banff Lesion Score	Description	0	1	2	3
Interstitial inflammation (i)	Proportion of unscarred cortex with inflammation	<10%	10–25%	26–50%	>50%
Tubulitis (t)	Inflammation consisting of mononuclear cells in the basolateral part of renal tubular epithelium, defined as number of mononuclear cells per 10 tubular epithelial cells of tubules in the most severely involved tubule	None	1–4	5–10	>10 or Foci of tubular basement membrane destruction with i $\geq$2 and t2 elsewhere
Intimal arteritis or endothelialitis or endarteritis (v)	Inflammation within arterial intima, defined by mononuclear cells in the subendothelial space of at least 1 artery	None	<25% of luminal area lost in the most severely affected artery	$\geq$25% luminal area lost in the most severely affected artery	Transmural arteritis and/or fibrinoid change, medial smooth muscle necrosis with lymphocyte infiltrate in vessel

Glomerulitis (g)	Inflammation within glomeruli, defined by the proportion of glomeruli showing complete or partial occlusion of 1 or more glomerular capillary by leukocyte infiltration and endothelial cell enlargement	None	<25%	25–75%	>75%
Peritubular capillaritis (ptc)	Degree of inflammation within peritubular capillaries, defined by the number of leukocytes within the most severely affected PTC. There must be at least 1 leukocyte in at least 10% of cortical PTC	<3 leukocytes/ PTC	3–4 leukocytes/ PTC	5–10 leukocytes/ PTC	>10 leukocytes/ PTC
C4d	Percentage of peritubular capillaries and vasa recta that has a linear, circumferential staining	None	<10%	10–50%	>50%

(Continued)

Table 55.8:   *(Continued)*

Banff Lesion Score	Description	0	1	2	3
	pattern for C4d by IF on snap frozen section or IHC on formalin fixated and paraffin-embedded tissue				
Interstitial fibrosis (ci)	Extent of cortical fibrosis	$\leq 5\%$	6–25%	26–50%	>50%
Tubular atrophy (ct)	Extent of cortical tubular atrophy, defined by tubules with a thickened basement membrane or a reduction of >50% tubular diameter	None	$\leq 25\%$	26–50%	>50%
Vascular fibrous intimal thickening (cv)	Extent of thickening of the arterial intima in the most severely affected artery	None	$\leq 25\%$ narrowing of luminal area	26–50% narrowing of luminal area	>50% narrowing of luminal area

Glomerular basement membrane double contours (cg)	Presence and extent of glomerular basement membrane (GBM) double contours in capillary loops of the most affected non-sclerotic glomerulus on PAS or silver stain	None	1a: GBM double contours seen only by EM 1b: 1–25% of peripheral capillary loops seen on LM	26–50% GBM double contours 26–50% of peripheral capillary loops	>50% GBM double contours > 50% of peripheral capillary loops
Mesangial matrix expansion (mm)	Percentage of nonsclerotic glomeruli with moderate mesangial matrix expansion, defined by expansion of the matrix in the mesangial interspace to exceed the width of 2 mesangial cells in the average in at least 2 glomerular lobules	None	≤25%	26–50%	>50%
Arteriolar hyalinosis (ah)	Extent of arteriolar hyalinosis, defined by PAS-positive arteriolar hyaline thickening	None	Mild to moderate PAS positive hyaline thickening in ≤1 arteriole	Moderate to severe PAS positive hyaline thickening in >1 arteriole	Severe PAS positive hyaline thickening in many arterioles

(Continued)

Table 55.8:   (*Continued*)

Banff Lesion Score	Description	0	1	2	3
Hyaline arteriolar thickening (aah)	Optional score, describing circumferential or noncircumferential hyalinosis of arterioles, which may be due to CNI arteriolopathy	None	1 arteriole without circumferential hyalinosis	≥1 arteriole without circumferential hyalinosis	Circumferential hyalinosis in many arterioles
Total inflammation (ti)	Extent of total cortical inflammation, including areas of interstitial fibrosis and tubular atrophy, subcapsular cortex and perivascular cortex	<10%	10–25%	26–50%	>50%
Inflammation in area of IFTA (i-IFTA)	Extent of inflammation in scarred areas (ci and ct)	<10%	10–25%	26–50%	>50%

Table 55.9: Banff Classification and Treatment of T-Cell Mediated Rejection

T-Cell Mediated Rejection (TCMR)		
TCMR	**Banff Criteria**	**Treatment**
Borderline or suspicious for acute TCMR	$t > 0$ and $i \leq 1$ or $t1$ and $i \geq 2$	• When there is elevated sCr, 51% of borderline rejection progress to acute rejection. So treatment is indicated if borderline rejection is associated with elevated sCr or proteinuria. • Treatment can be IV methylprednisolone 250–500 mg daily × 3d or PO prednisolone. • Optimise baseline immunosuppression, consider switch from CsA to TAC or AZA to MMF/MYF or if not on corticosteroids, start oral maintenance corticosteroids. • If there is no improvement in sCr following treatment, consider repeating biopsy. If there is persistent rejection on repeat biopsy, ATG treatment can be considered.
Grade 1A TCMR	$t2$ and $i \geq 2$	• IV methylprednisolone 500 mg daily × 3d. • Optimise baseline immunosuppression, consider switch from CsA to TAC or AZA to MMF/MYF or if not on corticosteroids, start oral maintenance corticosteroids. • If there is no improvement in sCr following treatment, consider repeating biopsy. If there is persistent rejection, ATG treatment can be considered.

(Continued)

Table 55.9: (*Continued*)

T-Cell Mediated Rejection (TCMR)		
TCMR	**Banff Criteria**	**Treatment**
Grade 1B TCMR	t3 and i ≥ 2	• IV methylprednisolone 500 mg daily × 3d. • Optimise baseline immunosuppression, consider switch from CsA to TAC or AZA to MMF/MYF or if not on corticosteroids, start oral maintenance corticosteroids. • If there is no improvement in sCr following treatment, consider repeating biopsy. If there is persistent rejection, ATG treatment can be considered.
Grade II TCMR		
Grade IIA TCMR	v1 regardless of t or i score	• IV Methylprednisolone 500 mg daily × 3d. • Start ATG 1.5 mg/kg/d up to a cumulative dose of 7.5 mg/kg. • If there is no improvement in sCr following treatment, consider repeating the biopsy.
Grade IIB TCMR	v2 regardless of t or i score	
Grade III TCMR	v3 regardless of t or i score	
CA-TCMR		
Grade 1A CA-TCMR	ti ≥2 + i-IFTA ≥2 + t2	• There is little data and consensus on the approach and treatment of CA-TCMR. • IV Methylprednisolone 500 mg daily × 3d ± IV ATG 1.5 mg/kg/d × 4d and augmented baseline immunosuppression may be used to treat CA-TCMR. • However, response to treatment, e.g., improvement in kidney function, is only seen in up to 20%. • Treatment may need to be withheld in biopsies showing significant glomerulosclerosis and IFTA.
Grade 1B CA-TCMR	ti ≥2 + i-IFTA ≥2 + t3	
Grade II CA-TCMR	Arterial intimal fibrosis with mononuclear cell inflammation in fibrosis and formation of neointima	

Antibody-mediated rejection

- Antibody-mediated rejection (ABMR) is mediated by antibodies produced from plasma cells, which are directed against antigens expressed on the KT. They can cause damage to the KT through complement dependent and independent pathways. The antibodies can already be pre-formed (detected prior to transplant) or developed de novo (detected only after transplant).

- Active ABMR occurs in approximately 5–10%, while chronic ABMR occurs more often in approximately 5–15% of KT. The frequency of ABMR is higher in individuals who are sensitised.

- Unlike TCMR, ABMR has a poorer prognosis, is associated with a GFR decline of 20% in the first 12 months following diagnosis, and is the most common cause of late graft loss.

- Risk for graft loss is determined by the degree of graft dysfunction and clinical and histological factors (Table 55.10).

- There are 3 diagnostic categories of ABMR — Active, chronic active and chronic inactive, each with a different approach to treatment (Table 55.11).

Table 55.10: Risk Factors for Graft Failure Following Antibody Mediated Rejection

Clinical	Histological	DSA
• Allograft dysfunction at diagnosis • Proteinuria • Time of diagnosis post-transplant • Non-adherence to medication	• cg >0 • cv >0 • IF/TA • Concomitant TCMR • C4d positivity	• Class II DSA • C1q positive DSA

Abbreviations: Glomerular basement membrane double contours cv, vascular fibrous intimal thickening; DSA, donor specific antibodies; IF/TA, interstitial fibrosis, tubular atrophy; TCMR, T-cell mediated rejection

Table 55.11:   Banff Classification and Treatment of Antibody-mediated Rejection

	Active Antibody-mediated Rejection (ABMR)	Chronic (Active) ABMR	Chronic (Inactive) ABMR
Histology	Acute tissue injury, at least one of the following: 1. g > 0 in the absence of GN and/or ptc > 0 in the absence of TCMR or borderline 2. v > 0 3. Acute TMA, in the absence of any other causes 4. ATN, in the absence of any other causes	Chronic tissue injury, at least one of the following: 1. cg > 0 if no evidence of chronic TMA or GN 2. Severe peritubular capillary basement membrane multilayering (≥7 layers in 1 cortical PTC and ≥5 in 2 additional capillaries) 3. Transplant arteriopathy (arterial intimal fibrosis of new onset)	Chronic tissue injury, at least one of the following: 1. Transplant glomerulopathy and/or 2. Severe peritubular capillary basement membrane multilayering 3. Significant loss of peritubular capillaries (capillaries no longer exist to show capillaritis)
Evidence of antibody interaction with the endothelium	• C4d2 or C4d3 (IF) or C4d > 0 (IHC) • MVI (g+pct >1) in the absence of GN, borderline or acute TCMR. If borderline or acute TCMR or infection is present, g+ptc >1 is not sufficient, and g must be >1	• C4d2 or C4d3 (IF) or C4d > 0 (IHC) • MVI (g+pct >1) in the absence of GN, borderline or acute TCMR. If borderline or acute TCMR or infection is present, g+ptc >1 is not sufficient, and g must be >1	• C4d negative • There may be prior evidence of antibody interaction with the endothelium

	• Increased expression of gene transcripts/classifiers in the biopsy tissue that is strongly associated with ABMR, if thoroughly validated	• Increased expression of thoroughly validated gene transcripts/classifiers in the biopsy tissue that is strongly associated with ABMR	
DSA	Detectable serum anti-HLA DSA. If anti-HLA DSA is undetected, non-HLA antibody testing should be considered. Otherwise • C4d2 or 3 (IF) or C4d >0 (IHC) • Increased expression of gene transcripts/classifiers in the biopsy tissue that is strongly associated with ABMR, if thoroughly validated	Detectable serum anti-HLA DSA. If anti-HLA DSA is undetected, non-HLA antibody testing should be considered. Otherwise • C4d2 or 3 (IF) or C4d >0 (IHC) • Increased expression of gene transcripts/classifiers in the biopsy tissue that is strongly associated with ABMR, if thoroughly validated	Anti-HLA DSA may be undetectable. However, there should be prior history of anti-HLA or non-HLA DSA
Clinical presentation	Abrupt increase in serum creatinine and oliguria ± proteinuria	Progressive worsening of kidney function with proteinuria in vintage patients, usually associated with a prior history of reduced immunosuppression	Progressive worsening of kidney function with proteinuria in vintage patients, usually associated with a prior history of reduced immunosuppression

(*Continued*)

Table 55.11: *(Continued)*

	Active Antibody-mediated Rejection (ABMR)	**Chronic (Active) ABMR**	**Chronic (Inactive) ABMR**
Prognosis	It may respond to prompt treatment by resolving completely or persist, progressing to chronic active AMR and chronic AMR	Typically, poorer response to treatment	Poor prognosis, almost universal graft loss
First-line treatment	TPE/DFPP+IVIG is considered standard of care for treatment of active AMR, but its efficacy is based only on observational studies of variable quality	No consensus on treatment and depends on chronicity and patient's comorbidities to tolerate augmented immunosuppression	Prognosis is guarded, regardless of treatment
Baseline immunosuppression	Augment — increase dose of existing immunosuppression, aiming for higher target drug levels or change to more potent agents, e.g., CsA → TAC AZA → MPA Add prednisolone	Augment — increase dose of existing immunosuppression, aiming for higher target drug levels or change to more potent agents, e.g., CsA → TAC AZA → MPA Add prednisolone	Augment — increase dose of existing immunosuppression or change to more potent agents, e.g., CsA → TAC AZA → MPA Add prednisolone
Methylprednisolone	IV 500 mg × 3d	IV 500 mg × 3d	Nil

Plasma exchange (PLEX)/ double filtration plasmapheresis (DFPP) and IVIG Immunoadsorption is used in place of PLEX/DFPP in some centres	4–$6 \times$ PLEX/DFPP + IVIG 100–200 mg after each PLEX/DFPP; 1–2 g/kg IVIG may be given at the end of treatment	May consider 4–6 x PLEX/DFPP + IVIG 100–200 mg after each PLEX/DFPP; 1–2 g/kg IVIG may be given at the end of treatment or Monthly IVIG 1–2 g/kg	Nil
Rituximab	± one dose of IV Rituximab 375 mg/kg/m² (space last dose of IVIG and Rituximab by 1 week)	± IV Rituximab 375 mg/kg/m² (space last dose of IVIG and Rituximab by 1 week)	Optimise baseline immunosuppression, counsel and prepare for return to dialysis if advanced CKD
Follow-up	Depending on the patient's condition and comorbidities, a repeat biopsy should be performed to assess the graft status before considering further treatments where they are expensive, potentially toxic, and the data on efficacy is limited (Table 55.9). In some patients, further escalation of immunosuppression is not appropriate, and the patient should be prepared to return to dialysis instead.		

Source: Modified from Rodriguez-Ramirez S, Al Jurdi A, Konvalinka A and Riella LV. (2022). Antibody-mediated rejection: Prevention, monitoring and treatment dilemmas. *Curr Opin Organ Transplant* **27**(5): 405–414.

Abbreviations: AZA, azathioprine; ATN, acute tubular necrosis; CKD, chronic kidney disease; CsA, cyclosporine; DFPP, double filtration plasmapheresis; DSA, donor specific antibody; GN, glomerulonephritis; HLA, human leukocyte antigen; IHC, immunohistochemistry; IF, immunofluorescence; IVIG, intravenous immunoglobulin; TMA, thrombotic microangiopathy; MPA; mycophenolic acid (e.g., mycophenolate mofetil, sodium mycophenolate); MVI, microvascular inflammation; PLEX, plasma exchange, TAC, tacrolimus

Table 55.11:   Second Line Treatment for Active Antibody Mediated Rejection

Second-line Treatment	Mechanism of Action	Investigated Uses
Eculizumab	• Anti-C5 mAb, inhibiting C5, thence blocking the complement final common pathway	Observational studies show variable results for active ABMR and may be less effective in chronic ABMR. No RCT has been performed.
C1 inhibitor or C1 esterase inhibitor	• Inhibits activation of the complement and intrinsic coagulation pathway	Observational studies as add-on therapy for active ABMR reported no significant change in histology but modest improvement in GFR. A RCT was terminated because of inefficacy.
Bortezomib	• First generation reversible proteasome inhibitor	Some observational studies for active and chronic active ABMR reported benefit but no efficacy demonstrated from BORTEJECT RCT for late ABMR.
Tocilizumab	• Anti-IL6 receptor mAb • Associated with rebound of IL-6 following discontinuation of tocilizumab	Numerous positive observational studies and case reports showing stabilisation or graft function, stable or improved histology, and sometimes lowering of DSA for active and chronic active ABMR. However, there is no RCT published. Main adverse effects were infections, but the frequency is comparable to that for standard of care.

Clazakizumab	• Anti-IL6 mAb • Unlike tocilizumab, less rebound of IL-6	1 phase 2 RCT in chronic active ABMR showed a small proportion (< 50%) stabilised graft function and improved histology. However, 25% developed serious infectious complications.
Imlifidase	• Endopeptidase cleaves 4 IgG Ab • Limitations cannot be given repeatedly because of the development of anti-imlifidase antibodies and the need to be coupled with other strategies, e.g., PLEX	No reports of its use for treatment of ABMR, but an RCT is being implemented.
Belatacept	• CTLA4-Ig binding to CD80 and CD86 receptors on APC and block CD28-mediated costimulation of T-cells	An observational study in active ABMR of belatacept combined with bortezomib showed improvement in the function/ molecular ABMR score and removal of DSA. Another observational study with withdrawal of CNI in chronic active ABMR showed improvement in eGFR, molecular ABMR score, and DSA but no change in histology.
Daratumumab	Anti-CD38 mAb, causing plasma cell depletion	Rare case reports of improvement in GFR, DSA and histology for chronic active ABMR but no RCT.

Source: Sethi S and Jordan SC. (2023). Novel therapies for treatment of antibody-mediated rejection of the kidney. *Curr Opin Organ Transplant* **28**(1): 29–35.

Abbreviations: ABMR, antibody mediated rejection; APC, antigen presenting cells; CNI, calcineurin inhibitor; DSA, donor specific antibody; eGFR, estimated glomerular filtration rate; IL, interleukin; mAb, monoclonal antibody; RCT, randomised controlled trial

Prophylaxis and monitoring after treatment of rejection

- Treatment of rejection is associated with potential morbidity and even mortality due to complications such as
  - Infection
  - Malignancy
  - Post-transplant diabetes mellitus
  - Increased cardiovascular risks factors — hyperlipidaemia, hypertension, obesity
  - Drug toxicities
- Prophylactic medications that are often prescribed (if not already on) during and following treatment of rejection include:
  - Nystatin mouthwash to prevent oral thrush
  - Co-trimoxazole prophylaxis
  - Valganciclovir prophylaxis for 1–3 months
  - Omeprazole for 1–3 months
- Patients should be monitored for the development of metabolic complications and opportunistic infections.

References

Beimler J and Zeier M (2009). Borderline rejection after renal transplantation — To treat or not to treat. *Clin Transplant* **23**(Suppl 21): 19–25.

Cabezas L, Jouve T, Malvezzi P, *et al.* (2022). Tocilizumab and active antibody-mediated rejection in kidney transplantation: A literature review. *Front Immunol* **13**, 839380.

Cooper JE and Wiseman AC (2013). Acute kidney injury in kidney transplantation. *Curr Opin Nephrol Hypertens* **22**(6): 698–703.

Doberer K, Duerr M, Halloran PF, *et al.* (2021) A randomised clinical trial of anti-IL-6 antibody clazakizumab in late antibody-mediated kidney transplant rejection. *J Am Soc Nephrol* **32**(3): 708–722.

Kung VL, Sandhu R, Haas M, *et al.* (2021). Chronic active T cell-mediated rejection is variably responsive to immunosuppressive therapy. *Kidney Int* **100**(2): 391–400.

Noguchi H, Matsukuma Y, Nakagawa K, *et al.* (2022). Treatment of chronic active T cell-mediated rejection after kidney transplantation: A retrospective cohort study of 37 transplants. *Nephrology (Carlton)* **27**(7): 632–638.

Reiterer C, Hu K, Sljivic S, *et al.* (2020). Mannitol and renal graft injury in patients undergoing deceased donor renal transplantation — A randomized controlled clinical trial. *BMC Nephrol* **21**(1): 307.

Roufosse C, Simmonds N, Clahsen-van Groningen M, *et al.* (2018). A 2018 reference guide to the Banff Classification of Renal Allograft Pathology. *Transplantation* **102**(11): 1795–1814.

Schinstock CA, Mannon RB, Budde K, *et al.* (2020) Recommended treatment for antibody-mediated rejection after kidney transplantation: The 2019 expert consensus from the Transplantion Society Working Group. *Transplantation* **104**(5): 911–922.

Sharif A and Borrows R (2013). Delayed graft function after kidney transplantation: The clinical perspective. *Am J Kidney Dis* **62**(1): 150–158.

Yakubu I, Moinuddin I and Gupta G (2023). Use of belatacept in kidney transplantation: What's new? *Curr Opin Organ Transplant* **28**(1): 36–45.

56 Post-Transplant Urinary Tract Infections

Carolyn Tien, Terence Kee

Introduction

- Urinary tract infection (UTI) is the most common bacterial infection after kidney transplantation (KT) — at SGH, it accounts for 35.5% of KT-associated infections requiring hospitalisation.

- UTI can occur any time after KT, but the peak incidence occurs in the first 6 months after KT (where many risk factors are present).

- Potential complications of post-transplant UTI include:

  - Bacteraemia (UTI is the most common cause of bacteraemia in KT)

  - Acute kidney injury (AKI)

  - Rejection

  - Interstitial fibrosis and tubular atrophy (IFTA)

  - Chronic Kidney Disease (CKD)

  - Graft loss

  - Emergence of multi-drug resistance uropathogens

  - Increased healthcare costs

  - Increased morbidity and mortality

- UTI occurs as an interplay of donor, recipient, and transplant-related risk factors (Table 56.1).

Table 56.1:   Risk Factors for Urinary Tract Infection

Recipient related	<ul><li>Advanced age</li><li>Female gender</li><li>Diabetes Mellitus</li><li>Malnutrition</li><li>Candiduria</li><li>Long period of dialysis before kidney transplant</li><li>Polycystic kidney disease</li><li>History of recurrent UTI prior to transplant</li><li>Lower urinary tract abnormalities — vesicoureteral reflux, bladder dysfunction, ureterostomy, ileal conduit, bladder augmentation</li><li>Renal calculi</li><li>Disused bladder (especially anuric dialysis patients)</li><li>Prolonged hospitalisation</li><li>Care in the intensive care unit</li><li>Infection of the native urinary tract</li></ul>
Donor-related	<ul><li>Deceased donor kidney</li><li>Infected donor kidney</li><li>Dual kidney transplants</li><li>Contaminated graft perfusion solution</li></ul>
Transplant-related	<ul><li>Retransplant</li><li>Delayed graft function</li><li>Use of thymoglobulin/mycophenolate mofetil</li><li>Recent augmentation of immunosuppression</li><li>Allograft rejection</li><li>Chronic allograft dysfunction</li><li>Urinary instrumentation such as indwelling urinary catheterisation, ureteral stent</li><li>Length of hospital stay</li></ul>

- UTI may be asymptomatic or symptomatic and can be stratified according to their symptoms, site, frequency, and presence/absence of functional and/or structural urinary abnormalities (Tables 56.2 and 56.3). All UTIs occurring in KT recipients are considered complicated UTIs due to immunosuppression and uretero-neocystostomy (Table 56.3).

Table 56.2:   Classification of Asymptomatic Bacteriuria and Urinary Tract Infections

UTI Category	Definition	Clinical Phenotype
Asymptomatic bacteriuria	• $>10^5$ bacterial colony-forming units per millilitre (CFU/mL) of urine • Urinary tract may be structurally and/or functionally abnormal	• No local and systemic symptoms or signs of UTI • Some authors do not always consider this a disease state
Simple cystitis	• $>10^5$ bacterial CFU/mL of urine • Urinary tract is structurally and functionally normal • There are no indwelling devices	• Infection of the lower urinary tract • Dysuria, urgency, frequency, suprapubic pain, haematuria • No systemic symptoms
Pyelonephritis	• $>10^5$ bacterial CFU/mL of urine • Urinary tract may be structurally and/or functionally abnormal	• Infection of the upper urinary tract • Pain over the allograft or costovertebral pain (if native kidney(s) are involved) • Systemic symptoms are present — fever, chills, malaise, haemodynamic instability, leucocytosis, bacteraemia (in 19–45%)
Recurrent UTI	≥ 3 UTIs in 1 year or ≥ 2 UTIs in 6 months — it includes relapses and reinfections	
Relapsing UTI	UTI with the same microorganism that caused the preceding UTI within 2 weeks after finishing the previous treatment for the prior UTI	
Reinfection	New episode of UTI and occurs 2 weeks after the end of treatment of a preceding UTI. It can be due to the same or different microorganisms	

Table 56.3:   Features of Uncomplicated vs. Complicated Urinary Tract Infections

Variable	Uncomplicated	Complicated
Typical patient	Otherwise, healthy, ambulatory, non-pregnant women with no history suggestive of structural, metabolic and/or functional abnormality of the urinary tract. There is no indwelling urinary devices.	Men, women, or children with structural, metabolic and/or functional abnormality of the urinary tract. There may be indwelling ureteric stents, bladder catheters or nephrostomy tubes.
Clinical spectrum	Mild cystitis to severe pyelonephritis	Mild cystitis to life-threatening urosepsis — increased risks of complications, e.g., bacteraemia, abscesses, prostatitis in men
Diagnosis	Easier to diagnose clinically	May be more difficult to diagnose — symptoms and signs may be subtle or atypical, e.g., impaired sensation, altered mental status, catheterised — urine FEME and culture always needed. Symptoms may also be mistaken for a gastrointestinal source of infection, e.g., nausea/vomiting, diarrhoea.
Response to treatment	Predictable with appropriate agent and treatment duration	MDRO more frequent, response less predictable, and may require invasive procedures for cure

Abbreviations: FEME, full examination and microscopy; MDRO, multi-drug resistant organism.

- In most cases, uropathogens causing UTI in KT recipients are usually gram-negative microorganisms (>70%). In 50–60%, *Escherichia coli* is responsible for UTI among KT recipients. Some uropathogens are associated with specific urinary conditions, e.g.:

Table 56.4: **Types of Uropathogens in Urinary Tract Infections after Kidney Transplantation**

Typical UTI		Atypical UTI
More Frequent	**Less Frequent**	
Escherichia coli	*Staphylococcus saprophyticus*	BK virus
Klebsiella spp.	*Streptococcus agalactiae*	Cytomegalovirus
Enterococcus spp.	*Staphylococcus aureus*	Adenovirus
Proteus spp.	*Citrobacter* spp.	*Candida* spp.
Pseudomonas aeruginosa	*Enterobacter* spp.	Tuberculosis
	Morganella spp.	*Ureaplasma* spp.
	Providencia spp.	*Corynebacterium urealyticum*
	Serratia spp.	

- *Staphyloccus aureus* — haemotogenous spread to the urinary tract

- *Corynebacterium urealyticum* — obstructive uropathy and/or encrusted cystitis

- However, there is an increased frequency of multidrug resistant organisms (MDRO) and extensively drug-resistant organisms (XDRO), especially among those who have been treated frequently for recurrent UTIs. This increases the risk of treatment failure and re-infection.

- Some other uropathogens are rarer and occur more often only in immunocompromised patients (Table 56.4).

Assessment of UTI

- Every KT recipient presenting with fever should be evaluated for UTI (Table 56.5). However, symptoms and signs may be subtle, e.g., presenting only with malaise.

Table 56.5:   Assessment of Urinary Tract Infection

History	Examination	Laboratory Tests	Radiological Tests
• Lower urinary tract symptoms — dysuria, urgency, frequency, haematuria • Pain over the KT • Systemic symptoms — fever, chills • Recent urological or gynecological instrumentation • Perineal hygiene practices • Sexual activity • Menstruation history	• Allograft tenderness or swelling • Bladder fullness • Flank tenderness for native kidney infection • Rectal examination for males to assess prostate • Vaginal examination for females	• Renal panel • Glucose • HbA1c • FBC • CRP • Procalcitonin • PSA (in males) • Immunosuppressive drug levels • Urine dipstick • Urine FEME • Urine C/S • Blood C/S • CMV PCR (to detect asymptomatic reactivation due to sepsis)	• Post-void residual urine volume measurement • US or CT KUB • Selected cases — cystoscopy, voiding cystourethrogram, urodynamic studies, MRI prostate • PET-CT scan may be required in difficult cases — native and polycystic kidney infections

Abbreviations: CMV, cytomegalovirus; CRP, C-reactive protein; CT, computer tomography; C/S, culture and sensitivity; FBC, full blood count; FEME, full examination and microscopy; HbA1c, haemoglobin A1c; KT, kidney transplant; KUB, kidney, ureter, bladder; MRI, magnetic resonance imaging; PCR, polymerase chain reaction; PET, position emission tomography; PSA, prostate specific antigen; US, ultrasound

- Unlike UTIs in the general population, UTI among KT recipients can be silent due to denervation of the transplanted kidney and masking of symptoms by immunosuppression — as a result, screening for UTI is mandatory whenever there is AKI of the KT, e.g., FBC, CRP, procalcitonin, urine FEME, and C/S.

- Diagnostic criteria for UTI include:

  - Inflammatory cells and/or microorganisms on urine examination — positive leukocyte esterase/nitrites on a urine dipstick and/or pyuria (≥ 10 wbc/hpf) or microorganisms on urine FEME

  - $>10^5$ colony-forming units (CFU)/mL of bacteria

  However, clinically significant UTI can still occur with a lesser degree of pyuria (e.g., <10 wbc/hpf) and bacterial colony count (e.g., 10^3–10^5 CFU/mL). The absence of pyuria should call the diagnosis of UTI into question.

- Urine samples should be midstream collections and performed after cleaning the perineum or glans penis. For urine collections from urinary catheters (especially those *in situ* >2 weeks), removal of the catheter and collecting urine by midstream voiding or after inserting a new urinary catheter is recommended.

- Not all patients may have a positive urine culture — yeasts, acid-fast bacilli, and *Corynebacterium urealyticum* (associated with urinary tract obstruction) may require special media to isolate and have longer incubation times. The yield of urine cultures is also lower when patients are pre-treated with UTI.

- For pyelonephritis and uropathogens associated with haematogenous spread, e.g., *Staphylococcus Aureus*, blood cultures should be obtained.

Prevention of UTI

- Routine urine C/S of kidney donors should be obtained prior to transplantation — for living kidney donors, positive urine C/S should be treated prior to transplantation, but for deceased kidney donors, transplantation may have to proceed without waiting for the result of the urine C/S.

- For deceased kidney donor transplantation, the donor's urine C/S should be traced in a timely manner to decide if post-transplant antibiotics need to be continued.

- All kidney transplant recipients should receive perioperative antibiotics prior to kidney transplant surgery.

- Trimethoprim-sulfamethoxazole (TMP/SMX) is often pre-scribed as a long-term UTI prophylaxis for KT recipients. Unfortunately, the prevalence of TMP/SMX resistance is high among uropathogens, and TMP/SMX prophylaxis is more important to prevent *pneumocystis jiroveci* instead.

- For patients who are unable to take TMP/SMX prophylaxis, alternative antibiotics can be prescribed, of which the duration depends on the risks for UTI. However, fluoroquinolones should be generally avoided as drug resistance easily emerges.

- Apart from antibiotics, other preventive measures may also be helpful, such as:
  - Minimising the duration/use of indwelling urethral catheters — if long-term urethral catherisation is required, intermittent self-catherisation is preferred
  - Early ureteral stent removal within 4 weeks of transplant surgery
  - Antibiotic treatment before and after ureteral stent removal (limited evidence)

- Maintaining adequate hydration to ensure an adequate urinary volume
- Avoid delaying micturition if there is a sensation of a full bladder — reflux may occur
- Frequent/timed voiding
- Wiping front to back for women
- Showers instead of bathtubs
- Minimising douching, sprays and powders in the genital area
- Avoiding sequential anal then vaginal intercourse
- Voiding after sexual intercourse
- Post-coital antibiotics if UTI is frequently associated with sexual intercourse
- Vaginal oestrogen for post-menopausal women to treat atrophic vaginitis
- Cleaning genital area after micturition for those on SLGT2 inhibitors
- Cranberry products (limited evidence)
- UTI vaccine like Uromune have been demonstrated to reduce UTI in KT recipients

Management of UTI

- Prompt diagnosis and treatment of UTI is essential to prevent spread to the upper urinary tract (pyelonephritis) and blood stream (bacteraemia).

- Antibiotics should be started as soon as a diagnosis of UTI is suspected (Table 56.5). If the patient has a history of previous UTI, then antibiotics may be guided by the history of previous uropathogens and sensitivities.

Table 56.6:   Management of UTIs

Type of UTI	Empirical Choice of Antibiotics (antibiotics should subsequently be adjusted to culture susceptibility results when available)	Duration of Antibiotics
Asymptomatic bacteriuria	Choice determined by culture susceptibilities	5 days
Simple cystitis	Amoxicillin-clavulanate (Augmentin) or 3rd-generation oral cephalosporins or Ciprofloxacin/Levofloxacin or Nitrofurantoin (if CrCL > 30 mL/min)	5–10 days
Pyelonephritis or complicated UTI	**Mild cases** IV Ceftriaxone (if no prior history of antibiotic resistance) **More severe cases** IV Piperacillin-Tazobactam or IV Carbapenem or IV Cefepime or Meropenem +/– Vancomycin (septic shock)	14 to 21 days

- Fluoroquinolones should be avoided as the empirical first choice whenever possible because of the higher probability for antibiotic resistance to develop.

- Definitive antimicrobial therapy should be directed at the organism isolated from urine culture, and the choice of antibiotic should be the most narrow-spectrum available. Duration of antibiotics is dependent on the type of UTI and risk factors that are present (Table 56.6).

- For those with a history or current multi-drug resistant UTI, treatment should be guided by an infectious disease physician.

- Imaging of the genitourinary tract is required in cases of recurrent UTI or severe infection. This is to exclude renal or perinephric abscess, obstruction, and emphysematous pyelonephritis (necrotising infection where gas in the renal parenchyma is detected on imaging).

- Immunosuppression generally do not need to be reduced or discontinued during treatment of UTI unless there is severe infection, e.g., septic shock.

Management of Asymptomatic Bacteriuria

- There is insufficient evidence at the time of writing to recommend or discourage screening and treating asymptomatic bacteriuria (ASB) in the first 1–2 months of KT. Treatment for 5 days can be considered if 2 consecutive urine samples grow $> 10^5$ of the same uropathogen. Treatment is not indicated if the 2nd urine culture shows clearance of the initial uropathogen or a different uropathogen is identified.

- Evidence is accumulating that screening and treating ASB after the first 1–2 months of KT may not be beneficial. Meta-analysis of 2 randomised controlled trials (RCTs) and one quasi-RCT of patients after the first 1–2 months of KT suggested no significant effect of antibiotics on the risk of symptomatic UTI or on graft related outcomes.

- Treatment for ASB may be appropriate in the following circumstances:

    - When there is a urinary catheter or DJ stent in the first month of KT

- Prior to invasive urologic procedures, e.g., DJ stent removal, cystoscopy, etc.
- Prior to a biopsy of the KT
- Prior to treatment or during treatment of allograft rejection
- When ASB is associated with a rise in sCr
- During pregnancy

ASB with multi-drug resistant bacteria will require a consult with an infectious disease physician to decide on the appropriate management. Treatment may be inappropriate as it may increase the risk of encouraging more antibiotic resistance.

- Asymptomatic candiduria may not need treatment unless prior to urologic procedures or when the patient is neutropenic — candida may be a coloniser of the bladder.

Management of Recurrent UTI

- It is important to identify and treat all risk factors for UTI in KT recipients with recurrent UTIs. Potential sources of recurrent infections include:
    - Urinary catheters
    - Ureteral stents
    - Nephrostomy tubes
    - Infected urinary stones
    - Infected kidney cysts
    - Native kidneys

However, no correctable risk factors may be identified in many patients (Figure 56.1).

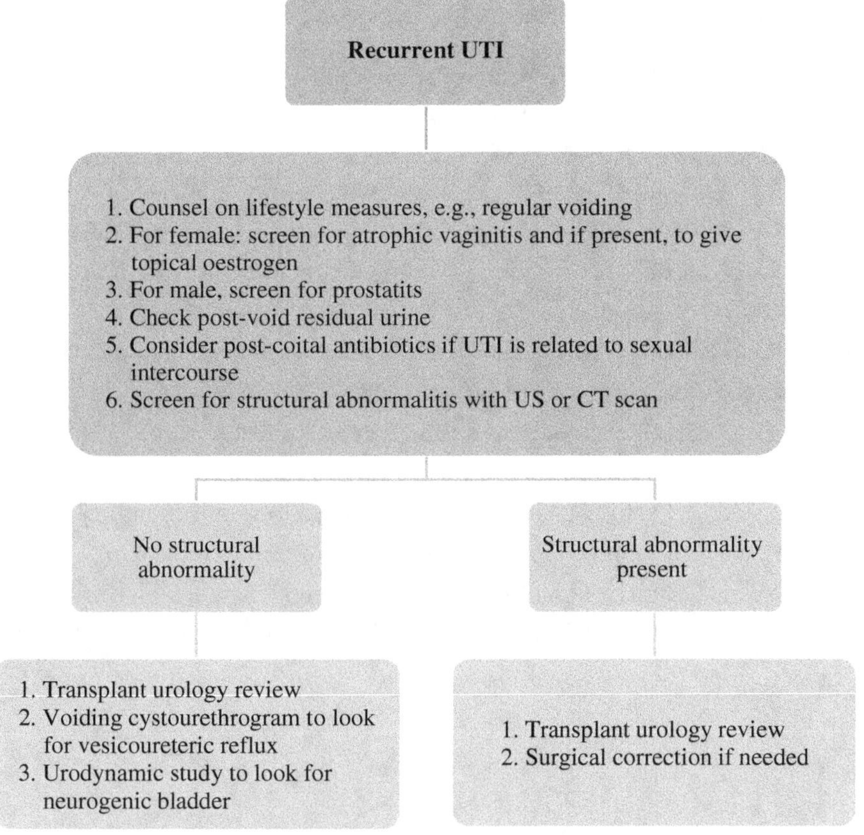

Figure 56.1:   Management of Recurrent Urinary Tract Infection

- In such cases, other measures may be considered as follows:

  - Extend the duration of antibiotics for the current episode of UTI, e.g., 4 to 6 weeks

  - Trial of long-term (e.g., 6 months) prophylaxis, but there is a risk of MDRO/XDRO

  - Consider reducing immunosuppression if it is immunologically safe to do so

  - Optimise glucose control in diabetics

References

Coussement J, Kaminski H, Scemla A and Manuel O (2020). Asymptomatic bacteriuria and urinary tract infections in kidney transplant recipients. *Curr Opin Infect Dis* **33**(6): 419–425.

Goldman JD and Julian K (2019). Urinary tract infections in solid organ transplant recipients: Guidelines from the American Society of Transplantation Infectious Diseases Community of Practice. *Clin Transplant* **33**(9): e13507.

Hollyer I and Ison MG (2018). The challenge of urinary tract infections in renal transplant recipients. *Transpl Infect Dis* **20**: e12828.

Hooton TM. (2012). Uncomplicated urinary tract infection. *N Eng J Med* **366**: 1028–1037.

Kee T, Lu YM and Vathsala A (2004). Spectrum of severe infections in an Asian renal transplant population. *Transplant Proc* **36**(7): 2001–2003.

Souza RM and Olsburgh J (2008). Urinary tract infection in the renal transplant patient. *Nat Clin Pract Nephrol* **4**(5): 252–264.

57 Cytomegalovirus

Terence Kee

Introduction

- Cytomegalovirus (CMV) is a ubiquitous beta-herpesvirus, which has significant clinical impact in KT as follows (Table 57.1).

- Primary CMV infections occur during childhood or early adulthood through contact with bodily fluids of CMV-infected individuals. Following primary infection, CMV establishes life-long latency, mainly in myeloid lineage cells.

- The 3 major mechanisms of acquiring CMV infection after KT are:

  a) Primary infection — seropositive donor kidney (CMV D+) to a CMV seronegative recipient (CMV R–), termed CMV D+R– KT or other sources (e.g., CMV D+ blood transfusion)

  b) Reactivation (of recipient CMV) or secondary infection (of donor CMV), termed CMV D+R+ or D–R+ KT

  c) Superinfection with a different strain of CMV that the recipient does not have (CMV D+R+ KT)

- CMV infection occurs mainly between 30 and 90 days after KT and is rare after 180 days, unless it is delayed due to the use of antiviral prophylaxis.

- Defects in CMV specific and innate immunity as well as the expression of proinflammatory cytokines leads to CMV

Table 57.1:   Effects of Cytomegalovirus Infection

Direct Effects	Indirect Effects	Non-clinical Effects
CMV Syndrome	Acute rejection	Increased total healthcare costs
Tissue invasive CMV Disease	Chronic rejection	Increased resource utilisation
	Opportunistic infections	Prolonged hospitalisation
	Arteriosclerosis	Repeat hospital admissions
	New-onset diabetes after transplantation	
	Cardiovascular disease	
	Malignancies	
	Mortality	

reactivation. Therefore, pharmacological immunosuppression, stress, and allograft rejection are risk factors for CMV reactivation (Table 57.2).

Table 57.2:   Risk factors for Cytomegalovirus Infections in Kidney Transplantation

- CMV D+R– kidney transplant
- Intense immunosuppression, e.g., exposure to antilymphocyte antibodies
- Severe lymphopenia, low CD4+ T-cell count
- HLA mismatches
- Genetic polymorphisms
- Allograft rejection
- CMV D+R– blood product transfusion
- Stress, e.g., critical illness, surgical procedures, bacterial and fungal sepsis

Definitions

- CMV DNAaemia — the detection of CMV DNA in blood

- CMV antigenaemia — the detection of CMV antigen in blood

- CMV viraemia — the detection of CMV in blood from viral culture

- CMV infection — evidence of CMV replication in tissue, blood or other bodily fluids (e.g., CMV DNAaemia), regardless of signs and symptoms. CMV replication is detected by (a) nucleic acid testing (NAT) via polymerase chain reaction (PCR), (b) antigen testing or (c) viral culture.

- Asymptomatic CMV infection — CMV replication without clinical signs or symptoms of disease

- CMV disease — evidence of CMV infection with clinical signs and symptoms. CMV disease can be classified as either (a) CMV viral syndrome or (b) CMV tissue-invasive disease (Table 57.3)

Table 57.3:   Definitions of Different CMV Diseases

Disease	Presumed Diagnosis	Confirmation
CMV syndrome	The presence of one or more of these signs: • Fever > 2 days • Malaise • Leukopenia • >5% atypical lymphocytes • Thrombocytopenia • Increased aminotransferases (>2-fold) • Evidence of active CMV infection	Clinical and laboratory evidence of CMV infection
Pneumonia	The presence of signs and symptoms of pneumonia plus evidence of CMV infection in the blood and/or bronchoalveolar lavage	Lung disease manifestations plus the presence of CMV in lung tissue based on immunohistochemistry with or without evidence of active CMV infection in the blood or bronchoalveolar lavage

(Continued)

Table 57.3:   (*Continued*)

Disease	Presumed Diagnosis	Confirmation
Gastrointestinal disease (esophagitis, gastritis, enterocolitis, colitis, pancreatitis)	The presence of signs and symptoms of gastrointestinal disease plus endoscopic signs of mucosal lesions and evidence of CMV infection in the blood	Gastrointestinal manifestations plus the detection of CMV in gastrointestinal tissues by immunohistochemistry
Hepatitis	An increase in liver enzymes and bilirubin levels (>2 fold) in the absence of other known causes plus evidence of CMV in the blood	The presence of increased live enzymes and bilirubin levels plus the presence of CMV in liver tissue, as determined by immunohistochemistry
Central nervous system disease	Neurological signs and symptoms in the absence of other known causes plus evidence of CMV (as detected by PCR) in the cerebrospinal fluid	Neurological signs and symptoms plus evidence of CMV infection in brain tissue, as detected by immunohistochemistry
Retinitis	Not applicable	Typical CMV lesions on the retina, as confirmed by an opthalmologist
Invasive disease in other organs, e.g., nephritis, myocarditis, pancreatitis	The presence of organ dysfunction in the absence of other known causes plus evidence of CMV in the blood	The presence of organ dysfunction, plus the presence of CMV in the target organ tissue, as detected by immunohistochemistry

- CMV tissue-invasive disease — evidence of CMV in tissue samples, e.g., inclusion bodies or viral antigens detected by immunohistochemistry except the central nervous system and retinal disease where CMV DNA in cerebrospinal or vitreous fluid suffice.

Pre-transplant screening

- Anti-CMV IgG should be performed for both the donor and recipient. The presence of CMV IgG does not protect against the reactivation of latent CMV or a new infection with a different CMV strain. Instead, the donor and recipient serostatus determines the risks for post-transplant CMV infection.

- An equivocal result for CMV IgG should be taken as a positive for the donor. For the recipient, it should be taken as a positive if the donor is seronegative or negative if the donor is seropositive.

- Recent blood transfusion or IVIG therapy may produce a false positive CMV IgG result.

- Donor or recipient with negative CMV serostatus should have their CMV IgG test repeated nearing or at the time of the kidney transplantation.

Post-transplant screening

- Either the CMV pp65 antigenaemia test or CMV DNAaemia test (using quantitative nucleic acid amplification testing or QNAT) can be used to screen for CMV infection after KT (Table 57.4).

- However, CMV pp65 antigenaemia or DNAaemia may not be present in compartmentalised CMV disease. For example, CMV DNAaemia may be absent in up to 50% of patients with CMV gastrointestinal disease. In such cases, histopathologic examination of tissue (for inclusion bodies) with immunohistochemical staining (for CMV antigen) or *in situ* DNA hybridisation (for CMV DNA) is required.

- Detection of CMV DNA in sites apart from cerebrospinal and retinal fluid may reflect viral shedding and thence needs to be interpreted in the context of clinical presentation and other

Table 57.4:   Comparison of CMV pp65 Antigen and CMV DNAaemia Test

	CMV pp65 Antigen Test	**CMV DNAaemia Test**
Description	• Detect pp65 antigen in CMV-infected peripheral blood neutrophils via immunostaining methods — this is a semi-quantitative measurement of viral load	• Detect CMV DNA in peripheral blood by quantitative real-time PCR
Units of measurement	• Number of polymorphonuclear cells infected	• Copies/mL or IU/mL
Advantages	• Less expensive • Does not require sophisticated and expensive equipment	• More expensive • More sensitive but may detect latent viral DNA (low-level CMV DNAaemia), which is not clinically significant • Broader linear range • Faster turnaround time • Higher throughput • Samples do not need to be processed immediately • World Health Organization International Reference Standard available
Disadvantages	• Labour intensive • Need to process sample within 6 to 8 hours of collection • Result interpretation is subjective, depending on the expertise of the laboratory technician	• Require expensive equipment and reagents • Less labour intensive • Not affected by leukopenia • Threshold of viral load to treat is not well defined — at the Singapore General Hospital, it is 1000 IU/mL.

Table 57.4:   (*Continued*)

CMV pp65 Antigen Test	CMV DNAaemia Test
• Threshold to treat is not well defined — at the Singapore General Hospital, it is 10 cells • Lack assay standardisation • Not sensitive when absolute neutrophil count < 1000/mm^3 • May not detect compartmentalised disease, e.g., retinitis, gastrointestinal disease	• May not detect compartmentalised diseases, e.g., retinitis, gastrointestinal disease

findings. For example, CMV pneumonia is defined by the detection of CMV DNA in bronchoalveolar lavage (BAL) fluid but combined with clinical symptoms and/or signs of pneumonia in the appropriate clinical setting.

CMV preventive strategies

- There are currently no effective vaccine against CMV for clinical use. Pre-emptive treatment, universal prophylaxis or a combination of both is used to prevent CMV disease after KT (Table 57.5).

- For CMV R– KT recipients who need blood product transfusion, the blood product should be from CMV seronegative donors (D–) or be leukocyte-depleted.

Pre-emptive treatment

- Pre-emptive treatment (PET) is scheduled monitoring for CMV infection (e.g., weekly CMV pp65 antigen or PCR test

Table 57.5:   Comparison of Pre-emptive Treatment vs. Universal Prophylaxis

Considerations	Universal Prophylaxis	Pre-emptive Treatment
Early CMV infection	Rare — as a result, it may be preferred for those at the highest risk for CMV, e.g., CMV D+R– and those receiving lymphocyte depleting antibodies	Common
Late CMV infection/disease	Common — need to monitor for CMV after discontinuation of prophylaxis, e.g., weekly for 3 months	Rare as CMV specific immunity develop earlier
Prevention of CMV disease	Good efficacy	Good efficacy only if weekly screening for CMV is performed
Drug resistance	Uncommon	Uncommon
Ease of implementation	Easy	More difficult
Patient adherence	Potential problem, especially if drug costs are an issue	Potential problem if the patient is not coming for a scheduled testing
Prevention of other herpes virus	Prevent herpes simplex and varicella zoster	Does not prevent
Other opportunistic infections	May prevent	Unknown
Costs	Drug costs	Monitoring costs
Safety	Drug toxicity	Less drug toxicity
Prevention of rejection	May prevent	Unknown
Graft survival	May improve	May improve

for at least 12 weeks post-transplant) and initiation of anti-CMV treatment at a pre-determined CMV pp65 antigen or DNA level (set by the individual transplant program). The aim is to prevent the progression of asymptomatic CMV infection to disease. Treatment is continued until the virus is no longer detectable or there is very stable low CMV DNAaemia on 2 consecutive weekly CMV tests.

Universal prophylaxis

- Universal prophylaxis (UP) is the administration of an anti-CMV drug around the time of transplantation for all at-risk patients to prevent CMV infection during a defined period where the risk for infection is the greatest, usually 3 to 6 months post-transplantation. It should be started within 10 days after KT. The duration of UP depends on the risks for CMV infection, e.g., 6 months for CMV D+/R− and those receiving lymphocyte depleting agents, otherwise 3 months for CMV D+/R+ and CMV D−/R+. Anti-CMV prophylaxis is not required for CMV D−/R− KT recipients.

Hybrid strategy

- A hybrid strategy is a combination of UP followed by PET to detect and treat post-prophylaxis delayed-onset CMV infection.

- PO Valganciclovir (VGCV) is the preferred drug for PET or UP, but it is costly, and its major toxicity is leukopenia (Table 57.6). IV Ganciclovir (GCV) is used early after transplantation when

Table 57.6: **Doses of Ganciclovir and Valganciclovir for the Treatment of CMV Infection or Disease**

Drug	>60 mL/min	40–60 mL/min	25–40 mL/min	10–25 mL/min	<10 mL/min
IV Ganciclovir	5 mg/kg BD	2.5 mg/kg BD	2.5 mg/kg/d	1.25 mg/kg/d	1.25 mg/kg after dialysis
PO Valganciclovir	900 mg BD	450 mg BD	450 mg OM	450 mg EOD	Not recommended

eGFR is < 10 mL/min or when there is a concern of gastrointestinal absorption. PO Valacyclovir can be used for UP but has a high pill burden and potential neurotoxicity. It is also not recommended for treatment of asymptomatic infection or CMV disease due to its lower efficacy.

- Anti-CMV prophylaxis should be given to patients treated for rejection for at least 1 to 3 months. Alternatively, a PET strategy may be employed to monitor and treat CMV infection as it arises.

Treatment of asymptomatic CMV infection

- Patients with asymptomatic CMV infection can be treated with PO VGCV. IV GCV should be used when gastrointestinal absorption is impaired (e.g., diarrhoea or vomiting) or when the viral loads are very high, where the risk of progression to symptomatic CMV disease is significant (Table 57.6).

- Renal panel, liver panel, FBC and CMV pp65 antigen or quantitative CMV PCR should be performed weekly.

- The patient should be monitored closely for the development of symptoms or laboratory abnormalities that may signify the onset of CMV disease.

- Treatment can stop once the CMV viraemia is undetectable or below detection limits on 2 consecutive weeks.

- Immunosuppression should be reduced to a degree appropriate to the severity of the infection or, if not possible, replace mycophenolate with everolimus while lowering the dose/ target level of the CNI. However, once the CMV infection is cleared, some immunosuppression may be increased but not to the previous doses, especially for those at high immunological a risk of rejection.

Table 57.7: Drugs Commonly Used for the Treatment of CMV Disease

Drug	Common Side Effects
Ganciclovir/valganciclovir	Myelosuppression
Foscarnet	Nephrotoxicity and electrolyte wasting
Cidofovir	Nephrotoxicity, Fanconi's syndrome, ocular toxicity
Immunoglobulins	Nephrotoxicity, thrombosis, haemolysis, transfusion-related acute lung injury

Treatment of CMV disease

- Patients with CMV disease (Table 57.7) should be admitted for IV GCV to quickly stabilise the infection and monitor for complications. Though PO VGCV has been used to treat mildly to moderately severe CMV disease, it has been associated with persistent viraemia at day 21 of treatment.

- Once the CMV disease is under control (e.g., symptoms are resolving or resolved, CMV viral load is reducing appropriately), it may be possible to switch to PO VGCV, provided the viral load is low and there is gastrointestinal absorption, e.g., no vomiting or diarrhoea.

- During treatment, patients are monitored once a week using CMV pp65 antigenaemia assay or CMV qPCR. The renal panel, liver panel, and FBC should also be monitored during treatment for the CMV disease so as to detect drug toxicity and myelotoxicity.

- With at least 2 weeks of appropriately dosed antiviral therapy, the CMV viral load should reduce by one-log.

- It is important that the antiviral drug dose be adjusted to changing the renal function but should not be reduced if leukopenia develops. Instead, the patient should be supported with GCSF (when the absolute neutrophil count is <1000/μL) and have other myelosuppressive drug therapies reduced or discontinued, e.g., bactrim, mycophenolate.

- Treatment should be continued for:

  a) a minimum of 2 weeks

  b) symptoms, signs and laboratory abnormalities of the disease is resolved and

  c) viraemia is undetectable or at very low levels on 2 consecutive measurements done a week apart

- IVIG or CMVIG may be given to patients who are CMV D+R– recipients or have severe CMV disease, drug-resistant virus, or hypogammaglobulinaemia, but the evidence for this is not clear. The dose and duration of CMV hyperimmune globulin should be discussed with an infectious disease physician.

- Immunosuppression should be reduced when there is CMV disease though this may be difficult in patients at high immunological risk of rejection or with recent rejection. In such cases, the physician may want to consider switching from mycophenolate to everolimus, which may also facilitate a lower target CNI level.

- Foscarnet and cidofovir are second-line alternative antiviral drugs for those who cannot tolerate VGCV or IV GCV. However, these drugs are nephrotoxic, and the patient should be forewarned. Letermovir may be an alternative in the future as it is not myelotoxic or nephrotoxic. However, the development of CMV resistance to letermovir is a limiting factor.

- After the completion of treatment, a 1–3-month course of secondary prophylaxis with PO VGCV may be given depending on the risks for relapse. Alternatively, the patient should be closely monitored for recurrent CMV viraemia after the discontinuation of treatment. This is because a recurrence of

CMV viraemia may occur in up to 35% of high-risk solid organ transplant recipients with CMV infection and disease.

- Once the CMV disease is cleared, immunosuppression may be increased but not back to previous doses, especially for patients at high risk of rejection due to the reduction of immunosuppression.

Refractory CMV

- Refractory CMV should be suspected if
  - (a) the viral load fails to decrease (<1 $\log_{10}$) or increases (>1 $\log_{10}$) despite 2 weeks of adequately dosed antiviral therapy
  - (b) clinical symptoms persist after 2 weeks of appropriately dosed antiviral therapy
- Risk factors for refractory CMV include:
  - (a) CMV D+R− recipients
  - (b) Over-immunosuppression — lacking CMV-specific T-cell immunity
  - (c) Ongoing active viral replication while on an antiviral drug
  - (d) Inadequate dose or absorption of an anti-CMV drug
  - (e) CMV resistance to an antiviral drug
  - (f) Prolonged antiviral drug exposure (usually >5 months)
  - (g) Exposure to antiviral drugs, which is a lower barrier to resistance
- Refractory CMV infection is associated with a higher rate of hospitalisation, increased length of hospital stay, higher health-care costs, increased rates of adverse events, rejection, graft loss, and mortality.

- Management of refractory CMV includes:
  - Ensuring that the calculated dose of GCV or VGCV is correct
  - If the patient was on PO VGCV, to ensure there is adherence to the antiviral therapy
  - Excluding GCV-resistant CMV
  - Reducing immunosuppression further or switching to an mTOR-inhibitor-based regimen
  - Converting to IV GCV if the patient was on PO VGCV

Ganciclovir-resistant CMV

- Ganciclovir (GCV)-resistant CMV should be suspected in patients
  - who fail to respond to at least 2 weeks of appropriately dosed antiviral treatment
  - whose CMV DNAaemia or disease recurs during prolonged antiviral therapy
- GCV-resistant CMV can develop in up to 3% of the cases — risk factors for GCV resistance include:
  a) Exposure to a prolonged subtherapeutic dose of antiviral drugs
  b) CMV D+R– recipient
  c) Intense immunosuppression
- GCV-resistant CMV possesses genetic mutations that reduce its susceptibility to anti-CMV drugs. It is usually associated with mutations in UL97 (code for a viral protein kinase that phosphorylates GCV into its active form) and UL54 (code for CMV DNA polymerase) genes.
- If GCV-resistant CMV is suspected, blood should be sent for genotypic testing of mutations in UL97 and UL54. Results are

more reliable when the CMV DNAaemia in the sample is at least 1000 IU/mL, and false negatives are possible.

- Immunosuppression should be cautiously reduced further, or a switch to a mTOR-inhibitor-containing regimen should be considered.

- An infectious disease specialist should also be consulted, as various types of mutations confer different degress of GCV resistance.

- The dose of IV GCV can be increased (up to 10 mg/kg BD, adjusted to renal function), or foscarnet (inhibit CMV DNA polymerase) can be given for GCV-resistant CMV. Subsequent antiviral therapy should be adjusted to the results of the genotypic testing when made available.

- Other agents that has been used to manage resistant CMV infection include cidofovir, CMV immunoglobulin or IVIG, maribavir, leflunomide, and artesunate.

- If available, an adoptive transfer of CMV-specific T-cells from autologous or allogeneic (organ donor or third party donors) has been used effectively for the treatment of resistant and refractory CMV after transplantation.

Very low CMV DNAaemia

- Current PCR assays can detect very low CMV DNA (<500 IU/ mL) in the absence of symptoms or signs of disease, which may clear with a slight reduction of immunosuppression or may eventually clear on its own.

- Very low CMV DNA may also persist following the completion of treatment for CMV infection or disease — newer guidelines suggest that treatment for CMV infection or disease can stop when very low CMV DNA is repeatedly detected a week apart.

Emerging CMV therapies where further studies are required

- Maribavir — inhibitor of UL97 kinase

- Letermovir — inhibitor of UL56 terminase

- Leflunomide — inhibit CMV virion assembly

- Artesunate — inhibit host cell function required for CMV replication

- CMV-specific T-cell therapy — autologous or third-party HLA matched CMV-specific T-cell therapy has been used as salvage therapy to clear CMV

- CMV monoclonal antibodies — Phase 2 studies of monoclonal antibodies like RG7667 demonstrate their effectiveness in reducing risk for CMV infection and disease, but further studies are required.

References

Kotton CN and Kamar N (2023). New insights on CMV management in solid organ transplant patients: Prevention, treatment, and management of resistant/refractory disease. *Infect Dis Ther* **12**(2): 333–342.

Kotton CN, Kumar D, Caliendo AM, *et al.* (2010). International consensus guidelines on the management of cytomegalovirus in solid organ transplantation. *Transplantation* **89**(7): 779–795.

Limaye AP, Babu TM and Boeckh M (2020). Progress and challenges in the prevention, diagnosis, and management of cytomegalovirus infection in transplantation. *Clin Microbiol Rev* **34**(1): e00043-19.

Razonable RR and Humar A (2019). Cytomegalovirus in solid organ transplant recipients — Guidelines of the American Society of Transplantation Infectious Diseases Community of Practice. *Clin Transplant* **33**(9): e13512.

58 BK Virus

Terence Kee

Introduction

- BK virus (BKV) is a DNA virus from the Polyomaviridae family. BK represents the initials of the patient where the virus was first isolated from the urine in 1971. BKV is the most common cause of polyomavirus associated nephropathy (PyVAN), but other polyomaviruses like John Cunningham (JC) and Simian Virus 40 (SV40) polyomavirus can also rarely cause PyVAN.

- Among 4 BKV genotypes, genotype 1 is the most common clinically encountered BKV. Infections with different genotypes may account for differences in responses to IVIG therapy.

- Primary BKV mucosal tract infection occurs during childhood in 90% and subsequently persists as a latent infection, predominantly in the renourinary tract. Occasionally, BKV can escape immune control and be detected in the urine.

- Immunosuppression and tissue injury can trigger BKV reactivation (in the donor or recipient uro-renal tract) (Table 58.1), leading to lytic replication in the tubular epithelium. As a result, tubular epithelial cell injury occurs, leading to inflammation and viruria (30%). If left uncontrolled, viraemia (15%) will occur 2–6 weeks later and may progress to BK virus associated nephropathy (BKVAN) (5%) in another 2–6 weeks. BKV infection can

Table 58.1:   Risk Factors for BKV Infection

Donor-related	Transplant-related	Recipient-related	Immunosuppression-related
• Deceased Donor • DCD • Donor viruria • BKV seropositivity	• Prolonged cold ischaemia time • DGF • Use of ureteric stent • ABO incompatibility • Higher degree of HLA mismatches • HLA A24, B55 • HLA-E genotype • Co-infection with CMV • ATN • Rejection episodes	• Older age • Younger age for children • Male gender • African-American • DM • Obesity • Haemoemodialysis • Antineutrophil cytoplasmic antibodies • Interferon-gamma gene polymorphisms • Re-transplant especially after graft loss due to PyVAN • Multiorgan recipient • BKV seronegativity • 1,25-dihydroxyvitamin D3 deficiency	• Depleting antibody therapies, e.g., thymoglobulin, Rituximab • Triple immunosuppression with Tacrolimus, Prednisolone and Mycophenolate • Higher tacrolimus levels • Higher steroid use

Abbreviations: ATN, acute tubular necrosis; BKV, BK virus; CMV, cytomegalovirus; DCD, donation after cardiac death; DGF, delayed graft function; DM, diabetes mellitus; HLA, human leukocyte antigen; PyVAN, polyomavirus associated nephropathy

also produce a cystitis or ureteric stricture. BKV may also be associated with a higher risk for urothelial malignancies.

- Both humoral and T-cell mediated immunity is important to suppress BKV infection. As a result, BKV infection is most common in the first year of transplantation when immunosuppression is the most intense. BKV seronegative recipients of seropositive kidney donor transplants have a higher risk of BKV infection than those who are seropositive, while those with adequate BKV-specific T-cell response have a lower risk for developing BKV viraemia.

- Some patients experience transient BK viraemia because their immune response is adequate to clear the virus. However, if immunity remains inadequate to clear BKV infection, up to 50% of patients may experience graft failure and return to dialysis. In the last 2 decades, graft loss is now less than 15% due to protocolised screening and preemptive reduction of immunosuppression.

Screening

- Screening for BKV is important because BKV infection is usually an asymptomatic infection, and by the time allograft dysfunction occurs, the infection has already progressed to a severe disease, manifesting with a high viral load, elevation in the serum creatinine, haematuria, and proteinuria. Therefore, earlier detection of BKV allows timely intervention and clearance of the infection before significant injury and fibrosis has occurred.

- Quantitative polymerase chain reaction (qPCR) testing for BKV in blood and urine is used to screen for BKV infection. Blood qPCR has a higher positive predictive value (50–82%) for

BKVAN than urine qPCR (31–67%). As a result, many transplant centres use blood qPCR for screening, but qPCR methods are not standardised, leading to intra- and inter-laboratory assay variability. In addition, most qPCR uses genotype 1 BKV DNA as the reference sequence and may be less sensitive for detecting other genotypes. This may account for a situation where the clinical course does not correlate with the viral load.

- When qPCR is not available, urine cytology can be obtained to detect BKV-infected tubular urothelial cells (called "decoy cells"). Decoy cells are identified by their large basophilic nuclei with ground glass intranuclear inclusion, but this finding is nonspecific and may also be found in uroepithelial cancer, JC polyomavirus, and adenovirus infection. Hence, their PPV is low. However, EM for cast-like polyomavirus aggregates (called "Polyomavirus Haufen or PyV-Haufen") in the urine has very high PPV (97%) and (100%) NPV. PyV-Haufen may also be useful for monitoring disease progression because levels of PyV-Haufen correlate better than qPCR for viral tubular injury, viral load, and disease classification.

- The American Society of Transplantation Infectious Disease Community of Practice (AST-IDCOP) recommends blood BKV qPCR monthly until month 9, and then every 3 months until 2 years, then reducing annually until 5 years, but individual transplant programs would have their own variations of this screening guideline. As 18% of BKVAN occurs after the 1st year of transplantation, blood BKV qPCR should also be episodically measured whenever there is allograft dysfunction, regardless of time after the transplantation.

- Probable and presumptive BKVAN can be diagnosed when the blood BKV viral load is persistently > 1000 copies/mL

(3 log 10 copies/mL) and >10,000 copies/mL (4 log 10 copies/mL), respectively, on 2 consecutive samples repeated 2 to 3 weeks apart. However, a definitive diagnosis of BKVAN requires a biopsy.

Diagnosis

- Biopsy of the kidney transplant is the gold standard for the diagnosis of BKVAN.

- The threshold to perform biopsy varies with individual transplant programs but should proceed if there is a concern for subclinical rejection or kidney dysfunction. It can also determine the extent of IFTA, which is prognostically important.

- The histological features of BKVAN include:

  - Cytopathic changes in the tubular epithelial cells (e.g., enlarged hyperchromatic nuclei with intranuclear inclusion bodies)

  - Inflammatory lymphocytic infiltrate

  - Interstitial fibrosis/tubular atrophy (IFTA)

  - Positive immunohistochemistry for Simian Virus 40 (SV40) Large T antigen (LTag) (expressed by the simian virus, JC and BKV). However, when there is an adequate immune response, clearance of SV40 LTag immunohistochemistry precedes the clearance of BKV viraemia by several weeks.

- AST-IDCOP 2019 recommends that histological findings of BKVAN be reported using the AST-IDCOP 2013 (Table 58.2) and Banff 2017 classification systems (Table 58.3).

- Acute rejection may co-exist with BKVAN histologically and can be suspected by the histological evidence of vascular and/or antibody-mediated rejection.

Table 58.2: American Society of Transplantation — Infectious Disease Community of Practice Histological Patterns of Polyomavirus Nephropathy (PyVAN)

Pattern	Description	Extent of Biopsy Score	Graft Function	Risk of Graft Loss
PyVAN-A				
Viral cytopathic changes	Mild	≤25%	Mostly baseline	<10%
Interstitial inflammation	Minimal	≤10%		
Tubular atrophy	Minimal	≤10%		
Interstitial fibrosis	Minimal	≤10%		
PyVAN-B				
Viral cytopathic changes	Variable	11–>50%	Mostly impaired	50%
Interstitial inflammation	Significant	11–>50%		
Tubular atrophy	Moderate	<50%		
Interstitial fibrosis	Moderate	<50%		
PyVAN-B1				
Interstitial inflammation	Moderate	11–25%	Slightly above baseline	25%
PyVAN-B2				
Interstitial inflammation	Significant	26–50%	Significantly impaired	50%
PyVAN-B3				
Interstitial inflammation	Extensive	>50%	Significantly impaired	75%
PyVAN-C				
Viral cytopathic changes	Variable	Variable	Significantly impaired	>80%
Interstitial inflammation	Variable	Variable	Progressive failure	
Tubular atrophy	Extensive	>50%		
Interstitial fibrosis	Extensive	>50%		

Table 58.3: Banff Working Group on the Polyomavirus Nephropathy Histologic Classification System

Class 1		Class 2		Class 3	
Pvl	Banff Ci Score	pvl	Banff Ci Score	pvl	Banff Ci Score
1	0–1	1	2–3	—	—
—	—	2	0–3	—	—
—	—	3	0–1	3	2–3

pvl 1: ≤1% of all tubules/ducts with viral replication
pvl 2: >1 to ≤10% of all tubules/ducts with viral replication
pvl 3: >10% of all tubules/ducts with viral replication

- Up to 30% of patients with BKVAN may have biopsies that do not show histological evidence of viral infection, especially when BKV viraemia is low and renal function remains stable. This is because BKV infection may be missed due to its multifocal distribution and initial medullary involvement in early disease. As a result, it is recommended that at least two biopsy core samples be obtained with at least one sample, including medullary tissue.

Management

- To date, there is no effective direct antiviral therapy for BKV infection. Drugs such as cidofovir, leflunomide and fluoroquinolones, which were purported to have anti-BKV properties, have not been shown to be beneficial in randomised controlled trials and/or systematic analysis.

- Reduction of immunosuppression is the first line of treatment. A usual trigger to reduce immunosuppression is when there is sustained BKV viraemia of more than 1000 copies/mL tested on 2 consecutive occasions performed 2 to 3 weeks apart or when 1 measurement is more than 10,000 copies/mL or when a biopsy shows BKVAN.

- Immunosuppression should be reduced in a stepwise fashion with a close monitoring of renal function and BKV viral load, e.g., 2 to 3 weekly serum creatinine and blood BKV qPCR. Donor-specific antibodies may also be measured to monitor for the risk of antibody-mediated rejection.

- Clearance of BKV infection is easier to achieve when viral loads are low, e.g., <10,000 copies/mL, but higher viral loads may take several months. Some patients may have persistent BKV infection despite substantial reduction of immunosuppression.

Approaches to reduction of immunosuppression

- There is no consensus on which is the best approach to reducing immunosuppression, and any of the following approaches may be effective. The choice of which component of the immunosuppression regimen to reduce depends on which drug is assessed to be contributing to significant immunosuppression (as measured by the drug concentration level or total daily dose) and/or which drug could be preferentially reduced without triggering a rejection.

- **Calcineurin inhibitor (CNI) first strategy** — The dose of CNI can be reduced to achieve trough levels (C0) values that are 1–2 ng/mL lower than previous target levels. If BKV persists despite stepwise reduction to lower C0 levels, CNI can be further reduced to achieve even lower C0 levels of less than 6 ng/mL for Tacrolimus or less than 150 ng/mL for Cyclosporine. However, CNI, whenever possible, should not be discontinued completely due to the risk of rejection. When very low C0 levels of CNI are desired, replacement of antimetabolite with an mTOR inhibitor may be required to mitigate the risk of rejection.

- **Antimetabolite first strategy** — Alternatively, a mycophenolate dose can be first reduced by 50% and then further reduced in a stepwise fashion according to the BKV viral load response. In many patients, the drug may have to be discontinued or replaced with Azathioprine or an mTOR inhibitor to avoid rejection.

- **Calcineurin inhibitor and antimetabolite first strategy** — This approach may be preferred when the viral load is very high or persistent. It may also be performed when doses of both drugs are very high, and there is an adequate buffer to reduce the dose without risk of rejection.

- If a patient is considered to be at high risk of rejection or where the dose cannot be reduced further, then a switch to a less potent immunosuppression is also possible, e.g., Tacrolimus to Cyclosporine, aiming for a C0 < 150 ng/mL, Mycophenolate to Azathioprine or MTOR inihibitor.

Intravenous Immunoglobulin

- Intravenous immunoglobulin (IVIG) has direct neutralising and immunomodulatory effects against BKV, especially to genotype I and II.

- May protect against acute rejection when immunosuppression is reduced, which may trigger the generation of donor-specific antibodies.

- Can be given when the BKV viral load is not decreasing with a reduction of immunosuppression or when further reduction of immunosuppression is associated with a high risk of rejection.

- The dose is 1–2 g/kg given over 24 to 48 hours on a monthly basis till BKV is cleared, or there is no longer a BKV clearance response.

BKV-specific T-cell therapy

- Infusion of a haplo-matched donor or off-the-shelf third-party BK-specific T-cells have been found to be effective and safe to clear BK viraemia. However, this therapy is expensive and limited to specialised centres.

Resumption of immunosuppression following the clearance of BKV infection

- Patients who had immunosuppression reduced for BKV are at higher risk of *de novo* DSA and rejection than those who had immunosuppression increased after the clearance of BKV.

- One protocol to resume immunosuppression following the clearance of BK is as follows:
  - After 4 weeks of undetectable viraemia, increase MMF by 500 mg/d every 2 weeks back up to its baseline pre-viraemia dosage, provided that the BKV remains undetected on every 2 weeks monitoring.
  - If BK viraemia remains undetectable for another 2 weeks, adjust the tacrolimus dose to achieve target trough levels of 5–7 ng/mL.

Prognosis

- Persistent BK viraemia is associated with progressive IFTA.
- High-level BK viraemia, deceased donor transplantation, late acute rejection, and renal fibrosis are associated with an increased risk of graft loss.
- Graft loss due to BKVN is not a contraindication to re-transplantation, but blood BKV qPCR should be negative prior to re-transplantation.

References

Cohen-Bucay A, Ramirez-Andrade SE, Gordon CE, *et al.* (2020). Advances in BK virus complications in organ transplantation and beyond. *Kidney Med* **2**(6): 771–786.

Hirsch HH, Randhawa PS and AST Infectious Diseases Community of Practice (2019). BK polyomavirus in solid organ transplantation — Guidelines from the American Society of Transplantation Infectious Diseases Community of Practice. *Clin Transplant* **33**(9): e13528.

Jahan S, Scuderi C, Francis L, *et al.* (2020). T-cell adoptive immunotherapy for BK nephropathy in renal transplantation. *Transpl Infect Dis* **22**(6): e13399.

Kant S, Dasgupta A, Bagnasco S and Brennan DC (2022). BK virus nephropathy in kidney transplantation: A state-of-the-art review. *Viruses* **14**(8): 1616.

Myint TM, Chong CHY, Wyld M, *et al.* (2022). Polyoma BK virus in kidney transplant recipients: Screening, monitoring, and management. *Transplantation* **106**(1): e76–e89.

Nelson AS, Heyenbruch D, Rubinstein JD, *et al.* (2020). Virus-specific T-cell therapy to treat BK polyomavirus infection in bone marrow and solid organ transplant recipients. *Blood Adv* **4**(22): 5745–5754.

Nickeleit V, Davis VG, Thompson B and Singh HK (2021). The urinary polyomavirus-haufen test: A highly predictive non-invasive biomarker to distinguish "presumptive" from "definitive" polyomavirus nephropathy: How to use it-when to use it-how does it compare to PCR based assays? *Viruses* **13**(1): 135.

Nickeleit V, Singh HK, Randhawa P, *et al.* (2018). The Banff Working Group classification of definitive polyomavirus nephropathy: Morphologic definitions and clinical correlations. *J Am Soc Nephrol* **29**(2): 680–693.

59   Long-Term Management of the Kidney Transplant Recipient

Liew Ian Tatt

Introduction

- Kidney transplant (KT) offers improved quality of life and survival for the patient with end-stage kidney disease (ESKD) for as long as the allograft function is maintained. Continued follow-up is required to maintain the allograft health, mitigate complications, and optimise outcomes for the patient.

- Cardiovascular disease, infections and cancers are the leading causes for mortality for kidney transplant recipients (KTRs) and require continued surveillance for early detection and treatment. Additionally, the recurrence of glomerulonephritis, gout and management of fertility are issues that need to be addressed.

Cardiovascular disease

- KT offers a survival benefit over remaining on dialysis, but the life expectancy of a KT recipient remains shorter than an age-matched individual from the general population. This is partly due to an increased incidence of cardiovascular disease (annual event rate of 3.5–5%) among KT recipients (though this incidence is lower than that among dialysis patients).

Table 59.1:　Cardiovascular Risk Factors for KT Recipients

Conventional Risk Factors	Non-conventional Risk Factors
• Hyperlipidaemia	• CMV infection
• Hypertension	• CKD, including mineral bone disease, chronic inflammation and uraemic milieu
• DM	
• Smoking	• Deranged neurohormonal axis, including renin-angiotensin-aldosterone system
• Obesity	
• Family history	• Endothelial dysfunction
• Age	• Advanced donor age
• Male gender	• Donor-recipient nephron mismatch
• South Asian and African American ethnicity	• Allograft dysfunction
	• Drugs, including steroids, CNIs

Abbreviations: CKD, chronic kidney disease; CMV, cytomegalovirus; CNI:, calcineurin inhibitors; DM, diabetes mellitus.

- KT recipients carry the burden of cumulative traditional and non-traditional cardiovascular risks factors through their lifetime with chronic kidney disease (CKD) (Table 59.1).

- All KT recipients should undertake lifestyle modifications to reduce their cardiovascular risks, such as:

  - Low sodium intake (<2 g/d)

  - Moderate intensity physical activity (≥150 min/wk)

  - Balanced diet

  - Maintaining a normal body mass index (18.5–24.9 kg/m^2) and waist circumference (<102 cm)

  - Reducing alcohol

  - Stopping smoking

Post-transplant diabetes mellitus

- Post-transplant diabetes mellitus (PTDM) is a common complication after KT — at Singapore General Hospital, the cumulative incidence was 15.8%, 22.8% and 24.5% at 1, 3 and 5 years following KT, depending on the prevailing risk factors (Table 59.2).

Table 59.2:   Risk Factors for Post-Transplant Diabetes Mellitus

Non-modifiable	Potentially Modifiable	Modifiable
• African-American	• Rejection (preventable)	• Obesity
• Hispanic	• Deceased donor (aim	• LDL-cholesterol
• Age > 45 years	for living donor)	• Corticosteroids
• Family history of DM	• Hepatitis C	• CNI
• HLA mismatches	• CMV	• mTOR inhibitor
• HLA A30, B27, B24	• Pre-transplant impaired	• Vitamin D
• Male donor	glucose tolerance	deficiency
• Donor liver steatosis	or impaired fasting	
• Genetic polymorphism	glucose	
• Polycystic kidney	• Proteinuria	
disease	• Hypomagnesaemia	

Source: Pham PT, Sarkar M, Pham PM, *et al.* (2000) Diabetes mellitus after solid organ transplantation. *Endotext*. MDText.com, Inc.

Abbreviations: CMV, cytomegalovirus; CNI, calcineurin inhibitor; DM, diabetes mellitus; HLA, human leukocyte antigen; mTOR, mammalian target of rapamycin; LDL, low density lipoprotein

- Potential KT candidates should be screened for DM through a review of medical/family history and laboratory tests (fasting plasma glucose, HbA1c). Those with prediabetes should be counselled on lifestyle modifications.

- Post-transplant hyperglycaemia is common, but the diagnosis of post-transplant diabetes mellitus (PTDM) can only be made 45 days after transplantation while on a stable dose of oral corticosteroids (Table 59.3).

Table 59.3:   The 2022 American Diabetes Association Diagnostic Criteria for Prediabetes and Diabetes

Test	Prediabetes	Diabetes Mellitus
HbA1c	5.7–6.4%	≥6.5%
Fasting plasma glucose	5.6–6.8 mmol/L	≥7 mmol/L
2-hour plasma glucose from oral glucose tolerance test	7.8–11.1 mmol/L	≥11.1 mmol/L
Random plasma glucose		≥11.1 mmol/L

- PTDM is associated with an increased risk of infections, cardiovascular disease, graft loss and mortality, so it is important to adopt preventive measures in routine post-transplant care, such as diet, physical activity, and weight loss. Some centres may initiate basal insulin for the treatment of post-transplant hyperglycaemia in an effort to "rest" the islet cells of the pancreas, which may reduce the subsequent development of PTDM.

- Screening for PTDM should be performed after KT (Table 59.4). Screening thereafter may be performed annually with fasting plasma glucose and HbA1c. Oral glucose tolerance test should be performed in those with suspected glucose disorders.

- Treatment of PTDM follows that of type II diabetes in the general population, with a target HbA1c < 7% for the general KTR population (Table 59.5). PTDM may be treated with oral anti-hyperglycaemic agents and/or insulin.

Table 59.4:   Screening for Post-Transplant Diabetes Mellitus

Time Post-transplantation (days)

Day 0–45	**Day 46–365**	**Day > 365**
Routine blood tests Presence of hyperglycaemia (do not diagnose as PTDM)	**Screening tests** 1. Fasting/ random glucose 2. OGTT 3. HbA1C	**Screening tests** 1. Fasting/random glucose 2. OGTT 3. HbA1C
Management of post-transplantation hyperglycaemia • Day 0–7: Insulin • Day 8–45: Insulin, oral anti-hyperglycaemic agents	**Management of post-transplantation diabetes mellitus** • Lifestyle modification • Oral anti-hyperglycaemic agents • Insulin	

Abbreviations: HbA1C, haemogloblin A1C; OGTT, oral glucose tolerance test; PTDM, post-transplant diabetes mellitus.

Source: Pham PT, Sarkar M, Pham PM, et al. (2000) Diabetes mellitus after solid organ transplantation. Endotext. MDText.com, Inc.

Table 59.5:   Screening and Management of Post-Transplant Diabetes Mellitus (PTDM)

Screening and Management	Comments
PTDM screening Baseline HbA1c at 3 months after KT, then at 6 and 12 months, and annual thereafter.	If screening HbA1c is in the prediabetic range, patients should be counselled on dietary and lifestyle modification and have HbA1c monitored every 3 months
Newly diagnosed PTDM Refer to dietician	Consider referring to an endocrinologist
Dietary modification Dietary modification with carbohydrate-controlled diet	Limit cholesterol intake to < 200 mg/d <7% of calories from saturated fats 2–3% of calories from trans-fatty acids ≤2400 mg of sodium per day >25 g of dietary fibre per day 2 servings of fish per week
Lifestyle modification Exercise, weight reduction or avoidance of excessive weight gain, smoking cessation	Define realistic goals, e.g., target weight loss of 5–10% of total body weight
Pharmacologic therapy Target HbA1c 7–7.5%, not to fall below 6% (particularly if hypoglycaemia is frequent) Treatment options — GLP-1 agonist, DDP-4 inhibitor, SGLT2 inhibitor, insulin	Acute, marked hyperglycaemia generally require inpatient management and IV insulin.
Adjustment or modification of immunosuppression Aim for a nadir prednisolone dose of 5 mg/d Routine corticosteroid withdrawal is not recommended Consider cyclosporine-based immunosuppression if multiple PTDM risk factors are present	Clinicians must be familiar with the patient's immune history before manipulating immunosuppression therapy. Immunosuppression adjustment to reduce PTDM risk in high immunological risk patients is not recommended.

Abbreviations: DPP-4 inhibitor, Dipeptidyl Peptidase 4 inhibitor; GLP-1 agonist, glucagon-like peptide-1 receptor agonist; HbA1C, haemogloblin A1C; IV, intravenous; KT, kidney transplant; PTDM, post-transplant diabetes mellitus; SGLT2, sodium-glucose cotransporter-2 inhibitor

Source: Pham PT, Sarkar M, Pham PM, *et al.* (2000) Diabetes mellitus after solid organ transplantation. *Endotext*. MDText.com, Inc.

Hypertension

- Hypertension (HTN) is common (>70%) amongst KT recipients due to essential HTN or secondary HTN risk factors (Table 59.6).

- HTN in KT recipients is associated with a higher frequency of graft dysfunction, cardiovascular disease, poorer graft, and patient survival. Each 10 mmHg increase in systolic BP is associated with an 18% increased risk of death. Lowering systolic BP to ≤140 mmHg has been shown to improve graft survival.

- Lack of clinical trial data limits our understanding on the optimal treatment targets of HTN for KTRs.

- Both calcium channel blockers (CCBs), angiotensin-converting enyzme inhibitors (ACEIs) and angiotensin receptor blockers

Table 59.6:   Risk Factors for Hypertension after Kidney Transplantation

Donor Factors	Recipient Factors	Immunosuppression	Allograft
• Age • Hypertension • Expanded criteria donor • Female to male KT • Pediatric to adult KT • Low donor/ recipient body weight ratio	• Age • Male gender • Smoking • Pre-existing hypertension • Obesity • Insulin resistance • Obstructive sleep apnea • Native kidneys • Hyperparathyroidism • Genetic factors • Polycynthaemia	• Corticosteroids • Calcineurin inhibitors	• Delayed graft function • Chronic kidney disease • Interstitial fibrosis and tubular atrophy • *De novo* and recurrent glomerulonephritis • Acute rejection • Anti-angiotensin II type 1 receptor antibody • Transplant renal artery stenosis

Abbreviation: KT, kidney transplant

(ARBs) have been shown to improve graft survival and are recommended as first-line treatment for HT in KT recipients.

- CCB are recommended as a first-line antihypertensive agent of choice based on several small trials demonstrating improved patient and graft outcomes. Biological explanations purported for the benefit of using CCB include its vasodilatory effects, which may mitigate the vasoconstrictive effect of calcineurin inhibitors (CNIs) in the allograft. A common adverse effect of CCB is leg oedema, which can be severe and does not improve with diuretics.

- Non-dihydropyridine CCBs (e.g., Diltiazem, Verapamil) inhibit CYP3A and P-glycoprotein, which lead to reduction of clearance of CNI and a corresponding increase in drug concentration levels. This drug interaction has been deliberately exploited to reduce doses of CNI and, thence, medication costs, especially for CYP3A5 expressors. However, if non-dihydropyridine CCBs need to be discontinued, the dose of CNI must be increased, and the drug concentration level should be closely measured to ensure adequate immunosuppression.

- ACEi and ARB may be used in particular if patients have other indications for it, e.g., proteinuria, cardiac disease. A doppler of the KT should be performed to exclude renal artery stenosis (RAS) prior to commencing ACEi/ARB. Common adverse effects of ACEi/ARB are anaemia and hyperkalaemia.

Dyslipidaemia

- Like HTN, dyslipidaemia is common (> 60%) among KT recipients who experienced elevations in total cholesterol, LDL-cholesterol and triglycerides.

- Dyslipidaemia after KT is associated with an increased risk of ischaemic heart disease and post-transplant mortality.

- Screening for dyslipidaemia should take place around 3 months when the CNI and corticosteroid dose are lowered and stabilised. Annual screening for dyslipidaemia is also recommended thereafter.

- Beta-hydroxy beta-methylglutaryl-CoA (HMG-CoA) reductase inhibitors (statins) are recommended to treat dyslipidaemia in KT recipients. This is based on benefits observed from the ALERT trial.

- The ALERT trial randomised 2100 stable KT recipients to fluvastatin or placebo. After a median follow-up of 5.1 years, the fluvastatin arm demonstrated a reduction in low-density lipoprotein (LDL) concentrations of 32%, with reductions in non-fatal myocardial infarction and cardiac death by 35%. However, the trial was inadequately powered for its primary composite outcome (cardiac death, non-fatal myocardial infarction, coronary intervention), and there were no significant differences between the groups with respect to this.

- CNIs, mammalian target of rapamycin inhibitors (mTORis) and statins share common hepatic enzymatic pathways, most importantly, the CYP3A4 enzymes. Co-administration of CNIs/mTORIs with a statin results in competition for these shared enyzmes of metabolism. This results in decreased enzymatic clearance of statins, which may result in statin-toxicity with rhabdomyolysis (Table 59.7).

Table 59.7: Recommended Daily Limits of Statin Therapy when Used in Combination with a Calcineurin Inhibitor or Mammalian Target of Rapamycin Inhibitor

Immunosuppression	Statin	Statin AUC Increase	Recommended Daily Limit
Cyclosporine	Atorvastatin	6–15 fold	10 mg
Tacrolimus	Fluvastatin	2–4 fold	40 mg
Everolimus	Lovastatin	5–20 fold	Avoid combination
Sirolimus	Pravastatin	5–10 fold	20 ng
	Rosuvastatin	7 fold	5 mg
	Simvastatin	6–8 fold	Avoid combination

Malignancy

- Malignancies after KT may be donor-transmitted, developed *de novo* or be a recurrence of a patient's pre-transplant malignancy. In general, malignancies that are more common among KT recipients are those associated with viral infections since immunosuppression impairs T-cell-mediated immunosurveillance of oncogenic viruses (Tables 59.8 and 59.9).

- At Singapore General Hospital, the incidence rate of malignancy was 3-fold higher than that in the general population, with the commonest malignancy being post-transplant lymphoproliferative disorder (PTLD). The cumulative incidence of malignancy was 1%, 4% and 10% at 1, 5 and 10 years, respectively. A diagnosis of malignancy was also associated with a poorer prognosis — the 10-year survival rate for KT recipients with malignancy was 64% compared to 83% for those without malignancy.

Table 59.8:   Standard Incidence Ratio of Cancers Following Kidney Transplantation

Standard Incidence Ratio*	Common Cancers Following Kidney Transplantation
>5	Kaposi's sarcoma Non-melanomatous skin cancers Post-transplant lymphoproliferative disorder Kidney Vulvar Penile Anogenital Liver Oropharyngeal
2–5	Cervical Thyroid Melanoma Oesophageal Multiple myeloma Leukaemia Oropharyngeal Bladder Colon
<2	Breast Ovarian Uterine Pancreatic Brain Prostate Testicular Lung

*The standard incidence ratio reflects the fold-increased risk of a malignancy in the kidney transplant recipient compared with the general population.

Source: Manickavasagar R and Thuraisingham, R (2020). Post-renal transplant malignancy surveillance. *Clin Med (Lond)* **20**(2): 142–145.

Table 59.9:   Viruses Associated with Post-Transplant Malignancies

Virus	Associated Post-renal Transplant Malignancy
Epstein–Barr Virus (EBV)	Post-transplant lymphoproliferative disorder Smooth muscle tumour
Human Papilloma Virus (HPV)	Squamous cell carcinoma
Human Herpes Virus 8 (HHV8)	Kaposi sarcoma, multiple myeloma
Human Immunodeficiency Virus (HIV)	Plasmablastic lymphoma, Merkel cell carcinoma
Hepatitis C Virus (HCV)	Hepatocellular carcinoma, plasma cell neoplasm
BK Virus (BKV)	Urothelial carcinoma

Source: Turshudzhyan A (2021). Post-renal transplant malignancies: Opportunities for prevention and early screening. *Cancer Treat Res Commun* **26**: 100283.

- All KT recipients should be counselled on general lifestyle modifications that may lower the risk of cancer, such as:
  - Smoking cessation
  - Limiting alcohol consumption
  - Dietary modifications — less red and processed meat, less refined grains and sweets, more poultry, fish, fruits, vegetables, beans, and other legumes
  - Maintaining a healthy weight
  - Remaining physically active with regular exercises
- Cancer screening after KT is extrapolated from the general population, with screening of specific cancers being of more value, such as skin, cervical, colorectal, and native kidney cancer (Table 59.10).

Table 59.10:   Common Cancer Prevention and Screening Tests for Kidney Transplant Recipients

Cancer	All Kidney Transplant Recipients	Prevention	Screening
Skin cancer	No age cut-off	Sunscreen, wear hats, avoid exposure to ultraviolet radiation during the sun peak hours.	Regular self-examination and skin examination by a physician at least annually.
Colorectal cancer	All aged 50 years and older	General lifestyle modifications	Faecal occult blood once every year or colonoscopy every 5–10 years. Those with a family history of colorectal cancer or personal history of colorectal polyp/malignancy or ovarian/endometrial cancer will need screening by colonoscopy.
Kidney cancer	No age cut-off	General lifestyle modifications, control BP	Screening for kidney cancer after KT is not universally practised across the world — at Singapore General Hospital, US screening is performed annually.
Hepatocellular carcinoma	No age cut-off	General lifestyle modifications, treat HBV/HCV	At least annual US and serum AFP for those with chronic HBV/HCV, cirrhosis and other liver disease.
Post-transplant lymphoproliferative disorder	No age cut-off	If possible, avoid EBV+ donor if potential recipient is EBV–. If EBV viral load rising in an EBV D+R– recipient, consider Rituximab.	Screen with quantitative EBV DNA if EBV D+R- monthly for 6 months and 3-monthly for 1 year.

Abbreviations: AFP, alpha-fetoprotein; D+, seropositive donor; DNA, deoxyribonucleic acid; EBV, epstein-barr virus; HBV, hepatitis B virus; HCV, hepatitis C virus; KT, kidney transplant; R+, seropositive recipient; US, ultrasound.

Cancer	Female Kidney Transplant Recipients	Prevention	Screening
Cervical cancer	All women who ever had sexual intercourse aged 25–69 years old	Risk of cervical cancer may be mitigated with HPV vaccinations, which are safe to be given even after KT. However, this does not confer 100% protection, and screening should still continue even amongst the vaccinated.	Papanicolaou (Pap) smear once every 3 years for women aged 25–29 years. High-risk HPV DNA testing once every 5 years for women aged 30–69 years. At age 69, women can stop screening if they have two consecutive negative HPV tests in the last 10 years, with the latest test done within the last 5 years.
Breast	All women aged 50–69 years of age	Breast feeding and limiting postmenopausal hormone therapy may be beneficial.	Mammogram every 2 years

Cancer	Male Kidney Transplant Recipients	Prevention	Screening
Prostate	All men aged 50–75 years of age	General lifestyle modifications	Annual digital rectal examination and prostate-specific antigen (PSA); notably, PSA levels may be lower in those on sirolimus.

Abbreviations: DNA, deoxyribonucleic acid; HPV, human papillomavirus; KT, kidney transplant; PSA, prostate specific antigen

- When a KT recipient is diagnosed with a cancer, reduction or withdrawal of immunosuppression is often attempted to restore some immune control over malignant cells. However, there is no consensus over this, and the approach is largely dependent on the physician's practice and individual patient's circumstances. Some considerations for adjusting immunosuppression after a diagnosis of cancer include:

  - Expected curability and prognosis — there may be no benefit if the cancer is advanced and the patient is for palliative treatment.

  - Immunologic risks of rejection — if the risks for rejection is high, it may be appropriate to minimise the dose of more oncogenic immunosuppressive agents and use immunosuppressive agents with anti-oncogenic properties, e.g., minimise calcineurin inhibitors with the use of mammalian target of rapamycin inhibitors instead of mycophenolate analogues (Table 59.11)

  - Type of cancer treatment — Some cancer treatments may be associated with significant myelotoxicity, and there may be a need to significantly reduce or stop specific immunosuppressive drugs. The use of immune-checkpoint inhibitors is associated with an increased risk of rejection. It is prudent to discuss treatment and anticipated adverse effects of chemotherapeutics with the oncologist to determine how the immunosuppressive regimen should be adjusted.

Hyperuricaemia and gout

- Hyperuricaemia (>416 μmol/L) and gout occurs in up to 80% and 28% of KTRs, respectively, due to risk factors such as

Table 59.11: Impact of Immunosuppressive Agents on Cancer Risk and Management

Immunosuppressive Agents	Cancer Risk	Cancer Management
Calcineurin inhibitors	Apart from T-cell suppression, it increases risk of cancer via TGF-β, p53 and IL-6 pathways.	Reduction of dose or withdrawal
Thymoglobulin	Increase risk of PTLD through impairment of T-cell immune surveillance	Avoid or minimise exposure
Azathioprine	Increase risk of skin cancer by sensitising the skin to ultraviolet radiation and DNA mutation	Reduction of dose or withdrawal or switch to other agents, e.g., mTOR inhibitors or mycophenolate
Mammalian target of rapamycin inhibitor	Inhibit cancer growth through cell-cycle arrest and initiation of apoptosis	Can replace azathioprine or mycophenolate to facilitate lower dose or withdrawal of calcineurin inhibitor

Source: Modified from Wong G and Chapman JR (2008). Cancers after renal transplantation. *Transplant Rev (Orlando)* **22**(2): 141–149.

metabolic syndrome, HTN, reduced GFR, calcineurin inhibitor (especially cyclosporine), diuretics, and other drugs associated with hyperuricaemia.

- Unlike the general population, hyperuricaemia has not been associated as a cardiovascular risk factor for KT recipients, but new-onset gout after KT is associated with graft loss and patient death.

- To reduce the risk of hyperuricaemia and gout, KT recipients should avoid alcohol, lose weight, and adopt a low purine diet, e.g., reduced consumption of seafood and meat.

- For acute gout attacks, NSAIDs and COX-2 inhibitors should be avoided whenever possible in KT recipients because of potential nephrotoxicity. Dose-adjusted colchicine can be given, but KT recipients are at a higher risk for colchicine myotoxicity (especially if on cyclosporine), presenting with muscle weakness and elevated creatinine kinase. As a result, an alternative may be to increase the dose of maintenance oral prednisolone (e.g., 20 mg for 5 days) or use IV hydrocortisone until the attack has resolved. The dose can then gradually reduce back to its baseline dose over a week to avoid a relapse of acute gout. If the patient is already on uric acid lowering therapy, this should not be discontinued during an acute attack of gout.

- Uric acid lowering therapy should be initiated for patients with hyperuricaemia and gouty arthritis, tophaceous gout, gouty erosive changes on X-rays, or recurrent attacks ($\geq$ 2 attacks/year). The starting dose should be low (according to GFR) and titrated to clinical response.

- If graft function is adequate (creatinine clearance > 30 mL/min), an uricosuric agent such as probenecid may be used to lower serum uric acid. However, urine volume should be at least 1500 mL/min, and the urine should be alkalinised (target pH 6.4–6.8) to avoid urate nephropathy and/or uric acid stones. Patients with a history of renal calculi and/or poor urine volume should not receive probenecid.

- Xanthine oxidase (XO) inhibitors such as allopurinol and febuxostat are alternatives and reduce the production of uric acid from purines. However, they should be avoided in KT recipients on azathioprine. Azathioprine is converted to its active metabolite 6-mercaptopurine (6-MP) in the liver, which is further catabolised by XO to inactive metabolites. As a result, XO inhibitors substantially inhibit the catabolism of 6-MP and the resultant accumulation 6-MP causes significant myelosuppression manifesting in potentially life-threatening pancytopenia.

- In KT recipients who are of Chinese, Thai or Korean ethnicity, they should be tested for the HLA-B*58:01 allele, which is associated with severe hypersensitivity reactions to allopurinol. HLA-B*58:01 positive patients should not receive allopurinol.

- For KTRs on azathioprine whose creatinine clearance is too low for probenecid, azathioprine may be switched to Mycophenolate Mofetil to allow the use of XO inhibitors.

- During the initiation of uric acid lowering therapy, patients should be on maintenance corticosteroids or low-dose colchicine to prevent gout attack. These can be discontinued while the target uric acid level is achieved or tophi have resolved.

- In difficult-to-control cases of gout, patients on tacrolimus may switch to cyclosporine with improvement in uric acid and control of gout. Another option is a switch to mTOR inhibitors. Anti-hypertensive therapy may also need to be adjusted. For example, losartan and amlodipine can increase uric acid clearance and reduce serum uric acid levels.

References

Acuna SA, Huang JW, Scott AL, *et al.* (2017). Cancer screening recommendations for solid organ transplant recipients: A systematic review of clinical practice guidelines. *Am J Transplant* **17**(1): 103–114.

Al-Adra D, Al-Qaoud T, Fowler K and Wong G (2022). *De novo* malignancies after kidney transplantation. *Clin J Am Soc Nephrol* **17**(3): 434–443.

Alexandrou ME, Ferro CJ, Boletis I, *et al.* (2022). Hypertension in kidney transplant recipients. *World J Transplant* **12**(8): 211–222.

Bee YM, Tan HC, Tay TL, *et al.* (2011). Incidence and risk factors for development of new-onset diabetes after kidney transplantation. *Ann Acad Med Singap* **40**(4): 160–167.

Dumanski SM and Ahmed SB (2019). Fertility and reproductive care in chronic kidney disease. *J Nephrol* **32**(1): 39–50.

Hecking M, Haidinger M, Döller D, *et al.* (2012). Early basal insulin therapy decreases new-onset diabetes after renal transplantation. *J Am Soc Nephrol* **23**(4): 739–749.

Kidney Disease: Improving Global Outcomes (KDIGO) Blood Pressure Work Group (2021). KDIGO 2021 clinical practice guidelines for the management of blood pressure in chronic kidney disease. *Kidney Int* **99**(3S): S1–S87.

Pham PT, Sarkar M, Pham PM and Pham PC (2000). Diabetes mellitus after solid organ transplantation. *Endotext.* MDText.com, Inc.

Teo SH, Lee KG, Lim GH, *et al.* (2019). Incidence, risk factors and outcomes of malignancies after kidney transplantation in Singapore: A 12-year experience. *Singapore Med J* **60**(5): 253–259.

Special Patients and Care

60 Pregnancy in Patients with Chronic or End-Stage Kidney Disease

Phang Chee Chin, Kwek Jia Liang

Structural changes in the kidney and urinary tract during pregnancy

- Functional hydronephrosis (dilation of ureters, kidney calyces, and pelvis) occurs in up to 80% of pregnant women and is more prominent on the right than the left. These anatomical changes increase the size of the kidneys size by 1 to 1.5 cm.

- Hormonal effects and external compression contribute to hydronephrosis and hydroureter observed during pregnancy. The dilated urinary tract results in urinary stasis and can potentially serve as a reservoir for bacteria, increasing the risk of pyelonephritis during pregnancy.

Functional changes in the kidney and urinary tract during pregnancy

- Functional changes also occur in response to the hormonal changes and metabolic demands of pregnancy (Table 60.1).

Table 60.1: Clinical and Laboratory Changes in Kidney Function During Pregnancy

Investigations	Non-pregnant State	Pregnancy
Plasma osmolality (mOsm/kg)	285	270–275
Serum sodium (mmol/L)	140	135
Serum creatinine (μmol/L)	62–88	35–53
Creatinine clearance (mL/min)	100	150
24-hr urine protein (mg/day)	<150	<300
Blood urea (mmol/L)	5–14	6–9
Arterial blood pH	7–40	7.44
Arterial PCO_2 (mm Hg)	40	30
Serum bicarbonate (mmol/L)	25	18–20
Serum uric acid (μmol/L)	178–356	119–297
Systolic blood presure (mm Hg)	100–120	90–110
Diastolic blood pressure (mm Hg)	60–80	50–70

- Kidney plasma flow increases by 80% by 12 weeks of gestation but decreases in the third trimester.

- With the increase in kidney plasma flow rate, the glomerular filtration rate (GFR) increases, peaking at 40–50% above baseline by the early second trimester and then declines slightly towards term.

- As a result of this physiological increase in the GFR, the serum creatinine concentration is lower (<77 μmol/L) and urinary protein excretion is higher (up to 300 mg/day) during normal pregnancy.

- Pregnancy also causes a fall in systemic vascular resistance, which is reflected by lower blood pressure (BP) and mean arterial pressure (MAP).

- There is also increased tubular excretion of glucose, amino acids, and uric acids. Erythropoietin, vitamin D and renin production are also increased.

Pregnancy in patients with chronic kidney disease

- Chronic kidney disease (CKD) at any stage increases the risk of pregnancy related complications, while pregnancy itself can hasten the progression of CKD (Table 60.2).

Table 60.2:   Complications During Pregnancy in Patients with Chronic Kidney Disease

Related to Chronic Kidney Disease	Related to Pregnancy
• Accelerated loss of kidney function • Worsening proteinuria or hypertension • Possible need for dialysis during pregnancy or the postpartum period • Urinary tract infections • Allosensitisation, which may increase difficulty in finding a histocompatible kidney donor for a kidney transplant	• Gestational hypertension • Pre-eclampsia • Intrauterine growth retardation • Spontaneous abortion • Intrauterine foetal death • Stillbirths • Polyhydramnios, especially in women on dialysis (due to foetal osmotic diuresis from high foetal blood urea levels) • Preterm delivery (<37 weeks gestation) • Small for gestational age/low birth weight • Caesarean delivery • Admission to the neonatal intensive care unit

- Pregnant women with CKD are at increased risk of worsening kidney function during pregnancy, with the risk being higher with worsening degrees of kidney dysfunction (Table 60.3).

- The risks of pregnancy-related complications increases with worsening severity of kidney dysfunction (Table 60.4) and other risk factors (Table 60.5).

- Urinary protein excretion increases during pregnancy due to increased GFR and glomerular basement membrane permeability. However, urinary protein excretion exceeding

Table 60.3:   Risks of Progression of CKD During Pregnancy According to Kidney Function

	Low Risk	**Moderate Risk**	**High Risk**
Description	Pregnancy may infrequently contribute to the progression of CKD	Potential pregnancy-related progression of CKD, especially with multiple risk factors present	Progression of CKD is very high and may require dialysis in pregnancy or within 6 months postpartum, especially with multiple risk factors present
Risk of increase in GFR stage	<15%	15–50%	>50%
Serum creatinine	124 μmol/L	124–212 μmol/L	>212 μmol/L
Blood pressure	<130/80 mmHg	130–139/80–90 mmHg	≥140/90 mmHg
Proteinuria	<1 g/day	1–3 g/day	>3 g/day

Abbreviations: CKD, chronic kidney disease; GFR, glomerular filtration rate

Source: Modified from Reynolds ML and Herrera CA (2020). Chronic kidney disease and pregnancy. *Adv Chronic Kidney Dis* **27**(6): 461–468.

Table 60.4:   Estimated Effects of Pre-Pregnancy Kidney Function on Pregnancy Outcomes

Mean Pre-Pregnancy Serum Creatinine (μmol/L)	**Effects on Pregnancy Outcomes**			
	Foetal Growth Retardation (%)	**Preterm Delivery (%)**	**Pre-Eclampsia (%)**	**Preinatal Deaths (%)**
<125	25	30	22	1
125–180	40	60	40	5
>180	65	>90	60	10
On dialysis	>90	>90	75	50*

* If conceived on dialysis, 50% of the infants survive. If conceived before introduction of dialysis, 75% of the infants survive.

Source: Williams D and Davison J (2008). Chronic kidney disease in pregnancy. *Br Med J (Clin Res Ed)* **336**(7637): 211–215.

Table 60.5:   Risk Factors for Adverse Outcomes in Pregnancy Among Patients with Chronic Kidney Disease

Proteinuria	• The risk of adverse outcomes increases as the baseline level of proteinuria rises. • Proteinuria > 1 g/day is associated with significant risks for adverse pregnancy and neonatal outcomes among women with CKD.
Chronic hypertension	Maternal chronic hypertension is associated with an increased risk of • Pre-eclampsia and preterm delivery, particularly before 34 weeks gestation. • Lower foetal survival when baseline BP is uncontrolled (>140/90 mmHg).
Baseline eGFR	• For women with early CKD (eGFR > 60 mL/min/1.73 m^2), the risk of progression is low in the absence of other risk factors. On the other hand, women with CKD experience increasing risk for progression of CKD as the baseline eGFR falls. • It is essential to counsel patients on the potential need to initiate dialysis during preconception counselling and pregnancy, especially among women with stage 4–5 CKD.
Aetiology of kidney disease	• The impact of the aetiology of CKD on pregnancy outcomes is less than the stage of CKD, proteinuria level, and chronic hypertension. • However, the presence of systemic disease is a significant predictor of adverse events, e.g., active lupus nephritis or previous nephritis predicts a worse pregnancy outcome with a significant increase in preterm delivery. Pregnancy itself increases the potential of a disease flare during any trimester or early postpartum. • Diabetic kidney disease has significantly higher rates of all adverse pregnancy outcomes, and uncontrolled diabetes is associated with a higher risk for congenital malformations and perinatal death.

300 mg/day is abnormal. Proteinuria occurring after 20 weeks is likely due to pre-eclampsia, while proteinuria developing before 20 weeks is likely due to an underlying kidney disease.

Principles of management

- Pregnancy in women with CKD is considered a high-risk pregnancy — both pregnancy (Table 60.6) and CKD (Table 60.7) aspects should be managed by a multidisciplinary team consisting of an obstetrician, nephrologist, expert midwife, dietician, pharmacist, and medical social worker, covering several areas of care.

Table 60.6: Management of Pregnancy in Women with Chronic Kidney Disease

Maternal Management	Interventions
Pre-pregnancy counselling	• Appropiate contraception in sexually active patients — avoid oestrogen containing contraceptives due to their cardiovascular risks. • Assess and stratify of risks for pregnancy complications and poor foetal outcomes. • Genetic counselling is required for those with genetic kidney diseases. • Determine timing for conception with consideration of age, fertility and activity of primary kidney disease.
Optimisation of maternal health prior to conception	• Stabilise primary kidney disease activity on minimal doses of medications that are appropriate for pregnancy (3–6 months observation period to ensure disease remains inactive is advised) • Control blood pressure • Optimise diabetes control • Address comorbidities • Provide adequate vaccination • Start folic acid — 0.4 mg daily for pregnancy at low risk for foetal neural tube defects (NTDs) and up to 5 mg for those at higher risk of foetal NTDs.

Table 60.6:   (*Continued*)

Maternal Management	Interventions
Review of medications	• Schedule time for withdrawal of ACEI or ARB • Discontinue or replace potential teratogenic medications • Monitor for disease relapse or flare after discontinuing or replacing medications, e.g., blood pressure, lupus activity
Diagnosis of pregnancy	• Use both serum β-HCG and US. β-HCG alone should not be used to diagnose pregnancy as levels may be low or high in non-pregnant women with CKD and ESKD. US confirms the presence of a viable foetus and estimates the gestational age for those with an elevated β-HCG.
Pregnancy care	• Pre-eclampsia prophylaxis with aspirin 75–150 mg/day if there are no contraindications before 12 weeks of gestation • Thromboembolic prophylaxis, as indicated
Dialysis	• Intensify dialysis during pregnancy (see Table 60.5)
Maternal surveillance	• Screen for gestational diabetes mellitus • Monitor for pre-eclampsia • Angiogenic markers (e.g., placental growth factor [PIGF], soluble fms-like tyrosine kinase [sFlt-1]) can be considered as an adjunct to diagnose superimposed pre-eclampsia but their exact role remains to be defined by future research.
Foetal surveillance	• Foetal surveillance – first and second trimester screening – growth scan after 28 to 30 weeks – doppler studies – cardiac monitoring in women with anti-Ro$^+$/La$^+$ antibodies
Plan delivery	• In the absence of an initiation for earlier delivery, plan the scheduling delivery by 39–40 weeks of gestation • Vaginal delivery is preferred, while caesarean delivery is performed for standard obstretric indications • If magnesium needs to be used to treat pre-eclampsia or eclampsia, levels need to be monitored — loading and continuous doses need to be reduced by 50% in patients on dialysis
Postpartum	• Breastfeeding is possible depending on the drugs that the patient is on • Provide contraception counselling

Abbreviations: ACEI, angiotensin-converting enzyme inhibitor; ARB, angiotensin receptor blocker; CKD, chronic kidney disease; ESA, erythropoietin-stimulating agents; ESKD, end-stage kidney disease; HCG, human chorionic gonadotropin; US, ultrasound

Table 60.7: Management of Chronic and End-Stage Kidney Disease During Pregnancy

Management	Approach
Frequency of clinic visits	• 1st trimester — monthly visit • 2nd trimester — fortnightly visit • 3rd trimester — weekly visit • Patients on dialysis will need to be monitored more frequently, e.g., weekly to 2-weekly, due to intensified dialysis and risks of electrolyte disturbances.
Routine tests for clinic visits	• Blood pressure • Weight • Electrolytes — renal panel, calcium, phosphate • Fasting glucose • Liver panel • Full blood count • UFEME • Urine C/S • Urine protein:creatinine ratio
Blood pressure	• Aim to maintain BP 110–135/70–85 mmHg on pregnancy appropriate medications • Too low a BP may cause foetal growth retardation, while too high a BP may cause progression of CKD • Avoid intradialytic hypotension in patients on HD
Proteinuria	• Non-dihydropyridine calcium channel blockers may reduce proteinuria to some extent during pregnancy • If there is significant oedema, loop diuretics, compression stockings, and elevation of the lower limbs may be advised. • To consider prophylactic anticoagulation (e.g., subcutaneous low-molecular weight heparin) during pregnancy and post-partum period for women with low risk of bleeding and nephrotic or subnephrotic range proteinuria with additional risk factors.
Dialysis initiation	• In patients with progressive CKD, consider initiating dialysis when the maternal urea concentration is 17–20 mmol/L, taking into account the gestational age, trajectory of kidney function decline, biochemical parameters, blood pressure, fluid status, and uraemic symptoms.

Table 60.7:   (*Continued*)

Management	Approach
Dialysis	• Intensify dialysis (to at least 36 hours/week) — increase duration and frequency of HD or increase number of exchanges in patients on PD. However, some have recommended women on PD to switch to HD in the first trimester so that adequate solute clearance can be achieved in the first trimester patients on PD. This is because there is a higher incidence for small gestational age infants born from women on PD compared to those on HD. • Aim for a pre-dialysis urea < 12.5 mmol/L, which has been associated with a lower risk of extreme prematurity (<30 weeks) and perinatal death. KT/V is not validated in pregnancy and cannot be used as an indicator of dialysis adequacy during pregnancy. • For HD, use a dialysis solution with higher potassium (3 mmol/L) and calcium (1.5 mmol/L) • Loop diuretics may be discontinued when there is intensified dialysis, which will achieve better fluid volume control. • Electrolytes will need to be monitored during intensified HD as hypokalaemia, hypocalcaemia and hypophosphataemia may develop. • Close monitoring and adjustment of dry weight because weight increases during pregnancy — avoid intradialytic hypotension, which may compromise uteroplacental perfusion.

Nutrition	• Refer to a dietician familiar with the nutritional needs of pregnant women with CKD or ESKD.
	• For patients with non-dialysis dependent CKD
	  ▪ Dietary restrictions may need to be adjusted because pregnancy is a hypercatabolic state while appetite may be reduced if there is worsening uraemia and metabolic acidosis.
	  ▪ Hyperkalaemia can be controlled with potassium-binding resins.

(*Continued*)

Table 60.7:   (*Continued*)

Management	Approach
	• For HD patients, adjust nutritional intake to meet the metabolic demands of pregnancy and intensified HD treatments: ■ Increase protein intake to 1.5–1.8 mg/kg/day and caloric intake to 25–35 kcal/kg/day ■ Increase water-soluble vitamins supplementation on intensified HD ■ PO_4 restriction may not be necessary with intensified dialysis ■ Electrolyte supplementation may be required — magnesium, potassium, phosphate
Metabolic bone disease	• Non-calcium-based phosphate binders should be switched to calcium-based phosphate binders because of safety concerns during pregnancy. • Among patients on intensified dialysis, phosphate control would be good and dietary phosphate restrictions may not be required. • Cinacalcet should be discontinued during pregnancy • Vitamin D analogues can be prescribed as appropriate • Aim for normal calcium and phosphate levels — avoid hypercalcaemia, which can cause foetal hypoparathyroidism
Anaemia	• Maintain a haemoglobin level of 10–11 g/dL, haematocrit 30–35% and ferritin 200–300 μg/mL • As haemoglobin falls during pregnancy, an increase in the dose of ESA is usually necessary • Maintain adequate iron stores using oral and/or intravenous iron sucrose as required
Postpartum care	• Monitor kidney function, which may deteriorate postpartum. • Monitor and manage kidney diseases, which may relapse. • Readjust medications as required, taking note of the drugs that are excreted in breast milk. • Patients on dialysis can return to their pre-pregnancy dialysis prescriptions. However, patients on PD who underwent caesarean section will have to wait

Table 60.7:   (*Continued*)

Management	Approach
	4–6 weeks for the wounds to heal before resuming PD.
	• Avoid excessive diuresis or ultrafiltration, which may impair breast milk production.
	• Patients should be closely monitored following delivery — serial monitoring of kidney function and proteinuria is required.
	• Medications should be reviewed and adjusted following delivery.
	• Patients should not be given nonsteroidal anti-inflammatory drugs for pain control.
	• Psychosocial support is important as the risks of postpartum depression is higher.

Abbreviations: CKD, chronic kidney disease; C/S, culture and sensitivity; ESA, erythropoiesis-stimulating agent; ESKD, end-stage kidney disease; HD, haemodialysis; PD, peritoneal dialysis; UFEME, urine full examination and microscopy

- At Singapore General Hospital, among pregnant patients on dialysis, the live birth rate was 82%. Severe hypertension occurred in 57%. Other complications included polyhydramnios (18%), premature rupture of the membranes (18%), obstretric cholestasis (18%), postpartum haemorrhage (9%), and foetal anomaly (9%).

- It is important to appreciate when assessing kidney function during pregnancy that a failure to see a physiological increase in GFR and/or fall in creatinine may reflect kidney dysfunction.

Medications in Pregnancy

- All child-bearing-age women who are started on medications with potential teratogenic effects should be counselled before starting the medication and offered the appropriate contraception (Table 60.8).

Table 60.8:　Management of Medications During Pregnancy

Drug	Pregnancy	Lactation	Considerations
Angiotensin-converting enzyme inhibitors and angiotensin receptor blockers	Unsafe	Safety data available for captopril and enalapril	Foetotoxic in 2nd and 3rd trimesters
Antihypertensive drugs			
Labetalol	Safe	Safe	Avoid if asthmatic
Nifedipine	Safe	Safe	Avoid if depression or if at risk of depression
Amlodipine	Limited data	Safe	
Hydralazine	Safe	Safe	
Methyldopa	Safe	Avoid in all: risk of postnatal depression	
Immunosuppressive drugs			
Glucocorticoids	Safe	Safe. Small amounts in the breast. If high dose, consider timing feeds to 4 h post administration	Potential maternal risks: Diabetes, hypertension, pre-eclampsia, infection, preterm rupture of membranes. Recent studies show no increased risk in orofacial clefts
Hydroxychloroquine	Safe	Safe	Risk of flare with discontinuation during pregnancy. It may reduce the risk of congenital heart block if there are maternal anti-Ro/SSA and/or anti-La/SSB antibodies.

Tacrolimus	Safe	Safe	Frequent monitoring during pregnancy and immediately postpartum. May require a higher dose during pregnancy
Cyclosporine	Safe	Safe	
Azathioprine	Safe	Safe. Low concentration in breast milk.	Check thiopurine methytransferase activity status before pregnancy or dosing
Cyclophosphamide	Unsafe	Excreted in breast milk. Discontinue breastfeeding during and for 36 h after treatment.	Effective contraception during and for 3 months after treatment. Risk of infertility, which is dose- and age-related
Mycophenolic acid analogues, e.g., Mycophenolate mofetil (Cellcept©) Sodium mycophenolate (Myfortic©)	Unsafe	Avoid use during lactation due to insufficient data	Effective contraception during and for 6 weeks after discontinuation of mycophenolic acid analogues
Sirolimus Everolimus	Unsafe	Avoid	Effective contraception during and for 12 weeks after discontinuation of the drug

- If a patient is deemed clinically stable to conceive, teratogenic drugs should be stopped or changed to pregnancy-safe medications when they express the wish for pregnancy.

- Patients should be monitored for at least 6 months after medication change for disease relapse or flare before attempting to conceive.

- Breastfeeding is not contraindicated in patients but needs to take into account the drug concentration in breast milk and impact on the neonate (Table 60.8).

References

Fitzpatrick A, Mohammadi F and Jesudason S (2016). Managing pregnancy in chronic kidney disease: Improving outcomes for mother and baby. *Int J Women's Health* **8**: 273–285.

Higby K, Suiter CR, Phelps JY, *et al.* (1994). Normal values of urinary albumin and total protein excretion during pregnancy. *Am J Obstet Gynecol* **171**(4): 984–989.

Hui D and Hladunewich MA (2019). Chronic kidney disease and pregnancy. *Obstet Gynecol* **133**(6): 1182–1194.

Jones DC and Hayslett JP (1996). Outcome of pregnancy in women with moderate or severe renal insufficiency. *N Engl J Med* **335**(4): 226–232.

Piccoli GB, Cabiddu G, Attini R, *et al.* (2015). Risk of adverse pregnancy outcomes in women with CKD. *J Am Soc Nephrol* **26**(8): 2011–2022.

Reynolds ML and Herrera CA (2020). Chronic kidney disease and pregnancy. *Adv Chronic Kidney Dis* **27**(6): 461–468.

Tan LK, Kanagalingam D, Tan HK and Choong HL (2006). Obstetric outcomes in women with end-stage renal failure requiring renal dialysis. *Int J Gynaecol Obstet* **94**(1): 17–22.

Wiles K, Chappell L, Clark K, *et al.* (2019). Clinical practice guideline on pregnancy and renal disease. *BMC Nephrol* **20**(1): 401.

Williams D and Davison, J (2008). Chronic kidney disease in pregnancy. *Br Med J (Clin Res Ed)* **336**(7637): 211–215.

Zhang JJ, Ma XX, Hao L, *et al.* (2015). A systematic review and meta-analysis of outcomes of pregnancy in CKD and CKD outcomes in pregnancy. *Clin J Am Soc Nephrol* **10**(11): 1964–1978.

61 Pregnancy in Kidney Transplantation

Liew Ian Tatt

- Infertility and sexual dysfunction in chronic kidney disease (CKD) and end-stage kidney disease (ESKD) is attributed to hormonal factors, medications and psychosocial factors (Table 61.1).

Table 61.1: Factors Contributing to Infertility in Patients with Chronic or End-Stage Kidney Disease

Men	Women
• Abnormal sex hormone levels — ↑ LH, FSH, PRL, ↓ oestrogen, progesterone	• Abnormal sex hormone levels — ↑ LH, FSH, PRL, oestrogen, ↓ Testosterone, AMH
• Loss of cyclicity of sex hormones	• Decreased sperm quantity and quality
• Anovulation	• Reduced libido
• Oligomenorrhea/amenorrhea	• Sexual dysfunction
• Abnormal endometrial morphology	• Medications
• Reduced ovarian reserve	
• Reduced libido	
• Sexual dysfunction	
• Medications	

Abbreviations: AMH, anti-Müllerian hormone; FSH, follicle-stimulating hormone; LH, luteinising hormone; PRL, prolactin

Source: Modified from Dumanski SM and Ahmed SB (2019). Fertility and reproductive care in chronic kidney disease. *J Nephrol* **32**(1): 39–50.

- A functioning allograft in women restores the hypothalamic-pituitary-gonadal axis, with regular menses and ovulatory cycles returning as early as 3 weeks after the kidney transplant (KT). This does not always occur in all women and may be due to allograft dysfunction, other comorbidities, and medications.

- Male KT recipients may also experience improvement in reproductive and sexual health, but spermatogenesis may be impaired with mammalian target of rapamycin inhibitor (mTORi) therapy.

- Pregnancy after KT is considered a high-risk pregnancy. Prenatal counselling, assessment and management by the transplant nephrologist and obstetrician is required to prepare for and, if possible, reduce possible complications during pregnancy (Table 61.2). Incidence of complications vary with centres, but at Singapore General Hospital, the reported complication rates are pre-eclampsia (50%) and preterm birth (70%). One graft loss (10%) was reported due to medication non-adherence.

Table 61.2: Complications of Pregnancy in Female Kidney Transplant Recipients

Recipient	Allograft	Foetus
• Hypertension	• Progression of pre-existing chronic kidney disease	• Miscarriages
• Pre-eclampsia		• Foetal growth restriction
• Gestational diabetes	• Worsening of proteinuria	• Intrauterine death
• Ectopic pregnancy	• Acute rejection during pregnancy	• Stillbirth
• Caesarean section	• Postpartum rejection	• Premature rupture of membranes
	• Pyelonephritis	• Preterm delivery
	• Graft loss	• Small for gestational age
		• Low birth weight
		• Birth defects

Pre-pregnancy

- Women are advised to wait at least 1 year after KT before trying to conceive, but the waiting period may be shortened or extended, individualised to the patient's condition. Prior to this, they should practise consistent contraceptive use. Some types such as oestrogen-containing contraceptives, may not be appropiate in women with specific risk profiles. Importantly, contraceptives are not always completely effective in KT recipients; e.g., mycophenolate can reduce oestrogen levels in patients on oestrogen-containing contraceptives, which will reduce their efficacy.

- Detailed review and increased level of monitoring is required before and after pregnancy (Table 61.3). Before embarking on

Table 61.3:   Transplant Screening and Monitoring Tests Before and During Pregnancy

Before Pregnancy	During Pregnancy
• Renal panel	• Visit schedule — every 3 weeks up to 20 weeks, every 2 weeks up to 28 weeks, then every week thereafter
• Glucose	
• Calculated GFR and CrCL	
• Liver panel	• BP daily
• $CaPO_4$	• Renal panel
• Uric acid	• Glucose
• HbA1c	• Calculated GFR and CrCL
• OGTT	• Liver panel
• Immunosuppressive drug level	• $CaPO_4$
• FBC	• Uric acid
• UFEME	• Immunosuppression drug level
• Urine C/S	• FBC
• Urine protein:creatinine ratio	• UFEME
• 24-hour urinary CrCL	• Urine C/S
• 24-hour urinary total protein	• Urine protein:creatinine ratio

(Continued)

Table 61.3:   (*Continued*)

Before Pregnancy	During Pregnancy
• Serologies — HBV, HCV, HIV, HSV, CMV, toxoplasmosis, rubella • Quantitative CMV PCR • Quantitative BKV PCR • US doppler kidney • RH status of patient and transplant, if possible	• OGTT each trimester • If seronegative at baseline, CMV IgM and toxoplasmosis IgM at each trimester • Quantitative CMV PCR at each trimester

Abbreviations: BKV, BK virus; Ca, calcium; CMV, cytomegalovirus; CrCL, creatinine clearance; C/S, culture and sensitivity; FBC, full blood count; UFEME, urine full examination and microscopy; GFR, glomerular filtration rate; HbA1c, haemoglobin A1C; HBV, hepatitis B virus; HCV, hepatitis C virus; HSV, hepatitis simplex virus; OGTT, oral glucose tolerance test; PCR, polymerase chain reaction; PO4, phosphate; RH, rhesus; US, ultrasound

conception, a female KT recipient should fulfill the following criteria:

- Allograft function must be stable — sCr $\leq$133 μmol/L

- There should be no or minimal proteinuria (<500 mg/d)

- No rejection should have occurred in the past 12 months

- Blood pressure must be well controlled ($\leq$140/90 mmHg)

- There is no active infection, especially fetotoxic ones, e.g., cytomegalovirus (CMV)

- Immunosuppressive drug levels are stabilised, and the patient is adherent to therapy and follow-up

- Patients should be suitable for conversion to azathioprine if they are on mycophenolate analogues or mTORi — in multi-ethnic Singapore where thiopurine methyltransferase (TPMT) activity may be variable in the asian population, TPMT activity should be determined prior to pregnancy.

- Absence of other comorbidities that are associated with poor pregnancy outcomes

- Apart from counselling, the medication regimen would also need to be reviewed and adjusted to remove or replace drugs with potential teratogenicity and/or fetotoxicity, e.g.:
    - Mycophenolate and mTORi should be replaced by azathioprine.
    - Atenolol should also be replaced as it is associated with foetal growth retardation. Other anti-hypertensive drugs (e.g., calcium channel blockers, labetolol, methyldopa, hydralazine) can replace angiotensin-converting enzyme inhibitors and angiotensin receptor blockers.
    - Trimethoprim sulfamethoxazole (TMP-SMX) should be discontinued during pregnancy.

  A washout period of at least 6 weeks (for mycophenolate), 8 weeks (for everolimus) or 12 weeks (for sirolimus) is recommended before attempting conception. Allograft and liver function should be closely monitored for at least 3 months to ensure the patient is tolerating drug changes before attempting conception.

- Female KT recipients should receive non-live vaccinations recommended for pregnancy in the general population, e.g., influenza, pneumococcus, hepatitis B, Tdap (diptheria, tetanus and pertussis), and COVID-19.

Pregnancy

- Aspirin (to reduce risk of pre-eclampsia) and folic acid (to prevent neural tube defects) should be started if there are no contraindications.

- Baseline oral glucose tolerance test should be performed to assess risks for diabetes mellitus, and a referral to the dietician should be made to ensure appropriate nutrition during pregnancy.

- Asymptomatic bacteriuria (ASB) during pregnancy increases the risk of pyelonephritis, preterm labour, low birth weight infants, and perinatal mortality. ASB should be screened at every visit and treated with the appropiate antibiotics according to sensitivities of the uropathogen and suitability of use during pregnancy. Kidney function and repeat urine culture should be repeated after the completion of antibiotics.

- For CMV R- women, CMV IgM and CMV PCR should be tested at each trimester, and if CMV infection is diagnosed, valacyclovir is preferred over valganciclovir/ganciclovir (VGCV/GCV) due to the latter's teratogenicity.

- Immunosuppressive drug levels should be monitored during every visit as levels may drop (especially 2nd trimester and thereafter) due to an increased volume of distribution, reduced protein/red blood cell binding, and increase in hepatic clearance. Dose of calcineurin inhibitors (CNI) may have to increase by 20–25% during pregnancy.

- Allograft dysfunction may occur during pregnancy, especially those with pre-pregnancy allograft dysfunction, proteinuria, hypertension, and recent (within 3 months of pregnancy) rejection. Rejection occurs in 1.3 to 9.4% and can be confirmed with a biopsy, preferably during the 1st and 2nd trimester. Treatment include high-dose corticosteroids and intravenous immunoglobulin, and some have reported the use of thymoglobulin, Rituximab and plasmaphresis.

Labour and delivery

- Stress dose corticosteroids are recommended if the patient is on maintenance steroid regimens.

- Vaginal delivery is possible in KT recipients, while caesarean section is performed for general obstetric indications. The risk of trauma to the KT and its ureter is 1–2%, and an ultrasound should be performed post-operatively to exclude unintentional injury.

- Postpartum, graft function, and immunosuppressive drug levels should be closely monitored till stabilisation is observed.

Lactation

- Breast feeding is not absolutely contraindicated if they are not on mycophenolate or mTORi (where there is insufficient data).

- Very low levels of immunosuppression has been detected in breast milk and appears safe for CNI, prednisolone and azathioprine.

References

Gonzalez Suarez ML, Parker AS and Cheungpasitporn W (2020). Pregnancy in kidney transplant recipients. *Adv Chronic Kidney Dis* **27**(6): 486–498.

Kham SK, Soh CK, Liu TC, *et al.* (2008). Thiopurine S-methyltransferase activity in three major Asian populations: A population-based study in Singapore. *Eur J Clin Pharmacol* **64**(4): 373–379.

Kwek JL, Tey V, Yang L, *et al.* (2015). Renal and obstetric outcomes in pregnancy after kidney transplantation: Twelve-year experience in a Singapore transplant center. *J Obstet Gynaecol* **41**(9): 1337–1344.

Lee EJ and Kalow W (1993). Thiopurine S-methyltransferase activity in a Chinese population. *Clin Pharmacol Ther* **54**(1): 28–33.

McKay DB and Josephson MA (2008). Pregnancy after kidney transplantation. *Clin J Am Soc Nephrol* **3**(Suppl 2): S117–S125.

62 Management of the Patient with a Failing Kidney Transplant

Ho Quan Yao

Introduction

- A failing kidney transplant (KT) can be defined as one where there is stable but low allograft function or declining function with anticipated graft loss within 1 year.

- Recipients with failing or a failed KT (RFKTs) are at a high risk of complications like infections, cardiovascular disease, and death. Dialysis after graft loss (DAGL) is associated with a higher mortality than those with a functioning KT or those who were on dialysis but transplant naive. There are many risk factors contributing to increased mortality (Table 62.1).

- The components of management include:
  - Diagnosis and management of the underlying causes(s) of the failing allograft
  - Optimising chronic kidney disease (CKD) care and associated risk factors
  - Planning for alternative kidney replacement therapy (KRT)
  - Management of immunosuppression
  - Considerations for a graft nephrectomy
  - Monitoring and management for graft intolerance syndrome

Table 62.1:   Risk Factors Associated with Mortality After Dialysis After Graft Loss

Delayed Dialysis	Allograft In-situ	Cardiovascular Risk Factors	Immunodeficiency
• Hyperkalaemia • Fluid overload • Metabolic acidosis • Psychosocial factors in response to graft loss and dialysis • Lack of permanent vascular access at initiation of dialysis	• Chronic inflammation • Malnutrition • Hypoalbuminaemia	• Renal bone disease • Increased sympathetic activity • Anaemia • Oxidative stress • Endothelial dysfunction	• Infections • Malignancy

Diagnosis and management of the underlying causes(s) of the failing allograft

- Investigation and management of the underlying cause(s) of the failing KT should be individualised with consideration to the patient's functional status, severity of allograft dysfunction, probability of response to intervention(s), co-morbidities that affect the potential tolerance to treatments, and the patient's preferences.

- The workup may include:

    - Review of the patient's history, such as the rate of progression of kidney disease, previous complications (e.g., surgical, infective, rejection), co-morbidities (e.g., control of diabetes mellitus), adherence to medications, exposure to nephrotoxins, and a physical examination

- ■ Urine full examination and microscopy
- ■ Urine protein:creatinine ratio or 24-hour urinary total protein
- ■ Ultrasound doppler of the KT
- ■ Immunosuppression drug levels
- ■ Cytomegalovirus/BK viral load
- ■ Donor specific antibodies
- ■ Secondary workup, including viral serologies, autoimmune markers, and myeloma screen, where appropriate
- ■ Biopsy of the KT, which may not be performed if the patient is assessed to be unable to tolerate augmented immunosuppression, or significant chronicity is expected on biopsy
- The cause of the failing KT may be multifactorial, and it is important to identify and prioritise which causes are the dominant drivers of KT failure. For example, there may be simultaneous non-crescentic IgA nephropathy and chronic active T-cell mediated rejection, of which the latter would require immediate treatment if deemed appropriate.
- Appropriate supportive therapy should be instituted, such as optimising ACEi or ARB, BP and glycaemic control.

Optimising CKD care and associated risk factors

- Management of CKD and associated risk factors, such as for cardiovascular disease, infection and malignancy, should be individualised and optimised (Table 62.2).
- Evidence that specific management for RFKT is lacking, and treatment targets are mostly extrapolated from non-transplant CKD patients.

Table 62.2: Areas to Address in Managing the Failing Kidney Transplant

Cardiovascular	Lifestyle	Metabolic	Infection and Malignancy
• Optimise – BP (<130/80 mmHg) – Anaemia – Proteinuria – Lipids – DM control	• Regular exercise • Stop smoking • Reduce or stop alcohol intake	• Achieve healthy weight • Appropriate diet restriction while maintaining adequate nutrition • Correct acidosis • Optimise secondary hyperparathyroidism	• Vaccinations especially HBV, pneumococcal, influenza and COVID-19 • Exclude RCC • Other age appropriate cancer screening • Examine skin annually for skin cancer • Avoid excessive immunosuppression

Abbreviations: BP, blood pressure; COVID-19, coronarvirus disease 2019; DM, diabetes mellitus; HBV, hepatitis B virus; RCC, renal cell carcinoma

Planning for alternative kidney replacement therapy

- The optimal time to return to dialysis or to re-transplant in RFKT is unclear — the timing should be individualised to the RFKT with considerations of the cause and trajectory of KT failure, complications related to KT failure or continuation of immunosuppression, comorbidities and the RFKT's preferences.

- Nevertheless, RFKTs are observed to be often uraemic and anaemic, initiating dialysis at a single-digit-estimated glomerular filtrate rate (eGFR) and hence experiencing high mortality. It is therefore important to start planning for re-transplantation (preferably pre-emptive KT) or return to dialysis at least 6–12 months before its anticipated need or when eGFR ≤20 mL/min.

- If a living donor kidney transplant (LDKT) is not possible, the physician should check if the patient is eligible for placement on the waiting list for a deceased donor kidney transplant (DDKT). There should also be plans for haemodialysis (HD) or peritoneal dialysis (PD); the choice would depend on the patient's suitability and preferences. There is no evidence that one dialysis modality is better than the other for patients with KT failure.

- Some patients, especially the elderly, very sick or with previous complications with dialysis, may choose only for kidney supportive care.

- Dialysis catheters should be avoided as much as possible due to the risk of infections in uraemic patients who are still on immunosuppression. It is, therefore, important to plan for timely creation of long-term dialysis access.

- There are often significant psychosocial distress accompanying the news of KT failure. Patients often have difficulties accepting the loss of the KT, and there may be depression, anxiety and other psychological problems. Prior to KT failure, patients have experienced recurrent admissions that may have caused them to lose their jobs and be financially strained. Involvement of the medical social worker and sometimes the psychiatrist is important to ensure a successful transition back to dialysis or re-transplant.

Management of immunosuppression following kidney transplant failure

- If the RFKT does not undergo a nephrectomy for KT failure, a decision will need to be made about maintaining or withdrawing immunosuppression. There are advantages and disadvantages of either approach (Table 62.3). Ultimately, the option needs to be personalised and based on factors such as:

Table 62.3: Advantages and Disadvantages of Maintaining Immuno-suppression in Patients with Kidney Transplant Failure

Advantages	Disadvantages
• Maintain residual kidney function	• Infections
• Minimise risk of allosensitisation	• Cancer
• Facilitate pre-emptive transplant	• Cardiovascular risks
• Avoid rejection/graft intolerance	• Metabolic complications
• Reduce risk for transplant nephrectomy	• Adverse effects of steroids
• Prevent steroid withdrawal syndrome	• Costs of immunosuppression

- Is there another functioning organ transplant (e.g., pancreas, liver) that requires continued immunosuppression?

- Possibility for re-transplant and the waiting time, especially for an LKD

- Tolerance to continuation of immunosuppression, e.g., infection, malignancy

- Whether there is still active rejection on a recent biopsy that may need some period of continued immunosuppression till urine output falls

- Residual kidney function (RKF), where modelling studies suggest survival benefits in those with RKF

• There is no consensus on how to wean off immunosuppression following KT failure, but a sequential monitored approach is appropriate in most circumstances. The general approaches used include stopping antimetabolite or tapering CNI first, while some would continue prednisolone indefinitely, especially if there are systemic autoimmune diseases that require suppression. It may be preferable to stop antimetabolite first rather than taper CNI because of a higher rate of transplant nephrectomy that may be associated with the latter.

• In general, there are several possible clinical scenarios that will guide the management of immunosuppression in patients with KT failure (Table 62.4):

Table 62.4:   Possible Approaches to Reducing Immunosuppression in Patients with Kidney Transplant Failure

Components of Immunosuppression	Transplant Nephrectomy	Re-transplant within a Year	No Re-transplant	
			Urine Output ≥500 mL/d	Urine Output <500 mL/d
Calcineurin inhibitor	Stop after nephrectomy	Maintain low-dose CNI with CsA C0 50–100 ng/L and TAC C0 3–5 ng/L	Maintain low-dose CNI while tapering off antimetabolite — then reduce dose of CNI by 25% per week till CNI is off	After stopping antimetabolite and observing for 2 weeks, reduce dose of CNI by 25% per week till CNI is off
Antimetabolite, e.g., mycophenolate azathioprine	Stop after nephrectomy	Reduce by 50% or stop completely	Reduce by 50%, taper off by 3–6 months of DAGL	Stop immediately
Prednisolone	May need to taper gradually, e.g., 1 mg/month depending on the duration of corticosteroid exposure and tolerance to steroid withdrawal — aim for discontinuation by 6 months	Continue low-dose prednisolone, aiming for nadir dose of 5 mg/d	Continue low-dose prednisolone, aiming for nadir dose of 5 mg/d — only start tapering when both CNI and antimetabolite are off	Continue low-dose prednisolone, aiming for nadir dose of 5 mg/d — only start tapering when both CNI and antimetabolite are off

- KT failure with nephrectomy performed — immunosuppression can be discontinued abruptly, but prednisolone may need to wean gradually, depending on the duration of corticosteroid exposure.

- Possible re-transplant with an LKD within a year — immunosuppression should be continued at a low dose to prevent allosensitisation, e.g., continue low-dose CNI and prednisolone but wean off MPA or AZA or mTORI if there is a delay in re-transplant.

- No LKD but significant urine output (>500 mL/d) — low-dose immunosuppression could be continued if there are no complications from remaining on immunosuppression. However, it should be weaned off gradually as urine output falls, with an aim for nil immunosuppression by 12 months.

- No LKD and poor or no urine output (<500 mL/d) — wean off immunosuppression gradually, aiming for nil immunosuppression by 6 months.

- During the reduction of immunosuppression, RFKT should be followed closely for graft intolerance syndrome and other complications. If graft intolerance occurs during tapering of immunosuppression, steroid therapy can be restarted with a view for transplant nephrectomy when the acute inflammation has subsided.

- For RFKT who experienced KT failure after receiving intense immunosuppression (e.g., treatment for active rejection), they should receive anti-microbial prophylaxis for a defined period until the perceived risk of opportunistic infections is lower.

Graft Intolerance Syndrome

- During immunosuppression withdrawal, chronic rejection and inflammation may develop in the failed allograft left *in-situ* and result in graft intolerance syndrome (GIS) (Table 62.5).

Table 62.5:   Clinical, Laboratory and Radiological Features of Graft Intolerance Syndrome

Clinical Findings	Laboratory Findings	Radiological Findings
• Fever • Gross haematuria • Allograft enlargement and localised oedema • Allograft tenderness • Malaise • Weight loss	• Haematological findings — thrombocytopenia, ESA-resistant anaemia • Elevated inflammatory markers — ferritin, CRP, ESR	• Radiological findings of graft inflammation, e.g., swelling, perinephric stranding

- GIS occurs in 30–50% of patients within 1 year of KT failure and is generally a diagnosis of exclusion, as signs and symptoms may mimic infection and malignancy.

- High-dose corticosteroids, e.g., IV hydrocortisone or prednisolone 1 mg/kg/day and NSAIDS (e.g., indomethacin) are first-line treatment and maintenance immunosuppression may be required for a period, e.g., 4–6 weeks, before being tapered. Antimicrobial prophylaxis is needed if high-dose immunosuppression is given for a prolonged period. Graft nephrectomy or coil embolisation may be required in refractory GIS.

- The risk for GIS may be lowered by a gradual reduction of immunosuppression or maintenance of low-dose immunosuppression.

Graft nephrectomy

- There are advantages and disadvantages of performing graft nephrectomies (Table 62.6), but they are not routinely required.

Table 62.6: Advantages and Disadvantages of Transplant Nephrectomy in Patients with Kidney Transplant Failure

Advantages	Disadvantages
• Avoid chronic inflammatory state • Avoid symptomatic acute rejection	• Increased levels of DSAs • Surgical morbidity and mortality • Loss of residual kidney function

- If KT failure occurs within the first year of transplantation, nephrectomy would be appropriate to facilitate the immediate withdrawal of immunosuppression — if the KT remains *in-situ*, symptomatic rejection is likely to occur during the weaning of immunosuppression, and there is an increased risk for infection and cancer.

- If KT failure occurs after the first year of transplantation, graft nephrectomy may be performed for:

  - Local complications

    - Severe rejection with pain and haematuria not responding to immunosuppression

    - Risk of graft rupture (e.g., vascular thrombosis, severe rejection)

    - Graft intolerance syndrome resistant to medical therapy

    - Recurrent or severe graft pyelonephritis not responding to antibiotic therapies

    - Malignancy within the graft

  - To create space for re-transplantation when the contralateral iliac fossa is not available

  - Facilitate rapid, complete withdrawal of immunosuppression because the patient is suffering from severe adverse effects to immunosuppression, infection or malignancy

- Some patients may be at high operative risk for nephrectomy, and percutaneous embolisation of the failed KT may be considered if there is no concern for infection or malignancy. However, embolisation may fail to induce graft ischaemia in 10–30% of cases. Post-embolisation complications are also common — abscess formation, migration of embolisation coils, puncture site complications, post-embolisation syndrome (fever, pain, malaise, haematuria, graft swelling).

Re-transplantation

- Re-transplantation following KT failure offers a survival benefit over remaining on dialysis. Unfortunately, only a minority of RFKTs would have an opportunity for re-transplantation as many would either have no LKD, or are too old or have accumulated significant comorbidities that preclude re-transplantation.

- If there is a LKD available, RFKT should be referred for re-transplantation when the eGFR is <20 mL/min so that by the time evaluation is completed, pre-emptive re-transplantation can be performed when the eGFR has fallen to 10–15 mL/min.

- As RFKT may be sensitised to the previous allograft and from other sensitisation events, the most compatible LKD should be sought.

- RFKTs with no living kidney donor can be placed on the waiting list for a DDKT if they are eligible.

- Antibody induction and the maintenance immunosuppression regimen should be individualised to the patient risk stratification for rejection and other considerations. However, for RFKTs who experienced graft loss due to BKVN, highly potent immunosuppression should be avoided while viraemia cleared before retransplantation.

- For RFKTs who experienced graft loss due to a recurrent primary disease that caused ESKD, there is generally a higher risk for another recurrence in the repeat transplant. This may influence the decision for a repeat transplant, and the perioperative immunosuppression may need to be different to reduce the risk of another recurrence.

References

British Transplantation Society (2014). Management of the failing kidney transplant. Guidelines and standards — British Transplantation Society. https://bts.org.uk/guidelines-standards. May 2014.

Kabani R, Quinn RR, Palmer S, *et al.* (2014). Risk of death following kidney allograft failure: A systematic review and meta-analysis of cohort studies. *Nephrol Dial Transplant* **29**(9): 1778–1786.

Lubetzky M, Tantisattamo E, Molnar MZ, *et al.* (2021). The failing kidney allograft: A review and recommendations for the care and management of a complex group of patients. *Am J Transplant* **21**(9): 2937–2949.

Sellarés J, de Freitas DG, Mengel M, *et al.* (2012). Understanding the causes of kidney transplant failure: The dominant role of antibody-mediated rejection and nonadherence. *Am J Transplant* **12**(2): 388–399.

63 Kidney Diseases in Cancer Patients

Tan Hui Zhuan

Introduction

- There is an increase in demand for medical care for kidney diseases associated with haemato-oncological disorders worldwide.

- This is driven by a higher prevalence of acute and chronic complications in patients with cancer, as well as the increased prevalence of cancer in patients with pre-existing kidney diseases.

- These complications can be contributed by

  - Malignancy and/or

  - Direct or indirect treatment toxicities from conventional chemotherapeutics, and more importantly, novel targeted, immune- or cellular therapies that are increasingly employed in contemporary cancer therapeutic regimens

- The combination of cancer and kidney impairment worsens patients' outcomes, prolongs hospitalisations, and complicates their management and treatment by limiting therapeutic options.

- A variety of kidney-related complications or clinical syndromes can occur among cancer patients, including:

  - acute kidney injury (AKI)

  - chronic kidney disease (CKD)

- glomerular diseases
- electrolyte disorders
- hypertension

- While it is beyond the scope of this handbook to cover the individual complications or clinical syndromes in detail, it is important to appreciate that novel therapies and/or treatment combinations with overlapping complications and clinical syndromes are increasingly used, confounding monitoring. Proactive, dynamic assessment, together with a high index of suspicion, remain paramount.

Acute kidney injury

- During critical illness, up to 50% of patients with cancer develop AKI.
- The risk of acute kidney injuries is exacerbated by pre-existing chronic kidney disease, a common comorbidity associated with increasing age and concomitant metabolic diseases.
- In general, the same aetiologies of AKI (pre-renal, intrinsic renal, post-renal causes) that occur in the general population can affect cancer patients.
- However, certain causes of AKI specific to the cancer patient population should be actively evaluated for (Figure 63.1).

Chronic kidney disease

- Patients with cancer may develop chronic kidney disease from cumulative and additive insults that are related or unrelated to the malignancy and its treatment.

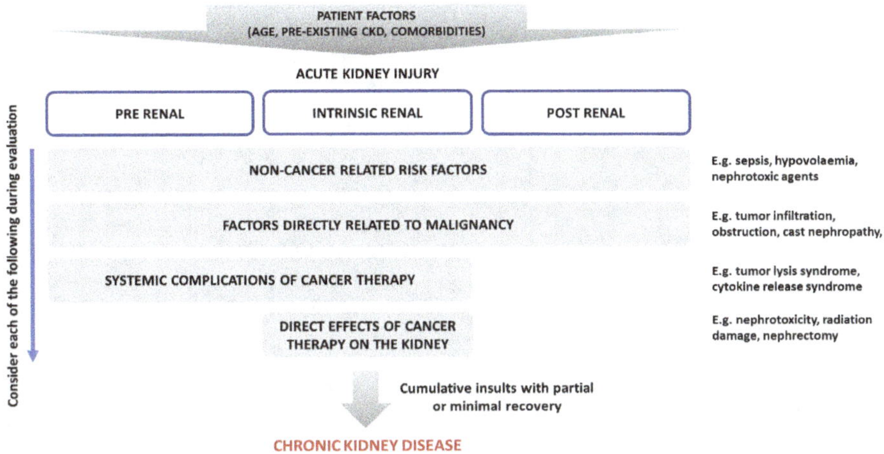

Figure 63.1:   Factors Contributing to Acute Kidney Injury and Chronic Kidney Disease in a Cancer Patient

Glomerular diseases and electrolyte disorders

- Patients with cancer may present with glomerular diseases and electrolyte abnormalities, which can be caused by the underlying malignancy (paraneoplastic) or its treatment.

- Therapy-associated glomerular diseases and electrolyte disturbances may present at various times during treatment, and patients receiving these drugs should be actively monitored for the development of proteinuria and/or kidney function impairment.

Reference

Christiansen CF, Johansen MB, Langeberg WJ, *et al.* (2011). Incidence of acute kidney injury in cancer patients: A Danish population-based cohort study. *Eur J Intern Med* **22**(4): 399–406.

64 Kidney Supportive Care

Lee Guozhang, Natalie Woong

Introduction

- Kidney supportive care (KSC) is a clinical approach that aims to improve the quality of life for patients with advanced chronic kidney disease (CKD) by integrating palliative care principles, knowledge and skills into routine kidney care.

- KSC can be provided at any part of the patient's journey, including those who choose dialysis or transplant (Figure 64.1).

- The Kidney Disease Improving Global Outcomes (KDIGO) recommended replacing "palliative care" with "supportive care" to avoid the misunderstanding that it is only limited to terminal care and reflect that it can be provided alongside life-prolonging measures. KSC is an umbrella term in which comprehensive conservative care is a subset (Table 64.1).

- KSC should be provided by a multidisciplinary team including physicians, nurses, medical social workers, pharmacists, and other allied health workers, aka Comprehensive Conservative Care (CCC).

- CCC is a holistic patient-centric approach that supports patients who opt for non-dialytic therapy.

- For patients who are unlikely to benefit from dialysis or kidney transplantation as a treatment choice, CCC is an option that should be provided.

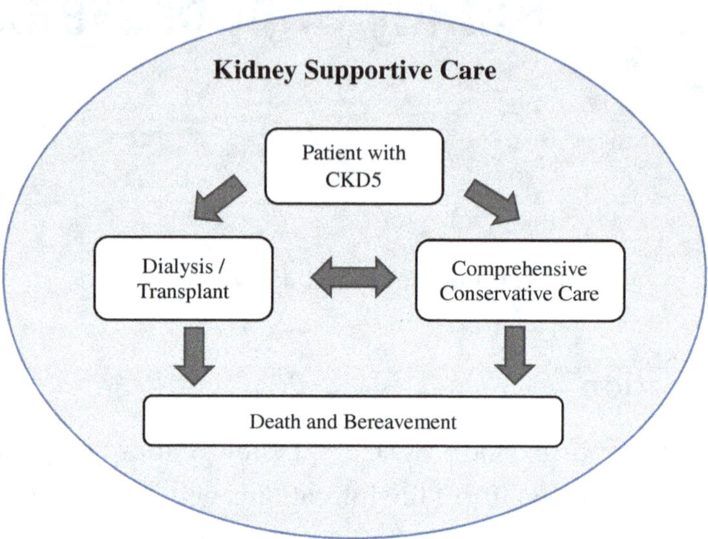

Figure 64.1: Kidney Supportive Care Encompasses All Parts of the Journey of a Patient with Stage V Chronic Kidney Disease

Table 64.1: Components of Kidney Supportive Care and Complete Conservative Care

1. Chronic Disease Management	• Interventions to delay progression of kidney disease and minimise risk of adverse events or complications • Medication review and de-prescribing as appropriate • Dietary counselling
2. Shared decision-making	• Discussion and decision for a long-term plan for dialysis or CCC
3. Active symptom management	• Monitor for worsening symptom burden and functional decline • Manage symptoms of CKD such as those from fluid overload and uraemia
4. Detailed communication, including advance care planning	• Prognosis sharing • Initiate and facilitate advance care planning, including goals of care discussion

Table 64.1:   (*Continued*)

5. Psychological and spiritual care	• Assess and manage for psychological and spiritual needs
6. Caregiver and family support	• Assess family and caregiver coping • Referral for appropriate caregiver support / services
7. End-of-life care	• Initiation of end-of-life care planning • Timely transition to community palliative and hospice services • Grief and bereavement support

- Patients are assured of continued medical care so that they do not go away with the notion that "nothing can be done" and receive treatment plans that are aligned with their priorities and values.

Prognostication

- Accurate prognostication is important to enable the patient to make an informed choice regarding ongoing care, to plan for the future, and to prepare for end-of-life care when appropriate.

- As prognostication is not exact, prognosis should be presented in terms of a range or time frame, for example, "3–6 months" or "months to less than a year", as well as to convey a degree of uncertainty. There is also the risk of sudden death in certain patients, e.g., with severe uraemia.

Prognostication for stage 5 chronic kidney disease patients on conservative care

- A systematic review showed a wide range of median survival from 6.3 to 23.4 months, partly due to differing populations and definitions. Factors predicting prolonged survival with conservative management include:

- Female gender
- Lower comorbidity score
- Albumin >35 g/L
- Referral to a nephrologist before reaching stage 5 CKD

- Other considerations when assessing prognosis include:
    - Rate of decline of kidney function and etiology
    - Functional decline or increasing symptom burden without an acute reversible event
    - Trajectory of functional status — the functional status remains stable during the last year of life but declines steeply in the last month of life
    - Increase in symptom burden towards the last month of life
    - Other comorbidities or concomitant life-limiting illnesses (e.g., cancer, advanced heart failure) that may affect prognosis

Prognostication for patients on dialysis who have dialysis withdrawn

- Consider the following factors:
    - Dialysis vintage (length of time since started on dialysis)
    - Residual kidney function
    - Dialysis modality, e.g., PD
    - Presence of concomitant life-limiting acute illness

- Prognosis is generally 1–2 weeks if patient is dialysis-dependent and anuric

- Reported median survival on withdrawal is around 8 days

Recognising dialysis patients at risk of deterioration

- Dialysis patients may have supportive and palliative care needs as they deteriorate, so they can benefit from a KSC approach. They can be identified through general and dialysis specific indicators (Table 64.2).

Table 64.2:   Indicators for Dialysis Patients at Risk of Deterioration

General Indicators of Poor or Deteriorating Health	Dialysis Specific Indicators
• Recurrent, unplanned hospital admissions	• Tolerating haemodialysis or peritoneal dialysis poorly, e.g., recurrent intradialytic hypotension with no/limited reversibility, recurrent access issues, tolerating poorly due to poor compliance
• Performance status is poor or deteriorating, with limited reversibility (e.g., in bed/chair more than 50% of the day)	
• Depends on others for care due to increasing physical and/or mental health problems; the person's carer needs more help and support	• Considering withdrawal of dialysis, e.g., due to poor quality of life, symptom burden
• Significant weight loss over the last few months or remains underweight	
• Persistent symptoms despite optimal treatment of underlying condition(s)	
• Concomitant life-limiting co-morbidities, e.g., advanced cancer, advanced dementia	

Goals of care discussion

- Assess informational preferences and explore how the patient and his/her family can make decisions

- Find out the extent in which he/she is aware of his/her conditions, how much he/she wants to know, and if he/she is ready for further discussions.

- Decision-making approaches may be patient or family-led. Others rely on physician recommendations, while some may desire shared decision-making.

• Eliciting goals, priorities and fears

- Explore what is/are the patient's goals/priorities, e.g., *"What are the things that are important for you to live well"*, *"what is the most important thing to you now"* or *"what is something so important to you that you cannot imagine living without"*.

- Explore any fears or worries and what may be considered as a form of suffering.

- Explore any sources of strength or motivation.

• Aligning treatment to stated goals

- Ask the patient what he/she hopes to achieve with a particular treatment, e.g., *"how do you hope dialysis will help you?"*

- Common treatment goals include life prolongation, maintaining independence, reducing symptoms, avoiding burden to family, etc.

- It is important to recognise potential trade-offs, e.g., hope for life-prolongation and avoiding the burden of treatment, and ask if the patient can accept the trade-offs in exchange for a potential benefit.

• Making recommendations to the patient and his/her family

- Initial recommendation should be based on the initial medical assessment and clinical indications, but the recommendation may vary according to the patient's values and stated goals.

- Present recommendations that are aligned to the patient's stated goals and priorities and what is acceptable to them.

- Consider the use of decision-making aids if available

- Consider goals of the care discussion guide, e.g., the Serious Illness Conversation Guide (SICG), which is available online for open access.

Principles of symptom assessment and management in advanced CKD

- Advanced CKD patients (both conservative care and on dialysis) have a high symptom burden, comparable to other advanced conditions such as cancer (Table 64.3).

Table 64.3: Symptom Prevalence in End-Stage Kidney Disease

Prevalence of Symptoms in End-Stage Kidney Disease	
Symptom	**Prevalence (%)**
Fatigue	76
Pruritus	74
Dyspnea	61
Pain	53
Constipation	53
Anorexia	47
Insomnia	41
Anxiety	38
Nausea	33
Restless legs	30
Depression	27

Symptom assessment

- It is important to always assess for the underlying cause(s) of the symptom
  - Consider factors related to (a) CKD itself, (b) treatment-related, (c) associated co-morbidities or (d) non-CKD related causes.
  - It may be difficult to distinguish from those attributed to co-existing conditions or side effects of medications.
  - Symptoms are often multifactorial and interdependent in nature, e.g., a patient may experience fatigue due to uraemia, anaemia, comorbid conditions (e.g., cardiac disease), psychosocial factors (e.g., depression), and medications (e.g., antihistamines).
- Symptoms can be multiple, with an average of 6–17 symptoms reported in the last month of life
  - Identify the most distressing symptoms for management first.
  - Treating one symptom may potentially exacerbate another symptom, e.g., diuresing a patient to dry can potentially elevate the urea and worsen uraemic symptoms and result in dry mouth/skin. In such cases, there is a need to find a balance.
  - Consider and identify psychosocial contributors, e.g., psycho-social distress impacting on the patient's pain experience.

Management of symptoms

- Consider treating the underlying cause(s) where possible and appropriate (Table 64.4). As a symptom may arise from multiple factors, treating a single cause may not completely alleviate the symptom, and all possible contributory factors may need to be addressed.

- Manage symptoms with specific goals or target in mind, such as improving quality of life or the function may be useful in managing the patient's expectations

- Optimising CKD management may improve symptoms, e.g., fluid status, anaemia

- If possible, consider the use of one drug with multiple indications in order to reduce polypharmacy and increasing the already high pill burden in CKD patients, e.g., mirtazapine may be used to treat a patient who reports insomnia, reduced appetite, and uraemic pruritus.

- Dose of certain medications excreted by the kidney will have to be adjusted or be avoided altogether

- Always consider non-pharmacological management options

Table 64.4:   Management Approaches for Common Symptoms in CKD

Symptom	Approach and Strategies
Fatigue	• Screen and address causes of fatigue — uraemia, fluid overload, anaemia, or other comorbid conditions such as heart failure • Optimise anaemia management with iron supplementation and erythropoiesis-stimulating agents • Advise on non-pharmacological measures, including energy-conservation strategies, pacing of activities, and exercise. May consider referral to physiotherapy or occupational therapy

(Continued)

Table 64.4:   (*Continued*)

Symptom	Approach and Strategies

Anorexia	• Assessment and addressing contributory factors
	  ■ Screen for depression, oral issues, e.g., thrush, taste disorders, gastrointestinal symptoms like nausea and constipation
	  ■ Review medications for polypharmacy and adverse effects
	• Non-pharmacological measures
	  ■ Dietary advice, e.g., small, frequent meals or caloric-dense food
	  ■ Nutritional counselling and supplementation as required.
	  ■ Loosen dietary restrictions if safe and appropriate
	• Pharmacological measures
	  ■ Treat gastrointestinal symptoms like nausea, constipation
	  ■ May trial prokinetics, e.g., domperidone 10 mg TDS pre-meal if having early satiety, bloating or suggestion of gastroparesis
	  ■ Consider antidepressants such as mirtazapine if there are other indications, e.g., depression, insomnia or itch
	  ■ Presently, there is no evidence for use of appetite stimulants such as megestrol in stage 5 CKD patients, and it is associated with fluid retention

Pruritus	• Treat reversible or contributory factors
	  ■ Assess for and treat dermatological causes such as eczema and xerosis with topical emollients, topical steroids
	  ■ Control calcium/phosphate levels and correct iron deficiency
	• Non-pharmacological measures
	  ■ Keep skin hydrated, e.g., avoid long and hot showers
	  ■ Avoid skin irritation, such as avoiding the use of irritating clothing, keeping nails clean, and use of non-soap, fragrance-free cleansers
	  ■ Topical emollients, e.g., QV cream, aqueous cream or menthol-based creams, which relieves pruritus
	• Pharmacological measures
	  ■ May consider a night dose of antihistamine, e.g., hydroxyzine 10–25 mg nocte for light sedation to reduce scratching if itch is mild

Table 64.4: *(Continued)*

Symptom	Approach and Strategies
	■ For moderate-severe itch and if patient has concomitant neuropathic pain, consider gabapentin 100 mg nocte (max. 300 mg nocte) or pregabalin 25 mg nocte (max. 75 mg nocte) for CrCl <15 (to dose post HD in dialysis patients) ■ Start at lower doses particularly in elderly patients, and monitor for adverse effects such as somnolence (4.5–18.5%) ■ May consider mirtazapine 7.5 mg nocte (starting dose) if the patient has concomitant insomnia, depression or anorexia

Pain	• Assess and treat cause of pain
	• Consider causes related to CKD, including treatment side-effects, comorbidities or unrelated causes
	• Pharmacological measures
	  ■ Avoid nephrotoxic medications such as NSAIDs
	  ■ Consider adjuvants such as gabapentin for neuropathic pain
	  ■ For mild pain, may consider paracetamol or anarex (if muscle relaxation is useful)
	  ■ Use weak opioids such as tramadol with caution. May start at 25 mg BD/TDS and limit dose to a maximum of 100–200 mg/day. Avoid codeine.
	  ■ Consider consulting palliative care physician for advice if strong opioids are needed. Fentanyl is the strong opioid of choice in CKD, and is available as a transdermal patch or injectable (IV/SC infusions). Oral morphine may be used in low doses with prolonged intervals between doses, e.g., 1–2.5 mg Q8H PRN.
	• Consider non-pharmacological measures if appropriate

Dyspnea	• Assess and treat reversible causes of dyspnea, e.g., fluid overload, anaemia
	• Non-pharmacological measures
	  ■ Supplemental oxygen if patient has hypoxia
	  ■ Use of hand-held fan blowing at the face, which reduces dyspnea by stimulating the trigeminal nerves
	  ■ Energy-conservation strategies, pacing of activities
	• Pharmacological measures
	  ■ Low-dose opioids may be considered if underlying cause cannot be reversed/optimised

When to refer to a specialist palliative care team

When to refer to specialist palliative care team
1. Difficult symptom burden and treatment
2. Challenges in decision-making for long-term treatment plan with complex clinical situations or psychosocial issues
3. Assistance in advance care planning and end-of-life care
4. Challenges in care planning in complex clinical or psychosocial situation
5. Multidisciplinary team support required
Note: In certain settings, specialist palliative care support may be integrated into the kidney service as a kidney supportive care service, with specific triggers for referral, such as a glomerular filtration rate cut-off or symptom management issues

References

Ariadne Labs. Serious illness conversation guide. https://www.ariadnelabs.org/resources/downloads/serious-illness-conversation-guide/

Davison SN, Levin A, Moss AH, *et al.* (2015). Executive summary of the KDIGO Controversies Conference on Supportive Care in Chronic Kidney Disease: Developing a roadmap to improving quality care. *Kidney Int* **88**(3): 447–459.

Ducharlet K, Philip J, Kiburg K, *et al.* (2021). Renal supportive care, palliative care and end-of-life care: Perceptions of similarities, differences and challenges across Australia and New Zealand. *Nephrology (Carlton)* **26**(1): 15–22.

Hole B, Hemmelgarn B, Brown E, *et al.* (2020). Supportive care for end-stage kidney disease: An integral part of kidney services across a range of income settings around the world. *Kidney Int Suppl* **10**(1): e86–e94.

Murtagh FE, Addington-Hall J and Higginson IJ (2007). The prevalence of symptoms in end-stage renal disease: A systematic review. *Adv Chronic Kidney Dis* **14**(1): 82–99.

Murtagh FE, Addington-Hall JM and Higginson IJ (2011). End-stage renal disease: A new trajectory of functional decline in the last year of life. *J Am Geriatr Soc* **59**(2): 304–308.

Murtagh FE, Addington-Hall JM, Edmonds PM, *et al.* (2007). Symptoms in advanced renal disease: A cross-sectional survey of symptom prevalence in stage 5 chronic kidney disease managed without dialysis. *J Palliat Med* **10**(6): 1266–1276.

Murtagh FE, Burns A, Moranne O, *et al.* (2016). Supportive care: Comprehensive conservative care in end-stage kidney disease. *Clin J Am Soc Nephrol* **11**(10): 1909–1914.

Murtagh FE, Sheerin NS, Addington-Hall J and Higginson IJ (2011). Trajectories of illness in stage 5 chronic kidney disease: A longitudinal study of patient symptoms and concerns in the last year of life. *Clin J Am Soc Nephrol* **6**(7): 1580–1590.

O'Connor NR and Kumar P (2012). Conservative management of end-stage renal disease without dialysis: A systematic review. *J Palliat Med* **15**(2): 228–235.

O'Connor NR, Dougherty M, Harris PS, *et al.* (2013). Survival after dialysis discontinuation and hospice enrollment for ESRD. *Clin J Am Soc Nephrol* **8**(12): 2117–2122.

SPICT. The SPICT™. 19 March 2021. https://www.spict.org.uk/the-spict/

65 Approach to Drug Dosing in Patients with Kidney Disease

Sim Mui Hian, Lee Puay Hoon

Introduction

- Patients may present with varying degrees of kidney dysfunction in clinical practice. Most drugs are cleared by the kidneys and kidney replacement therapies to varying extents. As a result of kidney dysfunction, the use of some drugs are contraindicated, whereas some may be used with caution.

- In most cases, this necessitates the clinician to adjust the drug dosing regimens to maximise efficacy and minimise the risk of toxicity. Failure to appropriately adjust the dosing regimen or avoiding it may result in significant toxicities (Table 65.1).

Pharmacokinetic Changes

- Kidney disease and uraemia affect the pharmacokinetics (PK) of many drugs (Table 65.2).

- In addition, there may also be altered pharmacodynamic responses of drugs in kidney dysfunction.

Table 65.1:   Significant Toxicities of Selected Drugs

Class	Drug(s)	Toxicity
Analgesic	Pethidine	Seizures
	Codeine, morphine	Central nervous system and respiratory adverse effects
Antibiotic	Cefepime, imipenem/cilastatin, ertapenem	Central nervous system toxicity
Antiviral	Aciclovir, valaciclovir	Neurotoxic
	Ganciclovir, valganciclovir	Myelotoxic
	Cidofovir	Myelotoxic, nephrotoxic
Antidiabetic agents	Glibenclamide, glimepiride	Hypoglycaemia
	Metformin	Lactic acidosis
Diuretic	Spironolactone, eplerenone	Hyperkalaemia
Low molecular weight heparin	Enoxaparin	Risk of haemorrhage

Table 65.2:   Effects of Chronic Kidney Disease on Drug Pharmacokinetics

Absorption	• Presence of uraemia-induced vomiting, diarrhoea and/or oedematous gastrointestinal tract can reduce drug absorption.
	• Commonly prescribed medications such as iron, calcium-based phosphate binders can form insoluble complexes with other medications and/or change gastric pH and alter absorption.
	• Presence of gastroparesis may delay absorption and prolong time to peak drug concentration and effect.
Distribution	• Changes to extracellular fluid have the greatest effects on hydrophilic drugs or drugs with low Vd (<0.7 L/kg). Presence of increased extracellular fluid, e.g., in fluid overload states may result in lower serum drug concentration.
	• Free fraction of acidic drugs may increase as a result of – hypoalbuminaemia – reduced binding sites or displacement from plasma protein due to competition by uraemic molecules and other organic wastes.

Table 65.2:   (*Continued*)

	Increased free fraction of drug may undergo biotransformation and result in reduced total drug concentration. • Free fraction of basic drugs may decrease as a result of binding to α-1 acid glycoprotein, which is often elevated in CKD.
Metabolism	Nonrenal drug clearance may be slower in patients with CKD than in patients with normal kidney function due to downregulation of activity of cytochrome P450 enzymes.
Elimination	For drugs excreted by the kidneys, elimination is reduced as a result of reduced glomerular and tubular function.

Abbreviations: CKD, chronic kidney disease; Vd, volume of distribution

Table 65.3:   Stepwise Approach to Adjust Drug Dosage Regimens in Patients with CKD, AKI and On Dialysis

Steps	Patients with CKD and AKI	Patients on Dialysis
Step 1 Obtain detailed history and relevant demographic/ clinical information	• Obtain demographic, past medical history, and complete medication list. • Assess for presence of conditions that may lead to increased extracellular volume. • Review laboratory parameters to assess renal function, liver function, and serum albumin levels.	
Step 2 Evaluate degree of renal impairment	• Use an appropriate tool to assess GFR or calculate Cl_{Cr} of the patient. The formula to use is dependent on guidance by drug labelling and established drug references. There is no reliable equation to estimate GFR or Cl_{Cr} in AKI. • GFR is estimated using the MDRD Study	• GFR or calculated Cl_{Cr} is not used here. • In HD, CKRT and hybrid therapies, drug removal is affected by – prescribed dialysis dose – modes of therapy (convection and/or diffusion) – types of filter used – types of replacement fluids given for CKRT and hybrid therapies

(*Continued*)

Table 65.3:　(Continued)

Steps	Patients with CKD and AKI	Patients on Dialysis
	equation or the CKD-EPI equation. In situations where both equations result in different dosing adjustments, rationalise dosing regimen based on the risk for toxicity versus the risk of undertreatment. • Cockcroft–Gault equation is used to calculate Cl_{Cr}.	• High-flux dialysis membranes may allow the passage of molecules up to 20,000 daltons. Additionally, drugs can also be removed via adhesion to the dialysis membrane. Among the factors of consideration, the prescribed dialysis dose is one of the most influential factor. • PD does not enhance drug removal to a significant degree for most typical PD prescription. Thus, drug dosing recommendations for GFR or $Cl_{Cr} < 15$ mL/min is applicable for most situations. • In general, drugs with high molecular weight, high degree of protein binding, and high Vd are less likely to be removed via dialysis.
<u>**Step 3**</u> Review current medications	• Identify drugs that require adjustments to the dosing regimen. • Choose drugs that have no or minimal nephrotoxicity whenever possible (unless already on long-term dialysis with no residual renal function).	
<u>**Step 4**</u> Determine individualised dosing regimen	• Determine if the desired treatment goal is to achieve a similar peak, trough or average steady-state drug concentration or achieve parameters such as time above MIC, peak/MIC ratio, or AUC/MIC ratio for drug classes such as antibiotics. • If there are no specific PK or pharmacodynamic targets, achieving an average steady-state drug concentration may be appropriate.	

Table 65.3:   (*Continued*)

Steps	Patients with CKD and AKI	Patients on Dialysis
	• Determine appropriate loading and maintenance regimens based on treatment goals, PK of drugs, and a patient's volume status and renal function. • Steady-state drug concentration is achieved after about 5 half-lives of a drug. A loading dose is often given to achieve therapeutic drug concentration rapidly. Consider a loading dose for drugs with long half-lives. Loading dose to be given is not affected by kidney function and, hence, is the same as in patients with normal kidney function. However, if there is a significant change in the Vd, there may be a need to modify the loading dose. Patient's loading dose = usual loading dose × the patient's Vd/normal Vd • Maintenance dose can be adjusted by reducing the dose and/or increasing the dosing interval to achieve the desired drug level for drugs with a reduced renal clearance. Refer to established drug references or drug labelling for recommendations.	
Step 5 Monitor	• Monitor for response and toxicity. • Perform therapeutic drug monitoring if available and/or applicable, especially for drugs with a narrow therapeutic index.	
Step 6 Revise regimen	• Adjust based on – response and/or toxicity – patient's clinical status – organ(s) function change and/or dialysis prescription changes. • For drugs with a clear dose-response relationship, the dose can be adjusted based on pharmacodynamic response.	

Abbreviations: AKI, acute kidney injury; AUC, area under the curve; Cl_{Cr}, creatinine clearance; CKD, chronic kidney disease; CKD-EPI, Chronic Kidney Disease Epidemiology Collaboration; CKRT, continuous kidney replacement therapy; GFR, glomerular filtration rate; HD, haemodialysis; MDRD, Modification of Diet in Renal Disease; MIC, minimum inhibitory concentration; PD, peritoneal dialysis; PK, pharmacokinetics; Vd, volume of distribution

Approach to dosing regimen adjustment

- A practical and stepwise approach to the adjustment of dosing regimens should be adopted for patients with chronic kidney disease (CKD), acute kidney injury (AKI), and those on dialysis (Table 65.3).

References

Hartmann B, Czock D and Keller F (2010). Drug therapy in patients with chronic renal failure. *Dtsch Arztebl Int* **107**(37): 647–656.

Hassan Y, Al-Ramahi R, Abd Aziz N and Ghazali, R (2009). Drug use and dosing in chronic kidney disease. *Ann Acad Med Singap* **38**(12): 1095–1103.

Matzke GR and Frye RF (2008). Drug therapy individualisation for patients with renal insufficiency. In: *Pharmacotherapy: A Pathophysiologic Approach*, 7th ed. DiPiro JT, Talbert RL, Yee GC, *et al.*, editors. The McGraw-Hill Companies, p. 833–844.

Matzke GR, Aronoff GR, Atkinson AJ, Jr, *et al.* (2011). Drug dosing consideration in patients with acute and chronic kidney disease — A clinical update from Kidney Disease: Improving Global Outcomes (KDIGO). *Kidney Int* **80**(11): 1122–1137.

Munar MY and Singh H (2007). Drug dosing adjustments in patients with chronic kidney disease. *Am Fam Physician* **75**(10): 1487–1496.

National Institute of Diabetes and Digestive and Kidney Diseases (2022). Determining drug dosing in adults with chronic kidney disease. U.S. Department of Health and Human Services. https://www.niddk.nih.gov/research-funding/research-programs/kidney-clinical-research-epidemiology/laboratory/ckd-drug-dosing-providers

Olyaei AJ and Steffl JL (2011). A quantitative approach to drug dosing in chronic kidney disease. *Blood Purif* **31**(1–3): 138–145.

66 Nutritional Care in Chronic Kidney Disease

Tan Sheau Kang, Pindar Yu

Introduction

- As chronic kidney disease (CKD) progresses, the nutritional requirements change significantly based on the patients'
    - Nutritional status
    - Laboratory results
    - Clinical conditions
    - Fluid status
    - Medications
    - Treatment for CKD stage 5, such as haemodialysis, peritoneal dialysis, kidney transplantation, or conservative management
- Protein-energy wasting (PEW) is common in patients with CKD. A meta-analysis reported the global prevalence of PEW was 11–54%, 28–54% and 28–52% among patients with CKD stages 3 to 5 (non-dialysis), patients on maintenance dialysis, and kidney transplant recipients, respectively.
- PEW is often associated with poor clinical outcomes, which include:
    - Increased mortality, cardiovascular disease, infections

- Reduced physical function with poorer quality of life
  - Increased hospitalisation rates and treatment costs
- Individualised medical nutrition therapy (MNT) provided by trained dietitians in close collaboration with physicians will help to:
  - Optimise nutritional status
  - Prevent or improve uraemic toxicity
  - Minimise risk imposed by comorbid diseases
  - Improve metabolic abnormalities
  - Prevent or treat renal bone disease
  - Address barriers to change and improve dietary adherence
- MNT comprises:
  - Comprehensive nutrition assessment
  - Determination of nutrition diagnosis
  - Implementation of nutrition intervention
  - Monitoring and evaluating a patient's progress

Nutrition assessment

- There are five domains in nutrition assessment (Figure 66.1).

Nutrition assessment tools

- Several tools have been validated for predicting malnutrition in patients with CKD, which are:
  - 7-point Subjective Global Assessment
  - Malnutrition-Inflammation Score
  - Handgrip strength

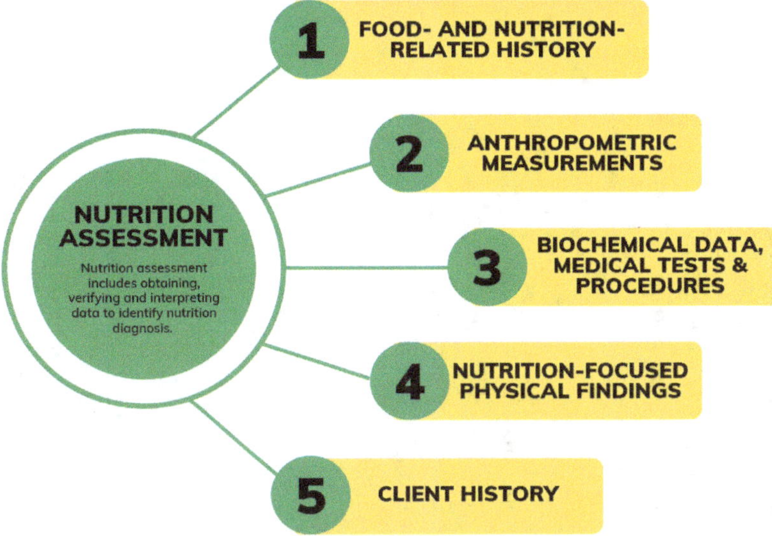

Figure 66.1:   Five Domains of Nutritional Assessment

Nutrition diagnosis

- Nutrition diagnosis is organised into three components (Table 66.1).

Table 66.1:   **Components of Nutritional Diagnosis**

Intake	Clinical	Behavioural-Environmental
• Energy • Nutrients • Fluids • Bioactive substances • Nutrition support	Nutritional problems that relate to medical or physical conditions	• Knowledge • Attitudes/beliefs • Physical environment • Access to food • Food safety

Nutrition intervention for CKD (non-dialysis) haemodialysis and peritoneal/dialysis

- Table 66.2 provides a summary of the dietary recommendations for patients with CKD (non-dialysis) and patients on maintenance dialysis (haemodialysis and peritoneal dialysis).

Table 66.2:   Nutrition Intervention for Chronic Kidney Disease (Non-Dialysis), Haemodialysis and Peritoneal Dialysis

Nutrients	CKD (non-dialysis)	HD	PD	Remark
Energy	25–35 kcal/kg body weight/day Energy requirements must be individualised based on metabolic stress, age, sex, comorbidities, physical activity levels, and weight status.			For PD patients, energy intake from dialysate should be taken into consideration.
Protein	**CKD stage 1 to 2** ■ Same as general populations **CKD stage 3 to 5 (non-dialysis)** ■ 0.8 g/kg body weight/day for metabolically stable patients ■ 0.28–0.43 g/kg body weight/day with keto acid analogues	1–1.2 g/kg/body weight/day		Protein requirements must be individualised for metabolic stress, comorbid complications, being overweight/underweight, and overall health goals.
Fat	Limit to 30% or less of total calories.			Emphasise unsaturated fatty acid sources in place of saturated fat and trans-fat.

Sodium	Less than 2000 mg sodium/day		Sodium restriction helps to lower blood pressure, improve cardiovascular disease, decrease fluid overload, reduce endothelial damage, improve proteinuria, and delay CKD progression.
Potassium	Individualise to maintain normal serum potassium levels.		Ensure adequate dietary fibre intake from fruits and vegetables.
Phosphorus	Individualise to maintain normal serum phosphorus levels.		Dietary education to identify inorganic sources and use of phosphate binders.
Calcium	800–1000 mg/day, including all sources of calcium.	Adjust calcium intake to avoid hypercalcaemia.	Sources of calcium include dietary calcium, supplements, binders, and dialysate.
Vitamins and other minerals	Recommended dietary allowances		If deficient, consider vitamins and minerals supplementation, as needed.

Abbreviations: CKD, chronic kidney disease; HD, haemodialysis; PD, peritoneal dialysis

Nutrition intervention for kidney transplantation

- Two phases of nutrition care for kidney transplant (KT) recipients are the acute post-transplantation recovery phase and the chronic post-transplantation maintenance phase (Table 66.3).

Table 66.3: Dietary Recommendations for Kidney Transplant Recipients

Nutrients	Acute Period	Chronic Period
Protein	1.2–2.0 g/kg/day	Same as general population. Adjust with chronic allograft dysfunction
Energy	30–35 kcal/kg/day or Basal energy expenditure × 1.3 to 1.5	25–35 kcal/kg/day Adjust to maintain or achieve ideal body weight
Nutrition support	In patients at risk of or with protein-energy wasting, nutritional supplement drinks are indicated if dietary counselling is unable to meet nutritional requirements	
Carbohydrates	Limit sugar and emphasise wholegrains and carbohydrate distribution to assist with glucose control and unwanted weight gain	
Fats	Limit to 30% or less of total calories. Emphasise unsaturated fatty acid sources in place of saturated fat and trans-fat	
Sodium	Less than 2000 mg/day to control hypertension and fluid balance.	
Potassium	2–4 g/day, if hyperkalaemic	Individualise to maintain normal serum potassium levels, depending on graft function and the effect of immunosuppressive therapy
Phosphorus	Individualise to maintain normal serum phosphorus levels, depending on allograft function	
Calcium	Individualise to maintain normal serum calcium levels	800–1200 mg/day to maintain serum calcium levels and normal bone metabolism

Table 66.3:   (*Continued*)

Nutrients	Acute Period	Chronic Period
Magnesium	Individualise based on allograft function and serum levels. If hypomagnesaemia, supplementation may be needed as dietary sources are usually not adequate to correct hypomagnesaemia.	
Other vitamins and minerals	Individualise, based on recommended dietary allowances.	
Fluid	Individualise, based on the allograft function. Generally unrestricted and encouraged. May be limited if oedema/fluid overload or requires dialysis.	Individualise, generally unrestricted and encouraged with an adequate allograft function.
Herbals	Contraindicated	
Drug-nutrient interactions	Avoid foods and drinks that inhibit the cytochrome P450 isoenzyme. Avoid grapefruit, grapefruit juice, pomegranate, pomegranate juice, and seville orange.	

- Acute post-KT recovery phase usually lasts 6–8 weeks (or longer if there are complications). The nutrition goals are to:
  - Optimise nutritional status to promote wound healing after surgery
  - Achieve acceptable electrolytes
  - Avoid foodborne illnesses
  - Avoid food-drug interaction
- Nutrition goals during the chronic post-KT maintenance phase are to:
  - Promote healthy eating habits to prevent or manage nutrition-related side effects from transplant medications

- Avoid foodborne illnesses

- Avoid food-drug interaction

- Food safety — immunosuppressed patients may have an increased risk of foodborne illnesses. Four basic principles in ensuring food safety include:

  - Washing and keeping your food, kitchen and hands clean

  - Separating raw and cooked food

  - Keeping food at safe temperatures

  - Cooking food thoroughly

Nutrition monitoring and evaluation

- Health outcomes and goals may change as patients move from one stage of CKD to the next or when there is a change in treatment modalities (e.g., HD, PD and KT).

- Regular follow-up sessions with dietitians are crucial for nutritional monitoring and evaluation. This is to assess the effectiveness of MNT and adjust nutrition intervention periodically, in consideration of laboratory results and nutritional status.

- Health outcomes that are used for nutrition monitoring and evaluation include:

  - Food and nutrition-related history

  - Changes in biochemical data, medical tests, and procedures

  - Changes in anthropometric measurements

  - Nutrition-focused physical findings.

References

Academy of Nutrition and Dietetics. (2023). The Nutrition Care Process (NCP). https://www.ncpro.org/nutrition-care-process

Carrero JJ, Thomas F, Nagy K, *et al.* (2018). Global prevalence of protein-energy wasting in kidney disease: A meta-analysis of contemporary observational studies from the International Society of Renal Nutrition and Metabolism. *J Ren Nutr* **28**(6): 380–392.

Fouque D, Kalantar-Zadeh K, Kopple J, *et al.* (2008). A proposed nomenclature and diagnostic criteria for protein-energy wasting in acute and chronic kidney disease. *Kidney Int* **73**(4): 391–398.

Ikizler TA, Burrowes JD, Byham-Gray LD, *et al.* (2020) KDOQI Clinical practice guideline for nutrition in CKD 2020 update. *Am J Kidney Dis* **76**(3 Suppl 1): S1–S107.

Norris H and Cochran CC (2022). Nutrition management of the adult kidney transplant patient. In: *Clinical Guide to Nutrition Care in Kidney Disease*. 3rd ed. Chicago: Academy of Nutrition and Dietetics, pp. 111–137.

67 Common Dermatological Manifestations of Kidney Disease

Denise Ann Tsang, Oh Choon Chiat

Dermatologic conditions are highly prevalent among patients with end-stage kidney disease (ESKD). Broadly, these may be grouped into:

(1) Cutaneous manifestations associated with the underlying aetiology of ESRD (i.e., diabetes mellitus, vasculitis)

(2) Cutaneous manifestations associated with ESRD

(3) Cutaneous manifestations associated with kidney transplant

The aim of this chapter is to provide an overview of the common cutaneous manifestations associated with ESRD.

(1) Pruritus

Pathophysiology

- Associated with protracted uraemia, although the exact mechanism is unclear

- Proposed hypotheses include increased systemic inflammation, imbalance in opiate receptors and a neuropathic process.

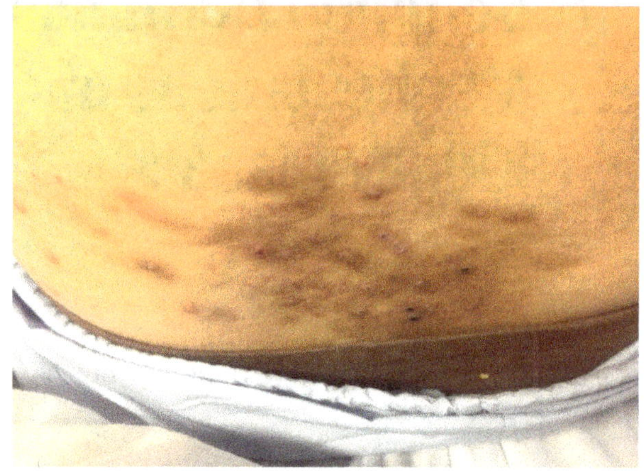

Figure 67.1:   Renal Pruritus. Hyperpigmented, Scaly Papules and Plaques over the Back Admixed with Excoriations

Clinical features (Figure 67.1)

- May be generalised or localised

- May or may not be associated with a rash

- Manifestations include excoriations, prurigo nodularis, lichen simplex chronicus (LSC)

Treatment (Table 67.1)

Table 67.1: Therapeutic Options for Uraemic Pruritus	
First line	Emollients e.g. White soft paraffin/liquid paraffin TDS, aqueous cream TDS
	Potent topical steroids for prurigo nodularis, LSC e.g. Mometasone furoate 0.1% ointment BD, beprosalic ointment BD
	Optimisation of haemodialysis prescription

Table 67.1:   (*Continued*)

Second line	Gabapentin
	■ Start at 100 mg OD and uptitrate gradually
	■ Maximum doses for patients on dialysis: 100 mg 3×/wk after dialysis (HD), 100 mg EON (PD)
	■ Pregabalin as an alternative
Third line	Phototherapy
	■ NB-UVB 3 times per week for 6 weeks
Fourth line	Mirtazapine
	■ Start from 7.5 mg ON, uptitrate to 15 mg ON slowly

Abbreviations: BD, twice a day; EON, every other night; HD, haemodialysis; OD, once a day; ON, once a night; NV-UVB, narrowband ultraviolet B; PD, peritoneal dialysis

(2) Xerosis

Pathophysiology

- Exact mechanism is unclear

- Proposed hypotheses include dehydration of the stratum corneum, eccrine gland dysfunction, decreased sebum and sweat production as a result of gland atrophy

Clinical features (Figure 67.2)

- Dry, cracked skin with scaling

- May or may not be associated with pruritus

- *Common sites*: Extensor surfaces of lower extremities, forearms

- *Associations*: Asteatotic eczema, acquired ichthyosis, LSC, contact dermatitis (to over-the-counter medications)

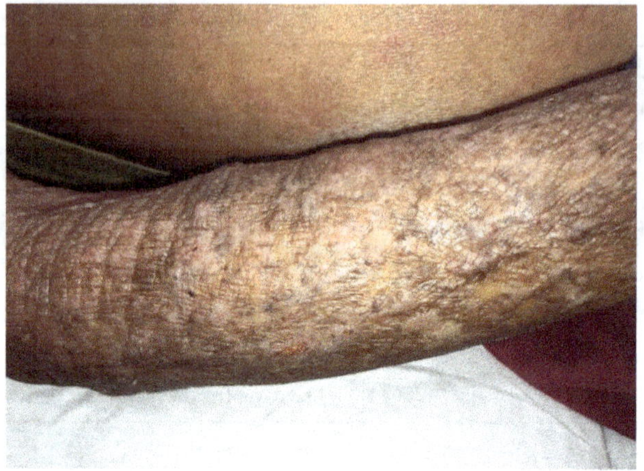

Figure 67.2: Xerosis. Dry, Scaly Skin over the Left Arm and Trunk, with Areas of Erythema and Post-inflammatory Hyperpigmentation

Treatment

1. Emollients e.g., White soft paraffin/liquid paraffin TDS, aqueous cream TDS

2. Treatment of associated dermatoses e.g., associated eczema or contact dermatitis will require treatment with topical steroids

(3) Acquired Perforating Dermatosis

Pathophysiology

- Pathogenesis is poorly understood
- It has been theorised that excessive scratching incites epithelial hyperplasia, follicular hyperkeratosis, and degeneration of dermal connective tissue, with subsequent elimination of degenerated elements through the epidermis.

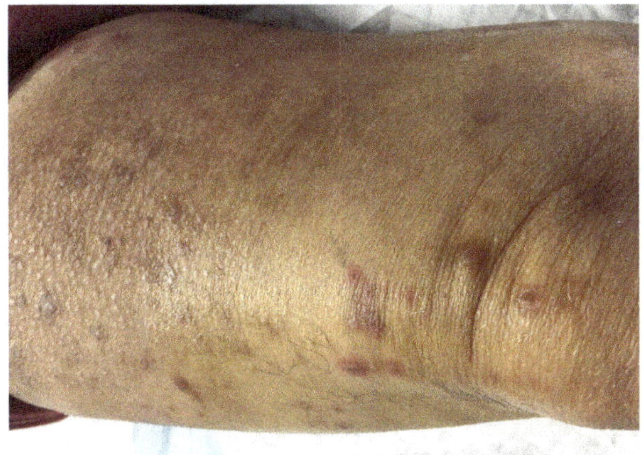

Figure 67.3:   Perforating Dermatosis. Discrete Erythematous Papules over the Knee with Crust-filled Craters

- Other proposed mechanisms include epidermal proliferation and differentiation mismatch, increased serum fibronectin, transforming growth factor-b3 overexpression and abnormal metalloproteinase reactivity.

Clinical features (Figure 67.3)

- Grouped dome-shaped papules or nodules, often umbilicated with a central crust-filled crater
- *Clinical course*: Spontaneous resolution of well-developed lesions with continued development of new lesions
- Treatment of extensive perforating dermatosis is difficult and various therapies have not produced consistent results.

Treatment (Table 67.2)

Table 67.2:   Therapeutic Options for Acquired Perforating Dermatosis (Yong *et al.*, 2014)

Topical	Corticosteroids e.g. Betamethasone valerate 0.05% cream BD, mometasone furorate 0.1% cream BD
	Topical retinoids e.g. Tretinoin cream 0.025% or 0.05% ON Keratolytics e.g. Salicylic acid
Physical	Phototherapy • PUVA • NB-UVB (Ohe *et al.*, 2004) • Photodynamic therapy Cryotherapy • *Frequency*: Weekly or fortnightly
Systemic	Antibiotics • *Examples*: Doxycycline, clindamycin Antihistamines • Fexofenadine 180 mg OD or BD, cetirizine 10 mg OD or BD Retinoids • Isotretinoin

Abbreviations: BD, twice a day; NV-UVB, narrowband ultraviolet B; OD, once a day; ON, once a night; PUVA, Psoralen plus ultraviolet A

(4) Calciphylaxis

Pathophysiology

- Not well understood

- "Sensitiser plus challenger" model has been proposed.

  - *Sensitiser (predisposing factor)*: Underlying metabolic dysfunction (e.g., secondary hyperparathyroidism, abnormal serum calcium and phosphate levels)

  - *Challenger (second incident)*: Trauma or increased calcium load eventually leads to calcium deposition and development of cutaneous necrosis

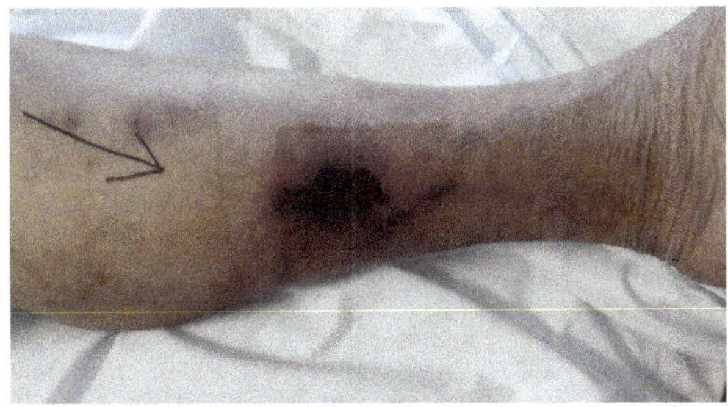

Figure 67.4:   Calciphylaxis. Cutaneous Necrosis with a Stellate Configuration (Proximally), Surrounding Retiform Purpura

Clinical features (Figure 67.4)

- Severe pain, burning, occasionally pruritic

- Most commonly occurs on the lower limbs

- Retiform purpura, livedo reticularis, stellate ulcers, cutaneous necrosis

Treatment (Table 67.3)

Table 67.3:   Therapeutic Options for Calciphylaxis (Bolognia *et al.*, 2017)

Underlying disease	Dialysis • Increase frequency or duration of dialysis • Low calcium dialysate Low phosphate diet, phosphate binders
Wound care	Intensive wound care • Appropriate dressings • Autolytic or chemical debridement Surgical debridement Management of wound infections

(Continued)

Table 67.3:　(*Continued*)

Disease-specific: Sodium thiosulphate	Dose • HD: 25 g thrice weekly (during the last hour of haemodialysis) • PD: 25 g weekly Route • Intravenous • Intra-lesional (for small lesions) Side effects • Nausea, vomiting, metabolic acidosis, QT prolongation, hypotension, volume overload, reduced bone density • May consider: Decreasing dose, increasing interval of administration, switching the diluent from saline to 5% dextrose (reduces nausea)
Others	Hyperbaric oxygen therapy, tissue plasminogen activator, anticoagulation and maggot therapy have been described in literature

Abbreviations: HD, haemodialysis; PD, peritoneal dialysis

(5) Pseudoporphyria

Pathophysiology

- Mechanism is unknown

- Uraemia has been proposed as a probable mechanism via decreasing the activity of uroporphyrinogen decarboxylase (catalyses the first decarboxylation pathway of the porphyrin pathway).

Clinical features (Figure 67.5)

- Vesicles and bullae with clear or haemorrhagic contents

- Develop after months to years of dialysis

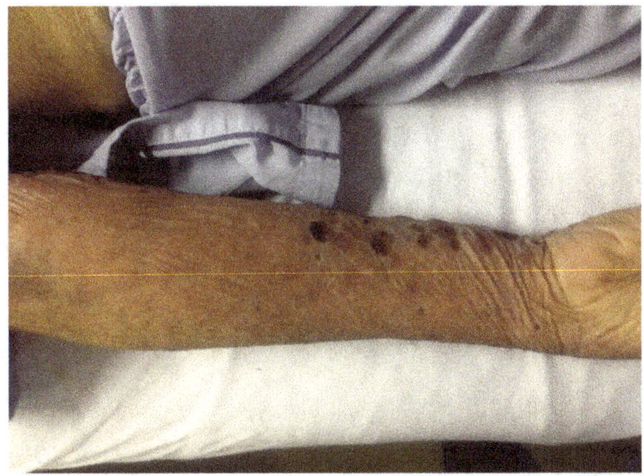

Figure 67.5:   Pseudoporphyria. Bullae and Erosions over the Forearm of a Patient Receiving Haemodialysis

- Exacerbated by sunlight
- *Common sites*: Dorsae of hands, scalp, face, and neck

Workup and treatment

1. Exclude true porphyria — plasma or serum porphyrin assay
   - Note that ESKD patient on HD or PD may have increased plasma porphyrin levels due to reduced excretion, in the absence of enzyme deficiency
2. Identify and stop photosensitising medications
   - Antibiotics: Tetracyclines, sulphonamides
   - Antifungals: Griseofulvin
   - Non-steroidal anti-inflammatory drugs: Ibuprofen, naproxen, piroxicam
   - Cardiovascular: Amiodarone, hydrochlorothiazide

3. Exclude aluminum toxicity

4. Sun protection

5. Oral N-acetylcysteine (600–1200 mg/day) led to the resolution of blistering and fragility within 3 weeks to 2 months in several cases of bullous disease of dialysis

References

Abdelbaqi-Salhab M, Shalhub S and Morgan MB (2003). A current review of the cutaneous manifestations of renal disease. *J Cutan Pathol* **30**(9): 527–538.

Bolognia JL, Schaffer JV and Lorenzo C (2017) *Dermatology E-Book*, 4th ed. Elsevier Health Sciences, Kindle Edition.

Combs SA, Teixeira JP and Germain MJ (2015). Pruritus in kidney disease. *Semin Nephrol* **35**(4): 383–391.

Gholyaf M, Sheikh V, Yasrebifar F, *et al.* (2020). Effect of mirtazapine on pruritus in patients on hemodialysis: A cross-over pilot study. *Int Urol Nephrol* **52**(6): 1155–1165.

Goel V, Sil A and Das A (2021). Cutaneous manifestations of chronic kidney disease, dialysis and post-renal transplant: A review. *Indian J Dermatol* **66**(1): 3.

Guiotoku MM, Pereira F de P, Miot HA and Marques MEA (2011). Pseudoporphyria induced by dialysis treated with oral N-acetylcysteine. *An Bras Dermatol* **86**(2): 383–385.

Ko M-J, Yang J-Y, Wu H-Y, *et al.* (2023) Narrowband ultraviolet B phototherapy for patients with refractory uraemic pruritus: A randomized controlled trial. *Br J Dermatol* **165**(3): 633–639.

Ohe S, Danno K, Sasaki H, *et al.* (2004). Treatment of acquired perforating dermatosis with narrowband ultraviolet B. *J Am Acad Dermatol* **50**(6): 892–894.

Yong A, Chong WS and Tey HL (2014). Effective treatment of uremic pruritus and acquired perforating dermatosis with amitriptyline. *Australas J Dermatol* **55**(3): e54–57.

68 Psychosocial Considerations in Kidney Disease

Faith Wong, Goh Soo Cheng

Patient's journey along the kidney disease illness trajectory

- Chronic kidney disease can be a long-drawn disease during which patients may oscillate between different time-phases of chronic illness before they finally reach their terminal phase.

- There are three time-phases of chronic illness within the Family System Illness (FSI) model developed by Rolland (1994):
  - The crisis phase
  - The chronic phase
  - The terminal phase

- Healthcare providers can use this model as a guide in providing care services and support.

The crisis phase

- The onset of end-stage kidney disease (ESKD) can be acute for some patients. This could be following an acute kidney injury or some patients being asymptomatic until the late stage of illness.

- Some patients may find it difficult to accept their diagnosis and procrastinate making plans for dialysis treatment.

- Even for patients who have made plans for treatment, the point of an ESKD diagnosis can throw them off equilibrium and into a crisis.

- During this phase, it is important to provide emotional and practical support to help patients and their families make sense of the diagnosis, understand various kidney replacement therapy (KRT) options, and decide on an appropriate treatment plan.

- Patients can experience a turmoil of emotions and thoughts as they grapple with the diagnosis and the deluge of information regarding their illness and treatment. Hence, healthcare providers should review patients' coping and assess if appropriate referrals to mental health services need to be initiated.

- Apart from validating patients' emotions and providing counselling to them, linking them to support group services or relevant community agencies for further assistance can be helpful for patients.

- Healthcare providers may also need to facilitate discussions between patients and their significant others, where appropriate, to derive at a shared decision on treatment and care plans for the patient.

- One of the tools to explore the patient's perception of the impact of their serious illnesses and treatment options is the Serious Illness Conversation Guide (SICG).

- At Singapore General Hospital, the renal medical social workers have adapted the SICG (Beddard-Huber *et al.*, 2021) to facilitate treatment discussions with renal patients (Table 68.1).

- Many patients are concerned about the financial burden of the treatment and their ability to afford it.

Table 68.1: Serious Illness Conversation Guide (Adapted from Canadian Version)

Set up the conversation	**Explain the role of healthcare provider** • I'm part of the team supporting patients with poorer kidney functions. • We want to understand your concerns and are here to support you. **Ask permission** • How are you feeling today? • Can we talk about your kidney condition today? Is this okay?
Assess understanding and information preferences	**Assess knowledge of own health and the available kidney replacement therapy options** • What do you know about your kidney condition so far? • What do you think is happening with your kidney condition right now? • How much information about your illness and treatment would you like from me? • What is your idea of dialysis treatment? • Do you have past experiences with family members/ friends on dialysis?
Share prognosis	**This is my understanding of where things are right now…** **Uncertain** • I'm worried that your kidney function could change quickly, and I think it is important to prepare for that possibility. Or **Time** • I wish we were not in this situation, but I am worried that you may reach end-stage kidney disease soon, and time may be as short as … (e.g., several months to a year). Or **Function** • I hope that your kidney function will remain stable as long as possible, but I'm worried that this may be as good as it will be, and things might get worse in the future.

(Continued)

Table 68.1:   (*Continued*)

Explore key topics	**Fears/worries** • When you think about your health worsening, what worries you? • What does "suffering" (use patient's term) mean to you? • How are you coping with the news of diagnosis? **Sources of strength** • What gives you strength through the hard times? • Who gives you strength? • Do you have a religion? • What do you pray for? Who do you pray to? **Priorities/Goals** • If your health gets worse, what's important to you? • Why is this important to you? • What do you hope dialysis can help you to achieve in life? **Critical abilities** • What abilities are so important for you that you can't imagine living without them? (e.g., functional independence, being able to take care of themselves, being able to work) **Trade-offs** • If your kidney function gets worse, how much treatment are you willing to go through to achieve _____ (based on what patient mention is important to them, e.g., functional independence)?
Explore social context	**Family background/Social support** • Is your family aware about what is important to you? • Can you tell me about your family? Who stays with you? • Who is supporting you financially? • How are you taking care of yourself? • If you need help with care, is there anyone in the family who can care for you? How is the level of commitment like?

Table 68.1: (*Continued*)

Close the conversation	**Summary and recommendation**
	• I've heard you say that _________ is really important to you.
	• Keeping that in mind, and what we know about your illness, I suggest that we ____ (e.g., refer you to community support / start the application for subsidised dialysis programme at our next meeting/ make a decision on your RRT modality at the next meeting). How does this plan sound to you?
	• If you think of anything else later, we can revisit the conversation another time.

- Sharing of information on healthcare financing options and assisting to apply for relevant subsidies and/or assistance for the patients can help to alleviate their financial burden and stress.

- Referrals can also be made to community-based care services to help patients access appropriate care support to manage and remain in the community.

The chronic phase

- Most patients take a while to adjust to the dialysis treatment regime and settle into a new routine as they enter the chronic phase.

- Depending on the patient's medical condition, the chronic phase can be short, or may stretch for years.

- During this phase, treatment fatigue may set in, and patients may find it challenging to maintain adherence to treatment regime. It is helpful to identify factors that influence patients' treatment adherence and enhance their motivation or remove barriers where possible.

- It is also a good opportunity to introduce Advance Care Planning (ACP) to ascertain and document patients' values and health-care preferences about treatment before they develop serious illness and become uncommunicative.

- Continual review of patients' values and preferences at this phase will ensure that their treatment goals are met and their treatment plan remains sustainable.

- Some patients may develop conditions that necessitate a change of treatment modality, which can then move them back to the crisis phase.

The terminal phase

- The transition to the terminal phase can present as either a gradual or sudden deterioration in the patient's medical condition.

- Intense emotional and existential concerns may arise, requiring healthcare providers to focus on goals of care conversations, psycho-emotional support, and end-of-life practical care needs.

- It is essential to educate and reassure patients that care and support continues during palliative care and that they are not abandoned.

- During the terminal phase, facilitating reconciliation with significant others, working on unfinished business, and providing a safe space to allow patients and their loved ones to talk about end-of-life issues are crucial to supporting patients.

- Collaboration with other allied health professionals like art or music therapists to conduct legacy work with the patients can also provide lasting memories for their loved ones.

- Referrals to community services for home care or inpatient hospice care will ensure that patients continue to receive appropriate care during this last phase of their life and alleviate their caregivers' care burden.

Understanding the impact of kidney disease through the Biopsychosocial-spiritual model

- The impact of chronic and ESKD is complex and multi-faceted.

- The illness can impact a person not just physically but also psychologically, socially and spiritually. Likewise, a person's psychological state, social situation, and spirituality can also impact how he/she copes with and adapts to the illness as well as the treatment.

- It is thus helpful to adopt the Bio-psychosocial-spiritual (BPSS) model in understanding patients and work with them on shared-decision-making in terms of their illness coping and treatment decisions.

- Engel (1977) developed the Biopsychosocial model, which was later expanded to include the spiritual domain (Hatala, 2013). Table 68.2 shows the four domains of the BPSS model, the possible impact, and suggested interventions for patients:

Psychosocial considerations for the different modalities of kidney replacement therapies

- KRT includes haemodialysis, peritoneal dialysis, and renal transplantation. Each therapy has its pros and cons.

Table 68.2:   The Four Domains of the BPSS Model

Domains	Possible Impact	Suggested Interventions
Biological	• Discomfort (e.g., nausea and bloatedness) or pain due to the condition or side effects of treatment • Body image issues — having a peritoneal dialysis catheter or bulging of vascular access • Decline in physical health and fatigue	• Provide psychoeducation on the medical condition and coping with illness • Clarify misconceptions • Explore kidney replacement therapy options • Collaborate with patient to review treatment goals and plan
Psychological	• Mental health conditions may affect decision-making, adherence to treatment or coping strategies (e.g., depression can result in a loss of motivation, or stigma and discrimination can worsen anxiety) • Inadequate/ineffective coping strategies may exacerbate mental health conditions • Greater appreciation for life and insights about self-care	• Validate the patient's emotions and affirm their resilience • Referral to mental health services for further assessment and intervention • Provide individual counselling or support group services • Provide psychoeducation on coping
Social	• Reduced employability due to a demanding treatment regime or deteriorating health condition. • Increase in financial burden due to treatment-related expenses (e.g., transport and medical reviews) • Changes in family roles, duties and responsibilities • Reduced opportunities and desire for socialisation due to a demanding treatment regime	• Review and encourage patients to enhance their social support network • Enhance access to financial subsidies or assistance • Referral to vocational services • Provide individual counselling or support group services for patient or family members • Referral to community services for support

Table 68.2:   (*Continued*)

Domains	Possible Impact	Suggested Interventions
	• Lifestyle changes like dietary and fluid restrictions and travel restrictions	
Spiritual	• Make meaning of their illness and suffering • Existential crisis and loss of hope • Questioning of values and beliefs	• Review the patient's spiritual resources and needs • Explore narratives and tap on their internal resources to help in their coping

- Patient and their family members should have a clear understanding what each KRT entails to make an informed decision and be committed to the long-term treatment.

- Firstly, patients need to understand which KRT is suitable for them based on their medical conditions and then consider the psychosocial factors relating to the treatment.

- Secondly, helping patients with their treatment decision-making involves understanding the BPSS aspects of their lives and how these factors can impact or be affected by their individual situations.

- Some psychosocial factors to consider includes the patient's lifestyle (e.g., how their daily routine or employment will be affected by the treatment regime), level of social support (e.g., commitment and competence of their caregiver to assist with treatment), financial situation (e.g., insurance coverage and eligibility for subsidies), and logistics arrangement (e.g., transport to and from the dialysis centre or storage space for PD solutions) for the treatment.

- After all, the aim of treatment is not just to extend life span but also, to maintain or enhance a patient's quality of life.

References

Beddard-Huber E, Gaspard G and Yue K. (2021). Adaptations to the serious illness conversation guide to be more culturally safe. *Int J Indig Health* **16**(1): 38–53.

Chueng SL, Chin E, Chua EC, *et al.* (2023). A bio-psychosocial-spiritual assessment guide for health and social work. https://sasw.org.sg/wp-content/uploads/2023/02/A-Bio-Psychosocial-Spiritual-Assessment-Guide-for-Health-and-Social-Work.pdf

Engel GL (1977). The need for a new medical model: A challenge for biomedicine. *Science* **196**(4286): 129–136.

Goh SC and Sim AGH (2021). Medical social work in Singapore: Context and practice. In: *Renal Social Work*. Lee GL and Goh SN (eds.). Singapore: World Scientific Publishing Company, pp. 127–145.

Hatala AR (2013) Towards a biopsychosocial-spiritual approach in health pyschology: Exploring theoretical orientations and future directions. *J Spiritual Ment Health* **15**(4): 256–276.

Mandel EI, Bernacki RE and Block SD (2017). Serious illness conversations in ESRD. *Clin J Am Soc Nephrol* **12**(5): 854–863.

Rolland JS (1994). *Families, Illness and Disability: An Integrative Treatment Model*. Basic Books.

69 Ethical Issues in Nephrology

Crystal Lim

- This chapter aims to provide clinicians with core concepts on clinical ethics to guide ethical decision-making. Its scope limits in-depth discussions of complex ethical theories and concepts.

The four meta-principles of bioethics

- Ethical theories provide a framework for thinking through ethical challenges; they do not necessarily provide answers. The most commonly used bioethics decision-making framework is the "four principles of bioethics" or "principlism" approach.

- This framework adopts a weighing and balancing of 4 core ethical principles to determine, through reasoning, which ethical principle should take priority (has more weight) or is most compelling in a particular ethical conflict or dilemma — hence, should be upheld.

- No ethical framework is adequate for addressing all ethical conflicts since these can be complex.

- When applying the principlism framework, one could additionally consider other principles and values relevant to the case, such as professional values of veracity (truthfulness), confidentiality and fidelity (promise-keeping) or virtues like compassion, trustworthiness and honesty.

- In ethical decision-making, our consideration is for an ethically *appropriate* course of action, not about what is the right or wrong action, since the latter may be hard to determine.

- Clinicians should be mindful not to impose their personal values when making ethical decisions.

- Beauchamp and Childress (2019) identified 4 core principles of bioethics: non-maleficence, beneficence, respect for autonomy, and justice. The following segment is derived from their work.

1. *Non-maleficence*

- Non-maleficence means to do no harm; it requires intentionally *avoiding* actions that will cause needless harm.

- Harm extends beyond causing physical injury or ill-doing.

- Harm is caused when there is "thwarting, defeating or setting back the interest — welfare condition of welfare advantage — of a person, whether intentionally or unintentionally" (Beauchamp & Childress, 2019).

- For example, the medical team assesses that a frail, elderly patient who lives alone has significant fall risk and wants her referred for nursing home placement, which is against this patient's wish. While the medical team means well because they want to prevent her from falling at home, which will then aggravate her condition (physical harm), their action causes her harm because they disregard her stated interest — to return to her home environment — which she values.

- Consideration for what constitutes harm takes into account the context.

2. *Beneficence*

- Beneficence means to do good — it involves taking actions to promote good, remove harm, or prevent harm in other persons.

- In contrast to non-maleficence which requires abstaining from actions that will cause harm, beneficence requires performing actions to bring about good.

- Beneficence can be obligatory or non-obligatory.

- Doing good requires resources or involves costs; hence, it is not always possible or justified.

- For example, a doctor is not obligated to provide clinically non-beneficial treatment to a patient who demands it because it will not offer the benefits that the patient is looking for.

3. *Respect for autonomy*

- The word "autonomy" is derived from Greek, and it means self-rule; it is about the liberty to act according to one's free will.

- In law and in ethics, it is deemed important to respect the autonomy of a capacitous person (that is, a person with mental capacity) because human beings should be allowed to choose their own course in life.

- Autonomy is not to be confused with individualism, which claims that a person's interest is more important than that of others or the community.

- The principle of respect for autonomy consists of:

  - *Positive autonomy*, which requires for actions that promote a person's liberty to act according to what he or she wants. Examples in healthcare include providing information to a patient so that the patient can decide on his treatment choice, providing justified medical treatment to patient who wants it, informed consent, maintaining patient confidentiality, and respecting the patient's privacy.

- *Negative autonomy* requires that a person is free from controlling interferences or constraints that will infringe on his liberty to act. In exercising his autonomy, for instance, a capacitous patient can reject medical information or medical treatment, including life-sustaining treatment.

- There are limits to respect for a person's autonomy, such as when a person's choice will:
  - cause harm to others
  - endanger public health
  - require scarce resources where funding is an issue
  - require substantial societal resources but achieve limited gains (that is, the costs disproportionately outweigh the benefits)

- An autonomous act must contain *all* three of the following:
  - The act is carried out with intentionality — A person either intends or does not intend a particular action.
  - The act is carried out with comprehension — complete comprehension is not required, and it is often hard to achieve anyway. Adequate comprehension or comprehension of what is pertinent and relevant suffices.
  - The act is carried out voluntarily — An act is voluntary if the person carrying out the act is not under the control of another person or the control of a personal psychological condition.

- An understanding of what constitutes an autonomous decision has implication for a doctor obtaining informed consent for treatment. Suppose an elderly patient was recently commenced on dialysis. She informs her doctor that she really does not want dialysis but relented because her adult children kept persuading her and used emotional blackmail tactics such that she felt pressured. The patient feels forced by her children to accept dialysis treatment and is unhappy. Her decision is not an autonomous one if it lacks voluntariness and can invalidate her informed consent. When confronted with such a situation, the renal team should further explore the patient's comprehension and preferences. If the patient indeed does not want dialysis treatment, a family conference to address the importance of allowing the patient her choice is advisable.

- In medicine, we use persuasion to influence patients towards positive change or to agree to certain actions, and this is acceptable, provided we do not go overboard. Excessive or undue influence is considered coercive — it renders a decision or action as lacking voluntariness, hence not autonomous. For example, if a patient has made an informed decision — that is, a decision made with adequate comprehension and with voluntariness — not to have chronic dialysis treatment, and a doctor repeatedly counsels the patient on the benefits of dialysis in the hope of changing the patient's mind. This is not acceptable because the doctor's undue or excessive persuasion can be experienced as coercive by the patient. In respecting a patient's autonomy, the doctor has a negative obligation to not impose controlling interferences on the patient's choice.

4. *Justice*

- In healthcare, we focus on distributive justice, which is about "fair, equitable and appropriate distribution of benefits and burdens determined by norms that structure the terms of social co-operation" (Childress & Beauchamp, 2019, p. 268).

- The principle of justice is complex, and fair allocation of resources is difficult to negotiate because of resource scarcity. Should we distribute to each person according to equal share, past contributions, merit, current need, or the potential to benefit from the treatment?

- Healthcare rationing or healthcare triaging is a reality that the practice of medicine cannot shun. A prudent response is to establish policy or guidelines that set priorities or criteria for access to treatment. Doing so reduces bedside rationing that tends to lead to decision-variability or inconsistency across decision-makers, and instead increases fair practice.

- Within the discussion of distributive justice is whether healthcare is a right, and public debate on this continues with no conclusion. Most societies agree on the right to basic or decent minimum of healthcare. However, constraining this right so that it does not burgeon to the provision of expansive and costly treatment is challenging. For example:
    - While living donor kidney transplant is deemed as basic healthcare, how should we regard expensive ABO-incompatible kidney transplant?
    - If the placement of a particular patient on chronic dialysis will only be feasible if this patient also receives nursing

home care and ambulance access for dialysis treatment — all of which will require full public funding because this patient does not have the financial means — should this patient then be considered for chronic dialysis given its other significant attendant costs?

- Should healthcare money be channelled to very expensive curative cancer treatment or on lifelong dialysis?

Case illustrations on the four bioethical principles

1. *Principles of non-maleficence, beneficence, and respect for autonomy*

A patient has previously made an informed decision not to have chronic dialysis when her kidneys fail. This patient is now admitted to the hospital. She is uraemic and has lost her mental capacity for treatment decision. The attending nephrologist decides that the patient should be commenced on dialysis because doctors have a duty to save lives, and extending a patient's life is an act of beneficence.

One could say that there are two types of harm here:

(1) The harm of patient dying imminently because patient is not dialysed.

(2) The harm that is caused to the patient when her wish not to be dialysed is ignored.

(Continued)

(Continued)

In this situation, because the patient has indicated her wish not to be dialysed, providing her with the treatment when she does not want it is not beneficence. On the contrary, it is maleficence (causing harm) because the doctor has set back her interest — which is not to have dialysis. While the intention of providing medical treatment is to alleviate symptoms and suffering and to postpone an untimely death, this may not be a goal that all patients seek. To provide treatment to a patient against the patient's wishes is a violation of the patient's autonomy. In this case, the doctor should respect the patient's decision that was made when she had capacity and not dialyse her. The ethical principles to be upheld here are non-maleficence: refraining from commencing dialysis for a patient who does not want it and respect for patient autonomy — since the patient has in the past expressed a wish not to be dialysed.

Now, let us tweak the above case scenario with this bit of new information: the patient's son informs that the patient mentioned to the family last week that she was having second thoughts about refusing dialysis because she realised that her kidneys were failing, and that she was not ready to die and be parted from her family. In this case, the patient should be provided dialysis with the aim of restoring her mental capacity, which would then allow the medical team to clarify directly with her if she has indeed changed her mind and now wants chronic dialysis treatment. Here, we are upholding the ethical principles of beneficence and respect for autonomy.

2. *Principles of justice and respect for autonomy*

A 62-year-old male who is an ex-smoker and on haemodialysis for the last four years has been admitted for critical limb ischaemia, necrotising fasciitis, and severe sepsis on a background of extensive peripheral vascular disease without revascularisation options. He is strongly advised for amputation as a life-saving procedure, but he refuses as he is adamant that he wants to keep his leg. However, he is afraid to die and wants "everything else" done for him, including intensive care, cardiopulmonary resuscitation, and mechanical ventilation. Without leg amputation, this patient will eventually die from uncontrolled sepsis regardless of ICU care. What is an ethically appropriate course of action here for the medical team?

The doctors have to respect the patient's negative autonomy — the right to refuse lower limb amputation. Hence, they cannot subject the patient to an amputation against his wishes; doing otherwise is a form of battery. However, the doctors are not obligated to fulfil the patient's positive autonomy by placing him in the ICU, should such a need arise, since ICU care is medically futile here: the patient will succumb to uncontrolled sepsis without a limb amputation. In this context, the principle of justice is the overriding principle: healthcare resources should not be expanded on medically futile interventions. Furthermore, beneficence is not always obligatory.

The four-box approach

- Understanding the 4 ethical principles is important for developing capability in ethical decision-making. However, clinicians often face challenges in prioritising these principles. Jonsen *et al.* (2022) developed a framework for organising information into 4 quadrants, and this has become commonly referred to as the "four-box" or "four topics approach" to ethical decision-making (Table 69.1). Each box suggests information to be obtained and deals with at least one of the 4 ethical principles, and collectively, all the 4 principles are considered in this framework.

Table 69.1:   The Four-Box Chart

Medical Indications	Patient Preferences
Principles: Beneficence and Non-maleficence	**Principle: Respect for Patient Autonomy**
1. What is the patient's medical problem? Is the problem acute? Chronic? Critical? Emergent? Terminal?	1. Has the patient been informed of the benefits and risks of diagnostic and treatment recommendations, understood this information, and given consent?
2. What are the goals of treatment?	2. Is the patient mentally capable and legally competent, or is there evidence of mental incapacity?
3. In what circumstances is medical treatment not indicated?	3. If the patient is capacitous, what is the patient stating about preferences for treatment?
4. What are the probabilities of success of various treatment options?	4. If the patient is incapacitous, has the patient expressed prior preferences? Does the patient have an advance care plan (ACP) to provide insight on the patient's likely values and preferences?
5. In sum, how can this patient be benefited by medical and nursing care, and how can harm be avoided?	5. Does the patient have a lasting power of attorney (LPA) donee or court-appointed deputy?
	6. Is the patient unwilling or unable to cooperate with medical treatment? If so, why?

Table 69.1:   (Continued)

Quality of Life	Contextual Features
Principles: Beneficence, Non-maleficence, and Respect for Patient Autonomy	**Principles: Justice and Fairness**
1. What are the prospects, with or without treatment, for a return to normal life, and what physical, mental and social deficits might the patient experience even if treatment succeeds?	1. Are there professional, inter-professional, or business interests that might create conflicts of interest in the clinical treatment of patients?
2. On what grounds can anyone judge that some quality of life would be undesirable for a patient who cannot make or express such a judgement?	2. Are there other parties other than the clinician and patient, such as family members, who have a legitimate interest in clinical decisions?
3. Are there biases that might prejudice the provider's evaluation of the patient's quality of life?	3. What are the limits imposed on patient confidentiality by the legitimate interest of third parties?
4. What ethical issues arise concerning improving or enhancing a patient's quality of life?	4. Are there financial factors that create conflicts of interest in clinical decisions?
5. Do quality of life assessments raise any questions that might contribute to a change of treatment plan, such as forgoing life-sustaining treatment?	5. Are there problems of allocation of resources that affect clinical decisions?
6. Are there plans to provide pain relief and provide comfort after a decision has been made to forgo life-sustaining interventions?	6. Are there religious factors that might influence clinical decisions?
	7. What are the legal issues that might affect clinical decisions?
	8. Are there considerations of clinical research and medical education that affect clinical decisions?
	9. Are there considerations of public health and safety that influence clinical decisions?
	10. Does institutional affiliation create conflicts that might influence clinical decisions?

Adapted from Jonsen AR, Siegler M and Winslade WJ (2022). *Clinical Ethics. A Practical Approach to Ethical Decisions in Clinical Medicine.* 9th ed. New York: McGraw-Hill.

- Good ethical decision-making begins with good facts. At times, what may appear as an ethical conflict is because there is insufficient information for the case.

- Ensure there is adequate relevant information to provide a clear and comprehensive picture of the case.

- Obtain and organise facts of the case and information according to medical indications, patient's preferences, quality of life, and contextual features. Then, consider the relevant guiding questions in each of the "Four Boxes" for the case in hand.

- Formulating an ethical question or a statement of the ethical problem is helpful in guiding the reasoning. An ethical question should contain salient information of the case. For example:

  - Is it ethically appropriate to withdraw dialysis in a patient who is minimally communicative, largely unaware of his surrounding, and ADL-dependent?

  - Is there an ethical obligation to provide dialysis for a capacitous patient who is bedridden and has two young children, and whose wish for dialysis will require nursing home placement but he is unable to afford these?

- Based on the medical facts and ethical considerations for the particular case, decide which box carries more weight. Since ethical principles underlie each box, determining the "weighty" box leads to deciding which ethical principle is the overriding principle for the case.

- Most ethical conflicts can be reasoned through using the ethics frameworks, and few are truly ethical dilemmas where one has to choose from 2 or more dire options.

Applying "The Four-Box" approach

This case example will demonstrate the use of "the four-box" approach.

A 79-year-old male is admitted for advanced chronic kidney disease requiring dialysis. His medical history includes severe

MEDICAL INDICATIONS **Principles: Beneficence and Non-maleficence**	PATIENT PREFERENCES **Principle: Respect for Patient Autonomy**
• 79-year-old male • Patient has severe kidney failure for which dialysis is indicated. • His severe dementia with recent food refusal and ischaemic heart disease with no further revascularisation options carry a very limited survival prognosis on dialysis. • Patient's primary nephrologist assessed that the patient would not benefit from dialysis and would be harmed by complications of dialysis	• Patient's wishes regarding dialysis are not known. • He has not made an ACP. • He has not appointed an LPA. • According to the Mental Capacity Act, a decision on life-sustaining treatment is a medical decision to be made by doctors (and not by family members) based on the best interests principle. • Doctors should enquire from the patient's family and caregivers what his likely wishes regarding dialysis might have been, although this cannot be the overriding determinant of the final medical decision.
QUALITY OF LIFE **Principles: Beneficence, Non-maleficence, and Respect for Patient Autonomy**	CONTEXTUAL FEATURES **Principles: Justice and Fairness**
• Quality of life is poor and likely to deteriorate even further due to progressive severe dementia on the background of bed-bound status from prior CVA and full dependency for activities of daily living.	• Family wants the patient to be dialysed. • The family has no difficulty with affordability of private dialysis and care of the patient. • No public funds will be used for the patient's dialysis and home care.

dementia with recent food refusal, ischaemic heart disease with no further revascularisation option, and poor functional status: he is bed-bound from prior CVA and fully dependent for activities of daily living. The patient has no prior advance care plan (ACP) or appointed lasting power of attorney (LPA) and has no capacity to decide on starting dialysis or any other medical treatments. His family members insist that he be started on long-term dialysis despite having been counselled against it by his nephrologist in prior clinic consultations. Patient's family is well-resourced and can afford dialysis and care of the patient at home.

In this case, although beneficence and non-maleficence are crucial elements, despite counselling, insist on dialysis. Doctors are not legally or ethically obligated to provide a treatment (dialysis) when they think doing so is in the patient's best interest. However, they are medically obligated to offer and facilitate the transfer of care to another physician who is willing to provide dialysis if this is the route the family persists on pursuing.

Mental capacity

- The law presumes competence of adults. Competence is a global concept, meaning that a competent person is deemed as capable to make decisions for all aspects of his/her life. As a matter of law, only a court can decide if a person lacks competence. It is impractical if every case of suspected impairment in decision-making is brought to the court. Therefore, the notion of mental capacity is applied in healthcare.

- According to the Mental Capacity Act (MCA) (2008), mental capacity is a clinical judgement on "the ability of a person to make a specific decision at the time the decision needs to be made. Mental capacity is not about a person's ability to make decisions in general but about making specific decisions.

- A patient is considered to lack mental capacity if he/she cannot perform <u>any one or more</u> of the following tasks in regard to the decision to be made (Table 69.2).

Table 69.2:   Tasks Required for Determination of Mental Capacity

Tasks	Requirements
1. Understand the information	• Ensure that information is communicated in a language and at a level where the patient can comprehend. • Use visual aids, videos, etc., to enhance the patient's comprehension, if needed. • Allow the patient time to process the information. • Encourage the patient to explain his condition in his own words. • If the patient shows adequate or material comprehension — that is, the essence of information relevant to the decision to be made — this suffices for demonstration of mental capacity.
2. Remember the information	The patient needs to remember the information at least until he can understand it, weigh the information, and communicate the decision.
3. Weigh up the information in light of one's values and preferences	• Patient is able to make use of the information and reason his decision. • Patient is able to compare treatment options and their implications and explain his choice. • Patient's choice demonstrates congruence with his values.
4. Communicate the decision	• Until the patient has communicated his decision, his mental capacity is yet to be demonstrated. • Steps must be taken to facilitate a patient's communication if he has difficulty. For example, for a patient who has lost his speech, writing or pointing to pictures may be ways to help the patient express his wishes.

The 5 statutory principles of Mental Capacity Act (2008)

- It is required of everyone who is managing or caring for a person lacking mental capacity to observe the following statutory principles.

  - Principle 1: A person must be assumed to have capacity unless it is established that he lacks capacity.

  - Principle 2: A person is not to be treated as unable to make a decision unless all practicable steps to help him to do so have been taken without success.

  - Principle 3: A person is not to be treated as unable to make a decision merely because he makes an unwise decision.

  - Principle 4: An act done, or a decision made, under this Act for or on behalf of a person who lacks capacity must be done or made in his best interests.

  - Principle 5: Choose the course of action that will least restrict the person's freedom.

When to assess for mental capacity?

- A patient should not be subjected to a formal mental capacity assessment simply on the basis that he is declining a medical intervention or care because his refusal could represent an autonomous choice (that is, one that is made with comprehension and voluntariness). However, if there are reasons to doubt the patient's mental capacity — such as incoherent speech, inability to comprehend his condition and/or treatment, or he is making decisions that are uncharacteristic of him — a mental capacity assessment is justified if this is in the patient's best interests.

- A patient can refuse a mental capacity assessment unless there is enough reason to believe that the refusal itself is made without decisional capacity. The MCA outlines a two-stage test of mental capacity:

<u>Stage 1</u>

Does the person have an impairment of the mind or brain, whether as a result of an illness or external factors such as alcohol or drug use?

<u>Stage 2</u>

If yes, does the impairment cause the person to be unable to make a specific decision when he needs to?

Who can assess mental capacity?

- Patient's caregiver can perform an informal assessment for day-to-day decisions because no training is required for this.
- For decisions on medical treatment, a mental capacity assessment is to be carried out by healthcare professionals. If uncertain about the patient's mental capacity, the healthcare professional should request a formal assessment.
- A registered medical practitioner or a mental health specialist can conduct a formal assessment on mental capacity
- For complex cases, assessment by a multi-disciplinary team should be considered.

Practical issues related to mental capacity assessment

- When there is doubt on a patient's mental capacity for serious or life-changing decisions such as nursing home placement, going for a major surgery or selling property, a formal assessment of mental capacity is required.

- In a situation where a patient has an underlying mental health disorder that complicates mental capacity assessment, it is prudent to have a psychiatrist conduct the mental capacity assessment — lest the assessment gets challenged subsequently — even though this is not a legal requirement.

- Do not assume that a patient lacks mental capacity on the basis that he suffers from a condition that affects cognitive functioning. Similarly, psychiatric diagnosis alone does not imply mental capacity.

- Since mental capacity is decision-specific, a patient may possess mental capacity for certain decisions (because it is less complex) but not others.

- Mental capacity is a threshold concept (or a sliding scale): information that is more complex to grasp or decisions that lead to grave consequences will require the patient to demonstrate a higher degree of capacity.

- At times, even experienced evaluators may disagree whether a patient has mental capacity. In such a situation, it is recommended that the evaluators discuss in-depth how they have assessed the patient, such as the actual questions posed to the patient and the patient's responses. This will provide a clearer, more comprehensive understanding with regard to the patient's likely capacity.

- Patient's consent and refusal for treatment and care can change over time and should not be regarded as a patient lacking capacity. Instead, this may warrant a careful examination for capacity.

- Mental capacity can be mercurial, changing from hour to hour because of the patient's medical condition, medication, fatigue, etc. Check the patient's medical diagnoses and medication list, and consider assessing the patient at different times of the day. Catch the patient when he/she is more alert to hold a conversation.

- A person with mental capacity is allowed to make decisions that others deem unwise. An unwise decision does not imply that a person lacks mental capacity.

- When a patient makes an "unwise decision", one should consider if it is an unwise decision by the patient's choice or it suggests that the person lacks mental capacity.

- Avoid a narrow focus on the patient's decision, that is, whether the patient agrees to treatment/care. Instead explore the patient's reasoning behind that decision. This is because a response of either "yes" or "no" does not necessarily equate a "reasoned response".

- Avoid stating, "Patient has full mental capacity" since the patient is being assessed for his ability to make a particular decision, and adequate capacity suffices. For example, one could write:
  - "Mr T has mental capacity for decision on renal replacement therapy."
  - "Madam A does not have mental capacity for decision on care placement."

- When it is unclear if a patient has mental capacity, we want to consider, on the balance of probability, is the patient more likely to have or lack mental capacity; it is not about demonstrating "beyond a reasonable doubt" whether the patient has capacity.

- If the decision is not urgent and there is a chance that the patient can regain mental capacity, postpone the decision until the patient has regained capacity to decide for himself.

- At the core of mental capacity assessment is to balance a person's right to make his own decisions and the need to protect him when he lacks the mental capacity for decisions.

Best interests principle

- The MCA requires that decisions made for a person lacking mental capacity must consider the best interests principle.

- Lasting power of attorney (LPA) and court-appointed deputy are not allowed to make decisions on a patient's life-sustaining treatment or treatment to prevent a serious deterioration.

- Decisions on life-saving treatment or treatment to prevent serious deterioration in a patient's condition is a medical decision to be made by a doctor by applying the best interests principle.

- The MCA offers no definition for the best interests principle since it is based on the context.

- Best interests cannot be determined solely on the basis of a patient's age, appearance, condition, and aspects of behaviour [section 6(1) MCA].

- The best interests of a patient consider various factors such as the patient's medical condition, circumstances, previously stated and current wishes, values, and preferences, if known.

- Patient's advance care plan (ACP), though not legally binding, can provide insights on an incapacitous patient's values and preferences, and these should be considered when evaluating the patient's best interests.

References

Beauchamp TL and Childress JF (2019). *Principles of Biomedical Ethics.* 8th ed. Oxford University Press.

Jonsen A, Siegler M and Winslade W (2021). *Clinical Ethics: A Practical Approach to Ethical Decisions in Clinical Medicine.* 9th ed. New York: McGraw-Hill.

Mental Capacity Act 2008. https://sso.agc.gov.sg/Acts-Supp/22-2008/Published/ 20100331?DocDate=20081017

70 Kidney Biopsy

Terence Kee

Introduction

- A percutaneous kidney biopsy is an invasive diagnostic procedure with potentially significant risks, including death (Table 70.1). A recent systematic review and meta-analysis of the literature on biopsies of native kidneys reveal that complications occur in 4.5% of patients.

Table 70.1: Risks of Percutaneous Kidney Biopsy

Complications	Frequency
Perinephric haematoma (mostly small <2 cm)	11%
Pain	4.3%
Macroscopic haematuria	3.5%
Bleeding requiring blood transfusion	1.6%
Interventions to stop bleeding	0.3%
Death	0.06%

Source: Poggio ED, McClelland RL, Blank KN, *et al.* (2020). Systematic review and meta-analysis of native kidney biopsy complications. *Clin J Am Soc Nephrol* **15**(11): 1595–1602.

- In a systematic review of kidney transplant biopsies, gross haematuria, bleeding requiring transfusion, and major complications occurred in 3.18%, 0.31% and 0.89%, respectively.

- Offering a kidney biopsy to a patient should only be performed if the biopsy can be performed without higher-than-expected risks and if the results of the biopsy will help decide on treatment options and/or prognostication (Table 70.2).

Table 70.2:   Risk Factors for Bleeding after a Kidney Biopsy

Variables	Risk Factor
Patient related factors	• Elevated sCr (>175 umol/L) • Hypertension (systolic BP >140 mmHg, diastolic BP >90 mmHg) • Age >40 years • Female gender • Low prebiopsy Hb (<12 g/dL) • Thrombocytopenia • Coagulopathy • Biopsy while on an antiplatelet agent • Biopsy for AKI
Procedural factors	• 14-gauge needle instead of a 16 or 18-gauge needle • >5 passes at biopsy • Lack of real-time ultrasound guidance • Lack of an automated biopsy device

Abbreviations: sCr, serum creatinine; BP, blood pressure; Hb, haemoglobin; AKI, acute kidney injury

- However, patients should be counselled that a biopsy could yield no kidney tissue, or there may be a sampling error, which may affect accurate interpretation.

- Patients should be assessed carefully ahead of time to confirm their suitability to undergo a biopsy (Table 70.3).

Table 70.3: Common Indications for a Kidney Biopsy

Indications	Comments
Haematuria	Biopsy may be considered in patients with haematuria associated with elevated sCr level or proteinuria. In some centres, a biopsy may be performed in potential living kidney donors to ascertain if haematuria has a glomerular cause before deciding on donation.
Proteinuria	Biopsy may be appropriate if there is significant (≥ 1 g/d) proteinuria confirmed on repeated measurements with or without elevated sCr or haematuria (especially if there is no other obvious cause for proteinuria, e.g., infection). Biopsy may also be considered in patients with diabetes: (1) if there is significant haematuria and/or pyuria without a cause of explanation, (2) when proteinuria is rapidly increasing over time or (3) when the kidney function is deteriorating rapidly. Patients with lower levels of proteinuria may also be offered a biopsy in the setting of a kidney transplant (where rejection or concern of recurrent glomerulonephritis) or when there is a systemic condition that is associated with kidney diseases, e.g., SLE.
AKI	Biopsy may be indicated if there is persistent AKI without an obvious cause or if the kidney function does not improve despite removal or adequate treatment of the cause. In cases where AKI is attributed to ATN, but the kidney function does not improve over 7–14 days, a biopsy may also be considered to confirm the diagnosis and exclude other causes of persistent AKI.
CKD	Biopsy may be considered in patients with pre-existing CKD where the trajectory of CKD progression accelerates or where there is new-onset haematuria or proteinuria. Sometimes, it may be offered to potential kidney transplant candidates where determining a cause of CKD would be important to determine the risk of recurrence after kidney transplantation.

(Continued)

Table 70.3:   (*Continued*)

Indications	Comments
Follow-up of treatment for kidney disease	Interval repeat biopsy may be performed to assess the response to the treatment of a prior kidney disease diagnosed on an earlier kidney biopsy. In kidney transplantation, a follow-up biopsy may be performed to confirm the clearance of rejection.
Pre-implant biopsy in kidney transplantation	Biopsies of kidneys from expanded criteria donors are performed to assess the histological quality of the kidney and determine if kidneys should be discarded or used as single or dual implants. In Singapore, implant biopsies are performed in standard criteria deceased donors to provide baseline histological assessment and prognostication of post-transplant function.
Protocol kidney transplant biopsies	In some centres around the world, protocol biopsies at specified time intervals after kidney transplantation are performed to assess for subclinical rejection. Treatment of subclinical rejection have been shown to reduce chronic damage detected on subsequent protocol biopsies.

Abbreviations: AKI, acute kidney injury; sCr, serum creatinine; ATN, acute tubular necrosis; CKD, chronic kidney disease; SLE, systemic lupus erythematosus

General approach to preparing a patient for biopsy

- Ensure that all possible non-invasive investigations have been performed to identify a possible reversible cause of kidney dysfunction, e.g., urinary tract infection, obstructive uropathy, renal artery stenosis.

- Counsel patient on the indication, risks and benefits, and expected journey of performing a kidney biopsy, as well as alternative options to obtain informed consent.

- In certain cases where a biopsy is critical, but the risks associated with a percutaneous approach is high, one could consider discussing with an interventional radiologist or a surgeon on

Table 70.4: Relative and Absolute Contraindications to a Kidney Biopsy

Contraindication	Comment
Increased bleeding risk	Significant uncorrected thrombocytopenia or coagulopathy, use of antiplatelet and anticoagulation medications that were not discontinued.
Anticoagulation concerns	Patients at a high risk of thrombosis if anticoagulation was suspended or had to be suspended for a prolonged period of time (because of a haemorrhagic complication from the biopsy), e.g., mechanical valve, active venous thromboembolic disease, high $CHADS_2$ score, LVAD, active APLS.
Uncontrolled hypertension	Systolic BP should be ideally <140 mmHg before proceeding to the biopsy.
Small echogenic kidneys	If the ultrasound shows small echogenic kidneys, the biopsy may not yield useful information (may only show extensive glomerulosclerosis, interstitial fibrosis, and tubular atrophy, which would not be amenable to any curative treatment).
Anatomical problems	Some kidneys may be structurally at the risk of complications if they are biopsied, e.g., horseshoe kidney, multiple cysts, hydronephrosis, arteriovenous malformation.
Solitary kidney	There may be risks of AKI or even nephrectomy triggered by a severe life-threatening haemorrhage. As a result, many would hesitate in performing a biopsy on a single function kidney. However, a biopsy of a solitary kidney may be essential and has been reported to be performed safely in experienced hands or via other approaches, e.g., surgical or transjugular.
Infection	Biopsy should not be performed over areas of skin that is infected or when there is ongoing pyelonephritis or a suspected/confirmed infected perinephric fluid collection.

(Continued)

Table 70.4: (*Continued*)

Contraindication	Comment
Patient unable to cooperate with biopsy or report complications	Patients who have psychiatric or neurological disorders that render them restless or uncooperative during a biopsy will be at a higher risk of complications if a biopsy is performed. A patient who has cognitive impairment may not be able to report symptoms of complications after a biopsy, which would then lead to delays in reporting and treatment.
Pregnancy	Pregnancy is not a contraindication to a kidney biopsy, but biopsies performed after 20 weeks of gestation is associated with a higher risk of bleeding complications.
Obesity	US may not render good images of the needle and kidney in obese patients, which theoretically may increase the risk of bleeding during a percutaneous kidney biopsy. Other approaches, such as transjugular or surgical (open or laparoscopic), to perform the biopsy have been performed.

Abbreviations: $CHADS_2$, congestive heart failure, hypertension, age ($\geq$65 years = 1 point, $\geq$75 years = 2 points, diabetes and stroke/transient ischaemic attack = 2 points); LVAD, left ventricular assist device; APLS, antiphospholipid syndrome; BP, blood pressure; AKI, acute kidney injury; ESKD, end-stage kidney disease; US, ultrasound

the option of a transjugular or surgical (open or laparoscopic) biopsy. However, a transjugular biopsy requires contrast while surgery require anaesthesia, which have their own specific risks.

- Review the medication chart to identify the use of antiplatelet and anticoagulant agents. If it is safe and possible to suspend the use of the drugs, the patient should be instructed to do so ahead of the biopsy.

  - Antiplatelet agents, e.g., aspirin, clopidogrel — stop 7 days before the date of the biopsy.

  - Anticoagulation — when to stop depends on the type of drug used and the pharmacokinetic clearance of the drug with the degree of kidney and liver dysfunction. Coagulation parameters should be normal prior to the biopsy.

The timing to resume antiplatelet and anticoagulation agents depends on whether there were any complications from the biopsy and the risk of complications from withholding the antiplatelet or anticoagulation agent for too long a time. In general, these agents can usually be restarted 48–72 hours after the biopsy.

- Tests to be performed just before proceeding with a kidney biopsy include:
  - Renal panel
  - FBC
  - PT/aPTT
  - Group and crossmatch to standby for blood transfusion
  - US Doppler to assess structure, vascular malformations, and areas of infarct (where tissue diagnosis may be unlikely)
- In patients with thrombocytopenia or coagulopathy, and where a kidney biopsy is important for the further management of the patient, platelets or fresh frozen plasma can be transfused to correct the thrombocytopenia or coagulopathy. The threshold to transfuse platelets should be lower in patients with chronic kidney dysfunction, where uraemia increases bleeding risks.
- For patients with significant uraemia, dialysis may be performed prior to the biopsy to reduce uraemic bleeding diathesis. Alternatively, IV or SC desmopressin (DDAVP) 0.3 µg/kg can be given 30 to 60 minutes prior to the biopsy. However, studies have not shown that it significantly reduces bleeding complications. Instead, it may be associated with severe hyponatraemia among patients with low eGFR.

- Blood pressure should be well-controlled prior to a biopsy. There is a 10-fold increased risk of complications if the systolic BP is >140 mmHg and diastolic BP is >90 mmHg.

- Each renal unit should have its own protocol on how biopsies should be performed, and hence, the readers should refer to their own hospital or renal unit's protocol. Some centres perform kidney biopsies as outpatient procedures, while others do it as inpatients. In general,

  - Patient would be placed in the prone (for native kidney biopsy) or supine (for transplant kidney biopsy) position to be cleaned and draped. Sometimes, a native kidney biopsy is performed in the lateral decubitus or a sitting position, e.g., pregnancy.

  - Adequate local anaesthesia should be given to ensure patient comfort and cooperation during the passage of the biopsy needle.

  - Biopsy is performed using real-time US to guide an automated spring-loaded biopsy needle device. The US should ensure that the needle passes through kidney tissue instead of adjacent organs, e.g., liver, spleen, intestines or unsuspecting fluid collections (where infections may be introduced).

  - Instead of US, CT is another modality to guide kidney biopsies in some centres, but it exposes the patient to the risk of radiation.

Post-biopsy management and follow-up

- Patient should be reviewed upon returning to the ward. Each renal unit should have its own monitoring protocol for patients undergoing a kidney biopsy.

- Patients should be monitored for signs and symptoms of bleeding, such as:

  - Hypotension

  - Hypertension — persistent hypertension after a biopsy could signify a capsular haematoma, which can be confirmed with a US or CT

  - Macroscopic haematuria

  - Pain over the biopsy site, e.g., flank for native kidney or iliac fossa for transplanted kidney suggesting haematoma

- Patient should be advised to rest supine in bed for at least 4 to 6 hours. Some centres discharge the patient after 4 to 6 hours, while others prefer to keep the patient overnight for observation.

- Patients should be advised to continue to monitor for symptoms and signs of post-biopsy complications, even after an overnight stay following a kidney biopsy. Late complications have occurred in over 10% of cases (Table 70.5).

Table 70.5: Cumulative Timing of Post-biopsy Complications

	n	≤4	≤8	≤12	≤24	>24
Total	91	42%	67%	85%	89%	11%
Minor complication	46	46%	67%	80%	87%	13%
Major complication	45	38%	67%	89%	91%	9%

Source: Whittier WL and Korbet SM. (2004). Timing of complications in percutaneous renal biopsy. *J Am Soc Nephrol* **15**(1): 142–147.

References

Bandari J, Fuller TW, Turner Ii RM, *et al.* (2016). Renal biopsy for medical renal disease: Indications and contraindications. *Can J Urol* **23**(1): 8121–8126.

Ho QY, Lim CC, Tan HZ, *et al.* (2022). Complications of percutaneous kidney allograft biopsy: Systematic review and meta-analysis. *Transplantation* **106**(7): 1497–1506.

Kee TY, Chapman JR, O'Connell PJ, *et al.* (2006). Treatment of subclinical rejection diagnosed by protocol biopsy of kidney transplants. *Transplantation* **82**(1): 36–42.

Lim CC, Siow B, Choo JCJ, *et al.* (2019). Desmopressin for the prevention of bleeding in percutaneous kidney biopsy: Efficacy and hyponatremia. *Int Urol Nephrol* **51**(6): 995–1004.

Luciano RL and Moeckel GW (2019). Update on the native kidney biopsy: Core curriculum 2019. *Am J Kidney Dis* **73**(3): 404–415.

Poggio ED, McClelland RL, Blank KN, *et al.* (2020). Systematic review and meta-analysis of native kidney biopsy complications. *Clin J Am Soc Nephrol* **15**(11): 1595–1602.

Whittier WL and Korbet SM (2004). Timing of complications in percutaneous renal biopsy. *J Am Soc Nephrol* **15**(1): 142–147.

71 Therapeutic Plasma Exchange

Riece Koniman, Manish Kaushik

Introduction

- Therapeutic plasma exchange (TPE) is an extracorporeal blood purification technique designed for the removal of high molecular weight substances.

- TPE has several therapeutic mechanisms of action, including:

  - Rapid removal of pathogenic substances to prevent ongoing organ damage, thus reducing morbidity and mortality.

  - Buying time for other therapies to suppress the production of pathogenic substances, which may take time, e.g., weeks to months. Moreover, some of these pathogenic substances also have long half-lives.

  - Replacing missing plasma components associated with some disease processes.

Principles

- TPE is a procedure whereby blood is passed through a plasma filter, which separates plasma from the cellular components. The plasma is subsequently discarded, which contains pathogenic substances in the plasma that are hence eliminated from the body.

- These pathogenic substances (e.g., immunoglobulins, immune complexes, proteins) have high molecular weight and cannot be removed from the blood by conventional methods, such as dialysis or haemofiltration.

- The plasma removed is replaced with an equal volume of an appropriate fluid, which is then returned to the patient to prevent haemodynamic compromise.

- The ideal target substance to be removed by TPE should have the following properties:

  - Target substance is identifiable
  - High molecular weight (MW) ≥15,000 Daltons (Da)
  - Slow rate of production
  - Low turnover
  - Low volume of distribution
  - High rate of transfer into the intravascular compartment

- The removal rate of any given substance depends on the plasma filtration rate and its sieving coefficient (ratio of the substance concentration between the filtrate and the blood side of the membrane). With the currently available plasma filters, the sieving coefficient of even the largest molecules, weighing >1 million Da, e.g., low-density lipoprotein (LDL) cholesterol, is approximately 1, which means that the concentration of these large molecules in the removed plasma is equal to that in the patient's blood.

- TPE can also be used for supplementation of certain substances, e.g., fresh frozen plasma (FFP) is used as replacement fluid to resupply coagulation factors in liver failure or ADAM metallopeptidase with Thrombospondin Type 1 Motif 13 (ADAMTS-13) in thrombotic thrombocytopenic purpura (TTP).

- Besides the removal of pathologenic substances and supplementation of deficient plasma components, other potential mechanisms by which TPE may exert its therapeutic effects include:

  - Stimulation of the proliferation of B cells and plasma cells, sensitising them to immunosuppressants

  - Removal of immune complexes and enhancing the macrophage/monocyte function

  - Removal of cytokines and adhesion molecules

  - Alterations in the immune system

Types of therapeutic plasma exchange procedures

- There are 2 separation techniques in TPE.

Membrane-based TPE

- A separation method that utilises a non-selective microporous membrane that allows for the passage of proteins across the membrane while leaving behind the cellular components.

- In membrane-based TPE, blood is drawn from the patient and is passed through a plasma filter with large pores (0.3–0.5 µm) before it is returned to the patient.

- The ultrafiltrate produced contains all the non-cellular components of the patient's plasma. Cellular components, such as red blood cells, white blood cells, and platelets are not filtered through the plasma filter and are returned to the patient.

- As plasma is filtered out, it is replaced simultaneously with the appropriate fluid (usually albumin or FFP) in equal volume to the plasma removed.

- When FFP is used as a replacement fluid, it can also be used for the supplementation of deficient plasma components, e.g., coagulation factors, ADAMTS-13.

- Plasma extraction ratio is limited to 30% to avoid clogging of the plasma separator. As a result, higher blood volume needs to be processed to achieve the desired plasma clearance.

- Advantage: Equipment is readily available — many continuous kidney replacement therapy machines have the capability to perform TPE.

- Disadvantages:

  - Less efficient in terms of plasma removal and requires longer treatment time (compared to centrifugal-based TPE)

  - Requires central vascular access

  - Non-selective removal of all plasma components

Centrifugal-based TPE

- A separation method using centrifugal force (produced by high-speed rotation) and specific gravity.

- Centrifugal force drives substances away from the centre of rotation according to their specific gravity. Substance with low specific gravity moves to the centre of the centrifugation bowl, whereas substance with high specific gravity moves to the edge of the centrifugation bowl. Selected blood components are then removed.

- Plasma extraction ratio can be as high as 80%; thus, centrifugal-based TPE can process a smaller blood volume to achieve the same desired plasma clearance as membrane-based TPE

- Advantages:
    - Greater plasma removal efficiency and requires shorter treatment time
    - Good separation of substances, allowing for the specific removal of pathological substances
    - Allows peripheral vascular access
- Disadvantage: Specific equipment is required

Indications for therapeutic plasma exchange

- The American Society for Apheresis provides a list of indications for therapeutic plasma exchange. Category 1 indications are disorders in which TPE is accepted as first-line therapy, either as a primary or adjunct therapy (Table 71.1).
- TPE has also been performed in other conditions, e.g., thyroid storm and hypertriglyceridaemia-induced pancreatitis.

Table 71.1: Category 1 Indications and Grading Recommendations (Based on Strength and Quality of Evidence) for Therapeutic Plasma Exchange

Disease	Indication	Grade
Acute inflammatory demyelinating polyneuropathy (Guillain-Barre syndrome)	Primary treatment	1A
Acute liver failure	(TPE-High Volume)	1A
Anti-GBM (Goodpasture syndrome)	Diffuse alveolar haemorrhage	1C
	Dialysis-independence	1B

(Continued)

Table 71.1: (*Continued*)

Disease	Indication	Grade
Catastrophic antiphospholipid syndrome		2C
Chronic inflammatory demyelinating polyneuropathy		1B
Focal segmental glomerulosclerosis	Recurrence in kidney Tx	1B
Hyperviscosity in hypergammaglobulinaemia	Symptomatic	1B
	Prophylaxis for Rituximab	1C
Myasthenia gravis	Acute, short-term treatment	1B
N-methyl-D-aspartate receptor antibody encephalitis		1C
Paraproteinaemic demyelinating neuropathies; Chronic acquired demyelinating polyneuropathies	IgG/IgA/IgM	1B
TMA, complement-mediated	Factor H autoantibody	2C
TMA, drug-associated	Ticlopidine	2B
TMA, TTP		1A
Liver transplantation	Desensitisation, ABO incompatible living donor	1C
Kidney transplantation, ABO compatible	Antibody-mediated rejection	1B
	Desensitisation, living donor	1B
Kidney transplantation, ABO incompatible	Desensitisation, living donor	1B
ANCA-associated vasculitis	MPA/GPA/RLV: RPGN, sCr >= 504 μmol/L	1A
	MPA/GPA/RLV: DAH	1C
Fulminant Wilson Disease		1C

Abbreviations: ANCA, anti-neutrophil cytoplasmic antibody; DAH, diffuse alveolar haemorrhage; GBM, glomerular basement membrane; GPA, granulomatosis with polyangiitis; MPA, microscopic polyangiitis; RLV, renal limited vasculitis; RPGN, rapidly progressive glomerulonephritis; sCr, serum creatinine; TMA, thrombotic microangiopathy; TTP, thrombotic thrombocytopenic purpura

Prescription of therapeutic plasma exchange

- Dose of TPE [processed plasma volume (PV)] is usually prescribed as 1–1.5x estimated PV.

- Removal of high MW substances during a single session of TPE is limited to the intravascular compartment due to the slow equilibration between the extravascular and intravascular compartments.

- The following formula can be used to calculate the reduction in concentration of the substance based on the PV exchanged during TPE:

$$X_1 = X_0 e^{-Ve/EPV},$$

where X_1 = final plasma concentration, X_0 = initial plasma concentration, Ve = plasma volume exchanged, and EPV = patient's estimated plasma volume.

- If the plasma volume exchanged (Ve) is equal to 1x EPV, the pre-treatment levels will be lowered by 63%.

- If Ve is equal to 1.5x EPV, the pre-treatment levels will be lowered by 78%.

- Increasing the plasma volume exchanged to >1.5x EPV during a single treatment yields a progressively smaller reduction in pre-treatment levels.

- Estimated PV = [0.065 × weight (kg)] × [1-haematocrit]

- Frequency of TPE is variable (depending on the disease and clinical condition, properties of molecule, etc.)

- IgM is largely distributed in the intravascular compartment (78%), and it has a half-life of 5 days; thus, IgM can be removed effectively with a few daily treatments.

- IgG only has <45% intravascular distribution, and it has a half-life of 21 days. As a result, more treatments with reasonable intervals (24–48 hours) to allow for a "rebound" (transfer from the extravascular to the intravascular compartment) are required.
- With 3 daily TPE sessions, it is estimated that the total body load for IgG will decline by ~70%, and the total body load for IgM will decline by ~80%
- Blood flow rate = 150–250 mL/min
- Plasma extraction ratio = 20–30%
- Replacement fluid
    - Volume of replacement fluid = Volume of plasma extracted
    - Most common replacement fluids are 5% albumin and FFP (depending on the clinical context) (Table 71.2)
    - Factors that may impact on the type of replacement fluid:
        - Underlying disease
        - Volume of plasma for exchange
        - Number and frequency of TPE
        - Risk of bleeding
        - Availability of supply
- Vascular access
    - Non-tunnelled or tunnelled dialysis catheter
    - Arteriovenous fistula/graft
- Anticoagulation
    - Unfractionated heparin
        - Initial bolus 1000–2000 IU
        - Maintenance infusion 500–1000 IU/h

Table 71.2: Advantages and Disadvantages of Fresh Frozen Plasma and Albumin as Replacement Fluid in the Therapeutic Plasma Exchange

Replacement Fluid	Advantages	Disadvantages
Fresh frozen plasma	• Replace certain deficient plasma components, e.g., ADAMTS 13, coagulation factors, immunoglobulins, plasma proteins	• Risk of viral transmission • Risk of allergic reaction or anaphylaxis • Citrate load • ABO compatibility • Frozen storage • Expensive
5% albumin	• No risk of viral transmission • Negligible risk of allergic reaction • Oncotic pressure is close to that of plasma • Less expensive than FFP • Room temperature storage	• Coagulopathy due to the removal of coagulation factors • Net loss of immunoglobulins and complements • Contains 4–24 mmol/L of aluminium (risk of aluminum toxicity in patients with renal impairment)

Table 71.3: Complications of Therapeutic Plasma Exchange

Complications	Causes

Hypotension	• Reduced cardiac output
	  – poor cardiac function
	  – decreased circulating volume
	  – extracorporeal blood volume
	  – insufficient replacement fluid (volume and/or oncotic pressure)
	  – dilution of proteins in fresh frozen plasma
	• Reduction in peripheral vascular resistance
	  – vasovagal reflex
	  – allergy
	  – autonomic neuropathy, e.g., in diabetes mellitus
	  – advanced atherosclerosis

(Continued)

Table 71.3:   (Continued)

Complications	Causes
Allergies	Plasma, e.g., fresh frozen plasma, cryoprecipitate Anticoagulant, e.g., heparin
Infections	Removal of immunoglobulins and complement factors Catheter-related blood stream infections Blood product transmitted infections, e.g., hepatitis B or C, HIV
Bleeding	Removal of coagulation factors, e.g., fibrinogen, factors V, VII, VIII, IX, X, prothrombin, antithrombin III — after a single TPE session with albumin as a replacement fluid, ~60% of coagulation factors and ~80% of fibrinogen may be removed Anticoagulation, e.g., heparin Underlying primary disease, e.g., acute liver failure
Electrolyte abnormalities	Sodium citrate in fresh frozen plasma causes hypocalcaemia and hypernatraemia Metabolism of citrate in fresh frozen plasma causes metabolic alkalosis Hypokalaemia occurs due to potassium removal and dilution by replacement fluid

Others	Thrombosis
	  – due to reduced levels of antithrombin III (if albumin is used as the replacement fluid)
	  – very low incidence of thrombotic events, but cases of pulmonary embolism, acute myocardial infarction, and ischaemic stroke have been reported
	Thrombocytopenia
	  – ~15% decreased in platelets due to the direct loss of platelets in the plasma extracted or by plasma filter clotting
	Transfusion-related lung injury (TRALI)
	  – infused antibodies from the donor's plasma to antigens on leukocytes of the recipient can cause leucoagglutination in the pulmonary circulation and systemic capillary leak
	Angiotensin-converting enzyme inhibitor-related complications (rare) — possibly due to decreased bradykinin breakdown

- Citrate — Citrate anticoagulation has been used for membrane-based TPE but must be performed under strict protocol and monitoring to mitigate the risks of citrate toxicity and hypocalcaemia.

- Monitor for complications (Table 71.3)

References

Ahmed S and Kaplan A. (2020). Therapeutic plasma exchange using membrane plasma separation. *Clin J Am Soc Nephrol* **15**(9): 1364–1370.

Daga Ruiz D, Fonseca San Miguel F, González de Molina FJ, *et al.* (2017). Plasmapheresis and other extracorporeal filtration techniques in critical patients. *Med. Intensiva* **41**(3): 174–187.

Kaplan A. (2012). Complications of apheresis. *Semin Dial* **25**(2): 152–158.

Kaplan AA. (2013). Therapeutic plasma exchange: A technical and operational review. *J Clin Apher* **28**(1): 3–10.

Padmanabhan A, Connelly-Smith L, Aqui N, *et al.* (2019). Guidelines on the use of therapeutic apheresis in clinical practice — Evidence-based approach from the Writing Committee of the American Society for Apheresis: The eighth special issue. *J Clin Apher* **34**(3): 171–354.

Index

atherosclerosis, 177–179

automated peritoneal dialysis, 426, 427

autonomy, 818–821, 823–827, 829

azathioprine, 591–593, 604, 606, 607, 609, 621

balance solution, 428

Banff lesion score, 650, 652, 654

BARKH acronym, 168

basiliximab, 584–586

beneficence, 818, 819, 823–827, 829, 830

beta blockers, 149

Bezold-Jarisch reflex, 355

bicarbonate, 91, 93, 94, 98–102

bioelectrical impedance, 337

bioimepdance, 132

bio-incompatible peritoneal dialysis solution, 429, 431

biopsychosocial-spiritual model, 813

BK virus, 697

BK virus associated nephropathy, 697

blood pressure, 144–146, 149

blood volume monitoring, 361

brachiobasilic transposition arteriovenous fistula, 368

brachiobasilic arteriovenous fistula, 368

breastfeeding, 735, 741, 742

bumetanide, 133

caesarean delivery, 731, 735

calcineurin inhibitor, 591–593, 596, 597, 600, 601, 615, 620

calciphylaxis, 158, 802, 803

calcitriol, 72–74, 76, 82

calcium channel blocker, 148

cardiac arrhythmia, 375, 378

cardiac evaluation, 578

carotid artery puncture, 376

catheter-associated urinary tract infection, 229

catheter malposition, 378, 379

catheter-related blood stream infections, 375, 379, 380

catheter tip kink, 448

catheter tip migration, 446, 448

cation, 83

central vein stenosis, 401, 402, 403, 413

centrifugal-based therapeutic plasma exchange, 852

charcoal haemoperfusion, 532

chronic kidney disease stage, 105, 107, 108, 110, 112, 114

chronic phase, 807, 811

chronic pyelonephritis, 4, 5

chronic rejection, 648, 649

chronic tubulointerstitial nephritis, 199, 200, 206, 208, 213, 214

CMV antigenaemia, 682

CMV disease, 682, 683, 685, 687, 688, 690–693

www.ingramcontent.com/pod-product-compliance
Lightning Source LLC
Chambersburg PA
CBHW071724150726
47998CB00005B/1498